Care of the Psyche

STANLEY W. JACKSON

Care of the Psyche

A HISTORY OF
PSYCHOLOGICAL HEALING

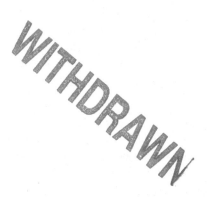

Yale University Press
New Haven &
London

Printed in the United States of America

Library of Congress Cataloging-in-Publication Data
Jackson, Stanley W. (date)
    Care of the psyche : a history of psychological healing / Stanley W. Jackson.
        p.   cm.
    Includes bibliographical references (p.   ) and index.
    ISBN 0-300-07671-1
    1. Counseling — History.   2. Psychotherapy — History.   I. Title.
BF637.C6J335   1999
616.89′14′09 — dc21   98-37512
                                                                                          CIP

A catalogue record for this book is available from the British Library.

The paper in this book meets the guidelines for permanence and durability of the
Committee on Production Guidelines for Book Longevity of the Council on
Library Resources.

10   9   8   7   6   5   4   3   2   1

To Joan — for many, many reasons

Seeing, Brutus, that we are made up of soul and body, what am I to think is the reason why for the care and maintenance of the body there has been devised an art which from its usefulness has had its discovery attributed to immortal gods, and is regarded as sacred, whilst on the other hand the need of an art of healing for the soul has not been felt so deeply before its discovery, nor has it been studied so closely after becoming known, nor welcomed with the approval of so many, and has even been regarded by a greater number with suspicion and hatred?

— Cicero, *Tusculan Disputations*

Contents

Acknowledgments

As I reflect on the origins and development of this book, I realize that there are quite a few bases for a sense of indebtedness. I am indebted to a great many authors from over the centuries, as one can tell from the numerous notes and references throughout this book; to an array of significant teachers, some of whom were never formally my teachers and some of whom I have never actually met; to many patients from whom I learned as they collaborated with me in their therapeutic undertakings; and to the students who have provided me with the privileges and satisfactions of teaching, not to mention the teacher's precious opportunity to continue learning.

Some of the chapters of this book have benefited from discussions with groups to which earlier versions had been presented — "The Healer-Sufferer Relationship," to the Department of Psychiatry, University of Western Ontario; "The Listening Healer" to the American Psychiatric Association as the Benjamin Rush Award Lecture in 1991, and to the Beaumont Medical Club of Connecticut; "Consolation and Comfort" to Professor Theodore M. Brown's seminar at the University of Rochester; "Persuasion" to the History of Psychiatry Section, Cornell University School of Medicine, and to the History of Medicine Colloquium, Section of the History of Medicine, Yale University School of Medicine.

The chapter on "the healer-sufferer relationship" benefited from being read, criticized, and discussed with me by Professor Robert U. Massey, internist, historian of medicine, and former dean of the University of Connecticut's School of Medicine, and by Professor John Harley Warner, historian of medicine at Yale University School of Medicine.

The whole manuscript was rigorously and constructively reviewed and criticized by Professor John C. Burnham, Departments of History and of Psychiatry, Ohio State University. Professor Burnham's comments and suggestions were helpful indeed and reflected the skills of a master editor; and, of course, residual defects are no fault of his.

Several of these chapters are based on earlier versions that were published as journal articles. I wish to express my appreciation for their helpful contributions to the editors and referees in each of these cases. And I thank the publishers of those journals for permission to draw on these materials — "The Use of the Passions in Psychological Healing," *J. Hist. Med. & Allied Sci.,* 1990, *45,* 150–75 [Copyright ©, 1990, Journal of the History of Medicine and Allied Sciences, Inc., adapted by permission]; "The Imagination and Psychological Healing," *J. Hist. Behav. Sci.,* 1990, *26,* 345–58 [Copyright ©, 1990, John Wiley & Sons, Inc., adapted by permission]; "The Listening Healer in the History of Psychological Healing," *Am. J. Psychiatry,* 1992, *149,* 1623–32 [Copyright ©, 1992, the American Psychiatric Association, adapted by permission]. "Catharsis and Abreaction" was written expressly as a chapter in this book, but, by invitation and with permission, a version of it was adapted and appeared as a chapter titled "Catharsis and Abreaction in the History of Psychological Healing" in a volume of *The Psychiatric Clinics of North America,* 1994, *17,* 471–91, Sharon Romm and Rohn S. Friedman (eds.). I wish to express my appreciation to those editors and to the publication's publisher, W. B. Saunders.

For generous and extensive assistance, I thank Ferenc A. Gyorgyey and Toby Appel, each in turn the Historical Librarian at the Historical Library, Harvey Cushing/John Hay Whitney Medical Library, Yale University, and their assistants. I am also indebted to numerous other librarians in the Cushing/Whitney Library; reference librarians, interlibrary loan librarians, and others. And my thanks to numerous other librarians in libraries throughout Yale University: Sterling Memorial Library, Cross Campus Library, Beinecke Rare Book and Manuscript Library, Classics Library, Divinity School Library, and the Seeley G. Mudd Library.

For her guidance, support, and other helpful contributions, I thank my editor at the Yale University Press, Gladys Topkis. For her superb contributions as my manuscript editor, I thank Susan Abel—truly a copyeditor par excellence.

As to Joan K. Jackson, she has, as always, helped me in ways beyond measure—typed the manuscript, served as in-house editor and critic, and continued to be my love and my friend as she has been for so many years.

PART ONE

Introductory Considerations

I

Introduction

Several decades of study and teaching in the history of medicine have left
me significantly impressed by the recurrent indications of psychological healing endeavors over many centuries. And many years as a practitioner and
teacher of psychotherapy have sensitized me to the problems inherent in comparing and contrasting the various approaches to psychotherapy. Why were
there such suggestive similarities between *this* approach and *that* approach,
and yet why did they still seem so different?

This book grew out of the realization that the similarities between approaches stemmed from shared ingredients and that the differences largely
derived from different approaches composed of varying combinations of a
relatively small number of ingredients. And so I undertook these explorations
into the history of a selection of basic elements that are found recurrently in
the twentieth-century psychotherapies, in the mental therapeutics of the nineteenth century, and in innumerable forms of mental healing over the centuries.
Although so many of our modern psychotherapies have relatively short histories — anywhere from a few decades to a hundred years — the elements out of
which most of them have been constituted date back many centuries.

This work is a study of the history of *psychological healing* in the care and
cure of human ailments. First, many and varied psychological measures have
been employed over the centuries in efforts to cure or relieve mental disorders or illnesses. Another rich tradition has been that in which psychological

treatment measures have been used to bring help, relief, or cure to those suffering from physical illnesses, including both those which we in the twentieth century would conceive of as having a clearly organic basis and those which we might term psychosomatic disorders. And some psychological ministerings have been directed toward easing the distress and suffering of the sick, without any particular thought that they might be curative.

By *healing* I refer to the various measures that have been employed by those social functionaries who can be classified as healers and who have made efforts to cure, to restore health, or to bring about recovery from sickness. Further, short of a cure, healing efforts have included many measures taken in striving toward such a goal, with an accompanying easing of the lot of the sick or a diminishing of their suffering. In short, salutary caring for the sick, as well as curing, is fairly included under the rubric *healing*. And by *psychological healing*,[1] I refer to the variety of efforts taken to minister to a person's ailments by psychological means or psychological interventions — whether or not they have been accompanied by medicinal or other physical interventions.

Psychological healing is used here as a generic term that includes processes and practices that have served, often in unarticulated ways, to resolve or ease psychological burdens that were to be found in many forms in different eras. With the increase in cultural and individual self-consciousness about such matters, these processes and practices came to be referred to as the cure of souls, pastoral care, mental healing, mind healing, mind cure, psychotherapeia, psychotherapeutics, and psychotherapy. That is to say, *psychological healing* is used to denote a broad range of mental, psychic, or psychological interventions that have served healing or ameliorative purposes over many centuries. The array of twentieth-century psychotherapies would be subsumed as species within the genus *psychological healing,* along with many other psychological interventions, old and new, that might not be categorized as psychotherapies.

Psychotherapy

As a further aid in orientation for the matters addressed in this study, it is useful to address here just what the term *psychotherapy* might be taken to mean. As the twentieth century began, *psychotherapy* and *psychotherapeutics* were employed as synonyms. Equivalents were *Psychotherapie* in German, *psychothérapie* in French, and *psicoterapeutica* in Italian. The thoughtful definition and summary of the views of the day in *Dictionary of Philosophy and Psychology* (1901) certainly reflected nineteenth-century developments and are not without relevance for our era. The discussion of psychotherapy was as follows:

The treatment of disease mainly or wholly by direct and indirect appeal to or utilization of mental conditions upon bodily states.

The term serves a useful function as the equivalent of the legitimate factor in the scientific treatment of disease, which utilizes and directs, examines and interprets such mental influences. There are many more or less extreme systems which depend upon similar principles, but present them under unwarranted and fantastic theories, or combined with irrelevant notions and practices. Some of these are noticed under Faith Cure and Mind Cure.

The recognition of the mutual influence of mind and body is one of the fundamental tenets of modern psychology. That bodily states condition mental processes is abundantly proven by the existence of mental diseases traceable to degenerations of specialized parts of the central nervous system, by the action of drugs, by the mental results of fatigue and ill health and of bodily injuries, by an endless series of every-day observations, and by the systematic experiments of the laboratory. That mental processes tend to have motor expression, and that concentrated attention or consciousness may interfere with the normal functioning of bodily processes, are evidenced in every-day matters by blushing, by the effect of embarrassment (upon speech), of fear (upon movement), of panic, of stage fright, of anxiety or nervousness (upon heart-beat or respiration), as in the moments preceding an appearance before the public. Witness the difficulty of swallowing a pill when too consciously intentioned. In extreme cases even death has been produced by fear or anticipation. Psychotherapeutics properly includes a recognition and utilization for purposes of treatment of all these factors.[2]

In this same context it was stated that there were both "(1) a general psychotherapeutic effect, and (2) special psychotherapeutic treatment; in both of which the methods may be in various degrees direct or indirect." Under the former were noted "any general influences which affect the success of medical treatment, such as the inducement of confidence in the physician on the part of the patient, the assuaging of unreasonable fears, the general tranquillization of the patient by sympathy and encouragement or, it may be, by stern counsel and masterful direction, and by a congenial and carefree environment." As for "special psychotherapeutic treatment," it was noted that "the associations of the term [*psychotherapy*] are in the main more specific." They included "definite systems and processes," along with "appeals to the imagination, . . . the impressive effects of mystic processes and elaborate procedures, . . . appeals to faith, . . . the efficacy of prayer, . . . and, in short, . . . the production, in a manner suitable for each individual, of an attitude of hopefulness and confidence of recovery, which undeniably contributes to a convalescent tone of the nervous system."[3]

Many scores of definitions have been offered in the years that have followed. Early on, as in the definition just cited, the emphasis was on treating disease through the influence of the mind on the body, already a prominent theme in nineteenth-century psychological therapeutics. *Psychotherapy* meant the use of psychological measures to influence the mind, with the mind in turn being the medium through which attempts were made to achieve therapeutic gains. At first, definitions emphasized that the goal was to employ the mind's influence gainfully for the treatment of bodily diseases. Then, with gradually increasing frequency, references appeared to the use of these psychological methods for the treatment of disorders of the mind. By 1909 the *Oxford English Dictionary* was defining *psychotherapy* in briefer, and somewhat broader, terms as "the treatment of disease by 'psychic' methods"; it then went on to quote as follows from the *Westminster Gazette* of 1904: "Though the word 'Psychotherapy' be new, and popular in America — the land of Faith-Healers — mental therapeutics acting through the 'unconscious mind' is no new thing."[4]

At the beginning of the twentieth century, definitions of psychotherapy were strongly influenced by the simple equation that psychotherapy was suggestive therapeutics; and suggestive therapeutics subsumed hypnosis as a significant adjuvant for the promotion of suggestive effects. Soon themes of education and guidance became elements in definitions, as they had long been elements in practice. Then, with the emergence of psychoanalysis, and the wide variety of psychodynamic psychotherapies derived from it, other features entered into definitional efforts.

While Sigmund Freud's (1856–1939) role was central in these developing influences from psychoanalysis, his views on psychotherapy in the 1890s tell us much about both his practices and the practices of the day, and, further, they speak to most psychotherapists across the years. From Josef Breuer's (1842–1925) hypnotically facilitated *catharsis* in the 1880s, Breuer and Freud evolved their *cathartic psychotherapy*, described in *Studies on Hysteria* in 1895. As Freud put it in his chapter "The Psychotherapy of Hysteria": "One works to the best of one's power, as an elucidator (where ignorance has given rise to fear), as a teacher, as the representative of a freer or superior view of the world, as a father confessor who gives absolution, as it were, by a continuance of his sympathy and respect after the confession has been made. One tries to give the patient human assistance, so far as this is allowed by the capacity of one's own personality and by the amount of sympathy that one can feel for the particular case."[5]

As one can readily see, Freud was already thinking of much more than catharsis when he used the term *psychotherapy*. From these roots, references to catharsis and abreaction came to be common; and terms such as *emotional release* and *expressive psychotherapy* eventually entered the picture. Discovering the hidden problem (or problems) and achieving an understanding of it (or them), along with the work of the psychotherapist as explainer, became increasingly common elements, and eventually terms such as *interpretation* and *insight*. The talking by the patient came to be emphasized, and, later, the listening of the psychotherapist. Many quite sophisticated definitions have come from these trends, yet their cardinal elements have continued to be talking and listening, expressiveness and emotional release, a search for understanding, interpretation and insight, and the context of a professional relationship in which a sufferer and a healer pursue a goal of cure or symptom relief. Some have focused more on the emotional life with an emphasis on catharsis or abreaction. Others seem to have favored the intellect as they stressed knowledge, rationality, interpretation, and insight.

As we shall see when we consider twentieth-century aspects of our story, these comments fall far short of exhausting the possibilities, even for quite reasonable definitions. But, for the moment, we shall mention further only the definitional summing up by one of the more thoughtful students of psychotherapy, Jerome D. Frank. As he expressed it, "Treatment always involves a personal relationship between healer and sufferer. Certain types of therapy rely primarily on the healer's ability to mobilize healing forces in the sufferer by psychological means. These forms of treatment may be generically termed psychotherapy." He then added that psychotherapy was characterized by

1. a trained, socially sanctioned healer, whose healing powers are accepted by the sufferer and by his social group or an important segment of it.
2. a sufferer who seeks relief from the healer.
3. a circumscribed, more or less structured series of contacts between the healer and the sufferer, through which the healer, often with the aid of a group, tries to produce certain changes in the sufferer's emotional state, attitudes and behavior. . . . Although physical and chemical adjuncts may be used, the healing influence is primarily exercised by words, acts, and rituals in which the sufferer, healer, and — if there is one — group, participate jointly.
   . . . sympathetic, time-limited contacts between a person in distress and someone who tries to reduce the distress by producing changes in the sufferer's feelings, attitudes, and behavior.[6]

The Term Psychotherapy

But just where did this term *psychotherapy* come from in the first place? It apparently emerged during a period of lively ferment in the development of psychological measures in medical treatment, toward the end of the 1880s, and had its roots in the Liébeault-Bernheim school of suggestive therapeutics at Nancy. It appeared in the title of a work by Hippolyte Bernheim (1840–1919) in 1891 — *Hypnotisme, suggestion, psychothérapie.*[7] But it had already been used by Frederik van Eeden (1860–1932) and Albert Willem van Renterghem (1845–1939), two Dutch physicians, both of whom had studied with Ambroise-Auguste Liébeault (1823–1904) and with Bernheim, and who in 1887 opened a "clinic in Amsterdam for the treatment of diseases by suggestion, according to Dr. Liébeault's method."[8] In a paper in 1895, Van Eeden said that in 1889 they had selected *suggestive psycho-therapy* as the name for their treatment, indicating that the first term reflected their indebtedness to Bernheim and the second term was "borrowed from Hack Tuke."[9] Later, in his autobiography, he claimed that this treatment method was "called *Psychotherapy* by us for the first time."[10] In Bernheim's writings we have views that were representative of these several authors. For him, psychotherapy meant "suggestive psychotherapy," "suggestive therapeutics," or "the *systematic and reasoned application of suggestion in the treatment of the ill.*" He defined suggestion as "the act by which an idea is introduced into the brain and accepted by it"; and "if an idea is accepted by the brain, and if the brain can realize it, then there is suggestion and an action caused by this suggestion."[11] It was suggestion, or suggestive therapeutics, that became the prevailing mode of psychological treatment around that time, for mental disorders in particular and for a wide variety of physical ailments. With arguments emanating from the Nancy school to the effect that suggestion was the essence of hypnosis, hypnotic suggestion was gradually replaced by suggestion in the waking state. The status of hypnosis became that of a useful adjuvant to suggestion.

By this time, a related term, *psychotherapeutics,* was already in use, and soon *psychotherapy* and *psychotherapeutics* were being used as synonyms. Like psychotherapy, psychotherapeutics usually meant suggestive therapeutics. In 1892, psychotherapeutics, with its synonym *psychotherapeia*, was listed in Daniel Hack Tuke's (1827–1895) *Dictionary of Psychological Medicine* and was defined as the "treatment of disease by the influence of the mind on the body."[12] Bernheim wrote the section "Suggestion and Hypnotism" in the same *Dictionary,* and there attributed to Tuke the introduction of the term *psychotherapeutics* to denote "the therapeutical use of suggestion" and referred to the said "therapeutical use" as "a most valuable application of suggestion, for which hypnotism is the most efficient adjuvant."[13] Indeed, in his *Influence of the Mind upon the Body* (1872), Tuke had devoted a chapter to "Psycho-therapeutics."[14] In that chapter he considered the "practical application of the influence of the mind on the body to medical practice." Borrowed from Tuke, this term — "Psycho-Therapeutics" — was used in publications by Frances Power Cobbe[15] in 1887 and by C. Lloyd Tuckey[16] in 1889.

As for the term *psychotherapeia*, noted by Tuke in his *Dictionary* as a synonym for *psychotherapeutics*, Walter Cooper Dendy (1794–1871) had used it as the title of a paper in 1853, and by it he meant the helpful influence of a healer's mind upon that of a sufferer. In his essay, he dealt with "prevention and remedy by psychical influence"; and he discussed various ways in which the physician might influence the emotions or the thoughts of the sufferer, with the mind in turn having a healing effect on bodily ailments.[17] The term was derived from the Greek words *therapeia* (tending, attending to, caring for, medically treating) and *psyche* (soul).

From Tuke's first writings on the subject of *psycho-therapeutics* to Bernheim's *suggestive therapeutics* and Van Eeden's and Van Renterghem's *psychotherapy* (and Dendy's brief essay), the emphasis was consistently and explicitly on two themes: the influence of the sufferer's mind on his own body, and the mobilization of that influence toward a goal of cure or relief of bodily ailments. Less clearly emphasized, yet always quite apparent, was a third theme: the physician's actions that were aimed at moving the sufferer's mind toward healing efforts. Tuke discussed this third theme under the "general influence of the physician upon the patient in exciting those mental states which act beneficially upon the body in disease."[18] Van Eeden, too, alluded to this theme — the actions of the healer, the influence of one mind on another — yet in a rather cryptic fashion. He defined *psycho-therapy* as "every method of healing which opposes disease by psychical means, or by the intervention of psychical functions." He made it clear that he meant "the psychical functions of the sufferer," that these functions could be mobilized by suggestion, and that suggestion was "the principal psychical process by which a sufferer can be aided." He added that "by suggestion . . . I understand every impulse given by one mind to another mind."[19]

Some Antecedents of Psychotherapeutics

Merely to appreciate the emergence of the terms *psychotherapeutics* and *psychotherapy*, we soon find ourselves dealing with the whole "Mesmer to Freud" era. In Tuke's views we have seen one of the tributaries that eventually flowed together to form the psychotherapy of the 1890s. Another flowed from Mesmer's magnetism and Puységur's artificial somnambulism through Braid's neurypnology and hypnotism to the hypnosis of Charcot and other late nineteenth-century practitioners. Although it, too, derived from magnetism and its successors, Liébeault's hypnosis took a rather different course in leading to Bernheim's suggestive therapeutics. The *moral treatment* derived from Pinel and the York Retreat was yet another influential stream. Each of these trends, and more, played a part in the development of the world of psychological healing in which Breuer and Freud crafted their still newer approaches and set the stage for so many of today's multitude of psychotherapies.

In considering the history of psychological healing, though, we are in a vast realm of themes and practices, many of which antedate Mesmer and some of which are as old as medicine itself (or, should I say as old as human-kind?). Confessing, in search of psychological relief, and confiding, to ease distress and meet the need for another person, have long histories. Various modes of persuasion have long been familiar. Consoling and comforting are as old as grief. Various supportive efforts are in all likelihood as old as the bonds between human beings. Charms, spells, incantations, and other magical uses of the spoken word in the interest of healing have a rich and lengthy history. The need to talk and the value of a good listener have long been recognized as instrumental in psychological healing. The idea of catharsis has its roots in ancient Greece. The various ways of using the passions or the imagination to promote healing have long been familiar as modes of psycho-logical healing. And placebos are nothing new. In fact, the majority of the psychological interventions that nineteenth- and twentieth-century psycho-therapists thought that they had discovered had long been known in some form or another.

Long before terms such as *psychotherapeutics* and *psychotherapy* were coined, methods were employed for treating or ministering to various forms of suffering — whether those were thought of as diseases, illnesses, ailments, dis-orders, syndromes, or other forms of sickness — through the use of psychologi-cal rather than physical measures. Troubled persons suffered and sought help; and healers of various stripes in various cultural contexts responded to the sufferers and their distress. Whether the healers were physicians, religious functionaries, philosophers, or practitioners of some other type, they re-sponded to the distressed persons who sought their help — with their tech-niques and interventions, with the rituals and structures associated with their approach to healing, with their concern and their version of an inclination to care, and with their very person.

In considering the history of psychological healing, some see the roots of such healing methods in various early works of the great philosophers. Others locate them in the wisdom and practices of shamans and medicine men, an-cient and more recent. Still others point to the traditions of priests and other religious functionaries who have responded to members of their flocks with concern, compassion, and practices that brought comfort and relief. Some have noted magical and magico-religious practices in the healing efforts of medicine men, priests, and others, and have given those practices a place in the history of psychological healing. And physicians and their medical traditions have often been accorded a significant place in accounts of the origin and development of psychological modes of healing. Whether the forms of distress were conceived of as diseases or some other form of human suffering, medical practitioners were sought out for comfort, caring, and consolation, in addition to the physical therapeutics of their moment in time. And various ethical systems and sets of values have served these differing healers in framing their explanations and guiding their practices.

Long before some physicians, in the nineteenth century, began to be designated as "psychiatrists" (*psyche* [soul] + *iatros* [healer]), there were philosophers who were referred to as "physicians of the soul," and, later, Christian confessors (priests) came to be called "physicians of the soul." Just as physicians have "ministered" to the psychologically distressed over many centuries, "the cure of souls" has had a long and rich tradition both in the history of philosophy and in the history of confession and pastoral care.[20]

In the traditions of philosophy, the power of the word has been central or primary in healing efforts.[21] Talking and listening have thus been particularly important, although reading the written word has also had its place. Suggestion and persuasion have long been significant, with the latter assuming a most important role from the time that rhetoric took its place in the interhuman activities of ancient Greece and Rome. The evocation of the passions and catharsis or abreaction have both long been significant. Consolation was a crucial mode of healing in the ancient world, and it has had a long history in philosophical healing traditions. Explanation or the offering of meaning has been important, and so has been the pursuit of self-understanding. And self-observation or self-examination has often been urged upon sufferers and practiced by them.

Among medicine men and shamans, so-called primitive theories of disease causation have tended to determine the techniques employed in treatment, and psychological factors have been prominent in both etiology and therapeutics.[22] The breaking of a taboo has led to confession and atoning for sins as means of dealing with the sufferer's guilt and fear, such atonement often being accompanied by a ceremony designed to reconcile the sufferer with his gods, his ancestors, and his community. The treatment of spirit or demon possession has involved driving out the offending entity through exorcism, purification rites, and magical maneuvers, or through extrusion, by transferring it to another living being. Where sorcery was considered the cause, the shaman's or medicine man's magic was used to counter the damaging magic that caused the illness. In the case of loss of soul, magico-religious interventions were undertaken to find and return the lost soul. These often involved the shaman's entering a trance state and allegedly traveling afar to seek, find, and return the lost soul to the sufferer. When the illness was attributed to intrusion of a disease-causing object, the alleged cause was extracted by the medicine man, magically or symbolically, often by apparently sucking it out of the sufferer's body and producing it through some sleight of hand.

Historical Writings on Psychological Healing

There is a considerable literature on the history of psychological healing, some of it very fine. Pierre Janet's *Psychological Healing,* though rather neglected, remains a valuable and interesting work. It deals mainly with various clinical approaches from Mesmer to the beginning of the twentieth century. George Barton Cutten's *Three Thousand Years of Mental Healing* took account of numerous magical cures, religious approaches, and a broad selection of irregular healing techniques. Walter Bromberg has traced modes of psychological healing over many centuries in his *Man Above Humanity*. Nigel Walker has written a brief history of psychotherapy that mainly tells the story of the emergence and development of Freud's psychoanalysis, with significant attention to the psychotherapies based on Adler's individual psychology and Jung's analytical psychology. He also touches briefly on the history of hypnosis and devoted some thoughtful attention to suggestion and conditioning. Jan Ehrenwald has provided an extensive series of quotations relevant to the history of mental healing, interwoven with editorial observations. Richard Chessick organizes a study around a selection of "great ideas" and the historical figures who embodied them; and he argues for the importance of having an integrated grasp of these ideas if one is to become a responsible and effective psychotherapist. Henri F. Ellenberger's magisterial study of dynamic psychiatry focuses on the era from Mesmer to the present, with emphases on the work of Janet, Freud, Adler, and Jung; and he includes an interesting background account of "the ancestry of dynamic psychotherapy." Dieter Wyss has written a critical history of depth psychology, beginning with Freud's work and including an almost endless array of subsequent "depth psychologists," all dealt with in careful detail. His emphasis, though, is rather on their theories than on their practices. James R. Barclay's *Foundations of Counseling Strategies* devotes considerable attention to philosophical origins of approaches to psychological healing, as well as accounts of more recent psychotherapeutic approaches. More recently, Donald Freedheim has edited a history of psychotherapy that concentrates on the last hundred years, with some attention to the earlier history of mesmerism and hypnosis, strong chapters on psychoanalytic theories of psychotherapy and on behavior therapy, and a series of essays on the modern psychotherapeutic scene.[23]

Other significant contributions to the history of psychological healing have been rather carefully focused. Adam Crabtree and Alan Gauld have made recent, valuable contributions to the history of mesmerism and hypnosis.[24] Other studies have concentrated on the history of psychoanalysis. Among them have been many biographies of Freud, from Ernest Jones' three-volume work to Peter Gay's fine study, each of which has included material on the history of clinical psychoanalysis. Reuben Fine contributed *A History of Psychoanalysis*. More recently, Lawrence Friedman's *Anatomy of Psychotherapy* is a specially valuable study of psychoanalysis and the related psychotherapies; and Robert S. Wallerstein's *Talking Cures* is a richly nuanced study of "the psychoanalyses and the psychotherapies," which deals with the development of both theory and clinical practice.[25]

Another realm that has produced works relevant to the history of psychological healing has been that of the cure of souls, religious healing, and pastoral care. John T. McNeill's *A History of the Cure of Souls* is an outstanding study in this category. Other representative volumes in the history of pastoral care have been written by Charles F. Kemp, William A. Clebsch and Charles R. Jaekle, and E. Brooks Holifield. Several multi-author volumes are very informative on the subject of healing and the religious traditions: *The Church and Healing*, edited by W. J. Sheils; *Caring and Curing*, edited by Ronald L. Numbers and Darrel W. Amundsen; *Healing and Restoring*, edited by Lawrence E. Sullivan. Leslie D. Weatherhead's *Psychology, Religion and Healing* combines attention to both religious healings and twentieth-century religiously informed psychotherapy.[26]

While the above selection is not exhaustive, it is quite representative. For the most part, these various works have traced the unfolding stories of identifiable clinical approaches to mental healing—how they emerged and developed; how they waxed and waned; how their associated schools of thought came and went; how some triumphed and others fell by the wayside; how one evolved from or followed on a predecessor. Often enough, invidious comparisons have been made between irrational and rational approaches; naturalistic approaches have been contrasted to supernatural approaches; competition has been portrayed; winners and losers have sometimes been declared; a progressivist stance has sometimes guided an account.

The Nature of This Study

Most of the writings just mentioned (and others) have interested me, in one way or another, and some have influenced me. In some contrast to these orientations, though, I have chosen to study a selection of basic elements or ingredients that have recurrently appeared as aspects of the many and varied approaches to psychological healing. I wish to emphasize something more sustained and continuous, less given to the comings and goings of different clinical approaches, than has usually been suggested. I address this array of elements in an effort to understand what psychological healing is and to understand its fundamental relation to being human. I have no intention of suggesting that *psychological healing* is all there is to therapeutic endeavors, but every intention of asserting that it is an essential aspect of therapeutics, and that we ignore it at our peril. Our remarkable technological advances will not replace it. "Woe to the medical man who has not learned to read the human heart as well as to recognize the febrile state!"[27]

Much of what is considered in this study has been drawn from medical writings over the centuries. Other relevant data have come from religious traditions, philosophical sources, and other writings. This work is rooted primarily in Western views and practices, with scattered references to the views and practices of other cultures. While non-Western healing contexts are not reported on in any detail in this work, scholars who have made a special study of such cultures indicate that many of the basic elements studied here are identifiable as significant ingredients in traditional healing approaches in non-Western cultures — for example, the significance of the healer-sufferer relationship, the role of hope, suggestion, persuasion, confession, catharsis or abreaction, explanation and interpretation, and conditioning.[28]

After a general account of psychological healing in ancient Greece and Rome, I will undertake a detailed study of the healer-sufferer relationship as a crucial factor in healing in general, and in psychological healing in particular, and chapters on the place of talking and listening. I will devote a chapter to the use of the passions and one to the use of the imagination. Attention will be given to catharsis and abreaction, and to confession — various forms of "getting things out," of expressiveness and release. Similarly, I will offer studies of consolation, of persuasion, and of suggestion (including placebo therapy). There will be a chapter on the emergence and development of animal magnetism, mesmerism, and hypnosis, as well as discussions of explanation and interpretation, and of insight, understanding, and being understood. The theme of self-observation will encompass attention to introspection. And a chapter will be devoted to conditioning and reward and punishment.

Whether in general medicine or in particular psychological healing contexts, some concepts and their related practices — wax and wane as they may, come and go as they do — seem to survive beyond changes of name or the rise and fall of their theoretical contexts or the social fads and fashions that constitute their support during various historical moments. Threads of continuing meaning survive from era to era, from one pattern of usage to another, in a way that suggests that there are at least a few elements basic to psychological healing.

Psychological Healing in
Ancient Greece and Rome

Three types of healing in the ancient world have often been differentiated — magical, religious, and empirico-rational — and these three have frequently been noted to have been inextricably interwoven with one another.
Each type has had associated with it a particular type of healer — the sorcerer-
magician, the priest, and the physician, respectively. Not infrequently, two or
more of these roles were interwoven and vested in a single person.

The ancients believed the world to be inhabited by demons, spirits, evil
forces, and gods who were potentially malevolent or potentially benevolent
factors in the life of a person and a culture. And disease and sickness were
among the burdens which these beings or entities might, if they were so disposed, visit upon human beings or relieve them of. Incantations, spells, and
charms, commonly with associated rituals, were employed with the aim of
influencing the various supernatural beings or forces in the interest of cure or
relief — to coerce them into favorable actions, to ward off their disease-induc-
ing actions, to persuade them to help, to influence them in some useful way.
Prayers were directed to the gods, petitioning them to use their powerful
influence in favor of better health for the sufferer. Frequently magical and
religious elements were combined in what can fairly be termed magico-religious healing. Supernatural forces, whether conceived of in magical or religious terms, were commonly thought to be factors in both the causing and the
curing of disease.

In the face of a relative powerlessness, human beings developed the measures noted above to counteract the powerful forces around them or to appeal to those forces to help them in their distress. The healer's experience and reputation, his status in the particular culture, his knowledge of the proper ritual, his use of the proper words with the proper tone and in the proper manner, and his belief in the efficacy of his words and actions all came together to calm and reassure sufferers, to soothe and comfort them, and to mitigate any sense of helplessness or hopelessness. Sufferers in need, and their willingness to believe and cooperate, completed the potentially healing situation.

Within this complex network of healing practices, the presence of psychological factors was implicit. Although it may be that only the changed perspectives of later times allowed such factors to be viewed as distinct elements in their own right, there is little doubt that psychological healing was a significant aspect of the healing practices of the ancient world, however explicitly recognized it was in those times.

Scholars, giving particular consideration to ancient Greece and Rome, have addressed these issues in terms of whether there was such a thing as "psychotherapy" in the ancient world. Although Chessick has stated that the "maieutic method of Socrates is certainly the first practice of individual intensive psychotherapy," several thoughtful students of the question have concluded that the practices of that era do not warrant being termed psychotherapy.[1] And Laín Entralgo has argued that, in medicine, this lack was crucially related to the Hippocratic physicians' dismissal of so much that might have allowed such a development.[2] Still, though, forms of psychological healing were certainly known and used.

In the literature of ancient Greece from the Homeric poems through the Aristotelian corpus, Laín Entralgo found much that spoke to him as a twentieth-century scholar who was pondering the question of whether there was any such thing as a systematic "verbal psychotherapy" in the healing practices of those times. Using the phrase "the therapy of the word" to differentiate psychological healing practices from surgical interventions, herbal remedies and other medicaments, and dietary measures, he found considerable evidence of the ancient world's versions of our perennial human efforts to influence the minds of our fellows, through psychic or mental means, in the interest of curing or ameliorating a wide variety of human ailments.

Ecstatic Ceremonies as Healing Rituals

In forms such as the Dionysian and the Corybantic rites, ancient Greece cultivated ecstatic ceremonies which, among their various functions, served as therapeutic approaches to mental disturbances, including madness. Variously referred to by scholars as mass ecstasies, ecstatic possession groups, and group cathartic rituals, they "belong to a family of religious rituals (of which Bacchic rites are another prominent example) which induce ecstatic or orgiastic experiences and so bring to the participants some kind of satisfaction and peace of mind."[3] Simon has noted that the Corybantic ecstatic ceremonies were explicitly represented by Aristophanes in *The Wasps* as one of a range of therapeutic remedies for madness.[4]

As E. R. Dodds put it, Dionysius the god "enables you for a short time to *stop being yourself* and thereby sets you free." Quoting the Scythians in Herodotus, he elaborated as follows: " 'Dionysius leads people on to behave madly' —which could mean anything from 'letting yourself go' to becoming 'possessed.' The aim of his cult was *ecstasis*—which again could mean anything from 'taking you out of yourself' to a profound alteration of personality. And its psychological function was to satisfy and relieve the impulse to reject responsibility." Dodds went on to say that "the essential similarity of the Corybantic to the old Dionysian cure" was that "both claimed to operate a catharsis by means of an infectious 'orgiastic' dance accompanied by the same kind of 'orgiastic' music—tunes in the Phrygian mode played on the flute and the kettledrum."[5]

Incantations, Spells, and Charms

Various magical uses of the spoken word, and associated rituals, constituted a significant theme in healing activities in the ancient world, as they have in so many cultures since. Faced with a relative powerlessness against the elements of nature and the diseases and miseries that have been their lot, human beings have continually sought ways to reduce that sense of being powerless and to ease their apprehensions. Magical practices have frequently served that purpose, as people strove to coerce the gods with conjurations or compel them to help with charms in the interest of curing or easing the various forms of suffering. These conjurations and charms were "verbal formulas of magic character, recited or chanted in the presence of the patient to achieve his cure."[6] Laín Entralgo cited an instance from the Homeric poems, which he viewed as reflecting traditions that long antedated the classical era, that were continuously present in popular medicine through the classical period, and that were to be found in so-called primitive cultures over many subsequent centuries.[7] Such a use of words can become "a conjuration [incantation, spell] with predominance of an intent to command or coerce the realities to be modified or avoided (such as a flow of blood or the action of a devil), a charm when its intent is predominantly entreaty or supplication." The efficacy of these magical practices depended on the verbal formula used, the power or virtue of the healer, and, in the case of the charm, the divine powers to whom the healer's words were addressed. At one end of a continuum of effort to obtain healing favors from the gods was the conjuration's effort to coerce, and at the other end was the charm's effort to win over by pleading. The charm, of course, had a certain kinship with prayer, but "one who prays . . . merely *asks* the gods for a favorable course of natural events."[8] Yet at times subscribers to a particular set of beliefs tended to call the efforts of others conjurations or charms and their own efforts prayers. Although in either case the frame of reference was a supernatural one, prayer was conceived of as nonmagical in nature.

Incubation and Temple Healing

Incubation was a practice common among the Greeks and Romans of antiquity in which they would sleep within the precincts of a temple in order to receive counsel and guidance in their dreams from a healing god. The guidance sought usually entailed remedies for ailments suffered by the sleepers, although it was not restricted to such misfortunes. In many instances, the cure occurred during the healing sleep itself. Preparatory purification rites and propitiatory offerings were common; catharsis was a significant theme. Although, often enough, the remedies were consonant with the medical practices of the day, the cures achieved frequently amounted to miracles and might fairly be said to have been instances of faith healing. But they were also akin to magic, in that ritual acts were employed to coerce the god into performing his healing function. This temple healing was most often associated with Aesculapius, in legend a hero and a physician, who was later said to have been the son of Apollo and viewed as the god of healing. The most famous Aesculapian temple was the one at Epidaurus, claimed by some to have been the birthplace of Aesculapius. Other notable Aesculapian sites were at Cos, the home of Hippocrates, and, during the time of the Roman Empire, at Pergamum, the home of Galen. While other cults and their shrines involved incubation and healing practices, the Aesculapian temples became the most prominent for that purpose. It was Aesculapius, with his staff and entwined holy snake, who would later become the symbol of the medical profession.[9]

The priest-healers associated with these temples mediated between sufferer and god, guided the sufferer's practices, interpreted his dreams, and often implemented remedies that came out of this process. Both standard medical cures and miraculous cures served to build the reputations of the healing centers; and the reputations drew the afflicted to them, and sustained or induced hope in the distressed sufferers. Frequently the patients brought chronic conditions or conditions that had been beyond the capacities of the physicians of the day. Bathing, diet, exercise, music, drama, standard medical remedies, and various magico-religious practices (such as prayers, self-abasement, propitiatory rites) were interwoven in the healing activities of the temples. Autosuggestion and self-induced trance have been proposed as explanations for many of the Aesculapian phenomena, but, whatever the case may have been, important psychological healing benefits seem to have been derived from the beliefs, the buttressed hopes, and the healing practices. Pilgrimages were made to these healing shrines in the sense that would become so familiar with later Christian centers, healing spas, and other sanatoria.

The original explanations for these healing phenomena were supernatural. The cures were attributed either to magic or, more often, to religious influences.[10] In either case, the significance of belief and of faith were recognized, the need to induce, to bolster, and to maintain such attitudes in the sufferer. "The faith that heals" was a central theme. Profound psychological experiences occurred, often accompanied by high emotionality. From the vantage point of more recent times, many have looked back at the temple cures and offered psychological explanations that accorded with later frames of reference — the influencing of the imagination or the stirring of the power of the imagination toward therapeutic ends, mesmeric effects, the results of somnambulistic states, hypnosis, suggestion, autosuggestion, or self-induced trance. Certainly the way was carefully paved for what we today might term the effects of suggestion. The sufferer came or was brought to the temple as a supplicant; there was a period of delay during which a priest informed the sufferer about the power of the god and the history of the temple's cures; also in this preparatory period, purification rites were carried out and propitiatory offerings were made; and only then was the person brought into the *abaton,* the sacred hall of the temple where incubation would take place. But, whatever one might favor among the more modern explanations, the inducing and sustaining of hope, the cultivation of confidence in the god, the site, and the practices, and the supporting and maintaining of the sufferer's morale seem to have been crucial. By whatever other name, these practices were, to a significant degree, forms of psychological healing.

Naturalistic Psychological Healing

In addition to the language of supplication and the language of magical influence, though, there was also the language of "pleasant speech" and "beguiling speech," naturalistic uses of speech to influence the mind of the sufferer favorably or therapeutically — *persuasive* and *strengthening* conversations: efforts to amuse, to cheer up, or to divert from distress or pain. While the speech in the previous two categories was addressed to the gods in the hearing of the sufferer, in the latter category the speech was addressed directly to the sufferer, with the thought that, through influencing the mind, it would affect the sufferer's very nature, including passions and bodily functions.[11]

A particularly important theme was the evolving place of *persuasion* in the curative use of the word. The psychological basis of the "efficacy of the word" received "the name of 'persuasion' (*peitho*)." Peitho, Persuasion, came to be "the goddess of the persuasive efficacy of the word." Later, rhetoric was referred to as the "demiurge of persuasion." And eventually "the rationalizing and secularizing spirit of the fifth century" transformed this persuasion that "once had been divine" into something "merely 'important.'" The persuasive word came to be viewed as "pacifying, gentle, beautiful, enchanting, and only very firm and keen minds can resist the power of its enchantment." Vigorous and persuasive words were "the key to interhuman relations."[12] The stirring of the other person's emotions by the persuader was recognized as a significant component in persuasion. Interestingly, with the growing recognition of "the persuasive power of the skillfully chosen word," persuasion came to be referred to metaphorically as charm or incantation.[13] The persuasive word had "the power to take away fear, banish pain, inspire happiness and increase compassion." Rhetoric, or the art of persuasion, was referred to by Plato (ca. 429–347 B.C.) as "*psychagogia,* the art of directing minds by means of speech." Gorgias (ca. 483–376 B.C.) thought that the persuasive word acted upon the soul as medicines did upon the body, but subject to the caveat that "the medicament of the persuasive word can be poison or remedy for other men, according to the intention with which it is used." Further, rhetoric was considered a means to persuade a sufferer to accept medical care.[14] In the work of Antiphon (fifth century B.C.) were further indications of the nature of curative persuasion. He believed that the painful could be eliminated, and that there was a definite technique for so doing, which involved "informing himself of the causes of the affliction and speaking to the patient accordingly. Verbal persuasion, acting according to the causes, succeeds in eliminating pain from the mind: the thought and the word of the curative rhetorician, his *logos,* set in order and rationalize the psychic and physical life of the sufferer."[15]

From the metaphorical use of the word *charm* to refer to beautiful speech and persuasive words, Plato completed a gradual process of secularizing the charm, of conceiving of it in naturalistic terms. Thus both the charm and the persuasive word were verbal expressions, and both produced "a *real and effective* change in the mind of the one upon whom they act[ed]." Further, this "real modification of the soul of the hearer consists in the production of *sophrosyne* . . . [in which] the mind of the hearer — and subsequently his body, to the extent possible — are calmed, enlightened, and set in good order. . . . And all this in a strictly natural way by the proper virtue of that which is said, and because of the personal frame of mind of the one who hears what is said to him." "So that the word of the physician may be persuasive and may engender *sophrosyne,* it must above all be subtly accommodated to the character and state of mind of the patient." It was that part of the soul in which the irrational or the element of belief predominated which was addressed by the charm and the persuasive word. And the crucial relation of persuasion and belief to human health required the patient's "deep and trusting confidence in the physician."[16]

The Hippocratic writers were apparently familiar with the potential of the persuasive word as a therapeutic agent, but they did not take up the potential for a verbal psychotherapy outlined by Plato. They restricted their use of the persuasive word to "winning the confidence of the patient and keeping the tone of his spirit at a good level."[17] It was only with Aristotle (384–322 B.C.) that the art of persuasion was taken a step further and a systematic technique developed, albeit the result was his *Rhetoric* rather than a primer on some form of verbal psychotherapy. As had Plato, he contrasted the logical, reasoned word serving to convince with the rhetorical word oriented more toward the passions and aiming to persuade. And, for Aristotle, the three crucial issues in successful persuasion were the character of the persuader, the disposition of the hearer which was associated with the proper recognition and influencing of the passions by the persuader, and the substance of what the persuader had to say.[18] It was this Aristotelian scheme which was to be the prototype for so much in the later history of rhetoric, and to have significant meaning for the later evolution of a therapeutically oriented persuasion.[19]

The contrast just noted between the logical use of words directed to the reason and aiming to convince, and the rhetorical use of words directed to the passions and aiming to persuade, was a recurrent theme for Plato. The structure underlying this was the basic dualism of reason and the passions, the *rational* modifiable by reasoning or dialectic and the *irrational* modifiable by education or psychagogia, through persuasion or rhetoric. In either case, the goal of these efforts was sophrosyne, the well-tempered balance and serenity in the person without which a healthful state could not be achieved and medications would not be effective. We have here the teacher-healer, the "physician of the soul," and two related yet contrasted modes that served his endeavors in psychological healing. And Aristotle developed these matters further in his attention to convincing *logic* and persuasive *rhetoric*.

In addition to the naturalistic modes of healing already mentioned, it is worth noting others that would appear recurrently in the history of psycholog-ical healing. "The timely word of the physician, and, in general, of a friend, can be *iatro logos,* and not only because it sometimes cures or relieves but also because it teaches and consoles."[20] As noted earlier, education was frequently interwoven with persuasion as a complex mode of "therapy of the word," a mode associated with the teacher-healer or "physician of the soul."

Still other forms of naturalistic psychological healing were catharsis in its secularized versions and consolation. From its religious roots in the interest of cleansing and purifying, catharsis gradually became a richer, more deeply meaningful medical catharsis, one with profound psychological overtones, a purification of the passions, a psychological healing mediated by the word (or by music). The comforting benefits of consolation were usually said to have been achieved by convincing the sufferer through reason, but it seems as though, at times, the persuasive word was being used to serve the purposes of consolation.[21]

The Philosopher as Physician of the Soul

Healing of the soul in the ancient world was originally the province of priest or religious functionary, and it was inextricably interwoven with moral counsel and guidance. This care and cure of the soul included such practices as advice, consolation, comfort, admonitions, and confession and the remission of sins. Spells, incantations, prayers, and magical charms were often crucial associated measures. In ancient Greece, significant among the numerous re-ligious cults was that of Apollo, with its oracular shrines, most notably the one at Delphi. Apollo's various functions included medicine, and he was the father of Aesculapius, the hero-physician who became the god of healing. Further, matters to do with individual morality were important concerns of the famed oracle associated with the temple at Delphi. Notable among the precepts of this tradition were "Know thyself" and "Nothing too much," which exhorta-tions were inscribed on the temple.

With the emergence of philosophy as a distinct vocation, although minister-ing to troubled souls was hardly abandoned by religious functionaries, the care and cure of souls increasingly became a concern of the philosophers. Prominent in this trend was Plato for whom "philosophy alone is the *therapeia* for sickness of the soul." And that therapeia that was philosophy was essen-tially an educative process for the psyche, for the soul or mind. He redefined "mental distress and mental illness as species of ignorance resulting from the excessive power of the appetitive over the rational." Man's soul suffered from a basic conflict between the desires and passions and the reason, between the irrational and the rational; and Plato's therapeutic goals for man were harmony, order, and self-control — the temperance that was sophrosyne. The ignorance was basically an "ignorance of oneself," and the resulting diseases of the soul included vice, ignorance, and madness. In Plato's early writings, the philosophical enterprise that was at once therapeutic and educative was *dialogue,* but it was gradually developed and refined to become *dialectic,* a method of questioning and answering that divided, defined, categorized, and abstracted. In contrast to dialogue's heavy reliance on persuasion and playing upon the passions, dialectic aimed "to discover and uncover truth, not to persuade or cajole." Rather than rhetoric, logic was to predominate, a process that involved ministering to the state of ignorance, developing and shaping character, and correcting or curing the person's disease of the soul, be it vice, ignorance, or madness. "Know thyself" was woven like a red thread through this process, and "nothing too much" was an essential feature of sophrosyne. For all that he was concerned with the liabilities and dangers of the irrational (the desires and passions) and favored the development of the rational (intellectual skills, self-control, and logic), Plato was also concerned to achieve "a proper balance between affect and intellect," to resolve conflict and bring about cooperation between them. He employed philosophy "as a way to put a man in touch with his true self, and truly help him to know himself" en route to these therapeutic-educative goals.[22] The idea of the philosopher as physician of the soul rested on these foundations. And Plato further asserted that physicians should treat the whole person, both body and soul, adding that "if the head and body are to be well, you must begin by curing the soul; that is the first thing." The cure was "to be effected by the use of certain charms," and those charms were "fair words."[23]

As had been the case with Plato, the Stoics placed a particularly high premium on reason where matters either moral or psychological were concerned.[24] Reason was considered supreme among the various classes of activity. Humanistically oriented, the Stoics "advocated integrity of character, devotion to duty, humanity toward fellow-sufferers, and the rigorous discipline of will."[25] Among their particular concerns were matters of the mind: sensation, imagination (phantasia), and the various aspects of understanding and reason. Taking a view akin to the sensationists of later times, they thought of the soul as a *tabula rasa* on which sense perceptions were written to build knowledge, a view eventually restated in terms of impressions on the imagination and then revised to include an active aspect to the process of perception. In addition, their inquiries into the realm of morals and ethics carried with it a special interest in the passions. The passions, or perturbations of the soul, particularly concerned them, for they were viewed as disturbers of a moral

approach and perturbers of reason's rule. A passion was defined as "an irrational and unnatural movement of the soul or impulse in excess."[26] The Stoics
argued that these perturbations should be controlled or eliminated by reason
and duty. The guiding principle in nature was universal reason, associated
with a divine being, and it was reflected in human reason. Reason could, and
should, operate to free the person from desires and passions. The *apatheia*
thus achieved should not be misunderstood as apathy. Rather, it was tranquillity of the soul, freedom (from the passions), peace of mind, happiness. To
facilitate this degree of psychological development — to be relieved of those
"diseases of the soul" that were the passions — the guidance of an older, wiser
man was advocated, one who knew the true good and had achieved mastery of
his own passions. Whether as a model or more directly as a teacher and
counselor, he played the role of assisting the person in developing his reason
and achieving control of his passions. Early in the Stoic tradition, the goal was
to be freed completely from passion, but later the severity of the doctrine was
modified somewhat to allow the idea that reason should be in control of the
passions. And this tradition came to include consolatory interventions, again
with a gradual mellowing in the severity of their tone. Philosophic guidance
brought knowledge, self-control, consolation, and peace of mind. The philosopher had come in yet another mode to serve as a healer of souls, a physician of the soul.

Marcus Tullius Cicero (106–43 B.C.) considered the healing of "diseases of
the soul" at some length and with considerable care in his *Tusculan Disputations*.[27] In many ways critical of the Stoic tradition in these matters, at the same
time Cicero appears to have been significantly influenced by that very tradition.
Judging the passions with a certain rigor and showing a certain Stoical firmness
in his suggestions, he nevertheless allowed that the passions were aspects of
being merely human and were thus neither to be judged too harshly nor to be
dealt with in terms of the Stoical goal of apatheia. Even so, critical of the
Aristotelians' respect for the passions, and their notion of "limit" or "mean," he
favored the approach of Socrates (469–399 B.C.) and the Academy whereby
reason was to be employed in combating the passions and ministering to the
distressing sicknesses of the soul. He repeatedly emphasized that the various
troubling conditions under discussion were "disorders" rather than "diseases"
in the sense of bodily diseases, yet he regularly wrote of them in terms of an
analogy to bodily diseases, and he periodically discussed them as though they
were no longer merely analogically related. These disorders, afflictions, or
"diseases of the soul" included fear, lust, anger, all manner of griefs and
sadnesses, various other passions, and unsoundness of mind. In modern terms,
any number of emotional disorders and states of psychological distress were

included, but not madness or our psychotic conditions. Although we might use "our own resources and strength . . . to be . . . our own physicians,"[28] the sick soul was not in a good position to prescribe for itself, and therefore the counsel and guidance of wise men, or philosophers, should be sought. In fact, philosophy was defined as "an art of healing the soul." Cicero went on to say that

> These . . . are the duties of comforters: to do away with distress root and branch, or allay it, or diminish it as far as possible, or stop its progress and not allow it to extend further, or divert it elsewhere. There are some who think it the sole duty of a comforter to insist that the evil has no existence at all, as is the view of Cleanthes; some, like the Peripatetics, favour the lesson that the evil is not serious. Some again favour the withdrawal of attention from evil to good, as Epicurus does; some, like the Cyrenaics, think it enough to show that nothing unexpected has taken place. Chrysippus on the other hand considers that the main thing in giving comfort is to remove from the mind of the mourner the belief [that is troubling him]. . . . There are some too in favour of concentrating all these ways of administering comfort (for one man is influenced in one way, one in another) pretty nearly as in my *Consolation* I threw them all into one attempt at consolation.

He then added, "But it is necessary in dealing with diseases of the soul, just as much as in dealing with bodily diseases, to choose the proper time." He outlined a series of classic consolatory interventions. He emphasized that "in the alleviation of distress . . . we have to consider what method of treatment is admissible in each particular case," and that different "words of comfort" were in order for different "disorders."[29] Treatment was to be individualized both according to the person and according to the form of the distress. Also, earlier he had noted that "distress . . . can be entirely rooted out when we have disentangled its cause."[30] Cicero summed up by observing, "But how far-reaching the roots of distress, how numerous, how bitter! All of them . . . must be picked out, and, if need be, by a discussion for each separate one. . . . A great undertaking and a hard one, who denies it? But what noble undertaking is not also hard? Yet, all the same, philosophy claims that she will succeed: only let us consent to her treatment."[31]

Finally, Cicero's comments on consolation merit some special mention. His reference to his own *Consolation* was to a work, now lost, that he wrote to console himself upon the loss of his daughter, and that was referred to and quoted from at several points in the *Tusculan Disputations*. And the theme of consolation and the mention of consolatory advice recurred frequently in the sections on the healing of sicknesses of the soul. Consolation was a crucial element in his psychological healing.

Essentially a Stoic and yet rather less harsh, Lucius Annaeus Seneca (ca. 4

B.C.–A.D. 65) took up similar matters within that "department of philosophy" which he termed "preceptorial." Philosophy, being practical, offered "precepts of advice" or guidance, while, at the same time "being theoretic," it had to have its "doctrines" as well. A doctrine was "a firm belief which will apply to life as a whole"; it was the matrix and integrative force that gave coherence and meaning to the precepts. These precepts were to be "appropriate to the individual case." As were other Stoics before him, Seneca was inclined to the use of a medical metaphor in dealing with states of distress and drew analogies between bodily diseases and the "diseases of the soul." Despite the significance he gave to "doctrines" in the regulation of conduct, he made it clear that precepts had to be added in order for the doctrines to have any useful effect; and "not only precept-giving . . . [but] even persuasion, consolation, and encouragement, are necessary." And he would add "the investigation of causes." Further, Seneca advocated that human beings treat one another with kindness. Emphasizing that "nature produced us related to one another," he urged, "let our hands be ready for all that needs to be helped," quoting Terence to the effect that nothing human should be considered foreign by another human being.[32]

In addition to the scattered consolatory comments in the letter just discussed, Seneca gave considerable attention to the theme of consolation. He dealt with the consoling of the bereaved, in particular, in several others of the *Epistulae morales ad Lucilium* and in two *consolationes* among his *Moral Essays*. Further, there was his *De consolatione ad Helviam* in which, in his own time of distress, he wrote to console his mother as she faced her grief on the occasion of his own exile.[33]

Then, in *De tranquillitate animi,* Seneca began by addressing the difficulties of a restless, dissatisfied, self-deprecating man, from whose distress with himself came "mourning and melancholy and the thousand waverings of an unsettled mind,"[34] and then went on to deliver an essay on achieving a tranquil soul in the face of life's trials and misfortunes. Quoting Lucretius, he commented that, in restlessly seeking distractions from his troubled state, "ever from himself doth each man flee."[35] He prescribed active involvement in public service or other constructive work. He especially recommended the benefits of a good friend: "What a blessing it is to have those to whose waiting hearts every secret may be committed with safety, whose knowledge of you you fear less than your knowledge of yourself, whose conversation soothes your anxiety, whose opinion assists your decision, whose cheerfulness scatters your sorrow, the very sight of whom gives you joy!"[36] For such a friend, "a wise man" would be best, but "in place of the best man take the one least bad!"[37] Advocating the application of reason to one's difficulties, he emphasized the consoling and comforting of a friend and reconciling him to his lot. He urged moderation in one's ways. And he recommended various recreational diversions.

A later reflection of the Stoic tradition of the cure of souls can be found in two works of Galen (131–201), *On the Passions of the Soul* and *On the Errors of the Soul,* in which he wrote as a moral philosopher and physician of the soul and outlined an essentially Stoic approach to the passions. Viewing a person's passions, flaws, and difficulties as "diseases of the soul" and noting the difficulty one has in discerning one's own problems and doing anything about them on one's own, Galen advised seeking the counsel and guidance of an older, wiser man, one who was "commonly considered to be good and noble," who had himself lived an excellent life, "who will help him by disclosing his every action which is wrong": "These overseers will be themselves well trained and able to recognize the errors and passions from which they have been set free and to see what they still require for perfection." The troubled person would set such a one "over himself . . . some overseer and instructor, who on every occasion will remind him, or rebuke him, or encourage and urge him on to cling to the better things by furnishing himself in all things as a good example of what he says and urges."[38] Further, he advised the person to go aside by himself, to consider the advice and admonitions, and to work at the task of changing himself.[39] And he recommended regular morning and evening reviews of the difficulties detected, and a pondering on the advice and exhortations received.[40] Whether or not these efforts can fairly be termed "psychotherapy," and scholarly opinion is divided on this question,[41] they certainly were forms of psychological healing.

There does not seem to be any doubt that psychological healing was known, accepted, and practiced in the cultures of the ancient world. However explained at the time — whether in magico-religious or in naturalistic terms — the gainful results of those practices are readily reconciled with modern notions of psychological or psychosomatic treatment. Whether in the form of healing rites that brought emotional release or catharsis and a valuable calming or through a magico-religious use of the word in spells, conjurations, and charms or through a naturalistic use of the word with a view toward healing or peace of mind, a great many psychological measures aimed at relieving, strengthening, or curing a person were practiced in ancient times.

Whether any of these practices might be fairly termed psychotherapeutic is quite another question. As already noted, some scholars have objected to the ancient practices' being referred to as forms of psychotherapy, and yet others have readily used the term *psychotherapy* for certain of the ancient world's healing practices. Perhaps the most judicious position has been that taken by

Laín Entralgo when he concluded that, although Plato had invented "a rigor-ously technical verbal psychotherapy," ancient medicine did not avail itself of the developmental possibilities thus offered. Laín Entralgo then chose "ther-apy of the word" as the generic term for a range of healing practices that were distinct from surgical, medicinal, and dietetic therapeutic interventions. These practices ranged from "prerational" modes of a magico-religious nature through the persuasive rhetoric of Gorgias the Sophist and the consolatory interventions of Antiphon the Sophist to the logotherapy outlined by Plato in his dialectic and on to the persuasion of Aristotle's *Rhetoric* and the catharsis of his *Poetics*.

As one might expect, a crucial issue is just what definition of psychotherapy to use as a point of reference. If one defines psychotherapy in accordance with many of the twentieth-century schools of psychotherapeutic endeavor, it can be very difficult to fit ancient healing practices into the definition. And yet many of these modern definitions would deny some twentieth-century psycho-therapies membership in that family of endeavors. At the same time, if one applies the *Oxford English Dictionary*'s definition of "the treatment of disease by 'psychic' methods" or *A Concise Encyclopaedia of Psychiatry*'s denotation, "the method of treating illness based on the use of psychological rather than physical techniques,"[42] one can readily gather in a very wide range of healing endeavors indeed. I have made a deliberate choice to use the term *psychologi-cal healing*, in an attempt to stand aside from these controversies and hope that this more neutral term may serve as the generic one to cover a wide range of healing approaches in which mental, psychic, or psychological interven-tions are the essentials of the practice.

Although one has to be somewhat tentative in portraying any sort of process of evolving psychological healing practices in the ancient world, the data surveyed in this chapter do suggest that they had a matrix of therapeutic practices and healing rituals of a magico-religious nature that had as their goal the removal of symptoms, reduction of tension, and attainment of a balanced state of mind. By a gradual process, practices associated with naturalistic explanations supplanted some of those associated with supernatural explana-tions, and an emerging tension developed between those who used and argued for naturalistic practices and those who continued to subscribe to super-natural practices. Along with this process went a trend within the realm of supernaturally based practices for advocates of some practices to argue that theirs were based on the true religion and that others were grounded in merely magical or pagan views. Eventually, sophrosyne, encompassing moderation, virtue, and sanity, came to be both an ideal manner of being and a sort of mental health goal.

Although often expressed in musical contexts as chants or songs, words were apparently a central feature of these practices. Originally it seems to have been the custom to address the words associated with healing efforts to supernatural powers in the interest of the sufferer, with the sufferer commonly hearing or knowing about them. Thus a psychological influence on the sufferer was at work, at least when considered from a modern perspective. Gradually a shift took place: the magico-religious overtones waned and the words were addressed directly to the sufferers in an effort to change them or influence them for their own good.

In the efforts toward improvement, the curative word was used in at least three different ways that involved the passions. For one, the word was used to remove or expel distressing symptoms or a distressing state, or to free the sufferer from distress. Not uncommonly, it was a passion or emotional state which was being relieved or dispelled. An analogy to the many evacuative physical remedies is to be noted here. Second, some uses of the word were aimed at strengthening, building up, or cheering up the suffering person. Frequently, the evocation of an emotional state was involved. An analogy to tonic physical remedies is to be noted here. Third, a complex mixture of modes of using the curative word might be employed. The first phase entailed an evocative use of the word to stimulate or stir up the passions; in the second phase an emotional release or catharsis led to peace of mind or an improved state.

In the curative uses of the word just noted, the comings and goings of the sufferer's passions played a crucial role. And the use of the persuasive word for curative ends entailed an influencing of the passions. But with Plato's vigorous espousal of rationality as opposed to irrationality (associated with passions and desires), there developed an increasingly clear dichotomy of a therapy of the word through an appeal to the rational as manifested in dialectic (logic) and a therapy of the word through an appeal to the irrational as manifested in persuasion (rhetoric).

With Aristotle, it seems fair to say that matters were more balanced. Certainly he recognized a clear place for the logical convincing of a person, and so the potential was there for guiding a troubled person, through reason, toward healthful change. But Aristotle took the passions into account in a quite different way. He respected their power, as Plato had, and he favored a careful management of them. Further, because he valued the contributions of the passions to human nature, he advocated moderation and balance, a position that stood in contrast to the Stoic view that the passions should be erased or suppressed. But he also developed instrumental roles for them that became a significant part of the curative use of the word. He articulated their place in the persuasive use of the word, and his views served for many centuries as a model for the use of the passions in healing according to the principle of *contraria contrariis curantur*. Further, he played a crucial role in the development of catharsis as another healing mode involving the word and bringing relief from emotional disturbances.

And so the various healing practices of a magico-religious nature had gradually been joined, and to some degree replaced, by curative uses of the word involving dialectic, persuasion, and catharsis. Consolation was yet another mode of psychological healing that took shape in ancient Greece and Rome, but it was really a derivative of the art of persuasion, for healing words developed as a means to persuade the grieving person away from his sadness.

In summing up, then, it is fair to say that various forms of psychological healing were practiced in ancient Greece and Rome. Nevertheless, there is little to suggest that psychological interventions constituted any sort of distinct category in the medical therapeutics of that era. Attention was given to being considerate and compassionate, to being trustworthy, to maintaining the patient's morale, to enhancing the patient's confidence in the physician and in the treatment, and to the therapeutic benefits of these factors; but these issues were apparently addressed as aspects of being a good person and an effective physician rather than as an aspect of psychological therapeutics. The Hippocratic writings indicate an awareness of the importance of the psychological factors in the physician's work with patients, including the use of suggestion in therapeutics; but they do not include any evidence of a developed mode of psychological healing. And, for all the contributions of Socrates, Plato, Aristotle, and other, later philosophers that might have served as the basis for developing a formal mode of psychological healing in medicine, the post-Hippocratic centuries brought little in the way of such a development prior to the second century A.D.[43]

In the early second century, the physician Soranus (fl. 98–138) included an emphasis on psychological interventions in his discussion of the treatment of mania and melancholia.[44] His therapeutic system called for treatment measures opposite in nature to the prevailing state associated with the disease, and that included efforts to induce in the mentally disturbed patient emotions opposite to those with which he was burdened in his sickness. His rationale was that "the particular characteristic of a case of mental disturbance must be corrected by emphasizing the opposite quality, so that the mental condition, too, may attain the balanced state of health"; and this was probably the earliest established advocacy of inducing passions as a healing measure in the medical treatment of disease.[45]

In the late second century A.D., Galen is said to have maintained that many were "cured by good counsel and persuasion alone"; and he left two case reports in which his interventions were shrewd examples of psychological healing.[46] As already noted, his treatises *On the Passions of the Soul* and *On the Errors of the Soul* outlined a mode of psychological healing, though these were not strictly medical treatises.

In spite of such indications that psychological interventions were part of therapeutics for some physicians, attention to psychological themes in Greco-Roman medical treatment was more often advocated as a means of engendering a rapport with the patient and to serve a general supportive purpose. Still, though, the induction of contrary passions, as recommended by Soranus, gradually became a recognized mode of treatment in mental disorders. And the use of persuasion, through therapeutic stratagems or "pious frauds," to free insane persons from their delusions was increasingly mentioned in medical writings. By the time of Alexander of Tralles (525–605) in late antiquity, what was to become a long tradition of citing such cases and suggesting such interventions was well established.[47]

Although this chapter has focused on the data from ancient Greece and Rome, the patterns and practices traced here are fairly representative of at least some other ancient cultures. Spencer L. Rogers, in writing about the healing practices of ancient Egypt, states that "the minds of the Egyptian people were . . . approached by psychotherapeutic suggestion through various channels: through the religious system and the priesthood, through the supernatural aspects of the medicinal treatment, and through the claims and performances of exorcists and magicians."[48] Incubation and temple healing were practiced much as they were in ancient Greece, and the Egyptian healing temples apparently influenced their later counterparts in Greece. Incantations were used for various healing purposes. And exorcism was employed for the casting out of evil spirits or demons that possessed the sufferer. As Heinrich von Staden has put it, "Spells, incantations, and charms . . . dominate many — and intrude upon all — Pharaonic medical papyri."[49]

Again, the evidence from ancient India indicates psychological healing practices of a similar nature. The oldest textual sources date from around the second millennium B.C. and are found scattered in the culture's principal religious literature, primarily in the *Atharvaveda*. This "Vedic medicine" was essentially a magico-religious system in which "external beings or forces of a demonic nature" entered the body of the victim and produced sickness. The removal of the evil spirits, demons, and other malevolent forces involved healing rituals that "required the recitation of religious incantations or charms." The healers were known for their skills in dancing and in the recitation of incantations. "Amulets or talismans . . . , usually of vegetal origin, were ritually bound to drive out demons and to act as prophylactic measures in preventing further attacks."[50] Among the array of charms against various diseases, some were particularly intended for use in cases of insanity. Given that insanity was considered to be "a state when the mind leaves the body," the healer undertook "to return the mind to the body." Various magico-religious healing rites were employed, including efforts to appease the gods through offerings, purifications, recitations of (Vedic) charms, and practices aimed at expelling the demon from the sufferer.[51] Somewhat later, probably around the beginning of the Christian era, more strictly medical works were written dealing with *ayurveda* (the science of longevity), the most prominent being the writings associated with the legendary physicians Charak and Susrut. Drawing on *Charaka Samhita* (Charaka collection) and *Susruta Samhita* (Susruta collection), K. C. Dube has identified psychological healing practices involving suggestion and autosuggestion, hypnotism, the use of charms, assurance and treatment with attention and care, confession and penance, and propitiatory offerings.[52] From *Charaka Samhita,* C. V. Haldipur has quoted the following verses to illustrate psychological healing in ancient Indian medicine: "The man who has become unhinged in his mind as the result of losing something that he dearly loves, should be consoled by the proffer of a substitute and by words of sympathy and comfort. As regards the mental derangement resulting from an excess of desire, grief, delight, envy or greed, it should be allayed by bringing the influence of its opposite passion to bear on the prevailing one and neutralize it."[53]

PART TWO

The Bedrock

3

The Healer-Sufferer Relationship

The ultimate basis for the practice of medicine, or healing by any other name, is the suffering of the patients and their explicit or implicit calls for help. Thus it is reasonable to assert that the primary function of a healer is to ease a patient's suffering, while striving to cure a disease or ameliorate its effects. And the healer-sufferer relationship has long been recognized as a crucial factor in healing — for better or for worse, depending on the extent to which it has been characterized by trust and confidence on the sufferer's part and a concerned, sympathetic, and humane response on the healer's part.

In the writings that have dealt with the healer-sufferer relationship over the centuries, three significant themes can be discerned. (1) In indicating how the healer should and should not respond to and behave with the sufferer, these writings have frequently taken a distinctly moral tone. Often enough, this moral approach has entailed assertions and urgings intended to guide the healer along an ethical path in the practice of healing. That is to say, such writings belong to the history of medical ethics. *What is morally right or wrong in a healer's treatment of and dealings with a sufferer?* (2) Sometimes these writings have dealt with how healers should present themselves and what sort of persons they should be; and, however subtly presented or however thinly veiled, the impression is that they are public relations tracts, or political statements, reflecting a profession's striving for prestige, social status, or authority. *What is good or bad in the interest of the profession or in the interest of the individual healer?* (3) This literature has frequently included arguments that such and such characteristics of the healer-sufferer relationship were crucial to healing or had a potential for this or that useful purpose in healing — or, by contrast, that certain characteristics of the relationship might interfere with healing. The relationship — and the attitudes and behaviors that characterized it — had therapeutic potential in their own right, as distinct from the treatment agents and procedures that the healer employed. *What in the relationship is beneficial or detrimental in the interest of the healing of the sufferer?* This third theme is central to this study, although these three themes are frequently interwoven in the literature.

As is clear in these three themes, several ideals were being enunciated for the guidance of a healer's behavior: behavior that was morally right or behavior that would be in the best interest of the particular healer or of healers in general or behavior that would be beneficial for the healing of the sufferer or behavior that would involve some combination of these three themes. Almost as clear, although usually not as explicit, is that the enunciation of these ideals usually reflected the recognized existence of contrary behaviors and that many of those behaviors constituted threats to the optimal treatment situation. In the case of the Hippocratic Oath, for example, we not only have instances of behavior that physicians were urged to avoid, but, by implication, such behaviors actually had occurred and were thought to have been detrimental to the best interests of patients. It seems likely that this was the basis for the injunction that the physician go into a patient's home only "to help the sick and never with the intention of doing harm or injury" and that he should not abuse his position by indulging "in sexual contacts with the bodies of women or of men, whether they be freemen or slaves." And the same may fairly be said regarding the injunction that the physician should hold in confidence those things that he learned in the course of treating patients.[1] The urging that the physician should adhere to a certain form in the relationship with a patient surely indicated that deviations from that form might well pose threats to the development of the most helpful type of relationship, to the trust and confidence in the physician that would be best for the treatment, and, ultimately, to the patient's best interests. In fact, throughout this study of the healer-sufferer relationship, more often than not the behavior that was urged or recommended was a direct reaction to behavior that had been unsatisfactory and a threat to optimal care.

Thoughts about the healer-sufferer relationship as somehow a factor in healing are hardly new, though considering it as perhaps the very matrix for the work of healing is a relatively modern approach. In the restricted version of doctor and patient, this relationship has been the object of considerable attention during the twentieth century. And, in recent decades, thought about psychotherapy has increasingly viewed the psychotherapist-patient relationship itself as a crucial factor in the gains (or losses, for that matter) from various psychological healing endeavors.

Discussions of, and comments about, the healer-sufferer relationship assume someone in the role of sufferer and someone in the role of healer, the sufferer afflicted by a disease or trauma and experiencing an illness, and the healer having some combination of experience, training, and social sanction as a healer. The sufferer brings a suffering self, or is brought, to the attention of the healer, who then is expected to mobilize experience and knowledge to diagnose the sufferer's disorder and implement a treatment plan. Questions arise about what, beyond the comments just made, is the nature of the relationship of these two persons in these two roles. And what factors of significance does each contribute to the relationship? In addition to bringing a suffering self and an illness, the sufferer also brings fears and hopes, attitudes toward healers in general and toward the particular healer, trust (whether great or small) in the healer and the healing context, pain and distress and their potential for influencing the healer. The healer brings experience, knowledge, the influence of a status, and healing capabilities, but also a capacity to sense and to resonate with the patient's suffering, which capacity has often been denominated sympathy and compassion over the centuries (with the notion of empathy introduced in many twentieth-century views of the clinical context). Complementary to the patient's trust is the healer's reliability and trustworthiness. And some form of friendship has often been considered an element in such a relationship.

Further, though, the healer-sufferer relationship has tended to be characterized by "a dependence-authority set" which has varied in degree and prominence from culture to culture and over time. The following description is especially apt and relevant: "One is . . . a patient because of what one needs, while one is a physician because of what one can give as a physician. Thus, in respect to their relationship, the physician is a resource to which the patient turns and is, at least potentially, an authority, while the patient, within the relationship and insofar as the patient is willing, accepts the other's authority as being, at least ostensibly, for the patient's good. Within the relationship the physician is in a position of strength, while the patient is in one of weakness and vulnerability, whether potential or realized."[2]

The Healer-Sufferer Relationship in Ancient Greece and Rome

In the writings from Greece of the fifth century B.C., one finds some indications of how the doctor-patient relationship was conceived of in that era, at least as an ideal. The patient sought the doctor's help in order to get well, and, in addition to whatever economic interests he had, the doctor was motivated by his desire to provide technical help to the patient. The Greeks referred to both these motives as bases for *philia*, or friendship, and the relationship that evolved out of them was thus conceived of as being based on friendship. In his *Lysis*, in a discussion of friendship, Plato said that the sick man loved his physician, essentially because he was sick.[3] And in the Hippocratic *Precepts*, in a discussion of the physician's approach to the patient, the author urged that the physician should feel love of humanity and then said, "For where there is love of man, there is also love of the art [of healing]. For some patients, though conscious that their condition is perilous, recover their health simply through their contentment with the goodness of the physician."[4] And, along these same lines, Galen asserted that "Hippocrates, Empedocles, Diocles, and not a few of the other early physicians healed the sick because of their love of mankind."[5] "Philia, as one of the generic forms of human relationships, was to the Greeks the basis of the doctor and patient relationship, specifically described as 'medical philia.'" For the doctor, "friendship with the patient consisted in a correct combination of *philanthropia* (love of man as such) and *philotechnia* (love of the art of healing). A doctor was thus a friend to his patient both as 'technophile' or friend of medicine, and 'anthrophile' or friend of man."[6]

It has been observed that two ingredients were blended in the friendship toward the doctor on the patient's part: "First, his confidence in medicine, and therefore in doctors as such; secondly, his confidence in the particular doctor who is looking after him, often followed by gratitude."[7] Further, while the physician might gain the patient's confidence and friendship mainly through his technical sufficiency, two of the Hippocratic writings, *Decorum* and *Physician*, indicated other sorts of measures that the physician might use to gain that confidence. These included appearance and dress, manner (serious and humane), way of life (regular and reliable), just conduct, control of himself, and social adeptness.[8]

And, scattered through the Hippocratic and Platonic writings are a few other comments that bear on the doctor-patient relationship. In *Epidemics*, the Hippocratic author stated, "The art has three factors, the disease, the patient, the physician." As central to his role, the physician was declared to be "the servant of the art"; and he was admonished "to help, or at least to do no harm." The author then commented on the patient's role: "The patient must co-operate with the physician in combating the disease."[9] In *Physician*, the author said that the physician should be "a gentleman in character," "grave and kind to all," and "fair" in all his dealings. Further, "the intimacy . . . between physician and patient is close."[10] Plato recognized in his writings that the physician had some self-interest regarding fees. And Plato referred to the doctor-patient relationship in terms of the ruler versus the subject and the stronger versus the weaker. But he also argued that medicine was invented "for the purpose of performing a service," that "the true physician" was "a healer of the sick" rather than "a maker of money," and that, "in so far as he is a physician," the doctor does not consider "his own good in what he prescribes, but the good of his patient."[11]

In reflecting on these various passages, one finds indications of what the doctor-patient relationship may have been like and what sort of influence it may have had on healing; but there tends to be an emphasis on what *ought* to be the nature of the relationship, what it might be in the *ideal*. Also, one finds a certain amount of advice on how the physician should behave in the interest of gaining the patient's confidence and trust, the implication being that these factors are important in the process of healing. At the same time, the clear indication is that there might be some conflict between philanthropic and mercenary motives on the physician's part, and that there may well be a certain tension between his acting in his own best interests and in the patient's best interests. In short, in addition to humane inclinations on the physician's part, effort was called for in order to achieve and maintain an optimal doctor-patient relationship, as the physician's self-interest could constitute a threat to an optimal relationship.

Further, though, in passages in some of the Platonic dialogues — *The Republic* and *Laws* — it becomes quite clear that the physician's relationship to the patient varied significantly according to the social status of the patient. In *Laws*, Plato differentiated two classes of doctors: (l) the true "doctors ... who have learned scientifically ... the art" and were freemen; and (2) "doctor's servants, who are also styled doctors," who might be "slaves or freemen," and who "acquire their knowledge of medicine by obeying and observing their masters." He then differentiated "two classes of patients ... slaves and freemen";

> and the slave doctors run about and cure the slaves, or wait for them in the dispensaries — practitioners of this sort never talk to their patients individually, or let them talk about their own individual complaints[.] The slave-doctor prescribes what mere experience suggests, as if he had exact knowledge; and when he has given his orders, like a tyrant, he rushes off with equal assurance to some other servant who is ill; and so he relieves the master of the house of the care of his invalid slaves. But the other doctor, who is a freeman, attends and practises upon freemen; and he carries his enquiries far back, and goes into the nature of the disorder; he enters into discourse with the patient and with his friends, and is at once getting information from the sick man, and also instructing him as far as he is able, and he will not prescribe for him until

> he has first convinced him; at last, when he has brought the patient more and more under his persuasive influences and set him on the road to health, he attempts to effect a cure.[12]

In other words, the routinized, impersonal relationship in the treatment of a slave was in sharp contrast to the personal, individualized approach in the treatment of a freeman. In the latter case, the physician would take the trouble to learn about the patient and his illness, to listen to him and be instructed by what he heard, to instruct him about his illness, and to use persuasion to enlist the patient's cooperation in the interest of a successful treatment outcome.

In *The Republic,* Plato referred to artisans who could not afford to neglect their work and thus, even if freemen, could not receive the careful, individualized treatment accorded the well-to-do freeman.

> When a carpenter is ill he asks the physician for a rough and ready cure; an emetic or a purge or a cautery or the knife, — these are his remedies. And if someone prescribes for him a course of dietetics, and tells him that he must swathe and swaddle his head, and all that sort of thing, he replies at once that he has no time to be ill, and that he sees no good in a life which is spent in nursing his disease to the neglect of his customary employment; and therefore bidding good-bye to this sort of physician, he resumes his ordinary habits, and either gets well and lives and does his business, or, if his constitution fails, he dies and has no more trouble.[13]

Several centuries after Hippocrates and Plato, the theme of friendship in the physician-patient relationship was again specially emphasized — by Seneca, the Stoic philosopher of first-century Rome. Reasoning that he owed little to the physician who perfunctorily looked after him along with numerous other patients, Seneca made it clear that he wished for a deeply personal concern from his physician. He wanted to have from him more attention than was professionally necessary; he wanted his doctor to worry about him in particular, to be concerned for him as a friend rather than for his own professional reputation. In fact, he would wish to be, "though a host of others call for him, . . . always his [the doctor's] chief concern." With this ideal realized, friendship would be at the heart of the physician-patient relationship, and "we [the patients] are under obligation to them, not because of their skill, which they sell, but because of their kindly and friendly goodwill."[14]

After a lengthy discussion of the orientation a medical practitioner should have in approaching patients with various ailments, the Roman encyclopedist Celsus (fl. A.D. 14–37) concluded that "it is more useful to have in the practitioner a friend rather than a stranger."[15]

Of special interest are the views of Scribonius Largus (ca. A.D. 1–50), a

Roman author who seems to have been influenced by Stoic beliefs and who wrote about how physicians should behave in the preface to his book *On Remedies*. The physician's heart should be " 'full of sympathy (*misericordiae*) and humaneness (*humanitas*), in accordance with the will (*voluntatem*) of medicine itself.' " Scribonius went on to say that the true physician "is not allowed to harm anybody, not even the enemies of the state (*hostibus*). . . . since medicine does not judge men by their circumstances in life (*fortuna*), nor by their character (*personis*). Rather does medicine promise (*pollicetur*) her succor in equal measure to all who implore her help, and she professes (*profitetur*) never to be injurious to anyone. . . . Medicine is the knowledge of healing, not of hurting. If she does not try in every way to help the sick with all means at her disposal, she fails to offer men the sympathy she promises."[16]

As Edelstein has stated it, "according to Scribonius, the sympathy and humaneness required of the physician are due to everybody in equal measure. Humaneness (*humanitas*) for him is not merely a friendliness of behavior, it is a 'proficiency and benevolence toward all men without distinction,' it truly is 'love of mankind,' " for *humanitas* is equivalent to the Greek *philanthropia*.[17] While sympathy and compassion had been considered by many to be desirable in a physician, Scribonius viewed such attitudes as obligatory.

A profound version of friendship — philanthropy — was urged on the physician dealing with a patient, in a work by Libanius (314–ca. 393), a distinguished Greek rhetorician and man of letters. "You desired to be one of the healers [of sickness], you had the benefit of having [good] teachers. Now, practice your art faithfully. Be reliable; cultivate love of man; if you are called to your patient, hasten to go; when you enter the sickroom, apply all your mental ability to the case at hand; share in the pain of those who suffer; rejoice with those who have found relief; consider yourself a partner in the disease; muster all you know for the fight to be fought; consider yourself to be of your contemporaries the brother, of those who are your elders the son, of those who are younger the father."[18] This passage, "the quintessence of pagan medical humanism,"[19] is "an address on the duties of the physician that is delivered to a doctor by a personification of the medical profession."[20] In addition to urging compassion, concern, benevolence, and a faithful practice of the art, this "love of man" seems to have advocated a resonance with the sufferer's state that was long referred to as *sympathy* and that contained the seeds of what the twentieth century would term *empathy*. Though heavy with rhetorical overlay, this idealized picture of the physician-patient relationship still reflects what some thought should exist, what some physicians strove for, what some physicians in all likelihood approximated, and what many patients probably wished for.[21]

Christian Influences on the Healer-Sufferer Relationship

As we have seen, the theme of friendship was a recurrent one in early writings about the healer-sufferer relationship; and often associated with it were direct or indirect references to compassion, concern, and sympathy, or even comments that we might reconcile with twentieth-century notions of empathy. Granted, these references most often appeared in contexts where an idealized version of the relationship was under discussion, or where how a healer *should behave* or *should have behaved* was at issue. Nevertheless, the value of friendship, compassion, and the like, for the clinical process was repeatedly argued, with indications that moral authorities thought the process should be influenced by these factors, that sufferers would prefer the process to be so influenced, that at least at times the process was so influenced, and that the clinical process went better when it was so influenced.

With the advent and spread of Christianity, a new language emerged for discussion of human relationships, and, some would argue, a new attitude was manifested in the theory and practice of philia. Two basic forms of benevolent relationships between one human and another were identified in the Christian frame of reference — neighborliness and friendship. Neighborliness involved concerns for the welfare of other persons just because they were fellow humans; and friendship involved concerns for a person's well-being because he or she was *that* particular human. In the Christian frame of reference, both forms of human relationship entailed an obligation to be concerned for and to act in the interest of the other person's health. As illustrated in the parable of the Good Samaritan and the wounded stranger, the Christian was urged to have compassion and come to the aid of the sick.[22] The Christian expectation of such behavior toward another person, whether friend or merely neighbor, whether known or a stranger, was based on the precepts, " Thou shalt love thy neighbor as thyself" and "Love thy neighbor as though he were Jesus Christ." Expected of Christians in general, these attitudes and values were expected to guide the Christian healer. And medical care came to be understood "*as going beyond the limits of the art itself,* and hence the *inclusion of consolation among a doctor's duties, along with the care of incurables and the dying.*"[23]

Further, "agape (Latinized as *caritas*), be it translated by charity, love, or benevolence, became a virtue that Paul (I Cor. 13) made a cornerstone of Christian ethics, placing it above faith and hope. Like the philanthropy of the Stoics, [and] the Hebrew love of one's neighbor," charity was urged toward both friends and neighbors, as a general attitude that could encompass feelings of "love and compassion toward those who suffered," including the sick. Whereas ancient Greek sources "attest that concern for the sick and for helpless strangers was expected of doctors, and that some doctors made it their compassionate concern," Christianity "was to make this expectation an obligation." Healing continued to be a good thing; "it was part of the love for one's neighbor."[24] Personal compassion, sympathy, and charity were recurrent themes in accounts of the attitudes that healers should have toward the sick for whom they cared, and there is evidence that, at least at times, these ideal values were realized in action.[25]

Significant reflections of this spirit are found in the writings of Benedict of Nursia (ca. 480–ca. 550) and in those of Cassiodorus (ca.485–ca. 580). St. Benedict, the "patriarch of Western monasticism," drew up the Rule of St. Benedict as a series of guidelines for both the spiritual and administrative life of a monastery. Among these guidelines are some important passages regarding the care of the sick. In outlining the duties of the cellarer, he included: "Let him have special care of the sick, of the children, of guests, and of the poor, knowing without doubt that he will have to render an account of all these on the Day of Judgement."[26] In "Of the Sick Brethren," he stated, "Before all things and above all things care must be taken of the sick, so that they may be served in the very deed as Christ Himself." The abbot should take care that the sick "suffer no neglect"; and the sick should keep in mind that "they are served for the honour of God, and not grieve their brethren who serve them by their importunity."[27] The theme of *philanthropia* as a cardinal element in the healer's activity was now given a Christian interpretation. And it is of special interest to note the reference to how the sick person should function in the healer-sufferer relationship.

Cassiodorus, a Roman official, adviser to Gothic rulers in Rome, and prolific author, later a monk, founded two monasteries on Benedictine lines at Vivarium. In writing to the supervising physician of the royal household, Cassiodorus advised: " 'Let your visits bring healing to the sick, new strength to the weak, certain hope to the weary. . . . Let the patient ask you about his ailment and hear from you the truth about it.' "[28] Later he wrote the *Institutiones divinarum et humanarum lectionum* for the instruction of the monks at his monastery. In the first book, the divine letters, he included a discourse *On Doctors* in which he was addressing those monks who were designated to care for the sick and who apparently were expected to possess medical knowledge and experience. "I salute you, distinguished brothers, who with sedulous care look after the health of the human body and perform the functions of blessed piety for those who flee to the shrines of holy men — you who are sad at the sufferings of others, sorrowful for those who are in danger, grieved at the pain of those who are received, and always distressed with personal sorrow at the misfortunes of others, so that, as experience of your art teaches you, you help the sick with genuine zeal."[29] Feeling distress in response to suffering was assumed to be part of the healer's role. Compassion and sympathy for the sick on the part of the healer were clearly expected to be aspects of the healer-sufferer relationship.

Concerning the medieval centuries that immediately followed, much has been made of an alleged deterioration in medical practice, and yet much has been said about the positive influence of Christian values regarding attitudes toward and care of the sick.[30] Sacramental healing efforts, miraculous healings associated with the cult of saints and relics, and other prayerful approaches to dealing with sickness were often the context for the healer-sufferer relationship; and concerns regarding the cure of the soul were often added to the traditional concerns regarding the cure of the body. The Christian emphasis on special consideration for the sick — and caring, compassion, and sympathy for the sufferer on the healer's part — continued to be the professed ideal, and often the actual practice.

Friendship was a theme of continuing significance. In the extant literature it allows us a perspective on the doctor-patient relationship through the medieval centuries. Various examples of advice to physicians indicate the importance given to gaining the patient's good opinion, overcoming the patient's doubts about the doctor or his procedures, bringing the patient to have confidence or trust in the doctor, and enlisting the patient's cooperation in the therapeutic enterprise, all of which had been elements of advice to physicians in antiquity and had implications for the influence on the healing process of the relationship between healer and sufferer. Further, "the gradual process of legal rationalisation of human relations" made it increasingly explicit that "the medical relation is a contract,"[31] an issue that brings up such questions as the degree of negotiation in the life of the healer-sufferer relationship and the extent to which collaboration might be one of its features.

Suffering, Compassion, and Sympathy

One need not explore the history of the healer-sufferer relationship for long before one meets up with references to compassion and sympathy. And differentiate, or try to differentiate, sympathy and compassion as one might, they have repeatedly been associated with each other — at times as synonyms, at times as parts of one another's definition, at times as ready referents for one another, and at times merely as closely related themes. *Sympathy*, which has its roots in Greek terms meaning "having a fellow feeling" and "suffering," is defined by the *Oxford English Dictionary* as "the quality or state of being affected by the condition of another with a feeling similar or corresponding to that of the other; the fact or capacity of entering into or sharing the feelings of another or others; fellow-feeling."[32] Eventually the Greek word gave rise to the Latin *sympathia*. As to *compassion*, the usages date back to the Latin of Tertullian and Jerome, meaning "to suffer together with, feel pity." The *Oxford English Dictionary* defines it as "suffering together with another, participation in suffering; fellow-feeling, sympathy." The following is then suggested to be a more modern meaning: "The feeling or emotion, when a person is moved by the suffering or distress of another, and by the desire to relieve it; pity that inclines one to spare or to succour."[33] Compassion and pity were for the most part used as synonyms in the Bible, both in the Old Testament and in the New Testament, although it has been noted that, in two places, "*compassion* retains its original meaning of *sympathy*."[34] Although compassion and pity are still often considered synonyms, the equivalence has been weakened because pity has come to imply sometimes a degree of condescension toward the person being pitied.

These sentiments of sympathy and compassion have repeatedly been put forward as the attitudes one person should have toward another, as the reactions a human being should have to distress and suffering on the part of a fellow human being. And the writings of Christian authors have played a significant part in the ongoing espousal of these sentiments. Augustine, for example, argued for compassion as a particularly notable virtue, and commented, "What is compassion but a kind of fellow-feeling in our hearts for another's misery, which compels us to come to his help by every means in our power?"[35]

These sentiments have long constituted an important theme in moral philosophy, or ethics. They have been referred to as ideals for human behavior toward friend, neighbor, and even stranger. They have been considered standards that humans should strive toward and be guided by as they soldier on in life and endeavor to be good, even when falling short of those ideals. Viewed another way, they have been considered natural attitudes and reactions for human beings, and those who have fallen seriously short of the mark have often been considered failed or defective human beings. And, as natural attitudes and reactions, it has been argued, they have been essential elements in the development of human societies and cultures and are important aspects of the essence of human relationships.

Thus it is not at all surprising that sympathy and compassion have been urged upon healers as optimal (perhaps even necessary) reactions to sufferers—that these sentiments which have been recurrently emphasized in the history of moral philosophy have so often been emphasized in medical ethics in particular. And no wonder they are hoped for and looked for by sufferers in their relations with their healers. In fact, it has been repeatedly suggested that healing prospers when its context is a healer-sufferer relationship character-ized by sympathy and compassion, and that it does not go so well when these sentiments are limited or absent. For example, Theophrastus Bombastus von Hohenheim, known as Paracelsus (1493–1541), argued that love is at the heart of the matter where the practice of medicine is concerned. "There are two kinds of physician — those who work for love, and those who work for their own profit. . . . The true and just physician is known by his love and by his unfailing love for his neighbour."[36] In another context, he commented that the physician's "office consists of nothing but compassion for others. . . . His office is . . . to cure the patient by the charity and love with which God has endowed man." He went on to say, "The art of medicine is rooted in the heart. . . . If your heart is just, you will also be a true physician. No one requires greater love of the heart than the physician. For him the ultimate instance is man's distress."[37] Once again, there are hints of the dangers that might interfere with being "a true physician": working for one's own profit, being less than just.

The seventeenth and eighteenth centuries brought a considerable attention to the nature of human beings, often couched in more secular terms. And the physician of that era learned and practiced in a context where those views were active and influential. Against a seventeenth-century background of Hobbes's work on human nature and morals, and Locke's theory of knowl-edge — and, around the turn of the century, Shaftesbury's more sanguine per-spective on human nature — the eighteenth century was associated with a sig-nificant increase in, and a somewhat new type of, attention to sympathy — into which some reference to compassion was often interwoven. The writings of a series of British moral philosophers emphasized sympathy as being of the essence in the so-called moral sense or as being crucial in the determining of moral behavior. It was argued that it was a central factor in human relation-ships and thus constituted "the cement of human society."

In the context of writing about human nature as entailing concern for others and an inclination toward social relations, as much as it entails self-interest, in 1726 Joseph Butler (1692–1752) — an English divine and philosopher — wrote about "such a correspondence between the inward sensations of one man and those of another." Further, he reasoned, "Men are so much one body, that in a peculiar manner they feel for each other, shame, sudden danger, resentment, honour, prosperity, distress; one or another, or all of these, from the social nature in general, from benevolence, upon the occasion of natural relation, acquaintance, protection, dependence; each of these being distinct cements of society."[38]

In *A System of Moral Philosophy*, published posthumously by his son in 1755, Francis Hutcheson (1694–1746) — a schoolmaster, and later professor of moral philosophy at Glasgow — took up and developed further Shaftesbury's notion of a *moral sense* by which a person perceived virtue and vice and was able to approve of the former and condemn the latter. After dealing with the external senses, an appetite for food, perceptions of pleasure and pain, and the "two calm natural determinations of the will," namely, self-love and benevolence toward others, Hutcheson considered six internal senses or *"finer Powers of Perception."*[39] Among the latter, he included a "sense of the soul we may call the *sympathetick*, different from all the external senses; by which when we apprehend the state of others, our hearts naturally have a fellow-feeling with them. When we see or know the pain, distress, or misery of any kind which another suffers, and turn our thoughts to it, we feel a strong sense of pity, and a great proneness to relieve, where no contrary passion with-holds us. And this without any artful views of advantage to accrue to us from giving relief, or of loss we shall sustain by these sufferings."[40]

With Butler's views and Shaftesbury's "moral sense" as part of his background, and particularly the influence of Hutcheson's views, in *A Treatise of Human Nature* in 1739, the Scottish philosopher and historian David Hume (1711–1776) gave considerable attention to the notion of sympathy. "No quality of human nature is more remarkable, both in itself and in its consequences, than that propensity we have to sympathize with others, and to receive by communication their inclinations and sentiments, however different from, or even contrary to our own." In explaining sympathy, he employed the principles of association and emphasized the role of the force of the imagination.[41] Further along in this work, he outlined "the nature and force of *sympathy*" as follows:

> The minds of all men are similar in their feelings and operations, nor can any one be actuated by any affection, of which all others are not, in some degree, susceptible. As in strings equally wound up, the motion of one communicates itself to the rest; so all the affections readily pass from one person to another, and beget correspondent movements in every human creature. When I see the *effects* of passion in the voice and gesture of any person, my mind immediately passes from these effects to their causes, and forms such a lively idea of the passion, as is presently converted into the passion itself. In like manner, when I perceive the *causes* of any emotion, my mind is convey'd to the effects, and is actuated with a like emotion.[42]

And, in another place, he added, "This principle of sympathy is of so powerful and insinuating a nature, that it enters into most of our sentiments and passions, and often takes place under the appearance of its contrary. . . . The sentiments of others can never affect us, but by becoming, in some measure, our own; in which case they operate upon us, by opposing and encreasing our passions, in the very same manner, as if they had been originally deriv'd from our own temper and disposition."[43]

In 1759, in *The Theory of Moral Sentiments,* the Scottish moral philosopher and economist Adam Smith (1723–1790) gave interesting attention to *sympathy,* his views being influenced by Hume and probably by Hutcheson. Smith addressed the question of a person's capacity to sense or appreciate the state of mind of another person as follows:

> As we have no immediate experiences of what other men feel, we can form no idea of the manner in which they are affected, but by conceiving what we ourselves should feel in the like situation. . . . By the imagination we place ourselves in his situation, we conceive ourselves enduring all the same torments, we enter as it were into his body, and become in some measure the same person with him, and thence form some idea of his sensations, and even feel something which, although weaker in degree, is not altogether unlike them. . . .
>
> That this is the source of our fellow-feeling for the misery of others, that it is by changing places in fancy with the sufferer, that we come either to conceive or be affected by what he feels, may be demonstrated by many obvious observations, if it should not be thought sufficiently evident of itself.[44]

He went on to note that it was not only "those circumstances . . . which create pain or sorrow, that call forth our fellow-feeling"; rather, "our sympathy with sorrow, though not more real, has been more taken notice of than our sympathy with joy. The word sympathy, in its most proper and primitive signification, denotes our fellow-feeling with the sufferings, not that with the enjoyments, of others."[45] But "sympathy, though its meaning was, perhaps, originally the same [as pity and compassion], may now, however, without much impropriety, be made use of to denote our fellow-feeling with any passion whatever."[46]

Smith took into account that "upon some occasions sympathy may seem to arise merely from the view of a certain emotion in another person. The passions, upon some occasions, may seem to be transfused from one man to another, instantaneously, and antecedent to any knowledge of what excited them in the person principally concerned." He pointed out that grief and joy are often thus quickly sensed, whereas anger, for example, is an emotion to which another person may be very slow to have a sympathetic response; and, even with grief and joy, there are instances enough when the other person has difficulty in sympathetically appreciating the nature of the affected person's state of mind. Sympathy with the person's emotions in these various instances takes time to develop and requires effort toward the goal of understanding why the person feels that way. Smith outlined a process characterized by curiosity and interest and involving questions and efforts to learn what has happened to the distressed person. He concluded that "sympathy, therefore, does not arise so much from the view of the passion, as from that of the situation which excites it." It is also significant that he recognized the need for "some disposition to sympathize."[47]

Still further, Smith indicated something especially important about the role of sympathy in coping with distress and troublement. He implied that the sympathetic response can bring consolation to troubled persons, be a distinct comfort to them, and serve to alleviate their distress. "Sympathy . . . alleviates grief by insinuating into the heart almost the only agreeable sensation which it is at that time capable of receiving." The sufferer is often relieved by finding a person to whom he can communicate the cause of his sorrow. On receiving another's sympathy, sufferers "seem to disburthen themselves of a part of their distress: he is not improperly said to share it with them. He not only feels a sorrow of the same kind with that which they feel, but as if he had derived a part of it to himself, what he feels seems to alleviate the weight of what they feel." These circumstances may well renew the sufferer's grief in the short run, but they commonly bring relief in the long run.[48] "The relief and consolation of human misery depend altogether upon our compassion" for the unfortunate person's distress.[49] It seems fair to conclude that Smith recognized the extent to which sufferers yearn for the sympathy and compassion of others, and find significant comfort in those sentiments when they are forthcoming.

During this same era a variety of other authors and critics employed the notion of sympathy in considering a person's capacity to understand another person, in seeking to understand the roots of moral behavior, in endeavoring to grasp the nature of poetic and other literary creativity, and in critical assessments of literary and other creative endeavors.[50] The basic reasoning was that the imagination was crucial and that, through the use of this faculty combined with sensibility, a *sympathetic understanding* of another could be gained. By the time of Samuel Johnson's *Dictionary* (1755), *sympathy* was defined as "fellowfeeling; mutual sensibility; the quality of being affected by affection of another"; and *to sympathize* meant "to feel with another; to feel in consequence of what another feels."[51] And thus, as these definitions implied, the passions or affects played a part in the activity of this *sympathetic imagination*. In an essay, "Of Sympathy," in 1776 James Beattie (1735–1803), a Scottish poet and writer on philosophy, provided us with a representative passage concerning how sensibility and imagination were thought to combine to bring about a sympathetic discernment or sympathetic understanding of another.

> When we consider the condition of another person, especially if it seem to be pleasurable or painful, we are apt to fancy ourselves in the same condition, and to feel in some degree the pain or pleasure that we think we should feel if we were really in that condition. Hence the good of others becomes in some measure our good, and their evil our evil; the obvious effect of which is, to bind men more closely together in society, and prompt them to promote the good, and relieve the distresses, of one another. Sympathy with distress is called Compassion or Pity: Sympathy with happiness has no particular name.[52]

A basic premise in this system of moral and psychological principles was that "there is a natural and instinctive sympathy for one's fellow man" which is of "primary importance in the constitution of man" and which serves, in concert with the imagination, to achieve an appreciative understanding of one's fellows.[53] As a modern scholar, Norman S. Fiering, has stated it, "eighteenth-century sympathy and humanitarianism" entailed notions of the naturalness of an "irresistible compassion."[54]

This theme of the sympathetic appreciation of another's distress also emerged as an active factor in considering the troubled, the melancholy, and the mad in the eighteenth century. "This emergent sympathy toward the mad—some of it authentic, some smacking of affectation—matched a growing preoccupation among the literati with the relations of self and society, the private and the public, the individual and the normal, the mazy motions of the mind." Increasingly, "affinities between the mentality of people at large and the insane" were being recognized, often to the end of bringing comfort to the troubled or mad, though sometimes to the discomfort of the not-so-mad.[55]

While the writings of eighteenth-century physicians do not tell us a great deal about their thought or practice on such matters, John Gregory (1724–1773) was a notable exception. As "Professor of the Practice of Physic" at the University of Edinburgh, Gregory included in his lectures to the students a thoughtful series on the physician-patient relationship, which was eventually published in 1772 as *Lectures on the Duties and Qualifications of a Physician* and became particularly influential. Gregory addressed at some length "the moral qualities peculiarly required in the character of a physician," with an emphasis on sympathy and compassion.

> The chief of these is humanity; that sensibility of heart which makes us feel for the distresses of our fellow-creatures, and which of consequence incites us in the most powerful manner to relieve them. Sympathy produces an anxious

attention to a thousand little circumstances that may tend to relieve the patient; an attention which money can never purchase: hence the inexpressible comfort of having a friend for a physician. Sympathy naturally engages the affection and confidence of a patient, which in many cases is of the utmost consequence to his recovery. If the physician possesses gentleness of manners, and a compassionate heart, and what Shakespeare so emphatically calls "the milk of human kindness," the patient feels his approach like that of a guardian angel ministering to his relief. . . . [But] physicians [who] are callous to sentiments of humanity, treat this sympathy with ridicule, and represent it either as hypocrisy, or the indication of a feeble mind. That sympathy is often affected, I am afraid is true; but this affectation may be easily seen through. . . . The insinuation that a compassionate and feeling heart is commonly accompanied with a weak understanding and feeble mind, is malignant and false. Experience demonstrates, that a gentle and humane temper, so far from being inconsistent with vigour of mind, is its usual attendant.[56]

Gregory contrasted such qualities with those of physicians who tended to be callous and noted that patients reacted poorly to such unfeeling doctors. He also mentioned that "a certain gentleness and flexibility" allowed a physician to be both patient and likelier to enlist the patient as a cooperative participant in his or her own treatment.[57]

A generation after Gregory, another eighteenth-century physician, the Idéologue Pierre-Jean-Georges Cabanis (1757–1808) gave significant attention to the theme of sympathy and compassion. Critically engaged in concerns about the nature of human beings and in social reform in Paris in the 1790s, Cabanis was familiar with the work of the Scottish moral philosophers (particularly Frances Hutcheson and Adam Smith) and their theory of moral sense, and he subscribed to a notion of moral sympathy. He wrote at length about sympathy, defining moral sympathy as follows: "The MORAL SYMPATHY consists in the faculty of sharing the ideas and affections of others, in the desire to make them share one's own ideas and affections, in the need to influence their will."[58] Then he commented on the physician's compassion and sympathy in *Coup d'oeil sur les révolutions et sur le réforme de la médicine.*

It is the duty of the physician to afford the sweetest and most soothing consolations to the patient couched on the bed of sickness; it is he alone, who can penetrate farthest into the confidence of infirmity and misfortune, and, therefore, it is he who can pour the most salutary balm into their wounds. But, for the same reason, he must not remain ignorant of the nature and destiny of these unhappy and too feeble mortals; he must not be void of compassion for those errors and miseries which may so readily become the lot of every one; but he must be indulgent and kind, as well as circumspect and reasonable.

Every one else may hate vice, and be revolted at folly: but the physician, if he knows how to observe and judge properly; if he possesses good sense, if he is just and liberal in his sentiments, can feel only pity for both, and can only redouble his zeal for the service of those degraded and unfortunate creatures, who ought to excite his compassion more forcibly, the more that they are insensible to their own unhappy state.[59]

"Magnetic Rapport" and Sympathy

During the late eighteenth century and the early decades of the nineteenth century, the emerging field of mesmerism, or animal magnetism, developed the concept of *magnetic rapport* as a key ingredient in another form of the healer-sufferer relationship. Gradually *sympathy* became part of the discussions of this intimate rapport. At times, these two terms were used more or less as synonyms; and at times sympathy was considered to be the essence of magnetic rapport.

Franz Anton Mesmer (1734–1815)—the physician whose research on animal magnetism eventually led to hypnosis—wrote "of sympathy, antipathy, of attraction, repulsion" as being among the "agents" in nature that reflected the presence of the "universal fluid" and accounted for a wide range of natural phenomena. He took sympathy to mean "nothing other than an inclination, a pleasant impulse we carry towards one another as two magnets are attracted to each other reciprocally."[60] And he thought of "animal magnetism" as a "sixth sense" whereby he sensed or perceived what went on in the patient.[61]

Understood as "a (real or supposed) affinity between certain things, by virtue of which they are similarly or correspondingly affected by the same influence, affect or influence one another . . . , or attract or tend towards each other,"[62] in the seventeenth century sympathy was thought to be the basis whereby wounds and illnesses could be cured. Over many centuries, it had been thought that injuries or illnesses in various organs or parts of the body might lead to similar disturbances in other organs or parts of the body—by virtue of a "consent" between bodily parts or a "sympathetic influence" from one organ to another.[63] During the Renaissance, *sympathy* came to refer also to putative actions at a distance between various bodies and parts of the universe. In the seventeenth century, this latter trend became the basis for healing efforts—such as Kenelm Digby's "powder of sympathy" and the "weapon salve"—referred to as *sympathetic medicine*. In pursuit of a natural rather than magical explanation, some conceived of this as *magnetic medicine*.[64] By the eighteenth century, such cures effected through "action at a distance" seem to have been abandoned in medicine. Medical explanations in terms of sympathy were once again confined to matters within the living body, and they were reasoned in relation to the nervous system.

This *sympathetic medicine* or *magnetic medicine* was a significant part of the heritage out of which Mesmer constructed his therapeutic theory: his magnetic healing was a descendant of the seventeenth-century's "sympathetic healing." As the notion of magnetic rapport developed, a sympathetic or animal magnetic influence was thought to operate as a healing influence transmitted from the magnetizer to the patient. Gradually, though, discussions of how the magnetizer sensed what was happening within the patient, and how he conveyed his healing influence to the patient, came to employ a magnetic rapport that entailed a sympathy understood more and more in the "fellow-feeling" tradition of the term, rather than in the sense of seventeenth-century sympathetic medicine.

In the 1780s, Armand Marie Jacques de Chastenet, marquis de Puységur (1751–1825), who had studied with Mesmer, discovered that some subjects fell into a sleeplike state when being mesmerized or magnetized; and he likened this state to sleepwalking. From this, he reasoned that the induction of this magnetic sleep (or magnetic somnambulism) brought about a special relationship between the magnetizer and the magnetized subject, which he termed *magnetic rapport;* and he viewed this relationship as having an important role in the healing process. For Puységur, the therapeutic work was based on this intimate rapport between the magnetizer and the subject, with no role for a magnetic fluid. This rapport brought with it "a trust of the magnetizer that is childlike in its intensity and extent."[65] Eventually, some magnetizers came to view this rapport as the basis for conceiving of magnetic healing in terms of suggestion.

In assessing Mesmer's rapport, Adam Crabtree, a historian of mesmerism and hypnotism, writes: "The mutual influence of magnetist and patient involved a kind of sympathy which Mesmer called the 'sixth sense.' Cures wrought by animal magnetism always had this empathic component strongly at the forefront. . . . Through his personal charisma Mesmer was able to set up a powerful empathic relationship with his patients."[66] Like Puységur, A. A. Tardy de Montravel—an early magnetizer and author on magnetic somnambulism—wrote at length in the 1780s about rapport, likening the nervous systems of the two parties in the relationship to "two musical instruments in such 'harmonic rapport' that a chord played on one creates a corresponding chord in the other." And this rapport was conceived of as "the result of the action of sympathy found everywhere in nature." He referred to "harmonic rapport as a kind of platonic love between magnetizer and patient." In his view, magnetic rapport was "identical with the state of sympathy that is at the heart of platonic love."[67] In this same period, Charles de Villers (1767–1815), a friend and associate of Puységur, viewed "harmonic rapport and love as essential to the healing process" and abandoned the idea of the involvement of a physical agent (magnetic fluid). "Healing . . . [was] produced through sympathy and harmonic rapport." For Villers, "the magnetizer must have 'moral affection' or 'sympathy,' brought about through a feeling of 'cordiality.' He equated this moral affection with what had been termed 'rapport' in magnetic writings. In magnetic healing, patients put their trust in the magnetizer and open themselves completely to his influence. He in turn exercises a familial benevolence toward them that is the means by which the healing action takes place."[68]

The view that sympathy was a critical factor in magnetic healing continued to be one of several viewpoints held by magnetic theorists. Because human beings were thought to share a common bond as members of the same species, the term *sympathy* was used to refer to this bond, and to explain the intimate communication that could occur between a magnetic healer and a patient. *Sympathy* used in this way reflected an explanatory tradition dating back to the magnetic healing of the seventeenth century; and, at the same time, this sympathy had a resonance with the familiar notion of sympathy as a "fellow-feeling" in response to the distress of a suffering person. References to "sympathy" occurred intermittently in later nineteenth-century animal-magnetic and hypnotic contexts, but by and large the usual term was "magnetic rapport," or merely "rapport."

Whereas rapport in the mesmeric-hypnotic tradition frequently implied a dependent, highly influenceable state in the patient and a dominant position for the magnetic healer from which he could influence the patient toward a healing goal, in the twentieth century *rapport* gradually shifted to a meaning quite independent of its mesmeric roots — namely, a harmonious relationship between a healer and a sufferer, characterized by sympathy, understanding, and a mutual confidence. Modern notions of a working alliance or a treatment alliance usually imply rapport in this sense.

Doctor and Patient in the Nineteenth Century

This theme of sympathy, compassion, and a sympathetic understanding of the *other* person remained significant on into the nineteenth century, in concerns about human relations in general and in discussions of the physician-patient relationship in particular. The imagination, through sympathetic intuition or sympathetic identification, was thought to perceive "the fundamental reality and inner working, the peculiar 'truth' and nature" of the *other*, whether that other was a work of art or literature, another person, or some other living being. So thought various philosophers, the romantic critics, and major literary figures of the early century;[69] and so, too, thought some among the physicians. The significance of sympathy continued to be argued through the rest of the century.

Those interested in the *moral treatment* of the insane that had emerged around the turn of the nineteenth century made repeated references to compassion and sympathy as essential elements in such treatment programs. In 1833, for example, the American reformer and educational pioneer Horace Mann (1796–1859) discussed the moral treatment program at Worcester State Hospital, Massachusetts, at some length. As someone who had lent crucial support to the founding of the hospital, he had become chairman of the hospital board of trustees; and, in the hospital's first annual report, he summed up matters as follows: "The whole scheme of moral treatment is embraced in a single idea — humanity — the law of love — that sympathy which appropriates another's consciousness of pain and makes it a personal relief from suffering whenever another's sufferings are relieved."[70]

Among the philosophers, Arthur Schopenhauer (1788–1860) held views that are particularly noteworthy. In 1840 he dealt with compassion and sympathy at considerable length in *On the Basis of Morality*, first published in 1841 along with another essay on ethics, in *The Two Fundamental Problems of Ethics*. Setting himself against the cold rationality of Kant's views that were in favor of *duty* as the basis for good deeds and moral behavior and that objected to "feelings of compassion and of tenderhearted sympathy," Schopenhauer grounded his theory of morality in those very feelings.[71]

Schopenhauer placed compassion at the heart of his moral system: "There are two clearly separate degrees wherein another's suffering can directly become my motive. . . . In the first degree, by counteracting egoistic and malicious motives, compassion prevents me from causing suffering to another. . . . In the second place, there is the higher degree where compassion works positively and incites me to active help." He identified "doing no injury" and "helping" as "cardinal virtues" — "justice" and "philanthropy" — and commented that "Both have their roots in natural compassion." He then added that "anyone appearing to be wanting in compassion is called inhuman, and so 'humanity' is often used as its synonym." And he used "loving-kindness, *caritas*" as synonyms for philanthropy.[72]

With regard to how compassion might operate, he wrote as follows:

> But now if my action is to be done simply and solely *for the sake of another,* then *his weal and woe* must be *directly my motive,* just as *my* weal and woe

are so in the case of all other actions. . . . Thus, how is it possible for *another's* weal and woe to become directly my motive, and this sometimes to such a degree that I more or less subordinate to them my own weal and woe, normally the sole source of my motives? Obviously only through that other man's becoming *the ultimate object* of my will in the same way as I myself otherwise am, and hence through my directly desiring *his* weal and not *his* woe just as immediately as I ordinarily do only *my own*. But this necessarily presupposes that, in the case of his *woe* as such, I suffer directly with him, I feel *his* woe just as I ordinarily feel only my own; and, likewise, I directly desire his weal in the same way I otherwise desire only my own. But this requires that I am in some way *identified with him*, in other words, that this entire *difference* between me and everyone else, which is the very basis of my egoism, is eliminated, to a certain extent at least. Now since I do not exist *inside the other man's skin,* then only by means of the *knowledge* I have of him in my head, can I identify myself with him to such an extent that my deed declares that difference abolished. However, the process here analyzed is not one that is imagined or invented; on the contrary, it is perfectly real and indeed by no means infrequent. It is the everyday phenomenon of *compassion,* of the immediate *participation,* independent of all ulterior considerations, primarily in the *suffering* of another, and thus in the prevention or elimination of it; for all satisfaction and all well-being and happiness consist in this. It is simply and solely this compassion that is the real basis of all *voluntary* justice and *genuine* loving-kindness. . . . As soon as this compassion is aroused, the weal and woe of another are nearest to my heart in exactly the same way, although not always in the same degree, as otherwise only my own are. Hence the difference between him and me is now no longer absolute.[73]

Among the physicians, Worthington Hooker (1806–1867), a Connecticut medical practitioner who from 1852 to 1867 was professor of the theory and practice of medicine at the Medical Institution of Yale College, in 1849 discussed sympathy at some length as a crucial element in the physician-patient relationship. He argued that this relationship optimally has the confidential nature of "an intimate friendship," which the physician needs to earn and to honor. Further, the physician "enters the dwelling of the sick as if he were one of the family, and the very office that he is to perform disarms all formality, and pre-supposes intercourse of the most familiar character. The patient is to speak to him not of a foreign subject, nor of some one else, but of himself, of his own body, of its pains and ailments, and that too with sufficient minuteness to communicate an adequate knowledge of his case. In so doing, he calls into exercise not only the scientific acumen of the *physician,* but, mingled with this the sympathy of the confidential *friend.*"[74]

Hooker then outlined his views regarding the naturalness and significance of the physician's "sympathy and kindness." In the process, he described the notion of "*active* sympathy," which involved the physician's management of his feelings of distress and sympathy in response to the patient's suffering by transforming them into constructive, healing actions — what in the twentieth century might be termed sublimation. In regard to the physician who develops the capacity for so managing his feelings, Hooker alluded to "the erroneous impression, that the practice of medicine and surgery necessarily subjects the heart to a hardening process." On the contrary, he maintained, while the physician "is acquiring this self-control, his sympathy with suffering is becoming all the time deeper and livelier, by the exercise of that active benevolence to which his profession calls him. It is only the physician who refuses to yield to this call, and pursues his profession as a mere trade for self-aggrandizement, that blunts his sensibilities, and hardens his heart."[75]

It was hardly novel to urge kindly feelings and humane sympathies toward suffering patients as significant for physicians. Young doctors just graduating from medical school testified to the prevalence of such values by emphasizing in their medical theses that the values should be characteristic of physicians.[76] Yet the notion that such sentiments were waning as components of clinical activities was bemoaned.

Much has been said about hardness, toughness, and "masculinity" as characteristics that were associated with devaluing sympathy and compassion. The argument was often that the physician should proceed, undeterred by a patient's suffering, on his appointed course to some valued medical end. Still, it is clear that patients, romantic and sentimental writers, and a scattering of medical spokesmen constantly decried scientific callousness and extremes of medical objectivity and wished for and, at times, demanded sensitivity to a sufferer's feelings through a kindly, sympathetic relationship.[77] There was considerable concern that physicians should "feel more emotional involvement with their patients" and that they should strive toward a feminine ideal in their relationships with them. "Assuredly it is not a pulseless, tideless being that is desired to officiate at the couch of sickness. Rather is the man most acceptable as a physician who most approximates the feminine type; who is kind, and gentle, and cautious, and sympathetic, and truthful, and delicately modest."[78]

These conflicting views became common concerns, and they continued to be significant aspects of discussions of the doctor-patient relationship during the rest of the century and on into the twentieth century — not to mention the fact that they are still lively concerns today. Such discussions about the doctor-patient relationship often involved and continue to involve three questions: what it ought to be, what it is, and what role it might have in healing.

The noted physician William Osler (1849–1919), speaking to a class of graduating medical students in 1889, urged in the most persuasive terms the value for the physician of "imperturbability" and "equanimity". He elaborated by saying that this meant "coolness and presence of mind under all circumstances, calmness amid storm, clearness of judgment in moments of grave peril, immobility, impassiveness, or, to use an old and expressive word, *phlegm*." While this might seem to suggest a certain aloofness or an unfortunate degree of detachment, this was clearly neither what Osler meant nor how he functioned. He certainly did respect and strive to promote "scientific medicine," and his era was the time in which scientific medicine was steadily evolving in ways that often tended to make an object of the patient and distance the physician from him or her. But, in the same valedictory address, Osler was arguing that this "equanimity" would have an important role in patients' coming to have confidence in the physician, that the physician's manner would have a calming effect, and that it would be "a comfort to all who came in contact with him." Osler went on to make it clear that he advocated adopting this calmness, this equanimity "without, at the same time, hardening 'the human heart by which we live.'" In further comment on patients, he mentioned "the need of an infinite patience and of an ever-tender charity toward these fellow-creatures."[79] Osler was here indicating the difficult fine line that a physician often needs to tread in managing both a degree of calmness and a degree of involvement, mixing a caring concern with a calming demeanor in the pursuit of therapeutic ends. Many who knew him as a clinician provide considerable evidence that Osler was not at all aloof or callous. He has been referred to as "the exemplar of humane practice" who manifested "'spontaneous, natural, and kindly interest in patients and students, and in people in general.'" He was "the humane, concerned physician," "the archetype of the humane physician," and "a master of the art of seeing always the human being who was ill, rather than seeing the illness as an interesting phenomenon that happened to be accompanied by a person."[80]

Sympathy, Women, and Medicine

The nineteenth-century struggles of women for entry into the medical profession constituted another context for the lively expression of views on sympathy as a significant factor in the healer-sufferer relationship. The pioneer American woman physician Elizabeth Blackwell (1821–1890) and others argued that women's natural traits or qualities especially fitted them for the practice of medicine. The kindness, gentleness, sympathy, and capacity for nurturance that were considered innate in women equipped them with a natural aptitude for the concerned caring that was essential to the role of physician.

Maternal inclinations were thought to be at the heart of the matter. And sympathy was frequently cited as being of the essence and as a crucial ingredient for the practice of medicine.[81]

Blackwell referred to the " 'intelligent sympathy with suffering' " which she considered "the mark of a good physician." She "emphasized sympathy and compassion" in the practice of medicine and particularly "identified such qualities with women."[82] Marie Zakrzewska (1829–1902), an immigrant German midwife and later a leading American physician, "frowned upon women who chose medicine out of female 'sympathy' ";[83] but she still held the view that "there are some qualifications . . . which form part of our affectional nature and without which no practitioner can succeed. Of these the most essential is sympathy."[84] Susan Dimock (1847–1875), a surgeon at the New England Hospital, "frequently commented that if she were asked 'to do without sympathy or medicine, I should say do without medicine.' "[85]

Sympathy and the Objectification of the Sufferer

Nicholas Jewson has argued that a traditional emphasis on the individual patient and the individual medical practitioner was considerably modified as the hospital began to assume increasing importance in the medical world of the early nineteenth century. With the emergence of *hospital medicine,* the attention of physicians began to shift from the diagnosis and treatment of complexes of symptoms in individual sufferers to the diagnosis and classification of cases. The focus was shifting from the "sick-man" as a small world unto himself to the patient as "a collection of synchronized organs, each with a specialized function."[86]

Then *laboratory medicine* began to take shape in German universities in the latter half of the nineteenth century. The theories and techniques of the physical sciences were introduced into the study of living organisms, and experimental physiology flourished. Cell theory entered the scene. The microscope and staining techniques brought to histology a new importance. Bacteriological investigations brought new perspectives on disease and led to new modes of therapeutic investigation. And clinical diagnosis was gradually reorganized around various "chemical tests of body substances designed to identify morbid physiological processes."[87] Attention gradually shifted away from the sick person to the case and then to the cell. Gradually the "distance" between the sick person and the physician increased, even when they were face to face. Or perhaps more accurately, the patient was gradually depersonalized in the doctor-patient relationship, and, all too often, the physician related to him or her more as an object than as a sufferer.

By the end of the century, these changes in medical knowledge and practice were becoming associated with the notion of *scientific medicine,* closely akin to the laboratory medicine described earlier. Emphasizing the "scientific" and "objective" in the treatment of patients, scientific medicine became the highly respected mode for the practicing physician. One gathered data from one's own examination of the patient, to which one added objective data from the "object" in question, namely the patient—such as reports of bacteriological examinations, various other laboratory test results, and so forth. As the scientific mode of gathering information, reaching a diagnosis, and planning a treatment increasingly took center stage in the clinical world, a humanistic mode of knowing patients, relating to them personally, and working with them as suffering persons often became less valued. For the physician, being scientific often came to be interpreted as being a detached observer who should be careful not to intrude on the reality being observed. "This is a conception of observation that was worked out in the study of purely physical objects. There was no question of trying to capture the subjectivity of those objects: they had none."[88] And so, in striving for the enhanced status of being a scientific physician, doctors often struggled to achieve the stance of the detached observer, only to lose something significant in their understanding of the very distress that brought their patients to them.

By the end of the century, the emerging technologies that brought such powerful assistance to the physician's diagnostic and therapeutic endeavors had frequently served to distance the healer from the sufferer, to transform the sufferer into more of an object and less of a person, and, all too often, to diminish the healer's capacity to provide "the tolerance and sympathy and forgiveness which only suffering can discover in a universe of fellow-sufferers."[89]

At the same time, throughout much of the century, there were reactions against this trend toward objectifying the sufferer. Complaints arose to the effect that sympathy and compassion were disappearing, or had disappeared, from the physician's approach to the patient. Much of the argument about the nature of the doctor-patient relationship involved concern about these sentiments: what the relationship was like and whether or not sympathy was a factor, what it should be like and the role of sympathy in the ideal relationship.

Doctor and Patient in the Twentieth Century

With the advent of the twentieth century, a growing tension emerged between medical science and clinical medicine. Encouraged and emboldened by the scientific developments of the latter half of the nineteenth century, medical scientists were arguing for and acquiring a larger place in the medical world, including an increased influence on what was done therapeutically. The "mere practitioner" was often striving to be more scientific in mode and manner, only to be perceived as maintaining an unsympathetic distance from the patient.

At the same time, though, the "old wine" of concern about kindly feelings and humane sympathies began to reappear in "new bottles" of concern about the importance and value of "the doctor-patient relationship" and "the patient as a person." And the twentieth century brought forth an extensive literature reflecting the concerns of physicians (and others) about these matters. Representative of the spirit of these writings, yet more eloquent than most, was the work of Francis Weld Peabody (1881–1927), a native of Cambridge and a notable physician and teacher at Harvard University who has often been cited for his comments about "the care of the patient." His essay of that title ends with the following sentences: "The good physician knows his patients through and through, and his knowledge is bought deeply. Time, sympathy and understanding must be lavishly dispensed, but the reward is to be found in that personal bond which forms the greatest satisfaction of the practice of medicine. One of the essential qualities of the clinician is interest in humanity, for *the secret of the care of the patient is in caring for the patient*."[90]

To a considerable extent "The Care of the Patient" constituted an urging to medical students and physicians to be moral, humane, and dedicated in carrying out their duties as healers, and ever mindful of the person while applying the science; and it urged serious, rather than dismissive, consideration of psychosomatic symptoms. Further, this essay contained significant elements that directly addressed the doctor-patient relationship. Peabody argued that "the practice of medicine in its broadest sense includes the whole relationship of the physician with his patient," and that "the significance of the intimate personal relationship between physician and patient cannot be too strongly emphasized, for in an extraordinarily large number of cases both diagnosis and treatment are directly dependent on it."[91] And he repeatedly emphasized the importance of "sympathy" on the physician's part.[92] The patient is looking for someone who will "take a human interest in him," in addition to having expert knowledge and therapeutic skills. These attitudes and this approach to the patient play a significant role in gaining his confidence, which, in turn, is so often critical in the therapeutic endeavor.[93]

Peabody urged physicians from the beginning to be doers of "friendly service," rather than merely questioners and gatherers of clinical facts. Doctors should get to know sufferers as persons, beyond their roles as a patients or clinical cases.[94] They should conceive of themselves as taking care of individuals rather than treating diseases. In summary, a significant part of the curing is in the caring.

Throughout "The Care of the Patient," Peabody was emphasizing the importance of psychological healing in the everyday practice of medicine; and he viewed such healing as an inherent potential in the physician-patient relationship. He was arguing for the actualization of this healing potential, irrespective of the nature of the illness.

Many medical authors and teachers in the twentieth century have expressed themselves along similar lines, and many more have merely shared his concerns and values (whether they have ever heard of Peabody or not); meanwhile, the remarkable advances of modern medicine and concerns about the efficient use of a clinician's time have brought an already familiar dilemma into sharper and sharper focus: Is it more critical to attend to the disease or to the sufferer? to treat disease or to treat the patient? In the twentieth century the focus has frequently oscillated between concerns about the science of the disease and the humanity of the patient. In fact, there appears to be a well-established tension between attention to diseases and attention to suffering persons.

The Healer-Sufferer Relationship in
Modern Psychotherapeutics

In the late decades of the nineteenth century, the centuries-old traditions of psychological healing, now interwoven with the influences of mesmerism and hypnosis, were gradually transformed into a variety of clinical approaches that came under the new generic term of *psychotherapy*. And attention began to be given to the healer-sufferer relationship in a newer form: the psychotherapist-patient relationship. Much of this attention was akin to the general physician's concerns about the doctor-patient relationship, but there were important new elements, often reflecting a more intensive examination of the relationship and its implications for healing.

In 1895, Sigmund Freud gave extended attention to the psychotherapy of that era. He emphasized the enlisting of the patient as "a collaborator" in the treatment process, and he mentioned several of the elements that constituted psychotherapy as he conceived of it. He then went on to say: "Besides the intellectual motives which we mobilize to overcome the resistance, *there is an affective factor, the personal influence of the physician, which we can seldom do without,* and in a number of cases the latter alone is in a position to remove the resistance. *The situation here is no different from what it is elsewhere in medicine and there is no therapeutic procedure of which one may say that it can do entirely without the co-operation of this personal factor.*"[95] Much more briefly, in 1913, Freud indicated that the basic "standpoint" of the psychoanalyst toward the patient should be that of "a serious interest in him" and "one of sympathetic understanding."[96]

Freud's erstwhile colleague Carl Jung (1875–1961) identified somewhat similar factors, in his own writings about psychotherapy. In 1921, in the process of considering "the therapeutic value of abreaction," Jung emphasized that the value could not lie in the replay of past experience alone. He argued that

> the intervention of the doctor is absolutely necessary. One can easily see what it means to the patient when he can confide his experience to an understanding and sympathetic doctor. His conscious mind finds in the doctor a moral support against the unmanageable affect of his traumatic complex. No longer does he stand alone in his battle with these elemental powers, but some one whom he trusts reaches out a hand, lending him moral strength to combat the tyranny of uncontrolled emotion. . . .
>
> For myself, I would . . . call it his [the doctor's] human interest and personal devotion. These are the property of no method, nor can they ever become one; they are moral qualities which are of the greatest importance in all methods of psychotherapy, and not in the case of abreaction alone.[97]

What are the essential themes in these views from two influential contributors to the evolution of modern psychological healing? There are clear indications of the significance of personal interest, attention, and concern. An affective tone is assumed to characterize the relationship; one finds no suggestion of cool detachment or emotional distance. A supportive element is made clear; the sufferer should not feel alone in his or her difficulties and struggles toward the goal of being healed. An atmosphere of collaboration is urged. And sympathy is expected to be a critical element; the healer needs to be a sympathetic presence for the sufferer.

Transference, Countertransference, and the Relationship

In addition to his comments on the psychotherapeutic relationship, Freud contributed two concepts of particular significance for our context: *transference* and *countertransference*. Developed in response to certain problems in the relationship, these two ideas facilitated an understanding of those problems, paved the way toward resolving them, served to prevent the relationship from deteriorating and becoming an obstacle to clinical progress, and provided an avenue to additional clinical information. After being introduced

by Freud, the notions evolved further in his work and in that of later generations of psychoanalysts; and they have had special meaning for the healer-
sufferer relationship, whether considered in terms of physician and patient in
the most general sense, or in the more particular instance of psychotherapist
and patient, or in the even more particular instance of psychoanalyst and
patient. They have served the relationship in a wide variety of twentieth-
century psychotherapies.

In 1895, Freud first mentioned *transference*, introducing the notion to explain certain affect-laden difficulties in the doctor-patient relationship that
interfered with the therapeutic work. He had alluded to "the trouble taken by
the physician and his friendliness" as compensating the patient for the burdens
of such work, particularly noting the distress and embarrassment often experienced on coming to thoughts and feelings that caused discomfort in the patient. Yet, in spite of this, it commonly happened that the discomfort became
too much at times, and the patient was no longer inclined to be cooperative in
the treatment procedure. Freud referred to the patient's experiencing a sense of
dread or anxiety in the face of these thoughts and feelings and eventually
concluded that these occurrences resulted from "transferring on to the figure
of the physician the distressing ideas which arise from the content of the
analysis. . . . Transference on to the physician takes place through a *false
connection.*" Troubling memories and their associated feelings, originally related to significant persons in the patient's earlier life, emerged in forms related
to the physician. The resulting alarm and discomfort affected the tenor of the
doctor-patient relationship, disturbing the needed cooperativeness and interfering with the therapeutic endeavor. From these experiences, Freud developed ways of helping the patient realize the nature and source of the difficulties; and so it became possible for both patient and doctor to learn from
these events, to re-establish a cooperative relationship, and to move on in the
therapeutic work.[98]

In 1901, Freud elaborated somewhat on the phenomena that he had named
"transferences." Of particular importance for considering the place of the
healer-sufferer relationship in therapeutic activities, he now added that, in
addition to affectionate transferences and the discomfort in facing distressing feelings and thoughts, frankly hostile transferences could also interfere
with the needed cooperativeness in the relationship.[99] Further, what was only
hinted at in 1901 became explicit in 1909. While transferences might be interferences in the treatment through their effects on the relationship, these very
effects could be examined and turned to constructive account as sources of
understanding of past relationships and conflicts.[100]

Then, in 1912, Freud referred to the affectionate and friendly transferences as instances of "positive transference" and termed the hostile transferences examples of "negative transference." He also emphasized that, when a friendly or positive transference took on an erotic character, it could affect the therapeutic relationship in ways that seriously interfered with the healing endeavor. That is to say, though a friendly transference frequently facilitated healing, in the case of both negative and positive transferences the nature of the doctor-patient relationship might come to be an obstacle to the healing endeavor.[101] Still further, in 1915, Freud pointed out that an affectionate transference, while it could become erotic in tone and seriously interfere with the therapeutic work, could also lead to a disappearance of symptoms out of love for and a wish to please the doctor.[102]

Somewhat later than had been the case with the phenomena in patients that led to the idea of transference, Freud realized that in certain instances feelings, reactions, and attitudes in the psychoanalyst could also affect the doctor-patient relationship in ways that interfered with the therapeutic work. That is, the psychoanalyst's clinical efforts might be disrupted by feelings toward a patient or conflicts aroused by a patient. In 1910, he introduced the term *countertransference* to denote these phenomena. Referring to it as an aspect of technique related "to the physician himself," he commented, "We have become aware of the 'counter-transference,' which arises in him as a result of the patient's influence on his conscious feelings, and we are almost inclined to insist that he shall recognize this counter-transference in himself and overcome it. . . . No psycho-analyst goes further than his own complexes and internal resistances permit."[103]

Although Freud did not develop this concept further, other psychoanalysts either changed or expanded its meaning, in several different ways. The phenomena thus accounted for were feelings and related problematic contributions by the psychoanalyst to the doctor-patient relationship, and usually the implication was that said contributions ran the risk of disrupting or interfering with the therapeutic enterprise. One alternative meaning, suggested by Adolph Stern (1879–1958) in 1924, was that countertransference referred to "the transference that the analyst makes to the patient." He stated further, "Theoretically, the countertransference on the part of the analyst has the same origin as the transferences on the part of the patient; namely, in the repressed infantile material of the analyst."[104] Others would later come to refer to such instances as the psychoanalyst's transference.

Some came to use the term *countertransference* to refer to any feelings or emotional responses that the psychoanalyst might experience toward the patient.[105] And still others began to use it to mean those feelings and attitudes in the psychoanalyst that were specifically reactions to the patient's transference.

Conceived of in these latter instances as a phenomenon complementary to the patient's transference, when carefully analyzed by the psychoanalyst it could lead to a valuable understanding of the patient. Nevertheless, if the psychoanalyst entered into the role being suggested by the patient's transference, it could blind him to understanding the patient.[106]

In the emergence and development of these two concepts — transference and countertransference — was a world of depth and detail regarding the healer-sufferer relationship. The richness of action and reaction in the emotions and attitudes of the two participants suggested in the use of these notions gave a further indication of why and how this relationship could be such a meaningful and effective factor in psychological healing, whether said psychological healing was explicitly the purpose of the therapeutic relationship or whether it was an unstated element in a general medical context. Though this range of phenomena might not be present in all therapeutic relationships and many such phenomena might not be attended to even when present in a clinical context, it was well to remember that these forces were potentially there, for good or for ill, in any healer-sufferer relationship.

The Therapeutic Alliance and the Relationship

While transference and countertransference came into common use to account for and deal with important aspects of the doctor-patient relationship, psychoanalysts increasingly took pains to give separate and distinct attention to other aspects of the relationship that have been referred to as the *therapeutic alliance, working alliance,* and *treatment alliance.* These terms reflected the recognition that there was much more to the relationship than undercurrents from the past, that two people were working together in a joint therapeutic endeavor, that many aspects of their relationship entailed complementary roles and cooperativeness, and that healing enterprises were increasingly being viewed as collaborations. Among psychoanalysts, the *treatment alliance* was defined as "the non-neurotic, rational, reasonable rapport which the patient has with his analyst and which enables him to work purposefully in the analytic situation";[107] but this notion was applicable in many clinical pairings beyond the limits of psychoanalysis. The detailed nature of the relationship between a healer and a sufferer could vary within a wide range, but one way or another an element of working together characterized the vast majority of such relationships. Quite apart from the sometimes problematic influence of those factors denominated *transference* and *countertransference,* the *treatment alliance* referred to the ways in which the two participants in a therapeutic relationship found common purpose in their joint endeavor and strove to work together for the sake of healing gains for one and a healer's satisfaction for the other.

Empathy and the Relationship

Another factor that came to be viewed as significant in twentieth-century healing contexts was *empathy*. The age-old concerns with sympathy and compassion constituted the matrix out of which this attention to empathy developed.[108] In those contexts, the term *empathy* came to refer to a type of person-to-person relatedness in which the empathizing person experienced the feelings, thoughts, and attitudes of the other person as if they were his or her own. The healer imaginatively entered the inner world of the sufferer, vicariously experienced the sufferer's experience, and then employed the empathic understanding thus gained, with healing intent on the sufferer's behalf. Empathy thus was one way in which a healer related to a sufferer, or a way of employing the healer-sufferer relationship toward healing ends.

Through the influence of the psychoanalysts' developing attention to empathy, and later through the influence of Rogers' client-centered therapy, empathy became a significant factor in considerations of the healer-sufferer relationship in psychoanalysis and in many twentieth-century psychotherapies.[109] The various notions of empathy that emerged under these influences varied somewhat in their details and in the way they were used. But, whatever was the case in a particular viewpoint, respect for the other person (the sufferer), a concerned effort to appreciate and understand the other, an attempt to turn that understanding to useful account for that other person, and the sustaining effect for the sufferer of the feeling that someone understood and was "with" him or her, were increasingly thought of as characteristics of the healer-sufferer relationship. And, in recent years, empathy has come to be emphasized more and more in writings about the doctor and the patient in general medical contexts.[110]

Healing and Hope

Apart from the various factors that have already been discussed, another that was crucial in healer-sufferer relationships was *hope*. Along with faith and charity (love), hope has been considered one of the three theological virtues in the Christian tradition, these having been originally grouped together by St. Paul in several places in his writings. Hope was also a common enough topic in the Old Testament. In Christian contexts, it has been defined as "the desire and search for a future good, difficult but not impossible of attainment."[111] While faith and love have had larger measures of attention in Christian literature, hope has certainly been taken into account. One of the more significant biblical references to hope speaks of it as "an anchor of the soul."[112]

As for contexts referable to healing, hope has not been frequently addressed, but it has hardly been ignored. As a timeless proverb has put it, "Hope is the physician of each misery." Galen commented, "Confidence and hope do be more good than physic." The famous French surgeon Ambroise Paré (1510–1590) said, "Always give the patient hope, even when death seems at hand."[113] And, a Scottish psychiatrist, W. A. F. Browne (1805–1885), emphasized, along with benevolent kindness and sympathy, the value of hope, quoting Coleridge: "In the treatment of nervous disease, he is the best physician who is the most ingenious inspirer of hope."[114]

In 1849, in *Physician and Patient,* Hooker commented that a medical remedy is often "essentially aided by the genial and animating influence of hope." Writing at length about the "influence of hope in the treatment of disease," he indicated the importance of the physician's hopefulness for both patient *and* physician, and the value of the engendering of hope in the patient for both ameliorative and curative ends.[115]

In considering "the influence of the mind upon the body in health and disease," in 1872 Daniel Hack Tuke, a British psychiatrist and descendant of the Tukes associated with the York Retreat, particularly noted the role of expectation and hope (in association with the imagination) in healing.[116] Freud seems to have said little, over the years of developing his own psychotherapeutics, about the place of hope, but he was clearly very aware of this factor, as can be seen from the following passage from an essay on "Psychical (or Mental) Treatment" in 1905.

> Our interest is most particularly engaged by the mental state of *expectation,* which puts in motion a number of mental forces that have the greatest influence on the onset and cure of physical disease. *Fearful* expectation is certainly not without its effect on the result. . . . The contrary state of mind, in which expectation is coloured by hope and faith, is an effective force with which we have to reckon, strictly speaking, in *all* our attempts at treatment and cure. We could not otherwise account for the peculiar results which we find produced by medicaments and therapeutic procedures.[117]

And James J. Walsh (1865–1942), an American psychiatrist, in 1912 in his compendious work on psychotherapy, took note of a crucial role for the "renewal of hope" in clinical endeavors.[118]

In more recent times, Jerome D. Frank has searchingly considered the place of hope and the patient's expectations in psychotherapy. From investigations undertaken in the 1950s, he concludes that a recurrent healing factor in a variety of psychotherapeutic approaches is "the potentiation and activation of the patient's favorable expectancies";[119] and he outlines his views that the patient's "favorable expectation" and "the patient's state of faith or hope" are critical factors in achieving a favorable outcome.[120] In 1968, in "The Role of Hope in Psychotherapy," he comments that hope or a "patient's positive expectations" are "closely linked to confidence or trust in the therapist." And they constitute "an important healing ingredient in all forms of medical treatment," a recognition that "came about through study of the so-called placebo response." He then proceeds to illustrate the point that "if hope can heal, lack of hope can delay recovery or even hasten death."[121] In 1974 Frank addresses this same theme in somewhat different terms. Conceiving of a significant portion of psychiatric disorders as entailing serious discouragement and diminished hope or even hopelessness ("demoralization"), he reasons that the essence of effective treatment lies in its capacity to enhance or arouse hope (the "ability to restore patient's morale").[122]

Among psychoanalysts, Thomas M. French (1892–1976) gave particular attention to hope — in general, as a central factor in the motivation of human behavior; and in particular, as a basis for therapeutic incentive. And he noted the critical significance of the loss of hope.[123] On the basis of clinical experience, he concluded that the psychoanalyst needs to be alert to and supportive of the patient's *"successively emerging hopes of a solution for his conflicts,"* and that *"we must depend on* the patient's *hopes as incentives for the therapeutic process."*[124] Gradually, the theme of hope became more common in psychoanalytic discussions, in implicit fashion in works such as Hans W. Loewald's (1906–1993) "On the Therapeutic Action of Psycho-Analysis"[125] and explicitly in such as Maxwell Gitelson's (1902–1965) "Curative Factors in Psycho-Analysis." Gitelson referred to the patient's *"optimistic* feeling," which entails a " 'hope' for, or 'expectation' of" the analyst's *"healing intention to 'maintain and support' the patient"*; and the analyst's commitment to provide a professional version of this healing support serves to open up the possibility of a "new beginning" for the patient.[126] To some degree, the psychoanalyst came to be seen as taking on a form of transmuted parental function in engendering and supporting hope.

From a context of concern for the mentally ill, in 1965 William F. Lynch — a Jesuit theologian, author, and student of the human imagination — wrote at length about being of help to the sick and about the place of hope in any such endeavor. He thought that "hope comes close to being the very heart and center of a human being." He defined hope as "the fundamental knowledge and feeling that there is a way out of difficulty, that things can work out, that we as human persons can somehow handle and manage internal and external reality, that there are 'solutions' . . . , that, above all, there are ways out of illness."[127] Lynch commented that, in general, "we humans, who need hope more than anything else in life, have written little about it."[128] Even where there is a considerable familiarity with hopelessness, as in psychiatry and psychoanalysis, he concluded that, until recent decades, there had been relatively little written about the engendering or sustaining of hope.

Also in the 1960s, emerging out of the study of diminished hope in psychiatric contexts, the work of Ezra Stotland — an American psychologist — gave sustained attention to "the psychology of hope" and reviewed an extensive literature on relevant experimental and field studies. He commented that "the importance of hope for man had long been known to layman and professional." He summed up a definitional discussion by saying, "*Hope* can therefore be regarded as a shorthand term for an expectation about goal attainment."[129]

On reviewing this historical account, it soon becomes clear that the themes that run through it are as old as time and yet as relevant to modern healers and sufferers as most of our prized medical discoveries. Today's discussions of the doctor-patient relationship frequently seem to be extensions of earlier accounts; and earlier discussions frequently seem applicable to modern contexts. For example, when we discuss hope — or compassion, or sympathy, or a healer's caring — we are addressing timeless issues in the relationships between healers and sufferers. At the same time, though, we are entering a realm that has come to be referred to as "nonspecific factors" and "relationship factors" in modern literature on psychotherapy.[130] And, in healing contexts in general, these factors have increasingly gained explicit recognition as being significant in what healers might crucially contribute and in how they might facilitate the potential benefits of their increasingly useful array of treatment possibilities — whether the primary psychological benefits of a psychotherapeutic endeavor, the placebo effect of an ostensibly medicinal or technological intervention, or the truly medicinal or technological agent, which so often is more successful when received from a sympathetic and concerned practitioner.

In the light of the necessary interdependence in most social relationships, it is hardly surprising to observe that the healer-sufferer relationship has commonly involved two persons endeavoring to influence one another. Traditionally, though, the emphasis has been on healers influencing sufferers; and only limited attention has been paid to just how natural, and probably common, it is for the two persons in this particular relationship to influence each other. Sufferers have clearly wished to influence healers toward curative or ameliorative actions; but, less obviously perhaps, they have also wished to influence healers to regard them favorably, to be respectful, or even to like them. Even less clearly associated with intention on the sufferer's part, the neediness and vulnerability of an ill or traumatized person has often enough induced a concerned, caring response in the healer, resulting in a beneficial atmosphere for the carrying out of the more obviously therapeutic activities. So, too, has a sufferer's trust and confidence been known to engender trust-worthiness and caring efforts in the healer. At the same time, the healer has wished to influence the sufferer toward cooperative behavior in the interest of a successful treatment outcome and an experience of meaning and reward for the healer in the carrying out of healing activities. Over time, this wish has manifested itself in efforts to get the sufferer to be a reasonably compliant recipient of prescriptions and other clinical advice, to be a loyal and not-too-difficult patient, to be an appreciative beneficiary of treatment interventions, and to behave in his or her own interest as a "good patient." While modern discussions have come to value a smoother process of negotiation and mutual influencing, mutual influencing is nothing new.

In what follows, I will briefly review the themes that have emerged in this study, despite differences in language and context, as both age-old and central to our modern healing efforts. First, the sufferer brings to the relationship the recurrent emphasis on the *trust* and *confidence* in the healer, and the further trust and confidence that can develop as they work at the healing enterprise. To quote (the seventeenth-century) Robert Burton, many a healer has achieved a strange cure "because the Patient puts his confidence in him, which Avicenna *prefers before art, precepts, and all remedies whatsoever.* . . . And he doth the best cures, according to Hippocrates, in whom most trust."[131]

This leads directly into the second theme: hope, and expectations of cure or of the easing of distress. Sufferers have approached treatment situations with varying degrees of hope that they would be helped. And a significant aspect of a treatment relationship has been the extent to which it supports the sufferer's hopeful expectations, or enhances hope where it was limited, or serves to arouse hope where the sufferer felt discouraged or even hopeless. And hope has been closely connected to faith, whether in the healer, in the remedies, or in the general healing context. Then there has been the healer's own faith in the healing enterprise. These are some of the modern implications of the historic phrase "the faith that heals." It has been in this realm that sufferers have found relief from a sense of hopelessness and helplessness, of feeling alone in the face of worrisome, threatening, and sometimes overwhelming situations.

Another theme is that of friendship. In his book *Doctor and Patient,* Laín

Entralgo deals with friendship in healing contexts from classical times to the present, arguing that it has been, and continues to be, a central factor in the healer-sufferer relationship.[132] From philia, or friendship, in the views of classical authorities, he proceeded to medical philia; then to *agape* or caritas as a Christian transmutation of philia, and how this characterized Christian views of what the healing relationship should be like; then, in recent times, the notion of medical comradeship, denoting the relationship between doctor and patient in seeking the better health of the patient; and then the more modern language that speaks of some sort of interpersonal bond between doctor and patient. All this is akin to what many others have discussed regarding the importance of benevolence, kindliness, and friendly support in the healer-sufferer relationship. In addition to the significance, in most healing relationships, of factors such as these, they have played a crucial role in clinical work, whether in the form of supportive psychotherapeutic techniques or of the medical practitioner's ministering over months or years to a chronically ill patient.

I have considered the sympathy and compassion that the healer could, and often did, bring to the healing context and the sustaining effect of such sentiments for the sufferer. This sympathy could be termed complementary to the yearning for sympathy and compassion on the part of sufferers. As Tolstoy stated it, the physician "satisfied that eternal human need for hope of relief, for sympathy, and that something should be done, which is felt by those who are suffering."[133]

And *empathy*: though the term is relatively modern, the phenomenon is nothing new, as we have seen; in large measure, it has emerged out of the traditional emphasis on sympathy and compassion in healing relationships. Empathy has so often been crucial: its role in coming to understand a patient; its role in tactfulness; its significance in the timing and phrasing of more technical activities that have been so highly regarded by the healers using them; and the sustaining effect it has had on the sufferer convinced that someone understood and was "with" him or her, that he or she was not alone in the healing struggle.

Where understanding and feeling understood have been concerned, empathy contributed crucially, but in numerous other ways the healer has brought knowledge and understanding to bear on the healing work. Despite the deeply meaningful experience of feeling understood, even the sense that someone was trying to understand, was working toward understanding, could be sustaining.

Apart from these various "ingredients" or "elements" in healing relationships, it may also be useful to think in terms of models of the relationship — a typology of healer-sufferer relationships. In antiquity the commonest model seems to have been that of a vulnerable person (a sufferer) in need and a healer as a figure of knowledge, healing capacity, and authority; in this model, the healer was regarded as more or less in charge, and compliance or obedience was expected of the sufferer. The sufferer as customer or client could modify this imbalance in authority and power, as the healer might well have needed the sufferer as client in order to earn a living. Insofar as the relationship involved a healer governed by sympathy, compassion, and other sentiments disposing toward care-taking, the needy, vulnerable sufferer was less at the mercy of the power and authority of the healer. At times, the overtones were clearly those of a child-parent relationship—sometimes a healer's tendency to be authoritarian suggested the stereotypical father and child of the day, and sometimes a healer's nurturant qualities suggested the model of mother and child. At other times, a pupil-teacher variant of this model seems to have been more the case. This general type has a long history, has probably been the commonest until very recent times, and is far from unknown today. That most people have some dependent inclinations may have disposed them toward this model; and it has been common for such inclinations to emerge during illness, even in patients not strongly inclined that way. And being in a position of authority could, with some physicians, bring out inclinations to be controlling, dominating, or authoritarian.

Nevertheless, certain factors served to modify this dependency-authority model. The recurrent indications that friendship was a factor suggest some tendency toward an equalizing of status in the relationship—indications that friendship was actually the case, or was wished for or sought by the sufferer, or was advocated by the community, or was valued as a standard by the healer. Also, the higher the social position of the patient, the more likely the relationship was to be of this more equal type. Further, in some instances, well-to-do patients were more than equal, to a physician whom they viewed more as an employee or retainer.

Under the influence of Christianity, there seems to have been an increased emphasis on care-taking sentiments on the healer's part, and a theme of Christian caring and friendship was often stressed. The emphasis on God as being the true or ultimate healer reduced the tendency for the physician to be perceived as a figure of authority and power, both in the eyes of sufferers and in those of physicians themselves. Frequently, though, this came to be the grounds for a role of dependency, obedience, and compliance on the part of the sufferer, with the physician professing humility (and perhaps feeling humble) while exercising authority.

Turning to more recent times, we find an increased concern with equality in the relationship, perhaps a reflection of the increasing tendency toward democratic values. Associated with this egalitarian trend, an element of negotiation increasingly entered into the determining of the relationship: whether to continue with this or that healer; what was the diagnosis all about and what would it entail for the patient; making a choice among treatment options; just who would be responsible for what in the healing effort; and various subtle features of just what behavior each participant would or would not put up with in the other. Although some sort of negotiation, frequently quite veiled or oblique, was hardly new, negotiation became a more important factor, and often a more explicit activity, in many twentieth-century instances.

Particularly in the latter half of the twentieth century, the model of two collaborators at work in the healing enterprise came to have a place. The mutual need for the other's contributions in order to achieve a good therapeutic outcome gained some recognition. Sometimes a patient's inclination to be independent was a factor here; sometimes a physician engendered a collaborative relationship, whether as a reflection of democratic values or out of a conviction that treatment progresses better as a result; and sometimes the patient's circumstances necessitated that he or she be more independent and assume more responsibility in the relationship, for example, in the case of certain chronic illnesses (such as diabetes). Further, collaboration tended to be associated with a more significant place for empathy in the healer's functions, although there is some question whether a collaborative mode led to a healer's being more empathic or whether an empathic healer tended to favor a collaborative mode.

While the modern literature on the doctor-patient relationship has indicated that various authorities favored one or another of these models of the relationship on this or that set of principles, it has also been argued that — depending on the patient's clinical state, the patient's basic nature, and the type of illness — different modes of relationship may well be preferable in different clinical circumstances. For example, certain acute illnesses — such as a cardiovascular emergency, a feverish state involving delirium, a trauma that has led to unconsciousness — might abruptly shift a patient from the way he or she was usually inclined to function in healing relationships and might, in the interest of responsible and effective care, demand that a physician "take charge" in ways that were quite at odds with his usual mode of relating to patients. In short, an inflexibility in relation to the possible models has been observed to be a poor thing. And, often enough, a pure version of any model has not been achievable, given the all-too-human nature of a particular sufferer or a particular healer, or the all-too-varying nature of the clinical circumstances.

Among twentieth-century students of healing relationships, Michael Balint (1890–1970), a Hungarian physician and psychoanalyst who settled in London, contributed some particularly thoughtful observations on how and why the nature of the relationship might vary. He commented, "In general, the greater the maturity of the patient, the better will be the results of a purely 'objective treatment' and the less will be the patient's need of 'subjective sympathetic therapy,' and vice versa."[134] After pointing out that the general practitioner or family doctor frequently had had a long-standing relationship with the patient, which had either started when the patient was well or had included significant periods of good health, he emphasized that, when an illness occurred, such a continuing relationship was of immeasurable supportive value as the doctor proceeded with what was usually meant by "treatment." Thinking in terms of a patient's dependency and a physician's support *versus* a patient's greater independence and responsibility in tandem with a more co-equal physician, he saw an acute illness as tilting the situation toward increased patient dependency and physician supportiveness; and then, with improvement or recovery, the relationship shifted back toward its usual balance. Where a chronic illness emerged, the two persons usually developed some type of compromise between these poles, with various forms of collaboration, depending on the particular illness and the nature of the particular persons.[135] Discussing the inherent psychotherapeutic potential within the general-practice relationship, he argued that *"every illness is also the 'vehicle' of a plea for love and attention."* It was frequently the case that the patient's "need of love, concern, sympathy and, above all, to be taken seriously must be accepted and to some extent gratified in the treatment."[136]

Still another issue that has been a basis for argument about what type of relationship would best serve the interests of healing — what was the optimal balance for the healer between the alternatives of clinical distance and emotional involvement? Despite all that has been mentioned about the unfortunate aspects of physicians' distancing themselves from patients, it has often been maintained that a degree of detachment may be advisable in clinical work. Such discussions have raised the following issues. Much of what physicians have been called upon to do has been disturbing, troubling, or anxiety-provoking. The surgeon has needed to have a cool head and a steady hand, no matter what seemed disturbing about the patient before him or merited a concerned response; most physicians have needed to learn ways to cope with their own distress in truly distressing situations, failing which their usefulness to patients might well have been impaired; and the psychotherapist has often needed to be able to call upon a certain objectivity, while remaining empathically attuned to the patient. Just as an extreme of detachment has sometimes led to an uncaring, overly mechanical view of the person (or body) being treated, so has a too intense degree of emotional involvement sometimes warped a physician's judgment in some unfortunate way in a difficult clinical situation. Often physicians need to look beyond the obvious signs and symptoms and the obvious suffering—even, as one physician expressed it, to "look through their patients to discover the underlying pure disease."[137] But if this were to become a matter of viewing the patient as transparent, the healer would risk losing sight of the suffering person. As has been so aptly said, "We are not here to see through one another. We are here to see one another through."[138]

4

The Listening Healer

Among other things, a healer is commonly a person to whom a sufferer tells things; and, out of his listening, the healer develops the basis for his therapeutic interventions. The psychological healer, in particular, is one who listens in order to learn and to understand; and, from the fruits of this listening, he or she develops the basis for reassuring, advising, consoling, comforting, interpreting, explaining, or otherwise intervening.

One author — an authority on communication — has said: "To be human is to speak. To be abundantly human is to speak freely and fully. The converse of this is a profound truth, also: that the good listener is the best physician for those who are ill in thought and feeling."[1]

Another authority — a psychological healer *par excellence,* the late Frieda Fromm-Reichmann — termed listening "a basic psychotherapeutic instrumentality." She said that, if she were asked to state in one sentence "the basic requirements as to the personality and the professional abilities of a psychiatrist," she would reply, "The psychotherapist must be able to listen." For her, this meant "to be able to listen and to gather information from another person in this other person's own right, without reacting along the lines of one's own problems or experiences."[2]

Others have approached the significance of listening, of being a good or useful or helpful listener, through statements about unfortunate tendencies in listening. For example, the German Protestant pastor Dietrich Bonhoeffer (1906–1945) commented, in his discussion of "the Ministry of Listening":

> Many people are looking for an ear that will listen. They do not find it among Christians, because these Christians are talking where they should be listening. But he who can no longer listen to his brother will soon be no longer listening to God either; he will be doing nothing but prattle in the presence of God too. This is the beginning of the death of the spiritual life, and in the end there is nothing left but spiritual chatter and clerical condescension arrayed in pious words. One who cannot listen long and patiently will presently be talking beside the point and be never really speaking to others, albeit he be not conscious of it. . . .
>
> Brotherly pastoral care is essentially distinguished from preaching by the fact that . . . there is the obligation of listening. There is a kind of listening with half an ear that presumes already to know what the other person has to say. It is an impatient, inattentive listening, that . . . is only waiting for a chance to speak and thus get rid of the other person. . . . Secular education today is aware that often a person can be helped merely by having someone who will listen to him seriously, and upon this insight it has constructed its own soul therapy, which has attracted great numbers of people.[3]

In speaking about *listening* to troubled or suffering persons, I am, of course, referring to listening in the superficial sense of hearing the words that they speak to healers; but, again of course, I am referring to much more besides. The listening healer who hears only the words would be effectively keeping the sufferer at a distance so that he or she, the listener, would be emotionally unaffected. Functioning in such a manner, and even if inferring distress and emotion from the sufferer's body language and tone of voice, a listener would miss a great deal. If this distancing operation is set aside, and the sufferer's affect is allowed to come through, the work of the listening healer is more difficult, *but* so much more is heard. He or she has a significantly different experience, learns a great deal more about the sufferer, and comes to understand a great deal more. The traditional plaint of the sufferer — "*hear me!*" — takes on the richer meanings that have always been inherent in it — that is to say, "hear me!" — yes — but also, "appreciate my distress, sense the depths and variations of my pain and troublement." "Hear me!" has always included a yearning to have one's plight empathically appreciated.

Seeing and Hearing in Knowing and Understanding

Visualism has held a primary position in the history of thought. Both the emphasis on direct visual referents and the predominant use of visual metaphors in the history of man's thinking about reality and experience were reflections of a primary emphasis on vision in studying natural phenomena and in developing explanations for how human beings know things. This emphasis on vision was a central theme in classical Greek philosophical thought. In large measure, what these Greek thinkers knew was what they had seen. As the five senses were gradually differentiated from one another as sources of information, seeing was accorded the predominant position in the acquisition of knowledge. From "insight" to "enlightenment," and beyond, our language continues to be replete with visual metaphors in the language of knowing.[4] Associated with this emphasis on vision was a relative inattention to hearing, and this was even more the case with the other external senses. As Aristotle stated it in his *Metaphysics,* "All men by nature desire to know. An indication of this is the delight we take in our senses . . . , above all others the sense of sight. . . . The reason is that this, most of all the senses, makes us know and brings to light many differences between things."[5] In his *Sense and Sensibilia,* he referred to "smelling, hearing, seeing" as senses that, to those animals that possess them, "are a means of preservation. . . . But in animals which have also intelligence they serve for the attainment of a higher perfection."[6] He then gave special attention to seeing and hearing. As he had in his *Metaphysics,* he emphasized that "seeing . . . is in its own right the superior sense"; but he added, "for developing thought hearing incidentally takes the precedence."[7] He went on to say that "it is hearing that contributes most to the growth of intelligence"[8]; and in *On the Soul,* he commented to the effect that hearing was necessary and crucial for the receiving of communication.[9] The other three senses—touching, tasting, smelling—came to be referred to as the "minor senses." Hearing continued to be accorded a special place as the sense that, by receiving speech, "mediated between minds"; and, through hearing, sound "as music" had "emotional quality" and could "be made a factor in the formation of the soul."[10] Still, though, seeing continued to be predominant in discussions of sensation and perception and to be emphasized in considerations of how knowledge was acquired. "In fact, throughout the Middle Ages, there was a tendency to ignore the other senses and concentrate on vision, while expressing the conviction that the general principles applying to vision should also hold true for the other senses."[11] And, at the end of the fifteenth century, Leonardo da Vinci (1452–1519) attested to the continuing primacy of seeing when he wrote, "The eye which is the window of the soul is the chief organ whereby the understanding can have the most complete and magnificent view of the infinite works of nature."[12] For centuries, seeing was thought to be the primary sense through which human beings attained knowledge about the world around them, although hearing was credited with a role in the development of intelligence and wisdom.

Listening and the Healer

In most of the recognized modes of psychological healing over the centuries, it is clear that the would-be healer, in some way or other, has taken some pains to learn about the sufferer's ailments or difficulties in the process of developing a basis for healing efforts. Sometimes the sufferer has presented himself and his difficulties to the healer who has mainly listened and, in so doing, has acquired the data needed in order to plan a helpful endeavor. Often enough, the listening has been supplemented by questions to bring out further data. Sometimes data have been conveyed to the healer by family members or friends of the sufferer, whether by word of mouth or by correspondence. Again and again, talking has clearly been an important aspect of the sufferer's activity in informing the healer about his ailments and difficulties, and in the ongoing interaction with the healer as a healing process has taken place. And so, complementarily, the healer's listening has been a crucial element as well.

These matters are obvious enough in examining historical materials about the distresses and ailments of sufferers and about the psychological healing endeavors undertaken in response to them, but it is almost totally by inference that this can be said. *Very* little is said about the listening aspect of these encounters and processes. It seems to have been quite taken for granted in the written accounts left to us.

Then the significance of listening can be inferred from another type of evidence, more obvious, albeit still somewhat indirect. This evidence comes from repeated indications to the effect that the troubled and the suffering have yearned for an interested and concerned listener. Particularly poignant instances of this yearning are found in the Book of Psalms, where particular Psalms and their place over many centuries make it clear that listening has been viewed by many as having the potential to ease a person's distress and suffering. "Hear my prayer, O Lord, and let my cry come unto thee. . . . Incline thine ear unto me."[13] "Lord, hear my voice: let thine ears be attentive to the voice of my supplications."[14] "Lord, I cry unto thee: make haste unto me; give ear unto my voice, when I cry unto thee."[15] "Attend unto my cry; for I am brought very low."[16] Recognizing this need for someone to listen with nurturant attentiveness, Paul R. Fleischman has aptly referred to "a God of listening" in discussing these yearnings. And he grouped such yearnings with "the need to be seen, known, responded to, confirmed, appreciated, cared for, mirrored, recognized, identified," as "the yearning for witnessed significance."[17] Further, this theme of the wished-for listener is an inherent aspect of the practice of prayer.

The significance of the listener is repeatedly present, albeit implicitly, in the long traditions of various psychological healing activities — such as consolation, persuasion, confession, or confiding — each of these being a long-established mode of ministering psychologically to distressed and troubled persons and of bringing healing relief. And here and there, there are clear indications of distress in the face of a listener's inattention or unsatisfactory listening.

In the case of confession, particularly in the form developed in the early Christian church, speaking and being listened to came to be of the essence. Out of a custom of public confession, there gradually emerged the tradition of the private, confidential form of confession; and the occasional latitude of being able to submit a written confession eventually gave way to the insistence that it should be an *auricular confession,* that is, "addressed to the ear; told privately in the ear."[18] Certainly the emphasis was repeatedly on the relief and comfort to be gained from expressing and acknowledging a wrongdoing, and on the benefits of carrying out a penance, being forgiven, and being reconciled with God; but there was also the implication that the confession was to be spoken "into the ear of" an attentive listener who was qualified to understand and authorized to forgive. While explicit references to listening were rare, the indications were clear that careful attention should be paid, that there should be an openness on the part of the confessor to the individual nature of the penitent, and, by implication, that the confessor should listen carefully. The confessor was to listen compassionately in order to understand and have the basis for a remedial response.

As with confession, in the traditions of persuasion and consolation, there seems to have been a developmental pattern — or perhaps a tension between two types of approach, a conflict that has never quite been resolved, rather than a development. In each tradition were traces of preset things that the healer, or listener, was to say or do in response to the sufferer or speaker. To a degree, if A was said by the sufferer, the healer's response was B; the response tended to be formulaic. Then, gradually, an emphasis on the individuality of the sufferer emerged, and a trend toward individualizing the responses accordingly. This trend demanded an increasingly careful and receptive listening to the *particular* sufferer.

Surveying the centuries of ministering to troubled souls, historians of pastoral care have assigned a place to listening among the modes of activity they subsume under the ministry of guidance and ranged those activities "along a continuum from advice-giving at one pole to an activity of listening and reflecting at the other pole."[19] They have noted listening to have had a significant role in three different ways in the history of pastoral care. First, "there is the listening which aims toward clarification under the simple idea that, unless the counselor restrains his temptation to do most of the talking, he will never know what the counselee is trying to say." Second, "under conditions in which the inner state of the troubled person is the key to a resolution of his difficulty, it becomes necessary for the counselee to unburden himself" to a concerned and attentive listener; and so, once again, the fact of listening and the nature of the listener become crucial. Third, listening may play a critical role in a counselor's learning what is troubling a person and then reflecting this back to him "in order that he may hear clearly his own thoughts."[20] As another historian of pastoral care stated it, "The Christian clergy have been a talkative lot. But for almost twenty centuries they have spent more time listening to people than preaching to them, and from the beginning they discovered that it was hard to listen, . . . [and] even harder to respond appropriately to what they were hearing."[21]

The Nineteenth Century

The nineteenth century brought even further emphasis on seeing rather than hearing, on looking rather than listening, in the realms of sickness and healing. The sufferer's appearance and visible behavior had always been thought to provide evidence to aid the healer in understanding the illness and to guide the healer toward appropriate treatment and accurate prognosis. Then, in the nineteenth century, when accumulating populations of mentally ill persons came under the observation of alienists and psychiatrists, a new tradition of seeing and looking developed which argued that significant correlations were there to be observed between the sufferer's appearance and his psychopathology. Physiognomy, or the study of human character through facial configuration, had long been considered a meaningful enterprise; and it had been especially furthered in the eighteenth century by the work of Johann Kaspar Lavater (1741–1801). Then, in the nineteenth century, Franz Joseph Gall (1758–1828) and Johann Kaspar Spurzheim (1776–1832) evolved the discipline of phrenology, according to which the bumps and contours of the head were thought to give evidence of mental faculties and character traits. Against this background, Alexander Morison (1779–1866) presented his *Outlines of Lectures on Mental Diseases,* in which he addressed the physiognomy of the insane and to which he added illustrative engravings; and, in 1838, he published *The Physiognomy of Mental Diseases,* which included more than a hundred plates of psychiatric patients, with the aim of demonstrating pictorially observable correlates of their mental illnesses. J. E. D. Esquirol (1772–1840) used illustrations of patients in his textbook *Maladies Mentales* in 1838. And, in the late nineteenth century, Jean-Martin Charcot

(1825–1893) and Paul Richer (1849–1933) published extensively on correlations between appearances and psychopathological states. Within this context, in the 1850s, Hugh W. Diamond (1809–1886), a psychiatrist who succeeded Morison at the Surrey County Asylum, developed the work that was to earn him the title of "father of psychiatric photography." Among the uses he made of his photographs of the insane, a primary one was the photograph as a diagnostic tool based on correlations of physiognomy and clinical states.[22]

Out of these activities and their associated assumptions emerged a groundswell of support for the notion that looking at insane patients was the essential avenue to knowledge of their psychopathology. Attention to the shape of the face and the head, to the facial expression, to gestures and postures, and to body build was thought to be of central significance. The primacy of seeing in knowing had received new support.

It is well to be reminded that these trends in looking in order to know about the mentally ill evolved in an era in regard to which Michel Foucault (1926–1984) could refer to the new clinical medicine as essentially growing out of an emphasis on seeing. In his *Birth of the Clinic,* he stated, "This book . . . is about the act of seeing, the gaze."[23] He went on to discuss "the clinical gaze" at some length and gave it a crucial place in the acquisition of clinical knowledge. By the end of the nineteenth century, the primacy of visual observation in medical knowledge in general was rarely questioned. It was against this background that listening gradually came to be attended to by healers in ways that it never had before.

The "Talking Cure" and Listening

An important reflection of the significance of listening in psychological healing is the famous case of Anna O., the patient who was treated by Josef Breuer in the early 1880s and whose treatment was so influential in the early development of the work of Sigmund Freud. The patient herself described the treatment, "speaking seriously, as a 'talking cure,' while she referred to it jokingly as 'chimney sweeping.'" In addition to the patient's term, *talking cure,* Breuer used such phrases as *talked through, talked away,* and *talking out* to indicate the nature of the therapeutic activity.[24] For all the emphasis on the patient's talking, though, it is consistently clear that the physician's role was also crucial and that his listening was a critical feature of that role. Yet neither *listening* nor any of its cognates were ever used in Breuer's report. In reading about this clinical work, one takes the listening for granted, and it is clearly reasonable to do so. It was only later, when thoughtful students of the Anna O. case were subjecting it to intensive study, that this theme of listening came to be made explicit. For example, Ellenberger aptly referred to "the tranquillising effect of Breuer's listening to the stories she told him" and observed that "he was able to soothe her by listening to her stories."[25] The emphasis on the therapeutic value of talking had always implied a meaningful listening as a complementary activity, but Ellenberger was identifying the further element of the soothing and healing effect of the listener's interested listening. Might it not, just as well, have been termed "the listening cure?"

Years later, with his own development of psychoanalysis well advanced, Freud had something to say about listening. In his "Recommendations to Physicians Practising Psycho-Analysis," he urged that one should not direct "attention to anything in particular" but maintain "the same 'evenly-suspended attention' . . . in the face of all that one hears."[26] In that essay he was advising against determined efforts to remember and was rather urging an unbiased, open-minded listening to everything the patient had to say. He explicitly indicated that the psychoanalyst would thus remember more and with less intrusion of bias; and he implicitly indicated that such a way of listening would lead to the psychoanalyst's hearing more. In an interesting metaphorical statement, he added: "He must then turn his own unconscious like a receptive organ towards the transmitting unconscious of the patient. He must adjust himself to the patient as a telephone receiver is adjusted to the transmitting microphone. Just as the receiver converts back into sound waves the electric oscillations in the telephone line which were set up by sound waves, so the doctor's unconscious is able, from the derivatives of the unconscious which are communicated to him, to reconstruct that unconscious, which has determined the patient's free associations."[27]

Freud said little else about the subject of listening, but this advice has influenced the manner of listening for many a clinician since that time. In fact, these recommendations of Freud's became central to considering listening in the teaching of psychoanalytic technique.[28] As Paul Ricoeur was to state it later, "Corresponding to the 'total communication' on the part of the patient is the 'total listening' on the part of the analyst."[29]

Theodor Reik (1888–1969) particularly emphasized this special approach to listening, though he preferred the term *free-floating attention* to Freud's *evenly-suspended attention*. But Reik's considerations of the listening healer went much further, and he offered some profound observations on the subject in his book on "the inner experience of a psychoanalyst," *Listening with the Third Ear*. Borrowing the term *the third ear* from Nietzsche, Reik used it to refer to a capacity that he thought a psychoanalyst needed to develop. The psychoanalyst needed "to learn how one mind speaks to another beyond words and in silence. He must learn to listen 'with the third ear.'" This "third ear . . . can catch what other people do not say, but only feel and think; and it can also be turned inward. It can hear voices from within the self that are otherwise not audible because they are drowned out by the noises of our conscious thought-processes."[30] Reik was discussing the notion of the analyst's sensing and resonating with feelings, and listening for nuances and meanings that went beyond, or lay beneath, the spoken words. These references to listening meant a sensitive, discerning use of the sense of hearing, but he was also using listening to stand for all the senses. The analyst was urged to open "all his senses to these impressions."[31] In his silence the analyst was to provide a receptivity that was freeing to the patient and that thus facilitated a more profound communication between sufferer and healer.

Empathic Listening

Empathic listening is a significant feature of modern thought on listening in healing contexts, but the term is a relative newcomer in the language of psychological healing. In order to appreciate how it came into use, though, one has to consider the history of the parent term, *empathy*. The roots of this latter term are to be found in the thinking of Theodore Lipps (1851–1914) and his use of the word *Einfühlung*. In 1872 Robert Vischer (1847–1933) addressed the question of an observer's attributing feeling and emotion to works of art and to forms of nature. He explained it as an unconscious process in which the observer endows such objects with vital content. And he named it *Einfühlung*. Then, beginning in the 1890s, Lipps studied this process extensively and effectively established the use of the term *Einfühlung*. His original view stemmed from the realm of aesthetics and concerned the attribution to or projection onto an art object of a viewer's feelings.[32] As Lipps defined it at one point, *Einfühlung* meant "feeling something, namely, oneself, into the esthetic object."[33] Later, he included one person's appreciation of the feelings and attitudes of another person as one of the ways in which *Einfühlung* might manifest itself.[34] The English word *empathy*, with its meaning of "feeling into," became the accepted translation for *Einfühlung* after it was suggested by Edward B. Titchener (1867–1927) in 1909.[35]

Various streams of development sprang from these origins, both in theory and in practice. But only slowly did the notion of empathy enter the clinical realm. Sigmund Freud was interested in Lipps' work and made several uses of the concept of *Einfühlung* in his *Jokes and Their Relation to the Unconscious* in 1905. Although these were not clinical applications of the concept, some of them did entail "putting oneself into" the psychical state of another person, the one producing the witticism.[36] Then, though it entailed empathy with a fictional person, a similar projection of oneself into the psychical state of another was mentioned in *Delusions and Dreams in Jensen's Gradiva* in 1907.[37] Perhaps more interesting to the clinician was Freud's use of the concept in his *Group Psychology and the Analysis of the Ego* in 1921. He referred to "the process which psychology calls 'empathy [Einfühlung]'" and which plays the largest part in our understanding of what is inherently foreign to our ego in other people"; and he invoked it to explain group members' appreciation or understanding of one another. In his brief discussion he associated empathy with identification and with imitation, stating, "A path leads from identification by way of imitation to empathy, that is, to the comprehension of the means by which we are enabled to take up any attitude at all towards another mental life."[38] Although not a clinical application of the concept, it was a use that had implications for clinical contexts.

The first study in the psychoanalytic literature to address empathy explicitly as a factor in the clinical process seems to have been "The Psycho-Analytic Method of Observation" by Theodore Schroeder (1864–1953) in 1925. Focusing on empathic insight, empathic understanding, and retrospective and inductive introspection, Schroeder wrote, "the psycho-analytic method makes experimental use of empathy as a means of reading something out of the psyche of another."[39] For the psychoanalyst or "empathist," this "empathic viewing of another's psyche involves a maximum of attention upon the associated affective tones, values and processes." Schroeder went on to say that "empathic insight implies a seeing (re-living) as if from within the person who is being observed. It is as if, by a conscious withdrawal of interest and by the exclusion from consciousness of all present relationship to everything else, one places one's own consciousness at the disposal of the unconscious determinants of another's personality."[40]

In 1926, Helene Deutsch (1884–1982) briefly discussed "intuitive empathy" in clarifying the nature of seemingly occult events in psychoanalysis; and she took it for granted that it was not an unusual phenomenon in the psychoanalytic process.[41] It is Sandor Ferenczi (1873–1933), though, who is usually thought to have been the first psychoanalyst to suggest explicitly that empathy is, and should be, an element in clinical work. In 1928, he introduced the notion of *tact* as a crucial factor in determining when the analyst should undertake an intervention, particularly an interpretation. He then raised the question, "But what is 'tact'?"; and he answered, "It is the capacity for empathy." He then elaborated: having succeeded, through empathy, "in forming a picture of possible or probable associations of the patient's of which he is still completely unaware, we, not having the patient's resistances to contend with, are able to conjecture, not only his withheld thoughts, but trends of his of which he is unconscious."[42] Ferenczi went on to say, "This empathy will protect us from unnecessarily stimulating the patient's resistance, or doing so at the wrong moment." Further, the analyst's empathy served to protect the patient from unnecessary pain.[43] Ferenczi used the term *the empathy rule* as a shorthand reference to these matters.[44] He noted that the analyst's mind "swings continuously between empathy, self-observation, and making judgments."[45] And he concluded by saying, "My principle aim in writing this paper was precisely to rob 'tact' of its mystical character."[46]

After Ferenczi, empathy was only rarely mentioned in the psychoanalytic literature over the next twenty-five years.[47] Then, in the 1950s, significant references to it began to increase.[48] A sea change was under way. The situation that had pertained earlier was aptly summed up by Roy Schafer, a significant contributor toward the 1950s increased interest in empathy. "Comparatively little investigation and conceptualization of empathy can be found in the psychoanalytic literature; despite persistent emphasis on its importance in the therapeutic process, not to speak of child development and personal relationships."[49] Particularly influential among the 1950s contributors was Heinz Kohut (1913–1981), whose work was to lead to the self psychology of today and whose emphasis on the role of empathy influenced psychoanalysis and psychotherapy in ways that brought empathy into the center of their clinical considerations.[50] Ralph R. Greenson (1911–1979), another member of this 1950s group, wrote in "Empathy and Its Vicissitudes" (1960):

> Most experienced psycho-analysts will agree that in order to carry out effective psychotherapy a knowledge of psycho-analytic theory and the intellectual understanding of a patient is not sufficient. In order to help, one has to know a patient differently — emotionally. One cannot truly grasp subtle and complicated feelings of people except by this 'emotional knowing.' It is 'emotional knowing,' the experiencing of another's feelings, that is meant by the term empathy. It is a very special mode of perceiving. Particularly for therapy, the capacity for empathy is an essential prerequisite. Although I believe these points are well known it is striking how little psycho-analytic literature exists on the subject of empathy. . . . There seems to be a tendency among analysts either to take empathy for granted or to underestimate it.
>   . . . To empathize means to share, to experience the feelings of another person. This sharing of feelings is temporary. . . . The main motive of empathy is to achieve an understanding of the patient.[51]

It must be much more than a coincidence that Schafer, Kohut, and Greenson, apparently working quite independently of one another, came out within a very short span of time with such vigorous espousals of the importance of empathy. Individually and collectively, they have had a significant influence on psychoanalysis and psychotherapy in the thirty years since then; and empathy has become a common topic in the literatures of those disciplines.

Although it was often unacknowledged in the psychoanalytic and psychotherapeutic literatures, in other scholarly traditions respectful attention was being paid to notions akin to empathy as ways of appreciating and knowing about the inner life of another person. As early as the beginning of the 1920s, social psychologists and sociologists were developing such ideas and studying their place in interhuman relationships. I would mention particularly Charles H. Cooley (1864–1929) and his "sympathetic introspection"[52] and George H. Mead (1863–1931) and his "role-taking."[53]

Turning again to clinical contexts, by 1951, when his *Client-Centered Therapy* was published, Carl R. Rogers' (1902–1987) psychotherapeutic approach recognized empathy as a central element in its operations. "It is the counselor's function to assume, in so far as he is able, the internal frame of reference of the client, to perceive the world as the client sees it, to perceive the client as he is seen by himself, to lay aside all perceptions from the external frame of reference while doing so, and to communicate something of this empathic understanding to the client."[54] During the 1940s, Rogers had gradually developed this viewpoint, and it became the essence of what, in his clinical work, he meant by "client-centeredness."

These various views of empathy varied somewhat, but they all entailed a coming to know about another through an imaginative experience of being in the world of his or her thoughts, feelings, and attitudes. One way or another, what was involved was a profound listening. The healer truly *hearkened* to the sufferer — that is to say, the effort was to hear *and* to know or understand.

While it has always been clear in the psychoanalytic literature that empathy entailed attentive listening to the patient, it was only after the increased, more focused attention to empathy in the 1950s that explicit references to listening became more frequent and even consistent. Greenson emphasized listening as a matter of course, but then made the point that "listening from the 'outside' " was insufficient, and that it had been crucial that he "shifted — from listening and observing from the outside to listening and feeling from the inside," that is, from an empathically attuned position.[55]

Gradually, out of the self psychologists' attention to empathy and the unavoidable, although often unstated, significance of the analyst's listening, there emerged an increasingly explicit emphasis on psychoanalytic listening and on empathic listening in psychoanalysis and psychotherapy. Although clearly indebted to and influenced by Kohut in her attention to empathy and in her mode of practice, Evelyne Schwaber seems to have played a critical role in bringing about the newer clinical practices. In a series of papers from 1979 to

1983, she discussed empathy as "a mode of analytic listening" and as "the listening perspective," in relation to self psychology.[56] She wrote about being used "as part of the core of the patient's self" by a pathologically narcissistic patient, and then went on to say, "I slowly came to recognize that listening in this way — having to place myself inside the patient's self experience — called somehow for another mode of listening, of perceiving, than one in which I would be positioned somewhat 'outside' — that is, as target rather than subject of the patient's affects, drives, and defenses."[57] Adding that "it is this listening stance which is what I mean by empathy," she referred to empathy as "a specific, scientific mode of perceiving — the matrix of depth-psychological observation."[58] This "quality of listening," this "subjective listening mode," was "the empathic mode," a "mode of psychological data gathering."[59] Schwaber argued that "each theoretical system may suggest a definition of the listening stance within its own framework," but that, as a method of gathering data, empathy has a certain independence from theories.[60] This listening mode or "listening stance attempts to minimize the introduction of an 'outsider' view." She termed this listening stance "empathic listening."[61] Parenthetically, it should be noted that listening is certainly at the heart of the matter in empathic listening, and yet the use of the term *listening* in such contexts is partly an effort to capture metaphorically a very complicated process.

Already well attuned to the significance of listening in psychotherapy, Richard Chessick has taken up the theme of empathic listening in a thoughtful and useful way. In his textbook of psychotherapy in 1974, he said that "it is clear . . . that listening, in a therapeutic sense, is an extremely active process. It occurs silently within the therapist and permits him fully to observe the patient's behavior, as well as his own association and emotional responses to the material presented by the patient."[62] Then, in his recent book on listening in psychotherapy, listening was the central, organizing theme in a study of five different "listening stances" that might be assumed by a psychotherapist; and he addressed "empathic listening" in some detail. Noting that Schwaber's approach introduced "an alternative mode of psychoanalytic listening from that of Freud," he categorized her "point of view as belonging to only one of the five models of theoretical understanding that must be used in a comprehensive listening process."[63]

Toward Listening

In the realm of psychological healing, during the twentieth century recognition of the significance of the healer's listening in the healing process has gradually increased. And there have been many indications of such a trend other than those just cited from psychoanalytic and psychodynamic therapeutic traditions. Turning to the context of a general physician's consultation room, we find proof that attentive, interested listening can turn an inchoate litany of complaints into a gradually coherent story of distress and discomfort. The patient has been the better for having told the doctor, whether it has been a confessing, a confiding, a catharsis, or a revealing of physical symptoms that would have otherwise gone undetected; and the doctor has been the better for having been *with* the patient in a healing endeavor rather than having rapidly gotten rid of him or her with the aid of a prescription pad. Often enough, the physician's listening has allowed the emergence of more private concerns and symptoms which have been the issues that were more crucially in need of therapeutic attention.

With regard to religious contexts, twentieth-century trends have relevance to considerations of confession. While it had always been the assumption that the confessor's attentive listening was significant, the extensive tradition of advice to confessors had not been noted for its references to that listening.[64] But our century's literature for confessors has been influenced by the trend toward explicit concerns about listening and its significance.[65] As to the penitents, it was not unknown in past centuries for a penitent to complain about the quality of a confessor's listening, but this has become an openly acknowledged issue in twentieth-century writings.[66]

Then, with regard to pastoral care, the authors of the following reflect twentieth-century trends in that realm. They were discussing what they termed "a listening presence." "Grief expressed is not grief heard unless someone is listening. Our being is validated in being heard. Standing by others at a time of loss means first of all to listen to them, to attend to their anguish, and to be present to them. We listen in order to stand in grief with another pilgrim, to transcend the barriers that isolate us from one another, to make the connections that diminish loneliness. . . . [And,] in order to listen, it is essential to be comfortable with silence."[67]

The following instance from a medical student's experience is a painful example of how a clinician struggled through a patient's off-putting distress to listen in a deeply meaningful, and useful, way.

> The . . . patient was a pathetic seven-year-old girl who had been badly burned over most of her body. She had to undergo a daily ordeal of a whirlpool bath during which the burnt flesh was tweezered away from her raw, open wounds. This experience was horribly painful to her. She screamed and moaned and begged the medical team, whose efforts she stubbornly fought off, not to hurt her anymore. My job as a neophyte clinical student was to hold her uninjured hand, as much to reassure and calm her as to enable the surgical resident to

quickly pull away the dead, infected tissue in the pool of swirling water, which rapidly turned pinkish, then bloody red. . . . I tried to distract this little patient from her traumatic daily confrontation with terrible pain. I tried talking to her about her home, her family, her school — almost anything that might draw her vigilant attention away from her suffering. I could barely tolerate the daily horror. . . . Then one day, I made contact. . . . uncertain what to do besides clutching the small hand, and in despair over her unrelenting anguish, I found myself asking her to tell me how she tolerated it, what the feeling was like of being so badly burned and having to experience the awful surgical ritual, day after day after day. She stopped, quite surprised, and looked at me from a face so disfigured it was difficult to read the expression; then in terms direct and simple, she told me. While she spoke, she grasped my hand harder and neither screamed nor fought off the surgeon or the nurse. Each day from then on, her trust established, she tried to give me a feeling of what she was experiencing. By the time my training took me off this rehabilitation unit, the little burned patient seemed noticeably better able to tolerate the debridement.[68]

Given these various instances of invaluable listening, what seem to be their main ingredients? The effective healer in the realm of psychological healing has tended to be someone who has been interested in talking with and listening to the other person. And these inclinations have been grounded in an interest in other people and a curiosity about them. Further, such healers have had a capacity for caring about and being concerned about others, particularly about those who were ill, troubled, or distressed. The sufferer has tended to seek out an interested, concerned healer responsive to the distress, who would minister to his or her ailments and bring relief, if not cure. Sufferers yearned to be listened to, to be taken seriously, and to be understood, crucial aspects of the healing process.

All this, in turn, has been set in a context of human need for connection with other persons, for the intimacy of a relationship with another person, for relationships as antidotes to aloneness or being isolated, for the closeness or meaningfulness associated with such connections (quite distinct from a sexual relationship or an erotic attachment). And these needs for such relationships have influenced both sufferers and healers. The sufferer has felt a yearning to be listened to, to be valued, and to be understood. And the healer has had his or her own need to listen, to understand, and so to bridge the divide between the two persons in the potentially healing dyadic relationship.

In situations such as these, the attentive listening of a concerned and interested healer has frequently had a compelling effect on the sufferer. The sufferer, often enough, responded by telling more about himself or herself, by revealing more. The very process of the sufferer's confiding, in turn, commonly has had a compelling effect on the listening healer. The listening and the talking, the talking and the listening, have had a mutual attachment effect. The relationship has been deepened—more has been said, more has been heard, more has been understood, more of a sense of being understood has been experienced. The term *the talking cure* has not been without its relevance to such situations, but at best the term was incomplete. The healer's listening was just as crucial; in fact, it was essential. While this listening has had to entail attentiveness and interest, the healer as listener was at the heart of the matter. The term, "the listening cure," would be just as pertinent. The sense that healers have been listening, that they have tried to appreciate sufferers' distresses or dilemmas, that they have been concerned and have tried to understand, that their listening may have led to understanding, these things have mattered profoundly to sufferers. These efforts have helped in healing interventions and may themselves have been healing in their effects. Perhaps we should say "the talking *and* listening cure."

Interferences with Listening

For all the increased recognition of the value of listening, anxiety has too often been experienced in the face of listening—perhaps I should say a fear of what might be heard and its disturbing, distressing effect on healers as listeners. What healers would hear, if they allowed themselves to listen, would be so disturbing, so terrible—be it about severe pain, about distress in the face of disabling disease, about panic, about the terror of inner disintegrative trends in a psychosis, about horrible rememberings or relivings of past traumas. Or some other communication might stir disturbing feelings in a healer—anger, shame, guilt, sexual feelings. These moments in the sufferer-healer interaction could interfere mightily in listening to a sufferer, in learning about his or her difficulties, in coming to appreciate and understand those difficulties. These sorts of effects could block listening that could be essential to acquiring the understanding necessary to treat the sufferer reasonably well. They could preclude the use of the healer's empathic capacities that might be essential to learning about the sufferer's difficulties and providing the necessary healing interventions. They could influence healers to interrupt, to change the subject, to talk instead of listening, to keep away somehow from such troubling effects.

Useful, even essential, listening may be avoided by modern healers for other reasons, though. Sometimes explained in terms of the efficient use of a healer's time, sometimes determined by the intrusions of modern diagnostic technology, and sometimes accounted for by strivings to be scientific or at least objective, the distance that modern clinicians have often put between themselves and their patients, or the distance imposed by a clinical structure, has seriously interfered with the valuable clinical listening that has come to be appreciated in the twentieth century. While anxiety or fear in the face of disturbing communications may be hidden within these other rationales, such communications are often distinct interferences in their own right.

In a thoughtful history of doctor-patient relationships entitled *Bedside Manners,* Edward Shorter has taken some pains to demonstrate "the informal psychotherapeutic power of the consultation," which power he has attributed to "the catharsis that the patient derives from telling his story to someone he trusts as a 'healer.'" But the recent trend in medicine has been "to steer the consultation toward a single, identifiable physical problem, the 'chief complaint.'" Physicians have developed question-and-answer techniques in history-taking that move patients toward a chief complaint, a recognizable pattern of symptoms, and then to a basis for a prescription. Often enough, this process has discovered a plausible excuse for the medical visit, while the real cause of the visit has remained undiscovered. What has occurred has been a shift from being patient-oriented to being disease-oriented. By reducing the opportunity for the patient to talk and avoiding the need for the doctor to listen, a type of efficiency has been achieved, but the cost has included the loss of healing opportunities, opportunities for psychological healing in the medical consultation itself. "One Dutch study showed that a *majority* of patients had some reason for seeing the doctor other than their 'chief complaint.'" As the author of another study (of a pediatric clinic) stated it, "'it is important to listen rather than to ask. . . . What the doctor should really be trying to do is to help the parents to talk.'" This erosion of careful listening has often meant the loss for patients of the chance to tell what was really troubling them and of the cathartic value of telling their stories. Shorter has pointed out that "listening is the main kind of informal psychotherapy the family doctor is able to conduct," that listening has been a crucial ally for the doctor in helping patients cope with psychological distress and mental disorders.[69]

As previously suggested, in still other ways, the significance of listening has often been lost sight of in contexts of sickness and healing. We are in an era of remarkable, almost incredible, advances in molecular biology in psychiatry — in medicine, in general. And various technological advances have allowed modern physicians to learn remarkable new things from patients that can guide their treatments. Yet these same technologies can also serve to distance them from patients. While seeing more, they are often at high risk of hearing less. Techniques from X rays to modern imaging have provided a comforting concreteness, a reassuring reliance on what can be seen. The readings derived from laboratory tests, too, so often have offered a reassuring sense of visualizable certainty about the numbers on the page of a report. What the sufferer has told the healer has not been viewed as being without significance, but, all too often, it has quickly moved the healer toward a category of things to check out with modern technologies and, sooner or later, to a category of concrete, material interventions: substances or procedures. Healers have listened in their special ways but, all too often, have heard mainly through the filters provided by their categories of investigative procedures, their diagnoses, and their technologically based interventions. And somehow sufferers have been put at a distance. Healers may listen more in narrowly categorized ways, and yet they will hear less, and are in serious danger of attending less to the person. As Howard Spiro has stated it, "The physician looks for disease rather than listens to the patient. Yet illness, the patient's complaint, can only be understood by listening to what he says." Although the detection of disease may come from the image, "the diagnosis of illness comes from listening." Moreover, "listening is much harder work than seeing; it takes time, concentration, and active participation. But physicians need to listen as much as to look, to make all senses work together."[70]

Even though the healer's listening has been an important mode for acquiring knowledge of the sufferer's sickness and distress, and thus for developing a basis for sound therapeutic ministrations, surprisingly little emphasis has been placed on the value and significance of clinical listening over the centuries. Even further, with the gradual emergence of modern clinical medicine in the nineteenth century, it was clinical looking that served to enhance the status of medicine and to strengthen its scientific underpinnings.

Somehow, though, around the turn of the twentieth century, a reaction took place to all this, and concern with listening to the sufferer came to the fore. In psychoanalysis and other depth psychologies, what the sufferer could and would tell the healer, the need to facilitate such telling, the need to listen carefully, and the emerging emphasis on empathy as a listening stance were aspects of an increased sensitivity to the person of the sufferer rather than to the disease from which he or she suffered. Parallel developments in general medicine in the first several decades produced increased concerns about sufferers that were reflected in catch phrases such as *the doctor-patient relationship* and *the patient as a person;* and listening carefully to their patients was urged on physicians as it had never been before. As William Osler put it, "Listen to the patient, he is telling you the diagnosis."[71]

Yet the same century that has brought more concern with and attention to listening than ever before has introduced more interferences with and rationales for not attending to listening than ever before. Patients have often complained that physicians were too busy, that they were not interested, or that they did not listen. As physicians strove to gather more data, to see more, to be more objective, to be more scientific, their patients' experience was often that the doctors were not listening.

There seems to be a natural tension between looking and listening as ways of knowing. But modern psychological healing has brought home the fact that the healer who really listens will hear the dejection and sadness that is so often at the heart of anger, the anger so often enmeshed in dejection and despair, the fear so often at the root of hostility, the strength in weakness and the weakness in strength, the more deeply felt in the apparently more prominently felt. It has become clear that listening is central to learning about and coming to understand sufferers, and that those steps are crucial to being a healer. The healer learns about the sufferer in direct proportion to the quantity *and* quality of his or her listening. And this is not to ignore looking, or to overlook disease, or to downgrade objectivity. It is fair to say of healing as of so much else, "To everything there is a season." A time to speak, and a time to hearken; a time to look, and a time to listen.

5

The Talking Cures

In psychological healing, as in much of human interaction in general, *talking* is of the essence. It is one of psychological healing's basic elements, serving the sufferer in conveying vital information about his or her ailments and general state to the healer and playing a crucial role in most of the healer's therapeutic interactions.

The term *talking cure* has been passed down to us from its original use in the 1880s by Bertha Pappenheim, the patient known as Anna O., through Josef Breuer's account of her cathartic therapy which will be discussed later in this chapter. This term has become a commonplace for referring to many of the twentieth-century psychotherapies, particularly those where expressiveness or a cathartic element is involved. The expression reflects the fact that, for the sufferer, in addition to serving communication and providing information, talking frequently leads to a sense of release and relief.

For the healer, talking serves the task of questioning a sufferer for information, conveying a diagnostic impression, providing advice and prescription, and implementing a wide range of interventions such as consolation, suggestion, persuasion, interpretation, and so on.

And so we use the term *talking cure* as one more way of referring to many of the modes of mental healing over the centuries and of highlighting that so many of them have crucially involved *talking*.

Talking and the Healer

"And therefore if the head and body are to be well, you must begin by curing the soul; that is the first thing. And the cure, my dear youth, has to be effected by the use of certain charms, and these charms are fair words; and by them temperance is implanted in the soul, and where temperance is, there health is speedily imparted, not only to the head, but to the whole body."[1] These "certain charms"—these "fair words" said by the healer, with healing intent, in the hearing of the sufferer—and their context here might fairly be termed the *locus classicus* for the potential significance of a healer's words, a healer's talking, in psychological healing. Often cited by physicians—and particularly practitioners of psychological medicine—as indicative of the importance of psychological healing, this passage comes from a Platonic dialogue in which sophrosyne was discussed at length and which has led to recurrent discussions of sophrosyne ever since. The virtue denominated sophrosyne by the ancient Greeks has variously been referred to as temperance; as self-control; as "the harmonious product of intense passion under perfect control"; and as "self-knowledge and self-restraint."[2] For Laín Entralgo, the implications of the *Charmides* are that the achieving of sophrosyne entailed rendering the mind of the sufferer "calmed, enlightened, and set in good order" by the use of "the psychologically effective word."[3] This temperance (sophrosyne) was achieved through the healer's use of "fair words" and was, in turn, a crucial element in the healing process, as Plato saw it. That is to say, these words—as elements of psychological healing—constituted an essential aspect of healing, whether of the soul or of the body. In fact, this achieving of sophrosyne amounted to acquiring "health of soul," which was "the true source of physical health."[4]

But of course the use of words to effect a healing influence on a person was not noted first by Plato. The therapeutic use of the word had a long history before Plato: charms, incantations, and various other magical uses of words had long had their place in healing efforts.[5] Out of these traditions gradually emerged the persuasive use of words in the interest of health. The word, without the addition of a magical power, came to be used to bring about the cure or the amelioration of sickness. Shorn of magical elements, the persuasive word found a place in the healers' efforts to achieve health for sufferers. The psychological and curative efficacy of the human word was now established in natural as well as in supernatural contexts.[6]

As Aeschylus expressed it, "Words are healers of the sick temper"; he added that timing and tact may also be significant in such a therapeutic use of words.[7] Or, as Cicero phrased the same passage, "Speech physician is to wrathful heart."[8] The soothing, calming use of words by a healer could console, ease a troubled state, or even cure.

In the emergence and development of persuasive techniques—in the traditions of rhetoric—words came to be used in a systematic way to influence another person. Among other purposes, persuasive words were used to influence persons in the interest of healing of their ailments.[9] Though it was recognized that persuasive words might be used for evil purposes or against a person's best interests, words could also be used to influence the reason of sufferers in ways that could benefit their health; and the evocative use of words to stir emotions became a mode of influencing a sufferer's state of mind in more healthful directions. Gorgias (ca. 483–376 B.C.) observed that words had the power " 'to take away fear, banish pain, inspire happiness and increase compassion,' " and he compared the influence of words to that of medications.[10] And Antiphon the Sophist (fifth century B.C.) developed a way of treating the grief-stricken by means of discourses. After informing himself of the causes of the affliction, he would unburden and console the sufferer; soothing recitations became part of his approach.[11]

With Plato, the transition from the magical use of words in charms and conjurations to their use in a psychological healing of an essentially rational nature can fairly be said to have been accomplished.[12] From magical words used on the basis of assumptions of a supernatural order, psychologically effective words gradually came to be employed on natural grounds to serve persuasive purposes; and healing became one of the goals of such persuasive efforts. In the *Phaedrus*, Plato had asserted that rhetoric was like medicine, and, as Laín Entralgo puts it in drawing on that same dialogue, "so that the word of the physician may be persuasive and may engender *sôphrosynê*, it must above all be subtly accommodated to the character and state of mind of the patient."[13]

In addition to those instances where an illness might be put right through a healer's persuasive words, Plato dealt with a healer's words as interventions that could lead to a verbal catharsis for the sufferer.[14] In this latter case, words were also brought forth from the sufferer in the process.

Then, in the *Laws*, Plato addressed once again the role of words in the realm of healing. He observed that the slave doctors who attended to slaves "never talk to their patients individually, or let them talk about their own individual complaints." In contrast, doctors who were freemen and attended to freemen encouraged their patients to talk and talked to them in turn, both getting information from them and instructing them—a much preferable course.[15]

But when one looks to the medical writings of classical antiquity, there is little indication that the physician's words were knowingly used for healing purposes. The Hippocratic writings contain nothing equivalent to the rhetoricians' or Plato's use of persuasive reasoning for therapeutic ends. Of course, words were used for communicative purposes by physicians in ways that were indirectly related to healing: as questions in the gathering of data in order to gain an understanding of the patient's illness; in the form of a prescription or other types of advice; in the form of explanation to the patient about his or her condition; and in the form of prognostic comments. And a patient's communicative use of words was significant in the presentation of a complaint and in response to some of the physician's verbal communications, particularly in what we would call history taking. Relevant here, although from a slightly later period, is an interesting recognition by Rufus of Ephesus (fl. 98–117) of the significance of talking in medical contexts, in his essay "On the Interrogation of the Patient."[16] In his advocacy of careful history taking, Rufus emphasized the importance of the physician's talk in the form of questioning the patient, "for thereby certain aspects of the disease can be better understood, and the treatment rendered more effective." And "in this way you can learn how far his mind is healthy or otherwise; also his physical strength and weakness; and you can get some idea of the disease and the part affected." Also, the patient's talking could provide clues regarding his physical strength or weakness, and "his speech" might well reveal whether "the whole thing is a matter of mental disturbance."[17]

Though these uses of words were only indirectly related to healing, the Hippocratic physician did, at times, use persuasive words in ways that were more directly related—persuading a patient toward confidence in the physician; supporting or enhancing a patient's morale. And an occasional example appears of what we might call a psychological intervention with healing intent in instances of facilitating improvement in apparently psychosomatic ailments through encouragement or the raising of hope.[18]

Further, though, the therapeutic use of words was an important element in the role of the passions in psychological healing.[19] Disturbances of the passions could be intimately involved in "psychosomatic" distress or might constitute disorders in their own right. "Among psychical symptoms are . . . griefs, passionate outbursts, strong desires. Accidents grieving the mind, either through vision or through hearing. How the body behaves: when a mill grinds the teeth are set on edge; the legs shake when one walks beside a precipice; the hands shake when one lifts a load that one should not lift; the sudden sight of a snake causes pallor. Fears, shame, pain, pleasure, passion and so forth: to each of these the appropriate member of the body responds by its action. Instances are sweats, palpitations of the heart, and so forth."[20] And a healer might induce a passion in a sufferer, either to replace a disturbing passion with a preferable one or to bring about bodily effects that changed the sufferer's symptoms for the better. The healer's use of words was a significant factor in these processes. But, although the Hippocratic writings clearly reflect an awareness of passion-related problems, they do not cite an instance of this type of therapeutic intervention.

Not long after the time of Hippocrates and Plato, Aristotle took up the discipline of rhetoric and further developed the art of persuasion. He gave careful attention to "the personal character of the speaker" and the task of "putting the audience into a certain frame of mind," yet he maintained that "persuasion is effected through speech itself."[21] Through his talking, the persuader worked to influence a person's emotions as a prelude to changing the latter's attitudes and thoughts. And so we have the outline of a crucial approach to psychological healing, with the healer's talking as a central factor. Although less clear and less certain than his contribution regarding the role of the word in persuasion, it has been vigorously argued that Aristotle also conceived of words as being used evocatively, and with healing intent, to stir up the emotions and bring about a verbal catharsis.[22]

Out of this background, a rich array of uses of speech — of words, of talking — came to play roles in psychological healing. Words were critical elements in contexts such as those already mentioned — the healing role the passions could be enlisted to play, persuasion in healing, cathartic healing, and various communicative activities that were auxiliary to healing activities — and in other activities with a healing potential, such as consolation and confession. In the words of Soranus (early second century A.D.) in his discussion of the treatment of mania, "By their words philosophers help to banish fear, sorrow, and wrath, and in so doing make no small contribution to the health of the body."[23]

The persuasive use of words served many purposes in psychological healing. It was common for educated persons in classical Greece and Rome to have had some exposure to rhetoric, whether or not they were formally trained as rhetoricians;[24] and there is much to suggest that medicine and rhetoric came to influence one another.[25] Against this background, it was quite natural that physicians would endeavor to influence and persuade their patients: to have confidence in, to cooperate with, and to think well of their physicians; to follow their physicians' advice and to strive to progress toward healthful goals. Persuasive words served in all these endeavors. Further, persuasion had a significant place in other modes of psychological healing: in the therapeutic induction of passions; in encouraging, exhorting, reassuring, advising, and instructing patients in the interest of their better health; and in facilitating patients' expressiveness, whether in the form of confiding, confessing, or merely providing relevant information.

Healers in the classical world employed words toward therapeutic ends in still another way. Whether philosophers, rhetoricians, or physicians, many made crucial use of speech in consoling many a sufferer. Although persuasion was often a significant factor in these efforts, consolation became a mode of healing in its own right. Evolving out of human sufferings and the natural responses of others to those sufferings, consolations were recorded early on in Greek literature. And the comforting use of words, whether spoken or written, was central to these efforts.[26]

In a sustained examination of the Hellenistic philosophers (Epicureans, Skeptics, Stoics), Martha Nussbaum has provided considerable further evidence of the significance of words in healing efforts in ancient times.[27] After citing Epicurus' statement, "Empty is that philosopher's argument by which no human suffering is therapeutically treated," she gave support to the Epicurean definition of philosophy: "Philosophy is an activity that secures the flourishing [*eudaimōn*] life by arguments and reasonings."[28] Philosophical arguments were conceived of as modes of psychological healing, and Nussbaum repeatedly made it clear that these arguments were crucially associated with words, whether spoken or written. It was "very natural, thinking about experiences of persuasion, consolation, exhortation, criticism, and calming, to feel that the art or arts in question would be arts of speech and argument, of *logos* somehow understood."[29] And so the philosophical arguments, employed toward healing ends, were conveyed in words, whether in a written treatise or letter, in a spoken lecture, or in more private conversation.

There is little evidence that over the subsequent centuries, and on into the nineteenth century, the role of talking in psychological healing was given much explicit attention. The various modes of healing activity already mentioned— such as persuasion or consolation on the part of healers, or confession on the part of sufferers—evolved and were given a fair share of attention. But the role of talking, whether for the healer or for the sufferer, was rarely discussed. Rather, its function was largely taken for granted. Yet it was significant, inherently essential, to most of these modes of activity, most of the time.

An interesting exception, though, was provided by Robert Burton (1577–1640), whose comments offer a useful perspective on talking in the interest of healing—very likely valid for the sixteenth and seventeenth centuries, probably valid for the Renaissance period, and very possibly representative of unspoken yet recognized sentiments over a far longer period of time. These comments are to be found in passages scattered here and there throughout *The Anatomy of Melancholy*. Burton noted that a sufferer's cares would be allayed by the "good words" and "fair speeches" of a friend's counsel. "Good words are cheerful and powerful of themselves, but much more from friends. . . . He pacifies our minds, he will ease our pain, assuage our anger . . . whose speech may ease our succourless estate, counsel relieve . . . our mourning." And Burton made these observations in a context where the value to the sufferer of a trusted friend in whom he could have confidence, to whom he could confide safely, to whom he could unburden himself and thus find relief — in short, to whom he could speak freely — was also being emphasized. And Burton makes the point that this helpful other person might be a friend or physician. It behooves such persons "by counsel, comfort, or persuasion" to ease or remove the sufferer's troubled state.

> Gentle speeches, and fair means must first be tried, no harsh language used, or uncomfortable words. . . . [The friend or physician should] ease him with comfort, cheerful speeches, fair promises, and good words: persuade him, advise him. Many, saith Galen, have been cured by good counsel and persuasion alone. *Heaviness of the heart of man doth bring it down, but a good word rejoiceth it. And there is he that speaketh words like the pricking of a sword, but the tongue of a wise man is health:* a gentle speech is the true cure of a wounded soul, . . . if it be wisely administered, it easeth grief and pain.[30]

He then cited the case of Plotinus who, on meeting Porphyrius in a suicidal frame of mind, "urged him to confess his grief: which when he had heard, he used such comfortable speeches, that he redeemed him from the jaws of Erebus, pacified his unquiet mind, insomuch that he was easily reconciled to himself. . . . By all means, therefore, fair promises, good words, gentle persuasions are to be used."[31]

In his discussion of the remedies for love melancholy, Burton emphasized the usefulness of "good counsel and persuasion." Although he granted that some thought that when the sufferer was in the grip of "head-strong passion," such efforts were of little use, he still asserted that "without question, good counsel and advice" were eminently helpful.[32]

Then, in his "Consolatory Digression," Burton again underscored the significant place of a healer's words in psychological healing. He prefaced his discussion by noting that he had "made mention of good counsel, comfortable speeches, persuasion, how necessarily they are required to the cure of a discontented or troubled mind, how present a remedy they yield, and many times a sole sufficient cure of themselves." Drawing on the "comfortable speeches" of the eminent consolers of the past, he outlined numerous consolatory interventions for a variety of losses and misfortunes; and words to influence the sufferer were clearly essential elements.[33]

In summary, Burton made mention of a healer's use of words in the raising of hope, the encouraging or exhorting toward improved spirits, the rectifying of the passions, the influencing of the imagination, the persuading of the sufferer toward a better state of mind and body, the consoling of the grief-stricken, and the providing of counsel and advice; and he referred to the benefit of the sufferer's speech in the process of cathartic release and in the form of confiding in a friend.

An Emerging Emphasis on the Sufferer's Talking

The significance of talking in psychological healing was often taken for granted, but it was hardly overlooked. As already noted, the crucial role of a healer's words was intermittently accorded explicit recognition. But it was relatively rare for the sufferer's words to be recognized as the crucial factors that they were. Galen provided one of those rare instances in his treatises *On the Passions and Errors of the Soul,* testifying to the value of the sufferer's talking. He recommended speaking of one's troubling passions — confiding in an older, experienced man about them and seeking his counsel and guidance.[34] In addition, discussions of cathartic moments, instances of confession, and sufferers' confidings often made clear the contribution made by a sufferer's words, albeit usually by implication.

Toward the end of the nineteenth century, though, the role of talking in psychological healing gradually came to be emphasized in a rather different way. Increased attention was given to talking in general as "psychotherapeutics" took shape as a distinct clinical endeavor. But what was novel was the emerging realization of the value of the patient's talking and the considerable attention that it began to receive. Although it was not new to recognize the significance of what the patient had to say, the patient's words began to be viewed as a crucial factor in psychological healing, in quite new ways.

A turning point was the case of "Anna O.," a patient whom Josef Breuer treated from 1880–1882 for a complex of difficulties that included various conversion symptoms, anxiety, and depression. This case was reported in detail by Breuer in *Studies on Hysteria,* which he wrote together with Sigmund Freud and published in 1895. The treatment had involved the patient's talking freely, in what was said to be an autohypnotic state, to an interested, attentive listener, her physician Dr. Breuer; and, later, Breuer would hypnotize the patient in the morning to facilitate her talking during the evening's autohypnosis. The talking would have a calming effect on the patient; and, as soon as the event which had given rise to a symptom was reproduced, she achieved relief from that symptom. The patient "described this procedure, speaking seriously, as a 'talking cure', while she referred to it jokingly as 'chimney-sweeping.'"[35] In describing the treatment, Breuer used such phrases as *talking through, talked away,* and *talking out* to indicate the nature of the therapeutic activity.[36]

Further examination of this case report soon makes it clear that this "talking cure" entailed a cathartic or abreactive experience and an element of confiding, purposes that were served by the talking. Then, from his association with Breuer, Freud developed his own approach to encouraging patients to talk: at first using hypnosis, later abandoning hypnosis and employing various suggestive measures to get patients to talk about their symptoms and the events associated with them, and eventually urging patients to talk freely about whatever came to mind, which came to be named free association.

In the late 1880s, Freud took up Breuer's cathartic method, using direct suggestion to a patient under hypnosis to promote the patient's talking freely, and he sought to alleviate the patient's symptoms through the recovery of hidden traumatic memories and the abreaction of strangulated affects. Essentially directed by a patient herself — Frau Emmy von N., probably treated in 1888 and 1889 — Freud employed a form of free association for the first time. This patient was spontaneously inclined to conversation which contained "a fairly complete reproduction of the memories and new impressions which have affected her since our last talk, and it often leads on, in a quite unexpected way, to pathogenic reminiscences of which she unburdens herself without being asked to. It is as though she had adopted my procedure and was making use of our conversation, apparently unconstrained and guided by chance, as a supplement to her hypnosis."[37] On one occasion, when Freud attempted to learn the meaning of certain symptoms through direct questioning, this patient said "in a definitely grumbling tone that I was not to keep on asking her where this and that came from, but to let her tell me what she had to say. I fell in with this, and she went on without preface."[38]

Influenced by the insistence of a patient — Anna O. to Breuer, Frau Emmy von N. to Freud — these two physicians adapted their therapeutic technique to their patients' inclinations. This process entailed a recognition that there was significant merit in thus adapting their technique; that collaboration with the patient was important; that the patient's putting her thoughts, images, and affects into words had a salutary effect; and that the patient's talking was vital, through both its *communicative* aspects (informing the physician and providing grounds for his interventions) and its *expressive* aspects (providing the release and relief of a cathartic experience).

While the notion that the doctor's words were significant in a healing process was well established, the view that the patient's talking might be a crucial part of the same process was taking on new and more profound meanings. At least implicitly, it had long been assumed that the patient's words were important in conveying the nature of the complaint and in answering questions so that the doctor might come to understand the illness and so prescribe usefully. But significant additional meaning for the patient's words was now being realized. On the basis of Breuer's work and Freud's own experience, Freud developed the formulation that the patient's talking would eventually allow the hidden memory of a traumatic experience to come into awareness once again; that, as the thoughts and images making up that memory were talked about, the accompanying affects would be evoked once again; that, gradually, through putting all this into words, a disturbing memory and its associated affects would be dissipated; and that, as a result, the symptom into which said hidden memory and strangulated affect had been converted would disappear.[39] "Once a picture has emerged from the patient's memory, we may hear him say that it becomes fragmentary and obscure in proportion as he proceeds with his description of it. *The patient is, as it were, getting rid of it by turning it into words.*"[40] Or, as he put it in more physicalist terms, "the excitation . . . [was led back] in this way from the somatic to the psychical sphere," and then "a discharge of the excitation by talking" was effected.[41] In either set of terms, the cure was brought about through words.

Parenthetically, during the years in which Breuer's experience was so influential for him and cathartic therapy was still central in his psychotherapeutic endeavors, Freud had occasion to contribute an essay that particularly underscored the importance of talking, but with the emphasis rather more on the healer's words. In a semipopular work on medicine, published in 1890, he said, "Words are the essential tool of mental treatment. A layman will no doubt find it hard to understand how pathological disorders of the body and mind can be eliminated by 'mere' words. He will feel that he is being asked to believe in magic. And he will not be so very wrong, for the words which we use in our everyday speech are nothing other than watered-down magic. But we shall have to follow a roundabout path in order to explain how science sets about restoring to words a part at least of their former magical power." And, further along in the same work, he added: "Words are the most important media by which one man seeks to bring his influence to bear on another; words are a good method of producing mental changes in the person to whom they are addressed. So that there is no longer anything puzzling in the assertion that the magic of words can remove the symptoms of illness, and especially such as are themselves founded on mental states."[42]

In the mid-1890s, Freud gradually gave up hypnosis and turned to the use of waking suggestions, in which he urged the patient to concentrate on the idea or issue at hand and at times applied the added influence of the pressure of his hand on the patient's forehead.[43] What resulted might fairly be called directed free association: the patient was urged to talk freely from the starting point of an idea or thought that had been raised by the patient in the first place.

By the late 1890s, Freud had essentially abandoned these suggestive techniques. In the process of his self-analysis, particularly in the analysis of his own dreams, Freud developed free association further. Whereas he had previously had his patients begin their free association from an idea or a thought, he now added free association that began from a dream element.[44] From this, he evolved the more developed form of free association — undirected free association — in which the patient was advised to speak of whatever came to mind, without any particular starting point. He urged that the patient renounce "All criticism of the thoughts that he perceives. We therefore tell him that the success of the psycho-analysis depends on his noticing and reporting whatever comes into his head and not being misled, for instance, into suppressing an idea because it strikes him as unimportant or irrelevant or because it seems meaningless."[45] And he noted that this state of mind bore "some analogy to the state before falling asleep. . . . As we fall asleep, 'involuntary ideas' emerge, owing to the relaxation of a certain deliberate (and no doubt also critical) activity which we allow to influence the course of our ideas while we are awake."[46]

As psychoanalysis developed, the role of the patient's talking continued to be recognized as significant, and yet it was not very often discussed as an activity in itself. In discussions of free association, the importance of the patient's talking — and talking as freely as possible — was assumed or hinted at, but only occasionally was it made the subject of explicit discussion. The patient's difficulties and hesitations in talking were commonly recognized. How the psychoanalyst might facilitate this talking was often mentioned. The value of talking as communication was recognized, as was the usefulness of verbal expressiveness. And the place of talking in confessing was noted. Yet the talking itself was rarely addressed. An interesting exception occurred in a public lecture which Freud delivered at the University of Vienna in 1915:

> Nothing takes place in a psycho-analytic treatment but an interchange of words between the patient and the analyst. The patient talks, tells of his past experiences and present impressions, complains, confesses to his wishes and his emotional impulses. The doctor listens, tries to direct the patient's processes of thought, exhorts, forces his attention in certain directions, gives him explanations and observes the reactions of understanding or rejection which he in this way provokes in him. . . . Words were originally magic and to this day words have retained much of their ancient magical power. By words one person can make another blissfully happy or drive him to despair, by words

the teacher conveys his knowledge to his pupils, by words the orator carries his audience with him and determines their judgements and decisions. Words provoke affects and are in general the means of mutual influence among men. Thus we shall not depreciate the use of words in psychotherapy.[47]

Although most psychoanalysts — and, indeed, Freud himself — might well have added that "nothing . . . but an exchange of words" was far too simple a description of psychoanalysis, they would have agreed that talking and words (both the sufferer's *and* the healer's) certainly constituted a necessary element in psychoanalysis and psychotherapy, albeit that element alone was not sufficient as a description.

Talking in Twentieth-Century Psychotherapy

Among the many twentieth-century forms of psychological healing that can be grouped together under the rubric *psychotherapy,* talking is a critical element in the vast majority of them. Verbal interchanges between a sufferer and a healer are central, necessary aspects of most psychotherapies. As already noted, as with most modes of healing, the sufferer usually brings his or her complaints, concerns, and array of symptoms to the healer in the form of words, as verbal communications. The healer, in turn, makes use of talking to ask questions and otherwise gather information, to offer explanations and advice, to provide a diagnosis and prognostic comments, and to outline a treatment plan. As the psychotherapeutic work takes place, words are essential elements in the activities of both parties.

For the various modes of psychotherapy derived from psychoanalysis, much the same can be said regarding the place of talking as has been said for psychoanalysis itself — whether they are considered variant forms of psychoanalysis, deviations from psychoanalysis, analytic therapies, psychoanalytically oriented psychotherapies, or psychodynamically oriented psychotherapies. Explicit attention to the role of talking has not been common in these treatment approaches. Rather, the assumption tends to be that it is desirable for the patient to talk freely; and so when explicit attention has been given, it has most often been to facilitate the patient's talking freely and frankly in the therapeutic context. Further, in addition to the basic communicative uses of words, the patient's talking was recognized as serving a range of expressive purposes such as catharsis or abreaction, confession, confiding, and, to varying degrees, free association or some modification thereof. As to the psychotherapist's talking, it too served basic communicative purposes; and, further, it was an essential element in clarification, confrontation, interpretation, and the conveying of empathy and understanding. Also, the therapist's words might serve purposes such as suggestion, persuasion, consolation, or reassurance, which might be elements in a particular instance of psychodynamically oriented psychotherapy.

For those psychotherapies that were developed more out of the traditions of hypnotherapy and suggestive therapeutics, the significance of the patient's words was rather less. There the emphasis was so much more on the psychotherapist's suggestions—the psychotherapist's words—that the patient often seems to have been some sort of malleable entity to be molded into healthier form. Yet, unstated though it tended to be, the patient's words were still crucial to the therapist's understanding—for gathering information about the sufferer's symptoms and difficulties, for acquiring the data on which to base appropriate suggestive interventions.

In the case of those modes of treatment that can be subsumed under the term *behavior therapy,* the situation has usually been similar to that of suggestive therapeutics. Basic communicative purposes have been served by both the patient's talking and the therapist's talking. In the unfolding process of the treatment, the therapist's words in the form of advice, guidance, and therapeutic instructions have been crucial. Patients' words have been important clues to behavioral changes or the lack thereof as treatment has progressed; but otherwise patients have generally allowed themselves to be directed and guided as their behavior was being molded or reshaped.

In those psychotherapeutic approaches termed *cognitive therapy,* verbal interchanges between patient and psychotherapist have been more common. Talking on the part of both patient and therapist has served the usual basic communicative purposes. Regarding the behavioral techniques that are part of cognitive therapy, the use of words has resembled that described for behavior therapy—primarily the therapist's words employed for guidance and therapeutic instructions, with a more limited role—reporting—served by the patient's words. But the various cognitive techniques have entailed a considerably larger role for talking by both parties—a good deal of verbal exchange has taken place, as the patient has revealed the nature of his or her various conceptions and assumptions, and as the therapist has guided the examination of them and the replacement of those which seem to be dysfunctional.

Certain clinical activities are grouped together as *supportive psychotherapy.* Here, again, talking has served basic communicative needs during the initial gathering of data and in prescribing. Beyond that, in some contrast to many other forms of psychotherapy, the ongoing endeavor has usually rested much more on what would traditionally be termed conversation. Such clinical work has included advice and guidance, instruction, suggestion, reassurance, comfort, and encouragement, without excluding some judicious use of many of the techniques associated with other psychotherapies already mentioned. Both the patient's words and the therapist's words have played a prominent and significant role.

Although many a journal article, book chapter, or whole book has been devoted to psychotherapy, little or no explicit attention has been paid to talking. But a scattering of serious students of the subject have given this aspect of the treatment careful attention. Some have shown concern with communication in psychotherapy, some have addressed the healing enterprise as dialogue, some have referred to it as *conversation,* and some have used the term *discourse.*

In very recent decades, though, psychotherapy has come to be studied in a new way, in which the participants' talking has been regarded as the very essence of the enterprise. The field in which these investigations have occurred, sociolinguistics, has been defined as the study of language in use; and psychotherapy as "an increasingly important type of conversation" has become one domain for this study of language in use.[48] William Labov and David Fanshel, in their *Therapeutic Discourse: Psychotherapy as Conversation,* investigate psychotherapy "as a form of conversational interaction," in which "the goals and techniques of therapy" are explored "through a close examination of the linguistic forms used by a patient and a therapist."[49] As these authors put it, "One of the most human things that human beings do is talk to one another";[50] and so it is little wonder that talking would be considered an essential element in psychotherapy. While one of their purposes in studying therapeutic discourse was "to extend the scope of linguistic analysis to conversation as a whole," another purpose was to study what took place in the verbal exchanges between patient and psychotherapist.[51]

In Kathleen Ferrara's *Therapeutic Ways with Words,* we have another sociolinguistic study in which the focus is on the talking that occurs in psychotherapy. Characterizing psychotherapy as a "speech event" and as "therapeutic discourse," this author has studied "how language is used by clients and therapists to create a therapeutic climate for change." She also makes mention of the commonplace that language is an essential element in both the diagnostic process and the treatment itself. She states that "the central theme of the book is that language and discourse are jointly constructed by interlocutions as they each take up portions of the other's speech to interweave with their own."[52] That language and discourse are interactive and jointly constructed is, the author concludes, "an outstanding feature" of psychotherapy and "one from which the greatest benefit is to be derived."[53] And such a view meshes well with the common realization that the patient is a crucial contributor to the psychotherapeutic enterprise and that said enterprise, when successful, is essentially a collaboration. The author then argues that the central importance of talking in psychotherapy rests on a certain bedrock: "The basic need of every human being for others with whom to share discourse is seen in the plaint, 'I just want someone that I can talk to.'"[54] Implied here, of course, is that listening is also of the essence.

The foregoing certainly testifies to the significance of talking in psychological healing, both in those activities which are aspects of the healer's role and those which are aspects of the sufferer's role. For all its significance in these various activities, though, the role of talking in healing has commonly been just taken for granted—assumed and left unstated—rather than explicitly addressed. Nevertheless, its importance has been repeatedly attested to in oblique ways. For example, there have been the many indications of how important it has been for the sufferer to be listened to in meaningful fashion. Among these indications have been yearnings to be heard in one's distress, to be able to confide and confess, to have accounts of one's suffering listened to and appreciated by another person, and to convey to another person one's neediness, whether as a way to feel less alone, to be comforted and consoled, or to be helped in some specifically clinical fashion. In these many ways, the importance of being listened to has implicitly emphasized the importance of a sufferer's words. And complementary to talking's role in seeking to be meaningfully listened to have been the myriad ways in which a healer's words have served to acknowledge such yearnings and to provide useful responses.

Not so indirect, though, were the observations of Brian Bird (1913–1992) who, in regard to healing contexts in general, captured particularly well the significance of talking.

> Of all the technical aids which increase the doctor's power of observation, none comes even close in value to the skillful use of spoken words—the words of the doctor and the words of the patient. Throughout all of medicine, use of words is still the main diagnostic technic, and while in therapy many mechanical and chemical aids are truly miraculous in their effectiveness, words continue to play a tremendous role.
>
> For these reasons, if medical skill is to reach its highest level, the technic of talking must be studied and developed. Talking cannot be left to accidental or incidental learning. The relationship between doctor and patient, which continues to be the central factor in good medical care, is directly based upon the talk that goes on between them. And the success of that talking is due, in

addition to the inherent qualities of the doctor, to the technical and scientific principles used in talking.[55]

In summary, talking in psychological healing serves several important purposes, just as it does in other interpersonal contexts. The need to communicate, to inform the other person, is significant; and complementary to this is talking in order to acquire information from the other person. The need to express oneself is natural, whether to communicate feelings, to unburden oneself, or to relate matters that have become too much to live with. People also feel the need to establish a relationship, to not be alone. And out of these needs emerges the more complex inclination to influence the other person in ways that are favorable to, gratifying for, comforting to, or reassuring to the speaker. In these various ways, talking serves the healer and the sufferer so that they can communicate, accommodate to one another, develop a collaborative mode of effort, and work together for the therapeutic benefit of the sufferer and the professional (and personal) benefit of the healer.

PART THREE

Expressiveness and Getting Things Out

6

Catharsis and Abreaction

The term *catharsis* was derived from the Greek *katharsis*, meaning purification, from *kathairein*, meaning to cleanse or purify. In the original edition of the *Oxford English Dictionary* in 1893, it was defined as "purgation of the excrements of the body; esp. evacuation of the bowels." In addition to this meaning, the adjective *cathartic* was given a second, more general, meaning of "cleansing, purifying, purging."[1] By the time the *OED Supplement* was published in 1933, the meanings of *catharsis* had been extended to include (1) "the purification of the emotions by vicarious experience, esp. through the drama (in reference to Aristotle's *Poetics* 6)," and, from the realm of psychotherapy, (2) "the process of relieving an abnormal excitement by re-establishing the association of the emotion with the memory or idea of the event which was the first cause of it, and of eliminating it by 'abreaction.'"[2] *Abreaction* was defined as "the liberation by revival and expression of the emotion associated with forgotten or repressed ideas of the event that first caused it. Hence *abreact*, to eliminate by abreaction."[3] Abreaction had not been mentioned in the original edition of the *OED*.

The original *OED* definitions recognized the roots of catharsis in both early Greek medicine and ancient rituals of cleansing and purification. The additions in the later *OED Supplement* took into account both the long tradition of discussions of Aristotelian thought regarding catharsis and tragedy and the relatively recent emergence of *catharsis* as a term referring to a mode of psychotherapeutic activity.

These two terms, *catharsis* and *abreaction,* intimately connected in modern thought, are often defined in conjunction with one another. For example, in her *Dictionary of Psychotherapy,* Walrond-Skinner defines *catharsis* as "the emotional release achieved by *abreaction.* . . . It produces release from repressed emotion and a subsequent feeling of relief and well-being."[4] And she defines *abreaction* as "the release of emotional energy which occurs either spontaneously or during the course of psychotherapy and which produces *catharsis.*"[5] Often enough, though, it is difficult to differentiate them, as many authors have used them as if they might be synonyms. The intimate relation of the two notions, and the difficulty in distinguishing between them, are nicely illustrated in the *Comprehensive Dictionary* by English and English where, under *catharsis,* the authors state, "*Catharsis* is the effect; *abreaction* is the method."[6] And yet, under *abreaction,* they say, "*Catharsis* is the method used, *abreaction* the result.[7] Although it is often difficult to differentiate them in a modern author's usage, the trend has been toward using *abreaction* in the restricted sense of the release or discharge of emotion and giving *catharsis* more complex meanings, including the emotional release.

In *The Encyclopedia of Philosophy,* G. B. Kerferd states,

> The most common meaning of the Greek word *katharsis* is purification, especially cleansing from guilt or ritual defilement. Virtually absent from the Homeric poems, such cleansings became important in the following archaic period. They were, above all, a feature of the mystery religions, including Orphism, through which they eventually influenced Christian doctrine and practice. . . . Plato in the *Phaedo* introduced the idea to philosophy by supposing that the soul must be purified by philosophy from contamination by things of this world in order to prepare itself for a better life. In the Hippocratic corpus we find the term used in the special sense of clearing off of morbid humors by evacuation, whether natural or induced by medicines.[8]

Then Aristotle took up the term,

> to express the effect produced by tragedy and certain kinds of music. Tragedy, by means of pity and fear, is said to effect a 'catharsis of such passions.' The conception of Aristotle, as seems clear from the passage relative to music in the *Politics* (v. 7), is that of exciting by art certain passions already existing in the spectator, viz. pity, fear, enthusiasm, in order that, after this homeopathic treatment, the person may experience relief from them and return to the normal condition. The cure is not wrought by the mere excitement, but by an excitement produced by an artistic agency, which at the same time brings order, harmony, and wholeness to bear. . . . The metaphor is primarily medical, but may quite possibly have reference also to religious purification.[9]

Around Aristotle's use of the term *catharsis* has grown up a rich scholarly tradition of interpretation and controversy over what his meaning might have been. The numerous interpretations, of which fifteen had already been developed by the end of the fifteenth century, "may be divided into three groups according as they interpret the term to mean (1) purification in the sense of refining; (2) a religious expiation or lustration; (3) a medical purgation and healing.[10]

Catharsis in Ancient Greece and Rome

As already indicated, catharsis had its roots in the purification rites of the ancient world. As a purification to free the person from uncleanliness due to sin or violation of a taboo, forms of catharsis were aspects of a variety of religious traditions. While these purifications entailed the washing of the body and thus a literal cleansing, often this cleansing also involved ridding the body of the impurities of a disease. Evacuative remedies found a place at the heart of ancient therapeutics: purgatives, emetics, blood-letting, diuretics, sudorifics, and so on. Further, though, a catharsis was frequently undertaken as a spiritual purification of a sinful uncleanliness, or as a prescribed preparatory act before prayer and sacrifice to appease the gods. Catharsis in the latter instances had a magical character and what we today would term a psychological effect on the person being cleansed. And so catharsis might entail a literal cleansing in the narrowest sense or involve a therapeutic cleansing in a medical sense or be a spiritual or moral cleansing with magical import or, often enough, constitute a complex combination of all three. That is to say, catharsis was associated with the goals of both bodily cleanliness and inner purity of a sacred or divine nature. Further, as Dodds has suggested, the literal and spiritual cleansing may well have passed "by imperceptible gradations into the deeper idea of atonement for sin," and have had a place in the evolution of confession.[11] As to the relation these bore to ancient medicine, Laín Entralgo has stated it thus: "In Greek society of the eighth to sixth centuries the physician was simultaneously a liberator from or a purifier of the physical stain in which the disease seemed to consist (a 'cathartist' more or less near to one or another religious cult) and an heir of some one of the 'first discoverers' to whom the source of medical knowledge used to be popularly and mystically referred."[12]

Plato developed, in addition to the meanings already noted, a catharsis that was in a sense at once ethical, psychological, and medical, addressed to the soul or mind.[13] Whereas catharsis of the body was "accomplished by gymnastics, which keep away ugliness, and by medicine, which frees it from illness," Plato evolved a special catharsis for "diseases of the soul," a catharsis of the soul for conditions such as wickedness, ignorance, sexual licentiousness, avarice, and scorn. Just as the physicians of the fifth century had transformed the physical and moral impurity of somatic illness into the disorder and imbalance of the material elements of the body, so did Plato transform the moral impurity that was a disease of the soul into an "imbalance or disorder of the beliefs, knowledge, feelings, and appetites that give the *psyche* its content and structure."[14] For these diseases of the soul, the traditional cathartic remedies were relevant only so far as they exerted "a suasive and educative effect upon the soul of one who undergoes them, for . . . the proper *katharsis* for moral disorder can be no other than the suitable and suasive word." The art of persuading through the word was conceived of as "verbal *katharsis*." This purification by the word entailed "the proper verbal reordering of the beliefs, knowledge, feelings, and appetites that give content to the 'soul' of man."[15] Plato had secularized catharsis.

As for Aristotle, in concerning himself with the catharsis of the passions, he emphasized pity and fear, through music and through tragedy.[16] And the *word* was the principal curative agent in the psychological healing that was tragic catharsis. Many scholars have argued about just how Aristotle was using the term *catharsis;* and there seems to be some basis both for the view that he intended it morally as a purification or cleansing of the soul through the arousal and release of passions, and for the view that he used it in a medical sense to indicate a purging and healing through the stirring and releasing, or modifying, of the passions. Enthusiastic music and the tragic spectacle served to excite and cleanse (based on the ritual cleansing of a magico-religious nature) and to stimulate, expel, relieve, and heal (based on the purgation of a medical nature). In seeking to bring about order, harmony, and calm, catharsis had elements of both purification and purgation. This was a psychic catharsis, or psychological purgation, of troubling passions from the soul, and it involved a psychosomatic process of relieving and calming that led to a healing result. While still drawing on its religious roots in the interest of cleansing and purifying, it had become a richer, more deeply meaningful medical catharsis, one with profound psychological overtones, a purification of the passions, a psychological healing mediated by the word (or by music).[17]

Another context in which catharsis seems to have had a place was the realm of Aesculapian temple healing. Within its traditions, the central practice of incubation (temple sleep) was associated with the purification of both body and soul through preparatory ablutions, other purification rites, and propitiatory offerings;[18] and drama and music were used at times. Catharsis was a theme in temple healing, although apparently not a central one.[19] As Brunius has noted, it is not clear whether the catharsis was strictly a purification or whether it was a medical purging. "At times the moral interpretation applies, at other times the psychological, and very often the religious as well as the medical."[20]

Catharsis over the Centuries

In the centuries after Aristotle, catharsis was a continuing factor, sometimes explicit and sometimes implicit, not always easily recognized nor readily reconcilable with its roots in antiquity. In assorted ways, and with associated rationales, emotions were evoked, heightened in intensity, and ultimately released or discharged. Existing emotional distress was addressed, through procedures for promoting emotional release and relief. And the tradition of Aristotelian catharsis continued, with many variations in rationale and in interpretation of Aristotle's alleged meaning.

Religious or magical ceremonies in many a social group and healing rituals within different cultures served to evoke lively emotions and led to emotional discharge; and catharsis and abreaction were an integral feature of many of those ceremonies and rituals. Dodds comments of the Dionysiac ritual in ancient Greece, "Its social function was essentially cathartic, in the psychological sense: it purged the individual of those infectious irrational impulses which, when dammed up, had given rise, as they have done in other cultures, to outbreaks of dancing mania and similar manifestations of collective hysteria; it relieved them by providing them with a ritual outlet." Later, by the fifth century B.C., the old Dionysiac cure had been largely succeeded by "a special ritual for the treatment of madness" developed by the Corybantes. Essentially similar, these two rituals "both claimed to operate a catharsis by means of an infectious 'orgiastic' dance accompanied by the same kind of 'orgiastic' music—tunes in the Phrygian mode played on the flute and the kettledrum."[21] And these magico-religious catharses have had their descendants over time in numerous cultures, both literate and preliterate.

Whether through rituals that evoked and released intense emotions, through orgiastic dancing, through the power of music, or through some combination of these, many societies dealt with both individual and group distress through procedures that induced cathartic experiences that brought release and relief. Exorcistic practices and Christian healing rites included ways of stimulating, intensifying, and, eventually, releasing emotions. Frequently, catharsis was interwoven with other techniques such as aspects of a mourning ritual, confession, suggestion, or persuasion.

Grieving and mourning have long been a context for emotional release. Many centuries of folk knowledge and practice make it clear that catharsis and abreaction, however named in a particular era or culture, have been inherent elements in the process of recovering from grief-ridden states. Supported by their culture's beliefs and rituals, assisted by those around them, grieving persons have been helped to cope with their distress through the expression of the feelings and concerns that have burdened them in the wake of a loss.

The process of confession, too, has over many centuries occasioned a cathartic reaction. As Dodds suggests, in discussing catharsis in ancient Greece, it seems that the earlier traditions of literal and spiritual cleansings from pollution, curse, and sin were gradually transformed into confession's "cleansing" relief from guilt and fear.[22] And the subsequent centuries of data on confession have frequently shown evidence of a cathartic element in the confessional experience.[23]

As to the Aristotelian tradition, the Renaissance brought an increased and enlivened interest in what Aristotle did and did not mean by his brief passage in *Poetics;* and this interest included some attention to the medical metaphor theme and to the medical implications of catharsis. In 1564, Antonio Minturno took such a view in his *L'Arte poetica.* In 1671, John Milton interpreted catharsis in a medically informed manner in his preface to *Samson Agonistes.* "Tragedy has the power, according to Milton, 'by raising pity and fear, or terror, to purge the mind of those and such like passions, that is, to temper and reduce them to just measure with a kind of delight, stirred up by reading or seeing those passions well imitated.'" Milton, applying the ancient medical principle *Similia similibus curantur* (like things cure likes), noted, "Nor is Nature wanting in her own effects to make good this assertion; for so in physic, things of melancholic hue and quality are used against melancholy, sour against sour, salt to remove salt humours." Later, Thomas Twining in 1789 and H. Weil in 1847 offered similar medical interpretations of catharsis.[24]

Scattered here and there are other hints that the notion of a "cathartic" release was in use, in relative independence of magico-religious traditions and Aristotelian perspectives. For example, in the late seventeenth century, Franciscus Mercurius Van Helmont (1618–1699) emphasized that weeping was "proper to Mankind," and that troubling ideas and images could be weakened and "reduc'd to rest" through tears:

> We find that when for the Death of a Friend, or other Cause, we are seized with extraordinary Sorrow, if we do weep freely, our Sorrow is by this means alleviated, and that the Image of our dead Friend, or the Thoughts of some other suffer'd Losses, will no longer be so strongly present with us. And on the contrary, Experience informs us, that Persons over-taken with some great grief or affliction, when they cannot discharge their Sorrow by Weeping, do often

fall into some Distemper or Sickness, because the Idea of the cause of their Sorrow, by this means encreaseth, and continues still present with them.[25]

And, in the early nineteenth century, Benjamin Rush (1745–1813) reported on a remedy suggested to him by "a madman in the Pennsylvania Hospital" who indicated that he kept a journal and commented: "Here (said he) I write down every thing that passes in my mind, and particularly malice and revenge. In recording the latter, I feel my mind emptied of something disagreeable to it, just as vomit empties the stomach of bile."[26]

Breuer, Freud, and Cathartic Treatment

From the mid-nineteenth century to the present, a goodly number of scholars have argued that the notion of a medical purgation and healing was a significant element in Aristotle's catharsis. Of particular importance in this trend was Jacob Bernays (1824–1881), who in 1857 argued effectively for such a view.[27] In addition to his influence on subsequent arguments regarding the implications of Aristotle's comments on catharsis, he was the uncle of Sigmund Freud's wife, and his views very likely influenced Breuer and Freud in the selection of the term *catharsis* for the mode of psychological healing that came to be associated with their names.

Bernays broke with "the moral interpretation of Aristotle's definition," and understood " 'catharsis of the passions' as a purging of the soul in the most purely medical sense of this term." He stated, " 'The word *katharsis* means one of the following two things in Greek: *either* the expiation of a guilt by means of certain priestly rites, *or* the suppression or relief of a distress by a purgative medical remedy.' " And he argued that Aristotle would have been using this second definition. Bernays' view was that Aristotle's tragic catharsis was based either analogically or literally on the notion of curing disease by the use of a purgative. According to Bernays, "Traditional medical doctrine in Greece taught that a purgative acts by first exacerbating and even bringing to a paroxysm the disease that it subsequently is to cure."[28]

Renewed interest in Bernays' work was stimulated when it was reprinted in 1880. Against this background, the term *catharsis* was applied by Breuer and Freud to a mode of psychological healing first used by Breuer in 1881 and then taken up by Freud. The term became associated with both their names through their joint publication *Studies on Hysteria* in 1895. During Breuer's treatment of "Anna O." for a complex of difficulties which included periods of anxiety, depression, hallucination, distraught behavior, paraphasia, and *absences*,[29] a pattern developed in which an hour's deep sleep in the evening would gradually evolve into an autohypnotic state during which the patient would tell "stories" to Breuer and become calm as a result; and Breuer eventually began to hypnotize the patient during the morning in order to facilitate the evening's "talking away" of her symptoms.[30] Breuer said of this procedure, "It took me completely by surprise, and not until symptoms had been got rid of in this way in a whole series of instances did I develop a therapeutic technique out of it."[31]

Out of this experience, Breuer (and later, Freud) developed the technique of hypnotizing a patient and then arousing "memories under hypnosis of the time at which the symptom made its first appearance."[32] Demonstrating the connection would then lead to understanding on the patient's part and the disappearance of the symptom. Breuer and Freud wrote, "*Each individual hysterical symptom immediately and permanently disappeared when we had succeeded in bringing clearly to light the memory of the event by which it was provoked and in arousing its accompanying affect, and when the patient had described that event in the greatest possible detail and had put the affect into words.*"[33]

Breuer and Freud thought of traumatic experiences as having distressing associated affects. If the disturbing event led to an affect-laden reaction — "from tears to acts of revenge" — the affects were discharged. Here they noted that "linguistic usage bears witness to this fact of daily observation by such phrases as 'to cry oneself out' [*sich ausweinen*] and 'to blow off steam' [*sich austoben*, literally 'to rage oneself out']." But, "if the reaction is suppressed, the affect remains attached to the memory." The discharge of affect was referred to as a " 'cathartic' effect" by Breuer and Freud; and it might be complete, partial, or suppressed, depending on the adequacy of the reaction — that is to say, it might be normal or potentially pathological. They then added, "But language serves as a substitute for action; by its help, an affect can be 'abreacted' almost as effectively. In other cases speaking is itself the adequate reflex, when, for instance, it is a lamentation or giving utterance to a tormenting secret, e.g. a confession." They then proceeded to explain hysterical symptoms as the outcome of "ideas which have become pathological" through persisting with "freshness and affective strength because they have been denied the normal wearing-away processes by means of abreaction and reproduction in states of uninhibited association."[34]

The treatment sequence began with hypnosis, then came the affectively charged re-experiencing of the traumatic memory, and, finally, the abreaction or discharge of the hitherto blocked affect. The re-experiencing and the discharge were named "the cathartic treatment." And this psychotherapeutic technique was an attempt to bring about a process modeled on the normal experience of discharging affects in reaction to disturbing events. This "psychotherapeutic procedure . . . *brings to an end the operative force of the idea which was not abreacted in the first instance, by allowing its strangulated affect to find a way out through speech; and it subjects it to associative correction by introducing it into normal consciousness (under light hypnosis) or by removing it through the physician's suggestion, as is done in somnambulism accompanied by amnesia."*[35]

Noting that the cathartic method had brought "considerable therapeutic advantages," he nevertheless entered the caveat that it was "a symptomatic and not a causal" method; and another problem with it was that many patients could not be hypnotized.[36] The latter point led him to the question of "how to by-pass hypnosis and yet obtain the pathogenic recollections." At this point, we see Freud moving beyond Breuer's method, and yet retaining the search for the pathogenic memories in the interest of promoting a cathartic discharge of them and their disturbing affects. He employed what he called insistence, or the pressure technique, in which he had patients lie down and close their eyes in order to concentrate; and then he would urge them to bring forward whatever thoughts were in mind. In some instances he used suggestion in the interest of the same goal. And, later, he began to use pressure on patients' foreheads while urging them to reveal their thoughts. These passages serve both as reminders of the suggestive psychotherapeutic techniques of that era and as foreshadowings of Freud's associative technique that was to come.[37]

From gradually using "the cathartic method" more and more without hypnosis as an essential accompaniment, Freud had gone on to abandon hypnosis, and then to evolve a complex of techniques in which catharsis was still to be found as an essential element. He still emphasized that "the patient only gets free from the hysterical symptom by reproducing the pathogenic impressions that caused it and by giving utterance to them with an expression of affect, and thus the therapeutic task *consists solely in inducing him to do so.*" He had shifted from "a cathartic treatment under hypnosis" to a cathartic treatment "under concentration." He concluded that the function of either hypnosis or the concentration technique was to remove resistances that were preventing the cathartic discharge or abreaction.[38]

Other Nineteenth-Century "Cathartists"

Particularly prominent among those who dealt in concepts and practices akin to "the cathartic treatment" was Pierre Janet (1859–1947), a French psychologist and psychiatrist who made numerous important contributions to the study of psychopathology. In 1889 *L'automatisme psychologique*, which had been his doctoral dissertation, was published; it included a case (Marie) in which an early trauma was relived under hypnosis and, aided by suggestions under hypnosis, a unilateral hysterical blindness was cured.[39]

In their "Preliminary Communication" in 1893, Breuer and Freud alluded to Janet's work; and, in their *Studies on Hysteria* in 1895, they frequently referred to his work, sometimes in reasoned disagreement and often in respectful appreciation.[40] Over the years that followed, Janet made many comments, increasingly critical as time went by, about Breuer and Freud's *Studies,* and, in particular, about psychoanalysis. On the one hand, he did not think that psychoanalysis amounted to much; on the other hand, he argued that those psychoanalytic notions that did amount to anything had been taken without proper credit from his own early work. Among the latter were the "cathartic treatment" and its related concepts. He maintained that he had discovered the cathartic treatment of the neuroses, and that psychoanalysis was merely an outgrowth of that work.

In his *Psychological Healing,* Janet brought to publication a series of lectures from 1904–1907 and added to that a chapter on psychoanalysis based on his presentation to the International Congress of Medicine in London in 1913.[41] In that chapter, he outlined his own early work on freeing patients from disorders through bringing them to express their traumatic memories that had been blocked from awareness; and he classified psychoanalysis, along with his own work, under the generic heading of "Treatment by Mental Liquidation." Criticizing some psychoanalytic concepts and asserting that others were nothing new, he argued that psychoanalysis was merely an extension of his "psychological analysis," and that the *cathartic treatment* was merely another name for his "mental disinfection by the dissociation of traumatic memories."[42] In Janet's view, these two approaches were both forms of "treatment by discharge"; in each case the traumatic memories were "liquidated." In his *Principles of Psychotherapy,* he again referred to "the liquidation of traumatic memories"; and he complained that Breuer and Freud had "baptized with the name of catharsis" what he had "referred to as a psychological dissociation, or as a moral fumigation."[43]

Under his heading of "Treatment by Mental Liquidation," Janet included a category "Treatment by Discharge" and, within this latter, a subcategory of "local discharge." There he dealt with matters such as catharsis and abreaction. Although critical of Freud's exposition, he found something meaningful in the notion of an event having been "charged with affect" or having "an emotive charge," along with the companion notion that this "charge" needed to be expended, that "abreaction" was in order, that "the aim of our treatment must be to facilitate the discharge." Preferring the terms *mental energy* and *psychological tension,* he found all of it to be rather similar to some of his own theories and practices. In his view, an event's occurring provoked the person's tendency to react. This tendency would be charged with a measure of vital energy and would press for activation; and it might then lose its charge, or discharge itself, in various ways. Or by contrast such tendencies might go undischarged, and the energies might accumulate, leading to some form of crisis. Janet then cited several cases in which one form or other of discharge (or abreaction) occurred with significant relief to the sufferer.[44]

Though the controversy between Janet and various psychoanalysts may have its own interest for many, its relevance in our context is the extent to which it suggests that the 1880s and 1890s constituted an era in which catharsis-like concepts and practices were very much "in the air." It does seem that Breuer and Janet *independently* evolved a clinical approach that identified traumatic memories that, having been somehow kept from awareness, lived on in people to cause various symptoms and could be identified and "discharged" through clinical endeavors that Breuer happened to term catharsis. In Vienna, the 1880s was a time of lively interest in catharsis, apparently stimulated by the republication in 1880 of Jacob Bernays' book on the Aristotelian concept. In Paris, Janet was only one among several French investigators of that era who were concerned with catharsis and similar notions.

In their *Studies on Hysteria,* Breuer and Freud not only recognized Janet's contributions, but they mentioned other similar work by Delboeuf and by Binet. Regarding J. R. L. Delboeuf (1831–1896), another physician who studied with Charcot, they commented that "the possibility of a therapeutic procedure of this kind has been clearly recognized by Delboeuf . . . , as is shown by the following. . . . 'We can now explain how the hypnotist promotes cure. He puts the subject back into the state in which his trouble first appeared and uses words to combat that trouble, as it now makes a fresh emergence.' "[45] Regarding Alfred Binet (1857–1911), a French psychologist whose many contributions included the Binet-Simon intelligence test, Breuer and Freud again noted an allusion to the possibility of a cathartic procedure: " 'We shall perhaps find that by taking the patient back by means of a mental artifice to the very moment at which the symptom first appeared, we may make him more susceptible to a therapeutic suggestion.' "[46]

Further still, two French physicians, Henri Bourru (1840–1914) and Prosper Ferdinand Burot, had developed "a technique very like the cathartic method" with a patient in 1887, and they reported on this work at the first International Congress of Experimental and Therapeutic Hypnotism in Paris in August 1889.[47] This patient presented a complex of hysterical symptoms rather like those of Breuer's patient Anna O. — paralyses, contractures, disturbances of vision, recurrent somnambulism, and so forth. At two junctures in her treatment, the authors used hypnosis to introduce "a hallucinatory state" in which the patient relived an important episode in her life, with lively bodily and emotional accompaniments; and remission of her symptoms followed. Bourru and Burot considered that these " 'beneficial reactive attacks . . . were above all hallucinations which produced in the patient a severe mental shaking, stirring up the affects associated with the thought which had originally disorganized the brain and caused the illness.' "[48] As L. Chertok stated it, "The main features of this account are, first, the return to the past, and second, the intense *hallucinatory revival of affect* or 'catharsis' proper, on which Breuer and Freud were later to insist so strongly."[49] The work of Bourru and Burot was known to Janet, and "Janet discovered his method in the process of verifying the findings described by Bourru and Burot in their *Variations de la personnalité*."[50]

In spite of these various claims, though, it is now clear that they all had a predecessor. Onno van der Hart and Kees van der Velden have brought to light an 1868 publication by a Dutch physician, Andries Hoek (1807–1885), who treated a young woman, Rika van B., from December 1850 through November 1851, with an "uncovering hypnotherapy" much like that later used by Janet, Breuer, and Freud.[51] By December 1850 this patient had been considered insane for five months; her symptoms included "periods of continuous talking and raving, dissociative symptoms such as amnesia, hallucinations and pseudo-epileptic seizures, depression, . . . suicidal urges . . . [and] several physical complaints such as pain in the left side of her body, headaches, and fever."[52] Using hypnotism, Hoek treated her nearly every day for eleven months.

During the first phase of treatment (December 1850 to May 1851), "Rika told Hoek her life story" which included "several traumatic experiences she had been unable to assimilate, including repeated abuse, rape, . . . the death by drowning of one of her uncle's servants," and the recent suicide by drowning of her ex-fiancé, following her breaking of their engagement. She experienced "serious relapses and 'attacks of madness,' " but, in the hypnotic state, she "was calm, and gave Hoek scrupulous instructions about the therapeutic strategy to be taken." During the second phase (May–August 1851), "while under hypnosis, she described in detail the traumatic experiences she was reliving," with a particularly important theme being the working through of the drowning of the uncle's servant when she was nine years old, "which [had] sensitized her to the ex-fiancé's suicide by drowning." During the third phase (August–November 1851), after initially doing much better, she experienced two very difficult days at the anniversary of her ex-fiancé's suicide. After working through this episode, she exhibited no further psychopathological symptoms.[53]

As van der Hart and van der Velden pointed out, the case of Rika van B.

reminds one of Breuer's case of Anna O. Not only was hypnosis used and a useful cathartic process achieved, but, in each case, the patient took an active role in determining the nature of the treatment and in guiding its course, with the physician respecting and accepting the patient's guidance. This case was apparently known neither to Breuer and Freud nor to Janet and the other French cathartists.

Catharsis and Psychoanalysis

By the time of *Studies on Hysteria* Freud had shifted from using the cathartic method under hypnosis to the promotion of cathartic effects by various means of facilitating, without hypnosis, the patient's expression of whatever thoughts came to mind. He continued to be guided by the idea of a search for pathogenic memories in the interest of achieving a cathartic discharge of them and their disturbing affects. Whether the technique involved hypnosis, concentration, or other modes of facilitation, the goal was to remove obstacles that were blocking the cathartic discharge or abreaction. During the 1890s, there was a gradual movement away from directed "free" association toward a more truly free form of association. As Freud explained in 1898, "Basing myself on the 'cathartic' method introduced by Josef Breuer, I have in recent years almost completely worked out a therapeutic procedure which I propose to describe as *'psycho-analytic.'* "[54] Still, though, he conceived of a cathartic process as an essential element in his emerging psychoanalysis. In fact, he continued to identify psychoanalysis closely with its cathartic roots. In 1903, he wrote, "The particular psychotherapeutic procedure which Freud practices and describes as 'psycho-analysis' is an outgrowth of what was known as the 'cathartic' method and was discussed by him in collaboration with Josef Breuer in their *Studies on Hysteria*."[55] In 1904, he wrote about "the method which Breuer called *cathartic,* but which I myself prefer to call 'analytic.' "[56] And in 1905, as optimal treatment for "psychoneurotics," he advocated "psycho-analytic investigation, which is employed in the therapeutic procedure introduced by Josef Breuer and myself in 1893 and known at that time as 'catharsis.' "[57] Nearly twenty years later, in 1923, Freud still could say, "The cathartic method was the immediate precursor of psycho-analysis; and, in spite of every extension of experience and of every modification of theory, is still contained within it as its nucleus."[58]

Subsequent to these various expressions of Freud's own views on the relation of catharsis to psychoanalysis, Sandor Ferenczi's *neocatharsis* was probably the most vigorous assertion in favor of a central role for catharsis. After agreeing to a place for an element of frustration and heightened tension in psychoanalytic work, he argued that, all too often, this led to apparently insoluble resistances, and so an element of indulgence and resultant relaxation should also have its place.[59] When "the principles of frustration and indulgence" were both allowed to govern his technique, he found that "miniature hysterical attacks" occurred.

> Unusual states of consciousness manifested themselves, which might also be termed autohypnotic. . . . One was forced to compare them with the phenomena of the Breuer-Freud *catharsis*. . . . [But] there is all the difference in the world between this cathartic termination to a long psycho-analysis and the fragmentary eruptions of emotion and recollection which the primitive catharsis could provoke and which had only a temporary effect. The catharsis of which I am speaking is, like many dreams, only a confirmation from the unconscious, a sign that our toilsome analytical construction, our technique of dealing with resistance and transference, have finally succeeded in drawing near to aetiological reality. There is little that the palaeocatharsis has in common with this *neocatharsis*.[60]

During the years since, however, opinions among authorities on psychoanalysis have varied a great deal regarding the relation of clinical psychoanalysis to catharsis, some asserting that clinical psychoanalysis was very far from including catharsis as any sort of significant element in its practices, and others maintaining that cathartic effects were still important in the clinical work of psychoanalysis. From the latter point of view, it can fairly be said that the reawakening of crucial memories and their associated affects, the reliving of those memories and the release from their influences, and the lively experience of those affects and their discharge or abreaction, were all to be found in most psychoanalyses. Although they were no longer considered to be the essence of psychoanalysis, the themes of discharge and release continued to have a place in the clinical process. Further, it could be argued that many patterns of repetition and working-through were very gradual, attenuated forms of catharsis. And, finally, transference themes were subtle reawakenings and relivings of crucial aspects of a person's past, often with lively associated affects; and so, in an oblique way, the working out of transference issues might also be considered an attenuated form of catharsis. But most psychoanalytic authorities thought of catharsis in more traditional terms, and, considering its gains temporary, deemed it not to have a significant place in psychoanalysis. They were more likely to emphasize the analysis of resistance and transference, working-through, interpretation, and insight as the important themes in technique.

In 1935, in a discussion of psychoanalytic technique, Franz Alexander (1891–1964) gave "emotional abreaction" a place in the complex of factors that brought about cure; but he emphasized that the mere expression of the unconscious tendencies and the associated affects which sustained a symptom were "not sufficient to secure a lasting cure."[61] More recently, in discussing "*abreaction* or catharsis," Ralph R. Greenson (1911–1979) has observed that abreaction gives patients a convincing, enlivened sense of what was unconscious or vague, and often brings a temporary sense of relief; but that it is not a central feature in psychoanalysis, and it is not one of the key curative factors.[62] Paul A. Dewald accords abreaction its place in psychoanalytic work in the following way:

> As pathogenic conflicts or traumatic experiences are recovered (either as transference responses or as memories), the affects associated with them are likewise reexperienced in the current analytic situation. This discharge of "strangulated affect" . . . is one necessary precursor to the ultimate resolution of conflict. By the repeated discharge of unpleasant affects associated with a particular conflict, relationship, or traumatic event, the memory becomes less distressing or painful to the patient's recall and thus can be accepted in consciousness more fully and with less accompanying psychic pain. As a result, the capacity of the patient to retain in consciousness the memory and understanding of the situation in question is enhanced, and having become conscious this material can now be subjected to new and more effective integrative and synthetic ego functions.
>
> In other words, abreaction is part of a process of desensitization to core conflicts, fantasies, experiences, or relationships which, because of their previously associated intensely painful affects, could not be accessible to conscious recognition and awareness and hence could not be resolved. . . . Abreaction is also an important element in the working-through process.[63]

But other psychoanalysts have not been so sanguine about catharsis. William A. Binstock has not only questioned the value of catharsis in the psychoanalytic process, but concludes, "The role of catharsis in human affairs is a most restricted and humble one. It is monstrously overvalued by people in general, by physicians in particular, and beyond all reason by mental healers and Americans."[64] And Bennet Simon has argued that "the concept of catharsis . . . in therapy . . . is an inadequate model for . . . the healing power of psychotherapy."[65]

Catharsis and Twentieth-Century Psychotherapies

Whatever its place in psychoanalysis might be said to be, the catharsis or abreaction of Breuer and Freud has, whether directly or indirectly, influenced a goodly number of other twentieth-century approaches to psychological healing. More often than not, though, these terms have not had quite the same meaning in their new contexts. As the term *catharsis* became more widely used in a variety of modern psychological healings and other psychological activities, its meaning became much more general in nature, and it was often rather vaguely defined. "It is generally understood to mean 'a process that relieves tension and anxiety by expressing emotions,' — emotions that have been hidden, restrained, or unconscious."[66] The connection with emotions, with their build-up or being dammed up, and with their release or discharge all tend to be retained; the purgation metaphor is still there; but the psychoanalytic notions of repressed traumatic memories and the reliving of them are no longer necessary implications.

One important context for cathartic or abreactive techniques emerged during World War I in the course of the development of treatment approaches to cope with the numerous casualties grouped together under the rubric *shell shock*. Particularly in the British army, both in France and in military treatment settings at home, a small number of physician-psychologists went against the traditional alternative military explanations of cowardice and malingering or organic disease. Instead, they conceived of most shell-shock victims as suffering from psychological disorders that would be amenable to psychotherapeutic interventions. While most physicians, whether military or civilian, were approaching these problems with physicalist modes of treatment or conventional exhortations such as "Put it out of your mind, forget about it" and "Pull yourself together, man," these more psychologically minded clinicians used suggestion and persuasion techniques in some instances, and in others they employed cathartic or abreactive techniques.

These shell-shock patients "displayed a bewildering range of physical and mental disabilities: paralyses and muscular contractures of the arms, legs, hands, and feet, loss of sight, speech and hearing, choreas, palsies and tics, mental fugues, catatonia and obsessive behavior, amnesia, severe sleeplessness, and terrifying nightmares."[67] Some among these sufferers were eventually recognized as having symptoms similar to hysteria, and others were thought to be afflicted with severe forms of neurasthenia. Gradually abreactive or cathartic techniques came to have a significant place in the treatment of these "war neuroses," and, by the end of the war, "squads of fifty RAMC officers were being given three-month courses on the techniques of 'abreactive' psychotherapy — including dream analysis."[68]

Prominent among those who influenced this trend was William Brown (1881–1952), a British physician and psychologist, who explicitly drew on Freud's work, using his earlier cathartic technique and borrowing a number of his concepts, while making it clear that he disagreed with Freud on some issues, such as the sexual etiology of the neuroses. From early in the war, Brown gave considerable attention to "the revival of emotional memories and its therapeutic value" and used hypnosis, reflecting the early Breuer-Freud orientation in striving to revive pathogenic memories and discharge their associated affects. As he stated it in a discussion in 1920, "It has been found again and again in the case of shell-shock patients, especially those seen in the field, that they suffer from loss of memory of the incidents immediately following upon the shell-shock, and that, if these memories are brought back again afterwards with emotional vividness—hallucinatory vividness, I might say—the other symptoms which they were showing tend to disappear."[69] Brown emphasized, however, that "the essential thing seems to be the revival of the emotion accompanying the memory," and the abreaction of this "excessive emotion." The "liberation of such pent-up emotion (known as 'abreaction') produces a resolution of the functional symptoms." This "excessive emotion" was "worked off by revival, with relief to the patient's mind (psychocatharsis)."[70] It is of note that, in discussing this presentation of Brown's, William McDougall (1871–1938) argued that "the discharge of emotional excitement plays no essential curative *role*." Instead, he would have it that "the essential step in bringing about relief was neither suggestion nor 'abreaction,' but just the abolition of the dissociation."[71] Again in response to Brown's views, Carl Jung took much the same position, maintaining that "the essential factor is the dissociation of the psyche and not the existence of a highly charged affect and, consequently, that the main therapeutic problem is not abreaction but how to integrate the dissociation."[72]

Quite similar disorders on the German side of the World War I lines led to similar clinical impressions and essentially the same therapeutic interventions. Ernst Simmel (1882–1947), a medical officer in the German army, has written about "war neuroses" on the basis of his experience with approximately two thousand cases. The symptoms included spastic or paretic conditions of the muscular system; compulsive, involuntary body movements; disturbances of speech, vision, and hearing; epileptiform attacks; various psychological disturbances, such as amnesia, emotional instability, and irritability; and sleep disturbances, such as sleeplessness and nightmares. Simmel developed a cathartic treatment approach in which he used hypnosis in order to lift the patient's amnesia and provide him with an "opportunity to repeat his traumas." At times, he used dream material "to induce hypnotic repetitions of traumatic war scenes"; and sometimes he used posthypnotic suggestions. A soldier would relive the traumatic experience and would "act out" terrifying hallucinations and fear-ridden memories. Further, this catharsis or emotional abreaction was facilitated by introducing, once the patient was under hypnosis, an "actual enemy" in the form of a stuffed dummy. After the patient's fear of the dummy had turned into rage, he would act out his rage on the dummy.[73]

Also, evidence indicates that other medical officers in the German and Austro-Hungarian armies during World War I objected to the mainstream views that explained war neuroses as malingering, cowardice, and weakness of the will. Mostly influenced by psychoanalytic writings, or trained in psychoanalysis, these physicians too employed cathartic methods in their efforts to treat the growing numbers of "shell-shocked" soldiers in the military settings in which they served.[74]

Among the medical officers who undertook these abreactive or cathartic treatments of war neuroses, some restricted their approach to the revival and reliving of the repressed traumatic experiences under hypnosis and tended to emphasize the release of dammed-up emotions. Brown's approach was an important example of the efforts of this group of clinicians. Others used similar cathartic methods but proceeded to discussion in the waking state of the relived experiences, and sometimes to dream interpretation, in the interest of understanding and resolving the underlying conflict and undoing the dissociation. Simmel belonged to this latter group.

Although clinical catharsis and abreaction were not forgotten during the 1920s and 1930s, they fell into relative disuse during those decades. As the impact of the large numbers of sufferers from shell shock gradually faded, the use of such techniques became much less frequent. But World War II brought another rash of casualties in which a mixture of physical and psychological symptoms occurred without any direct influence from the usual causes of the wounds of war. Associated with this new wave of traumatic reactions to the stress of war was a lively reawakening of interest in and use of catharsis and abreaction in treatment. Considering "the symptomatology of war neuroses, as precipitated by World War II," Simmel emphasized that it was "in no way different from the picture of war neuroses during World War I."[75] He also noted that "in modern warfare military psychiatrists are on duty at the front lines, or in close contact with the fighting units," and thus "a kind of *short psychotherapy*" could be used. In such work, " 'talking' gives the soldier the opportunity for catharsis and for mastering his emotional reactions *intellectually*. The soldier can 'get off his chest' impressions which otherwise would crush his spirit."[76]

Even as the abreactive and cathartic techniques employed with the "battle neuroses" of World War II gave clear indications of their heritage — Breuer and Freud's catharsis, psychoanalytic notions of dammed-up affect and the value of its release and the reintegration of repressed memories, and the use of catharsis and abreaction with the war neuroses of World War I — other, more recent influences gave many of these abreactive undertakings a new coloration. Familiar approaches were employed in which a hypnotic trance was established to achieve an emotional catharsis or release and to recall the hitherto repressed memories; and subsequent efforts were aimed at working through and reintegrating the painful combat experiences.[77] But the 1930s had seen the emergence of certain barbiturates as adjuvants to various forms of psychotherapeutic work.[78] Although such approaches were not yet prominent during that decade, they rapidly became so during World War II. Under the rubrics *narcoanalysis* and *narcosynthesis,* agents such as sodium amytal and sodium pentothal were used in a manner roughly analogous to hypnosis.[79] And various other wartime clinicians undertook similar clinical efforts with agents such as ether,[80] a chloroform and ether mixture,[81] and nitrous oxide.[82] The narcotized state was considered an equivalent to the trance state for achieving abreactive release and access to repressed traumatic material. Although some of these approaches focused on the abreactive release of emotion as the essence of the therapeutic action, many of them also emphasized the recall of traumatic experiences and their eventual integration, in the waking state, with the rest of the person's experience.

In the wake of World War II, interest in psychological healing methods increased significantly. Various modes of catharsis and abreaction were aspects of many of these treatment approaches, and, in some instances, they became the very essence of the treatment. For many of these, the established definition of catharsis or abreaction was relevant: that is, gaining access to repressed memories of traumatic experiences, a modified reliving of those experiences, becoming aware of associated painful emotions, and experiencing a release of and relief from those emotions. Whether this was achieved in a hypnotic state, a narcotized state, or a waking state was usually not essential to the definition. In some approaches, the integration of the attendant memories with the rest of the patient's experiences was a significant element; in others, the emotionally charged recall and the emotional release were considered sufficient. Further, catharsis or abreaction was often more broadly — even loosely or casually — defined. Merely expressing emotions, communicating them to an interested listener (or listeners), often came to be referred to as catharsis or abreaction. Often this was not a question of gaining access to repressed emotions and memories. Rather, these matters had been suppressed; the sufferer had been afraid, ashamed, or otherwise hesitant to acknowledge them fully but had been distinctly aware of them. They were "bottled up," but not unavailable to awareness. The term *ventilation* came into use: it was considered a therapeutically useful process to "get things out," "get things off your chest," "talk about it," "talk things out," without particular attention to whether something might remain repressed. The boundaries of meaning for catharsis and abreaction became very loosely defined indeed.

Although many psychoanalysts had either dismissed catharsis or abreaction or minimized any role it might have in their clinical work, in 1954 Edward Bibring (1894–1959), a leading psychoanalyst, took a more measured view, recognizing both its continuing place in various psychotherapies and the problem of the broader or looser definitions. In discussing the psychotherapeutic principles inherent in clinical psychoanalysis and the psychotherapies derived from it, he considered in detail the technical and curative application of these principles. Defining abreactive techniques as those which brought about "relief from acute tension through emotional discharge," he included them as one among five groups of basic psychotherapeutic techniques, the others being suggestive, manipulative, clarifying, and interpretive techniques.[83]

Noting that "some therapists emphasize its [abreaction's] value in the belief that plain abreaction, as such, cures in a kind of automatic or mechanical way as a one-act treatment," Bibring related much of the controversy about abreaction to the fact that three different etiological conceptions had been presented together in the original discussions of the Breuer-Freud cathartic therapy. These were "the conceptions of hypnoid hysteria (Breuer-Freud), of retention hysteria (Freud), and that of defense hysteria (Freud)." He then went on to say that "abreaction as a one-act therapy referred only to the 'pure' retention hysteria" in which an emotional discharge had not occurred, "but without causing any dissociation of the mind." In contrast, in the other two forms of hysteria, the therapy involved two steps: "a complete abreaction of the affects, in form of verbalization, simultaneously with the reminiscence of the events"; and "the necessity that the pathogenic 'idea' be dealt with," either by bringing it "into normal consciousness" and "into associative readjustment" or by dispelling it "by means of the physician's suggestion," whether under hypnosis or not. This more complex psychotherapeutic process required remembering the split-off experiences, an emotional discharge that transformed "an emotionally strong idea into a weak one," and then the associative readjustment of the idea. Bibring argued that strictly speaking, abreaction referred only to the emotional discharge and yet it was often used to refer to both the remembering and the emotional discharge. In his scheme, abreaction was only one phase of a complex psychotherapeutic process. Bibring also pointed out that in many instances in psychoanalysis, abreaction had come to provide a "sense of 'emotional reliving,' " and thus conviction, in the process of acquiring insight, rather than functioning as a curative agent."[84]

Prominent among the postwar treatments in which catharsis and abreaction had a significant place was *psychodrama,* in which a release from internal conflict was sought through role-playing which facilitated a cathartic experience. Developed by Jacob L. Moreno (1889–1974) in the 1920s and 1930s, this approach flourished after the war in the United States as a wide variety of group psychotherapies were developing. In psychodrama, efforts were made to re-enact critical past conflicts to facilitate emotional expression and cathartic release. The goals of the catharsis thus achieved were the gaining of insight and, ultimately, behavioral change. With its cast of director-therapist, protagonist-patient, other persons taking up roles from the patient's life, and still others serving as auxiliary egos, psychodrama emerged as a special form of group psychotherapy.[85]

Among the many other group psychotherapies, a good number used cathartic techniques as aspects of their therapeutic work. And in the plethora of quasi-therapeutic groups, such as encounter groups and sensitivity groups, cathartic or abreactive methods often had a significant place. Regarding these quasi-treatment groups, in 1973 Binstock observed: "The doctrine of catharsis, gradually and reluctantly expelled from its secure position in the fundament of psychoanalysis, is once again becoming entrenched in today's America. In the many forms of the sensitivity training–encounter–human potential movement, we are confronted anew with the vitality of the notion that Western man must approach his emotions through elaborate and ritualized exercises."[86]

In the realm of the individual psychotherapies, a number of approaches — *Reichian therapy, bioenergetics, gestalt therapy,* and *primal therapy,* among others — had significant cathartic elements. Although catharsis was given little explicit attention in some of these, the achievement of emotional release, the discharge of pent-up emotions and energies, and expressive efforts toward a freeing up of energies were common themes, with a clear kinship to more explicit cathartic or abreactive measures.

A variety of clinical endeavors derived from the character analysis, vegetotherapy, and orgone therapy of Wilhelm Reich (1897–1957). Evolving out of his earlier character analysis, Reich's later work undertook to break down the person's character "armor" with the aim of freeing up his (orgone) energy and making it available for more productive purposes. This approach developed into direct efforts to loosen up muscular "armor" through breathing exercises, massage, and other forms of physical work. Emotional release was a central aspect of this freeing up of energy, this undoing of restrictions on both physical and psychological energy.[87]

Out of long experience as Reich's student, Alexander Lowen gradually developed his own clinical approach, which he termed *bioenergetics.*[88] Continuing the emphasis on work with the body, and addressing concerns about the need for bound-up energy to be freed, Lowen thought of energy in broader terms than Reich's focus on sexual energy and orgastic potency. Defining bioenergetics as "the study of the human personality in terms of the energetic processes of the body,"[89] he concerned himself with activating sources of energy in the patient, freeing up energies bound up in and by bodily restrictions, the expressive use of those energies, and the removal of chronic tensions. In implicit fashion, emotional discharge or release was repeatedly apparent as a theme in his work. For all the emphasis on the body, though, Lowen's approach included the process of self-discovery and the resolution of long-standing conflicts and traumatic memories.

Drawing on Gestalt psychology, making use of some of the techniques from the Reichian tradition, and influenced by psychoanalysis but emphasizing the here and now rather than historical data, Fritz Perls (1893–1970) developed gestalt therapy, with applications in both group psychotherapy and individual psychotherapy contexts.[90] Having the goals of "liberation from *psychopathological* unfinished business" and "catalyzing and nurturing undeveloped or unrealized *human potential*,"[91] this approach included considerable attention to emotions, to becoming aware of them and to expressing them freely. Once again, it included little explicit reference to catharsis but a prominent implicit theme of emotional release. But gestalt therapy both recognized the limitations of mere catharsis and retained the value of identifying and working though conflicts.

Primal therapy was a particularly notable example of a treatment in which cathartic or abreactive experiences were at the very heart of the therapeutic work. With minimal explicit reference to catharsis or abreaction, Arthur Janov developed his highly emotive mode of treatment termed the primal scream, or primal therapy.[92] In this clinical approach, patients were urged to relive core experiences from their early past. These "primal" experiences were those in which the person found reality too painful and so developed a neurotic adjustment that eventually led to the clinical condition and symptoms that had become his or her illness. Emboldened by dramatic cathartic moments in his patients' treatments and arguing that suppression, repression, and psychological defenses in general were against the patient's best interests, Janov promoted the reliving of early traumatic experiences in vivid fashion, including the re-experiencing and expressing of the deeply disturbing affects that were associated with those experiences. Frustrated basic needs and the associated feelings that had been warded off were said to be reawakened and released through cathartic outpourings, and, in episodes of particularly lively reliving, the traumatic memories recaptured. "The disease," Janov asserted, "is the denial of feeling, and the remedy is to feel."[93] For all his claim to total originality and his avoidance of the terms *catharsis* and *abreaction,* Janov's treatment approach was constructed on a cornerstone of cathartic experience that was somewhat reminiscent of the early Breuer-Freud cathartic therapy.

These various accounts point to a significant place for cathartic or abreactive methods among the array of practices in the realm of psychological healing, in spite of the psychoanalytic tradition of serious reservations in the wake of Freud's disenchantment with cathartic treatment; but controversies abounded where catharsis/abreaction was concerned. Further, those controversies were made the more complicated by the fact that the protagonists, while using similar terms, were frequently not talking about the same thing.

From its earlier meanings of purification and cleansing to the notion of purging and, eventually, to the idea of an emotional release, catharsis has implied getting something out, getting rid of something, becoming freed from something through some sort of evacuative mode, whether literally or metaphorically. Then, with the emergence of the cathartic therapy of the late nineteenth century, catharsis came to mean the lively remembering of a traumatic experience, *in addition to* the experiencing of its accompanying affect leading to an emotional release. Further, starting from Breuer and Freud's notion of subjecting the pathogenic idea or recovered memory to "associative correction," another addition was gradually made to this cathartic work: namely, along with the emotional release and the remembering, the recovered traumatic memories needed to become integrated with the rest of the patient's mental life — what was eventually conceived of by some as the undoing of dissociation. In these few sentences, we already have the potential for three different definitions of catharsis.

There have been controversies about mere emotional release: was it or was it not useful, in and of itself? should it or should it not be a goal in itself? Some have argued that the emotional release and the vivid remembering were both necessary, and were enough for a gainful therapeutic experience. Then this view was challenged by still others who considered the integration of the traumatic memories with the rest of the person's mental life to be necessary.

Many psychoanalysts, among others, have argued that catharsis brought only temporary relief and that symptoms soon returned. And yet, with the general value accorded to the free expression of emotions and attitudes in many twentieth-century psychotherapies, and with the common psychotherapeutic experience of useful abreactive moments, it has also been argued by many that catharsis is still a gainful aspect of treatment in a wide variety of psychological healing modes, including those influenced by psychoanalysis.

While some were minimizing the place of catharsis, the waves of psychological casualties in both World War I and World War II brought dramatic increases in the use of and respect for cathartic/abreactive treatment measures, with no small psychoanalytic influence at work in each instance. And, each time, the post-war period brought increased interest in and use of such methods with disorders that were not war-related.

The years between the two World Wars, and particularly the experiences with "war neuroses" in World War II, further enlivened many of the controversies. Some emphasized the emotional release and the remembering of repressed traumatic experiences, and others strongly urged that further work to reintegrate the previously dissociated memories was essential. But there were those who maintained that the emotional discharge alone was sufficient. Then, as catharsis increasingly became an aspect of various newer psychotherapies after World War II, the meaning of catharsis often became much more general in nature. It frequently came to mean no more than the relief of tension through the lively expression of emotion — a beneficial emotional release. And various neocathartic psychotherapies took the view that "the work of psychotherapy is to bring about a discharge of a blocked affect." In these approaches, psychotherapy came to be viewed as essentially "an affective purgation."[94] Parenthetically, it should be noted that these simpler meanings — mere emotional release or "ventilation" of feelings[95] — were similar to the sense of what catharsis was in many instances during earlier centuries.

Arguments about the proper place of catharsis in psychological healing have continued unabated in the years since World War II. In 1953, Percival M. Symonds (1893–1960), an American psychologist, reported on an extensive survey of reports on psychotherapeutic treatment in an attempt to determine what might be the crucial factors in useful clinical change; and he concluded that "an overwhelming number of the changes were due to abreactions." From this, he advanced the hypothesis that "all [favorable] changes in behavior and adjustment occurring as a result of psychotherapy follow abreaction in the therapeutic context."[96] Although he asserted that "abreaction is the central therapeutic agent," he also thought that this abreaction was dependent on, first, "an accepting and permissive relationship set up by the therapist" and, second, insight or a significant change in perception.[97] It is not clear, though, whether Symonds' view of abreaction was that it was essentially an emotional release or that it also included the remembering of the traumatic experiences or the reintegration of the recaptured memories.

In contrast to Symonds, others who argued from clinical data were far from sanguine about the place of catharsis in psychological healing. Frederick H. Lowy, a Canadian psychiatrist and psychoanalyst, for example, raised serious questions. Without dismissing the possibility of a useful role for catharsis within a larger psychotherapeutic context, he emphasized the relatively frequent, simplistic use of catharsis by, in particular, inexperienced or poorly trained psychotherapists and the various "abreactive-experiencing therapies" associated with the human potential movement. Noting the dangers of proceeding as though "the major objective of treatment" was "the direct expression of repressed affects" or "the discharge of strangulated affects," he argued that any abreactive activity needed to take place within a larger framework of "the understanding and resolution of conflicts, the strengthening of adaptive ego defences and the improvement of internal and external object relations."[98] Without significant attention to these latter themes, he maintained, any benefits from catharsis were likely to be merely temporary. It should be noted, however, that Lowy was arguing against an implicit definition of catharsis and abreaction that entailed only a simple emotional release, rather than the more complex meaning that included the reintegration of the disturbing, dissociated experiences.

If further evidence was needed to indicate the continuing significance of catharsis in psychological healing, the work of Michael P. Nichols and Melvin Zax would certainly provide it. In a thoughtful study of the subject, they differentiated two ways in which catharsis continues to have a role in modern psychotherapies. On the one hand, catharsis may be merely one element in a larger complex of psychotherapeutic activity; on the other hand, in some psychotherapeutic approaches catharsis is a central element.

While recognizing the dangers inherent in the thoughtless promotion of abreactive techniques, these authors maintained that catharsis can play a useful role in many psychotherapies. They recognized that the term *catharsis* is commonly used to mean "a process that relieves tension and anxiety by expressing emotions," but their view was that it "includes but goes beyond tension reduction." They effectively argued that "catharsis is not a simple, unitary phenomenon, but a complex process, involving two related, but separate, components: one, cognitive-emotional, the other somatic-emotional. The former consists of the contents of consciousness during the re-experiencing of an emotional event. The latter consists of the physical discharge of emotion, such as the tears and sobbing of grief, or the trembling and sweating of fear."[99] And they concluded that catharsis is most effective when it includes both components.

Thomas J. Scheff, who has also written at length about catharsis, argues that it is "a necessary condition for therapeutic change." And he maintains that "the theory of catharsis further argues that unresolved emotional distress gives rise to rigid or neurotic patterns of behavior and that catharsis dissipates these patterns."[100]

Although the many caveats regarding catharsis cannot be ignored — for example, the risks of mere emotional release *without* the context of an understanding listener or supportive social situation, or the concerns about

emotional release without attention to the psychological stability of the troubled person—cathartic or abreactive measures cannot be dismissed out of
hand. Such events tend to occur in psychological healing contexts, and they
can be useful or employed to useful ends. Simple "ventilation" may well have
limited merit or may even be counterproductive, whereas emotional release as
an element in a larger healing context may be eminently beneficial.

7

Confession and Confiding

The term *confession* is defined as "the disclosing of something the knowledge of which by others is considered humiliating or prejudicial to the person confessing: a making known or acknowledging of one's fault, wrong, crime, weakness, etc." Although this definition encompasses matters of special importance in the traditions of both law and religion, it is the religious association that is relevant to the history of psychological healing. In that tradition, it has been considered "a religious act: the acknowledging of sin or sinfulness." More specifically, it became "auricular confession": that is, "addressed to the ear; told privately in the ear."[1] As to the subjective aspects, whether the person is deemed a penitent or a sufferer, the following statement from an early twentieth-century historian of confession captures the matter well: "The uneasiness of thought concealed, the pain of having something 'on one's mind,' the relief when one is rid of it — these rank surely among our most familiar mental sensations."[2]

Closely akin to confession is *confiding*. Without the overtones of sin associated with confession, confiding — the imparting of personal and private matters to a trusted other person — can have a similar significance to the confider, bringing a sense of release, relief, unburdening, and perhaps a meaningful sense of reduced aloneness. With confiding, though, an accompanying easing of guilt is not at issue.

Twentieth-century authorities on cross-cultural healing practices have noted confession to be nearly omnipresent in such contexts. And during this century, it has been repeatedly noted that confession has been a significant element in many psychotherapeutic endeavors.

The Judaeo-Christian Tradition

Though evidence exists of confessional practices in the classical world of Greece and Rome, the early history of the confession of sins is associated more with early Assyro-Babylonian and Asiatic customs: "Confession of sins, in the Greek world as well as among the other Indo-european peoples, did not belong originally to the Indo-european element."[3] Thus the ideas associated with confession antedate by many centuries their more familiar connections with the Roman Catholic Church. These ideas entailed "the acknowledgment of sin or of wrongdoing on the part of one who felt himself thereby out of favour with the deity whom he worshipped, or in danger of that disadvantage. The sin or wrongdoing might affect a fellow-man, or might be an offence against religion, justice, or morality, for which the deity, jealous with regard to the due observance of right, exacted a penalty and inflicted punishment." One of the means of righting such a situation was "the making of confession — self-humiliation and abasement by the acknowledgment of the sin. Humiliation was evidently regarded as being acceptable to the deity, and acknowledgment of wrongdoing as paving the way to forgiveness." Ancient inscriptions indicate that the penitent made "his confession directly to the deity, without the intermediary of a priest or any other person."[4] In some cases, though, a priest apparently spoke for the penitent, and petitioned on his behalf for pardon, peace, or comfort.

It was with the Hebrew and the Christian religions, however, that a deep sense of the guiltiness of sin and a deep contrition for it became significant. For Jews, "it was ordered that on the Day of Atonement the high priest should make confession of sins in the name of the whole people, and the day is still kept by the Jews with fasting and confession of sins. The Jews were also enjoined to confess their sins individually to God, and in certain cases to man."[5] The Old Testament contains numerous indications that both individual and public confession were strongly urged and that the advice was followed. It is of special interest to note that the Hebrew words *Yom Kippur* that have been translated as *Day of Atonement* in English were translated in Spanish as *el Dia de Perdon,* meaning *day of forgiveness.* The word *kippur* was derived from the Babylonian, and in that language combined both meanings: atonement for sin by the penitent and forgiveness of the sin by God. It was in this heritage of combined atonement and forgiveness that Christian confession had its roots.[6]

The forerunners of the term *confession* as we know it today emerged in the language of the Christian Church. *Confession* and very similar terms in French and Italian were all derived from the Latin *confessio* (confession, acknowledgment) and *confiteor* (to confess, admit, acknowledge). There were two important uses of these terms: (1) confession of faith, which meant a profession of belief; (2) confession of sins. It is the second of these traditions of Christian usage that is of particular relevance for this study. Used in this sense, public confession before the brethren or congregation existed in an earlier tradition. This confession entailed repentance, atonement, the seeking of a forgiving reception, and a resolve to turn away from the sins, wrongdoings, or ungodly ways that were being confessed. Later, the more frequent practice would be private, or auricular confession, to a priest, which became one of the essential elements of the Sacrament of Penance in the Roman Catholic Church. Although often used as a term for the whole penitential procedure, confession more accurately was only one aspect of it, along with the assigning and carrying out of penance, and the receiving of absolution or forgiveness.

The Christian view of confession was derived from statements of Jesus that bestowed on his apostles the authority to forgive sins; and this bestowal became the basis for the priest's role in this regard. Sinners' misdeeds could alienate them from God and from their fellows, but their sincere repentance, confession, and atonement could lead to forgiveness and reconciliation with God and with their brethren.

A papal ordinance in the fifth century contributed to the diminishing role of public confession; the pope in question (Leo I) demanded a strict confidentiality on the part of the confessor, a view that eventually developed into "the seal of confession." The early medieval penitential handbooks, or guides for confessors, further influenced the regulation of confession and penance. There were variations in the catalogues of sins, and in what could and could not be forgiven through just what forms and durations of penance. And the severity of judgment and of penitential exercises waxed and waned from one era to another.

Confession continued to be a common but not notably regular practice. It was only with the Fourth Lateran Council of 1215 that the place of confession was reaffirmed with enough authority to establish it as a regular and obligatory practice, though enforced confession was to be recurrently a source of considerable conflict.[7] The Sacrament of Penance received noteworthy and influential attention in the decrees of that Council.[8] In Canon 21 it was declared that everyone who had reached the age of reason was required to confess his or her sins to the parish priest at least once a year and was to receive the Sacrament of the Eucharist at least at Easter.[9]

In the wake of the Reformation in the sixteenth century, the variations in the practice in the various other Christian denominations became considerable. Some continued to adhere to views much like those of the Roman Catholic Church; some retained the practice, while denying its sacramental character in consequence of the Protestant concept of justification by faith alone; some replaced private confession with a general confession followed by a general absolution; and some retained the private confession as an option. In times of religious revival, it has frequently been employed much as it was in the early Church, with the converted or repentant relating or confessing their experiences.[10] In the 1920s and 1930s, a new Christian religious group, the Buchmanites, or Oxford Group, revived the tradition of a public and detailed confession, regarded as the first step toward a sincere conversion; this custom was drawn upon in developing the practices of Alcoholics Anonymous.

Confession and Healing

The healing of disease and the priestly ministering to a sinful soul were often closely intertwined in Western cultural contexts. The Old Testament had repeatedly associated disease with punishment for sin, and so sickness and sinfulness were readily associated with one another. And in the traditions of Christianity, confession, in association with penance and absolution, was often an aspect of healing a sufferer from a disease, the procedures being handled by a priest. Also, even when no disease was at stake in the ordinary sense, Christian confession often entailed the use of a medical metaphor, sometimes explicitly and sometimes with an apparent lack of awareness that suggests how natural such an intertwinement was. In these latter regards, confession was thought of as "medicine for the soul," was an aspect of "the healing of souls" or "the cure of souls," and was the basis for referring to the priest-confessor as "a physician of souls."[11]

But prior to the emergence of the Christian confessor as "a physician of souls," in the classical world there had been the tradition of the philosopher as "a physician of souls," as a person thought to be specially equipped to minister to "diseases of the soul." That the philosopher might deal helpfully with spiritual (psychological) matters was discussed in analogy to the physician as the person who treated diseases of the body, and at other times a medical metaphor was employed to refer to such activities. Galen thought that the ideal physician should also be a philosopher.[12] Medicine and philosophy were intimately related in these ways for many in classical antiquity and would continue to be well into the medieval era. Out of these historical intertwinements, and with the model of Christ as healer, teacher, and philosopher, the early Church Fathers "formulated an image of the ideal spiritual leader based upon a likeness to an ideal physician." Christian teaching had "replaced philosophy as the medication of the sick soul. The actual attributes of the physician and pastor were held by the Fathers to be almost identical." And, further, for the Christian world the concept of disease came to comprise "essentially any deviation from standards of human health, belief, or behavior."[13]

The various traditions that contributed to the use of a medical metaphor in the discussions on confession in the medieval Church came together to make medical phrasings seem perfectly natural. The convention of the philosopher as "a physician of souls" was there to be drawn upon. The image of Christ as healer in a literal sense played a significant part. And the early Church Fathers had frequently reflected a knowledge of and an interest in medicine in their writings and had readily adopted a medical manner of speaking.[14] Probably a particular influence, though, was the sustained use of a medical metaphor by John Cassian (ca. 360–435), whose writings came to be "much used as an authority by the framers of the early penitentials." The penitential handbooks that were developed over the next several centuries frequently implied that confession was a form of healing and that sins were afflictions for which penitents should be treated and cured. This literature frequently involved "the conception of penance as medicine for the soul," in which the medical principle of contraries curing contraries was the commonest governing notion.[15] The processes of confession and penance were conceived of

> as constituting a treatment in itself effective toward the recovery of the health that has been lost through sin. . . . The authors of these handbooks . . . had a sympathetic knowledge of human nature and a desire to deliver men and women from the mental obsessions and social maladjustments caused by their misdeeds. . . . 'Not all are to be weighed in the same balance, although they be associated in one fault' but there must be discrimination according to cases. The physician of souls must . . . identify himself as far as possible with the patient. . . . [Despite a severity of prescription at times,] the penitentials often reveal the considerateness of the experienced adviser of souls, wise in the lore of human nature and desiring to 'minister to the mind diseased.'[16]

The custom of conceiving of the sin-confession-penance cycle in medical terms was to continue into the later medieval centuries with many interesting examples, including pastoral manuals, such as Robert Grosseteste's (c. 1170–1253) *Templum Dei* (also known as *Templum Domini*), and confessional manuals, such as the anonymous *Manuel des Pechiez* of the late thirteenth century and Robert Mannyng of Brunne's (c. 1280–1340?) *Handlyng Synne*, based on *Manuel des Pechiez*.[17] Comforting those in spiritual distress and ministering to the overburdened conscience had long been thought of as crucial aspects of the pastoral role, and these sorts of writings illustrate just how central confession and penance were deemed to be in such activities and just how natural it was to conceive of the clergy as engaged in the healing of troubled souls. And the deep meaningfulness of a medical metaphor in dealing with the soul's unease is further illustrated through its sustained use in Henry of Lancaster's (c. 1310–1361) devotional treatise, *Le Livre de Seyntz Medicines*.[18]

When we turn to early medical writings, though, we find no indication that their treatment recommendations included any form of confessional practice, whether for mental disorders or physical disorders. As E. R. Dodds put it, "*confession* of sin, auricular or public, is foreign to the Greek tradition." At the same time, it was "not peculiar to Christianity."[19] Raffaele Pettazzoni has identified numerous instances of confessional practice in the literature of antiquity, but only one of these, Ovid's account of King Midas' unquenchable thirst, might possibly be conceived of in terms of treatment of a disease; and that story had its roots in ancient Phrygia rather than the classical Greece and Rome of the extant medical literature from antiquity.[20]

Although neither the medicine nor the philosophy of the classical world had included a tradition of confession in its healing practices, developments in early medieval Christian thought set the stage for confession to become connected with traditional medical healing in the Western world. The Bible, and particularly Christ's healing miracles, provided a basis for seeking cures through the faith of the sick person and the supportive mediation of the religious functionary. Prayers by and on behalf of the sick person, the visiting of a saint's relics, the petitioning for a saint's intervention on behalf of the sufferer, and the proper management of healing rituals by a priest were all thought to play their part in the cure of disease. And, as sinfulness was often at issue, confession was frequently involved in seeking a cure. Often enough the sinfulness was thought to have brought about a disease as punishment; but sometimes "the diseased state" was merely a manner of speaking about the state of sinfulness itself, and sometimes a burdened state of inner distress or guilt was termed a disease in a metaphorical sense.

Drawing on a Judaic tradition for the practice of confession itself and on a Greco-Roman tradition of the philosopher as teacher-healer for its rationale, early medieval Christianity gradually developed its own healing tradition in which confession was of central significance. And, with disease as a divine punishment for sin on the one hand and the care of the sick as an occasion for good works on the other, the notion of the priest as someone who ministered to the sick was strengthened further.[21] Then, as the medieval centuries wore on, many a priest became trained as a physician, and the intermingling of confession for the sick soul with the physician's remedies for the sick body became quite common. To a significant extent, early medieval medicine came to be centered in monasteries and practiced by monks. And it was nothing very strange for a priest without formal medical training to view himself (or to be so viewed by others) as a healer in the broadest sense.

In Canon 21 of the decrees of the Fourth Lateran Council of 1215, it was enjoined that the priest be "discreet and cautious that he may pour wine and oil into the wounds of one injured after the manner of a skillful physician, carefully inquiring into the circumstances of the sinner and the sin, from the nature of which he may understand what kind of advice to give and what remedy to apply, making use of different experiments to heal the sick one."[22] And it required of the confessor that he hold in confidence what he had learned from the penitent. The use here of a medical metaphor was very much in the tradition already established in the penitential literature,[23] and it made quite clear the extent to which confession was conceived of as part of a healing process. On the other hand, Canon 22 soon made it equally clear that the religious practice and the priest were primary, no matter how much "a skillful physician" might serve as a model for aspects of the priest's function. This latter canon, after noting that "bodily infirmity is sometimes caused by sin," commanded the "when physicians of the body are called to the bedside of the sick, before all else they admonish them to call for the physician of souls, so that after spiritual health has been restored to them, the application of bodily medicine may be of greater benefit, for the cause being removed the effect will pass away."[24] Severe religious penalty was threatened if the physician were to "transgress this decree." The reaffirmation of this decree by later popes suggests ongoing efforts to maintain a degree of central control over members of the church and to use the physician and the moments of sickness as agents[25]; but it also indicates the continuing concern with the notion of disease as punishment for sin and with confession as an element in healing, however much it also testifies to doubts and differences of opinion about the decree itself.

In the medical literature of the later medieval centuries, there was no indication that this precept from Canon 22 was guiding the practice of physicians, or at least that anything akin to it was formally advocated in the medical world; and neither does this literature reflect any significant place for the idea of disease as a punishment for sin. Thus it seems probable that the decree was honored more in the breach than in the observance. On the other hand, John Mirfeld (d. 1407), an English cleric and medical compiler of the late fourteenth century, wrote in the spirit of that decree in the following extract from his "Physicians and Their Medicines," a chapter in his *Florarium Bartholomei*: "The physician, when called in to attend the sick, ought, before everything else, to warn them, and to persuade them at the outset to call in physicians of the soul, that is to say, Confessors; and then, when provision has been made for their spiritual health, he may lawfully proceed to apply his remedy to the body and make use of medicine. And if any physician shall disobey this ordinance, let him be forbidden to enter a church until he has made due amends for his fault."[26] Mirfeld was here drawing on canon law, and he went on to cite as authority Christ's first forgiving a sick man his sins before curing him of the palsy.

Confession continued to serve the cause of psychological healing in subsequent centuries through its place in the church-related activities of confession, penance, and absolution. With the advent of the Reformation, though, practices such as confession and exorcism were decried and largely abandoned by most Protestant denominations. But confession retained its significant role as a means of psychological healing for the Roman Catholic Church, and this has continued to be the case into modern times.

With the abandonment of auricular confession, Protestant congregations and their clergy met the desire (and need?) for some form of psychological healing through spiritual counseling, consolation, and prayer and fasting. Many Protestant clergymen saw themselves as "physicians of the soul" and actively campaigned among those who would listen to the end that they should repent and convert (as a form of "rebirth") in order to be saved from perdition.[27] Confession was only occasionally mentioned in such contexts, but some form of confession or something akin to confession must have been common in the process of repenting. Nevertheless, conventional medicine of post-Reformation times did not recognize any place for confession in its healing practices. Psychological healing in the late sixteenth and seventeenth centuries was left largely to the clergy, although some physicians probably made useful psychological interventions on the basis of humane, intuitive efforts, without formulating their activities as medical therapeutics.

The following are two examples, from the first half of the seventeenth century, of British clergymen who recognized confession as a useful factor in coping with mental disturbances. These instances lacked the relatively formal structure associated with confession in Roman Catholic contexts; and they were not at all similar to the medical practices of the day. The two men, Robert Burton (1577–1640) and John Sym (1581–1637), addressed severe problems of psychological distress and included confession among the means that might usefully be called upon in the treatment of those conditions. Burton, the great scholar of melancholy, advocated confession in an extensive discussion of religious melancholy. For the anguish, fears, and despair that could beset a person, he commented, "Faith, hope, repentance, are the sovereign cures and remedies, the sole comforts in this case; confess, humble thyself, repent, it is sufficient."[28] While Burton's language gives this passage a somewhat religious tone, these comments were not formally related to a religious context. Sym, a Scottish Calvinist minister who presided over a parish in Essex, was greatly concerned with the significant incidence of suicide. In his *Lifes Preservative Against Self-Killing,* he developed a psychological therapeutics whose purpose was to save the suicidally inclined person from that sinful inclination. Associating such states of mind with melancholy, often related to ill health, loss, or dishonor, Sym advocated a form of spiritual counseling and encouragement. He would urge a godly way of life, support ways of diminishing a sense of guilt and despair, urge the avoidance of various temptations and means that could incline one toward self-murder, and encourage a hopeful outlook.[29] Among his "antidotes for prevention of self-murder," Sym included confession.

> When all his other private endeavours prove ineffectuall, (or rather in the first place, when he feels his soule troubled) . . . *then* is hee to open his estate, and *confesse* the same to others, who can and may help him. . . . *For,* both the worke is easily one, and the burthen lightly borne, that hath the help of many hands: *and* also vent of the minde, by *confession,* doth often give ease to an oppressed heart. . . .
>
> *Touching* this *confession,* in this case *fower* things as *Caveats* are to bee carefully observed; that men under such temptations may have good by this course.
>
> *First, they are to bee circumspect and warie whom they choose to open their state, and confesse themselves to.*
>
> *That* they be not people undiscreet; *or* of *weake* judgments, and little experience in such cases of conscience. . . .
>
> *Neither* must such a man make choice of *blabs* of their tongues. . . .
>
> . . . such as, in this case, wee are to make our *spirituall Physitians,* should bee *advised, grave, sober-spirited persons,* and *reserved* from needlessly divulging mens *secrets* to others.[30]

By the eighteenth century, secularized explanations of mental disorders were well established in medicine, and orthodox medical treatment of such ailments "repudiated all manner of religious therapy for insanity until the early nineteenth century."[31] While various Protestant denominations continued with psychological healing practices that at times included confession in the spirit of Burton's or Sym's views, medical contexts, although they became more and more the locus for treatment of the mentally ill, did not develop much in the way of psychological healing until the emergence of moral treatment at the end of the eighteenth century with the work of Pinel at the Salpêtrière in Paris and of the Quaker Tukes at the York Retreat.

Relevant here is an interesting chapter in the history of confession as a healing activity, namely, the story of "the pathogenic secret" as outlined by Henri F. Ellenberger.[32] By this term he referred to a range of burdensome feelings such as thwarted love, jealousy, hatred, or ambition; ailments or infirmities of which the person is ashamed; a wide range of moral offenses; memories of traumatic events; and burdensome knowledge regarding other persons. While a strong sense of guilt may be crucially involved, that is not necessarily the case; keeping the secret may be associated more with shame or fear. But Ellenberger noted that "there is always an element of hopelessness in it."[33] Against a background of the long history of auricular confession, certain Protestant clergymen evolved their own version of "the cure of souls" that involved obtaining confession of the distressing secret and, often, also helping the sufferer resolve an associated dilemma. Gradually this knowledge of the pathogenic secret and this healing activity were taken up by laymen, that is, nonclergy. In the late eighteenth and early nineteenth centuries, instances of this pattern of activity began to be noted by various animal magnetists or mesmerists, and later by their descendants, the hypnotists. Later in the nineteenth century, this knowledge and the treatment practice were systematized by Moritz Benedikt (1835–1920), a Viennese physician whose work became known to Josef Breuer and Sigmund Freud. And Carl Jung, too, addressed the subject of pathogenic secrets. This tradition must have had some role in the emergence of psychoanalysis, but it is important to note that those pathogenic secrets were all quite consciously experienced by those who were burdened with them. In contrast, psychoanalysis was often dealing with unconscious pathogenic secrets that needed to be brought to awareness before they could be communicated to a healer or have their associated dilemmas resolved. As sin and guilt were so often aspects of the sufferer's distress, this tradition is certainly a part of the history of confession; but many instances of a pathogenic secret did not involve sin and guilt and were, instead, associated with shame and fear. In these latter instances, it was more a matter of confiding in a sympathetic listener and finding relief and comfort.

Anthropological Data on Confession

In addition to this evidence of the significance of the practice of confession over the centuries, there is much to indicate its significance across cultures. Confession has been shown to be a widespread and deeply meaningful practice in various African and American Indian cultures, quite apart from the influence on those cultures of the Christian churches; and anthropological and folkloric data have demonstrated its presence in still other groups.[34] In many of these cultures the belief persists that some transgression is the likely cause of a sufferer's disease or of some calamity within the social group, and confession of that transgression is considered crucial in the search for cure or relief. Common among the critical sins are murder, eating of forbidden food, and sexual activity with a forbidden person or of a forbidden sort.[35] And confession appears to relieve the psychological distress, whether through easing of a fear of danger, retribution, or punishment, or through easing of guilt.

In his studies of the confession of sins among "uncivilized peoples," Pettazzoni has suggested a less internalized sense of distress than is thought to be the case in the Christian framework or in modern depth psychology. He reasons that the advent of misfortune causes individuals or groups to look within themselves, to accuse themselves, and to confess in order to ease the misfortunes that they believe they have surely brought upon themselves. Confession "is not in its essence an expiation, satisfaction of reparation directed to Deity." Rather, Pettazzoni argues, confessions "aim at being and essentially are deliverances"—deliverance from the distress which overwhelms an individual with the advent of misfortune or which weighs down a community plagued by misfortunes. An "irresistible need of self-accusation" serves "to deflect an evil which threatens to attack" the individual or the community; and the confession brings "deliverance from an unbearable anxiety." That "it is on this experience of deliverance and consolation that the deep and intimate value of confession rests" is true irrespective of the degree of civilization that characterizes a culture. This "primitive fear of misfortunes which threaten and the pressing anxiety to avoid them" may be transformed into profound remorse and "an anxious need to make one's peace with God." As this distress "becomes more and more internal and subjective," with varying modifications from culture to culture, "the fundamental feature of the practice of confessing sins will still be that essential function of deliverance, which is the indwelling justification of its existence, because in it consists its universal human worth."[36]

Some of these cultures have had a tradition of public confession; in others it has been a private confession, at times with the assurance that secrecy will be maintained. In some settings, "sin in itself is . . . conceived of as an entity—a living creature which may be material or spiritual. In either case a confession of one's sins, in oral manner, seems to operate in such a way that the hidden or harbored devil is expelled from the body, soul, or mind, of the repentant person; and then, as a result, he improves in health or escapes death."[37] The confession is usually made to a social functionary recognized for his or her role in such a practice, perhaps a priest, perhaps a medicine man, in some instances by a woman to a midwife at the time of childbirth. In some societies the rituals associated with confession and the relief of psychological distress take the form of symbolic vomiting, sometimes of actual vomiting, and in some instances the very act of speaking (confessing) is conceived of as symbolic vomiting. The theme of getting something out, or expelling it, is often quite apparent. To term it an emotional catharsis frequently seems quite appropriate. Pettazzoni has made some comments that are especially relevant here.

> The declaration in confession of a sin is the evocation of that sin. Thanks to the mystical power of the spoken word, the sin is magically recalled when declared. In savage confessions, it is the magic of the spoken word which is in play. As pronouncing the name of a person is magically equivalent to evoking that person, so when declaring a sin one calls it back, so as to say, from the past occasion when it was committed, tears it away in a manner from the person who committed it, brings it out from within that person, in short *expresses* it in the proper sense of the Latin *exprimere,* to press out, to extract by pressure. . . . Once the sin is put into words, that is to say, evoked, the harmful influences which come from it are themselves brought back from the realm of the past into that of the present. They are in a way set within arm's reach, and now it is possible to submit them to some physical treatment suitable for getting rid of them, by means of water, smoke, fire or what not. Confession is continually linked to eliminatory practices because, as an evocation of sin and only as such, it really plays a part in the whole process of elimination.[38]

In many preliterate cultures, a sufferer's confession of wrongdoing has been the first step toward recovery from a disease, and facilitation of confession has been a crucial aspect of a healer's work to relieve or cure a sick person of a disease. Confession has been an important element in the medicine of the culture. It must be kept in mind, however, that in many of these settings the functions of healer and those of priest have been less differentiated than is the case in the Western world today. The committing of a sin was the way in which someone came to have a disease, and the confessing of that sin was a necessary undoing in the process of being healed from that disease. Further, the same social functionary heard the confession, served as the intermediary with a deity in seeking relief from the punishment represented by the disease, and presided over the process of healing from that disease. That is to say, sin and disease were inextricably intertwined, and priest and healer were one.

As to psychological healing in particular, from his extensive survey of North American native cultures, Weston La Barre concludes, "The virtually pan-American distribution of the trait of confession, in one cultural context or another, leaves little doubt that it is a genuinely aboriginal psychothera-peutic technique. Indeed, we are probably dealing here with a custom already old in Asia, for the Paleo-Siberian Kamchadal of Kamchatka had a very simi-lar conception of sin."[39] In a survey of cross-cultural healing practices, E. Fuller Torrey concludes, "Confession and suggestion are the two most impor-tant psychological therapies used in other cultures."[40] And he points out how very different cultures tend to use similar psychotherapeutic techniques — such as confession — in spite of holding very different beliefs about the causes of sicknessess.[41]

Confiding

Akin to the confessing of sins is the confiding of fears, worries, sorrows, and other distressing burdens. Confession is associated with the relieving of a guilty conscience and the seeking of forgiveness; in confiding, the person seeks relief from the burdens of grief, worry, fear, and the like, through talking about them to an interested listener, to someone who will be attentive, who will care, and who can be trusted. The very term *to confide* means to trust, to have faith in, or to repose confidence in someone.[42] Rather than forgiveness and the easing of conscience, what is sought is relief from being alone with an overwhelming sense of being burdened. Confiding may entail a search for understanding, or a yearning to have sadness and grief appreciated, or a wish to be consoled or comforted, or an effort to feel less alone. As Francis Bacon (1561–1626) stated it in his essay, *Of Friendship,* "Communicating of a man's selfe to his Frend . . . cutteth Griefes in halfes." And he observed that "the second Fruit of Frendship" is that "it maketh daylight in the Understanding, out of darknesse & confusion of thoughts. . . . Whosoever hath his minde fraught with many thoughts, his wits and understanding doe clarifie and breake up, in the communicating and discoursing with another."[43]

Not too many years after Bacon, Burton wrote about confiding, in *The Anatomy of Melancholy.* He advised that, if the sufferer was unable to control his own fears, griefs, and troublesome imaginings, then "the best way for ease is to impart our misery to some friend, not to smother it up in our own breast." He advocated confiding in and seeking the counsel of "some discreet, trusty, loving friend." The sufferer would find "ease in complaining" and his cares would be allayed by the "good words" and "fair speeches" of the friend's counsel. "The simple narration many times easeth our distressed mind, & in the midst of great extremities; so divers have been relieved, by exonerating themselves to a faithful friend: he sees that which we cannot see for passion and discontent, he pacifies our minds, he will ease our pain, assuage our anger." This friend would be someone to whom we could "freely and sincerely pour out our secrets; nothing so delighteth and easeth the mind, as when we have a prepared bosom, to which our secrets may descend, of whose conscience we are assured as our own, whose speech may ease our succourless estate, counsel relieve, mirth expel our mourning, and whose very sight may be acceptable unto us." For those "distressed in mind" and "much perplexed," he advised: "First pray to God, and lay himself open to him, and then to some special friend, whom we hold most dear, to tell all our grievances to him; nothing so forcible to strengthen, recreate, and heal, the wounded soul of a miserable man." He then added the sufferer's "Physician" to those in whom he might confide and from whom he might receive counsel, if he were not able "to resist or overcome these heart-eating passions" by himself.[44]

In identifying friendship as a context for confiding, and confiding as a means toward relief, comfort, and an improved perspective on one's troubles, Bacon and Burton were not introducing anything new to psychological healing. They were just saying it better. Friendliness in the healer-sufferer relationship, and the associated significance of trust, sympathy, and compassion, had long been recognized as providing a context that facilitated confiding in a healer, and such confiding had long been recognized as serving the therapeutic process well.[45] And these matters have continued to be the case since the time of Bacon and Burton.

In the nineteenth century, along with the increasingly explicit concern about sympathy in the doctor-patient relationship, reflections recurred of the view that physicians should contribute to that relationship in such a way that they would be trusted and that patients would confide in them. Yet it is only with the twentieth century that we find any significant amount of explicit attention paid to the value of confiding in psychological healing, although this attention has usually been embedded in a discussion of the value, in such healing, of confession. Confiding has occurred in a context of confessing; confessing has been used loosely to include what most people would call confiding; and confessions and confidings have been grouped together without significant differentiation. In addition, some discussions of the benefits of catharsis have implicitly been referring to the value of confiding; and, more generally, the constant emphasis in psychotherapy on expressiveness has often implied that confiding was beneficial.

The Twentieth-Century Psychotherapies

A scattering of comments have suggested that confession is an element in clinical psychoanalytic work or that psychoanalysis actively borrowed from the confessional tradition or that it was only natural that the Roman Catholic practice would have influenced this emerging form of psychological healing in Catholic Vienna. In fact, both Josef Breuer and Sigmund Freud mentioned the Roman Catholic tradition in their *Studies on Hysteria* in 1895, although they acknowledged some similarity rather than suggested an indebtedness. Breuer commented on excitation and conflicts associated with sexual feelings and ideas, and he mentioned that it was "a normal, appropriate reaction" to be inclined "to communicate them by speech." He then added, "We meet the same urge as one of the basic factors of a major historical institution — the Roman Catholic confessional. Telling things is a relief; it discharges tension even when the person to whom they are told is not a priest and even when no absolution follows. If the excitation is denied this outlet it is sometimes converted into a somatic phenomenon, just as is the excitation belonging to traumatic effects."[46] In the same work, Freud made more or less the same point. Speaking of the activity of the psychotherapist, he said, "One works to the best of one's power, as an elucidator (where ignorance has given rise to fear), as a teacher, as the representative of a freer or superior view of the world, as a father confessor who gives absolution, as it were, by a continuance of his sympathy and respect after the confession has been made."[47]

As the cathartic technique was abandoned and psychoanalysis took shape, Freud made less and less reference to catharsis and little allusion to confession. But in 1926 in *The Question of Lay Analysis,* he employed an imaginary dialogue in which his interlocutor commented that the principle of having the patient communicate freely to the analyst was "the principle of Confession, which the Catholic Church has used from time immemorial." To this, Freud replied, " 'Yes and no!' Confession no doubt plays a part in analysis — as an introduction to it, we might say. But it is very far from constituting the essence of analysis or from explaining its effects. In Confession the sinner tells what he knows; in analysis the neurotic has to tell more."[48]

Carl Jung, Freud's erstwhile colleague, also addressed the question of the relation of confession to psychoanalysis and to his own analytical psychology. Parenthetically, it should be noted that he was much more ready to associate psychological healing with religious ministering than Freud had been. In fact, he maintained that "religions are systems of healing for psychic illness."[49]

In 1936, Jung commented, "My method, like Freud's, is built upon the practice of confession."[50] By that time he had already made it clear that he conceived of confession as a basic element in his clinical work. Viewing the practice of analytical psychology as composed of "four stages, namely, confession, elucidation, education, and transformation," he went on to say, "The first beginnings of all analytical treatment of the soul are to be found in its prototype, the confessional. Since, however, the two have no direct causal connection, but rather grow from a common irrational psychic root, it is difficult for an outsider to see at once the relation between the groundwork of psychoanalysis and the religious institution of the confessional."[51] Referring to the early cathartic method out of which psychoanalysis developed, Jung stated: "The goal of the cathartic method is full confession — not merely the intellectual recognition of the facts with the head, but their confirmation by the heart and the actual release of suppressed emotion." He then commented that "our psychology" lays a "systematic emphasis . . . upon the significance of confession." Interestingly, he added that "the new psychology would have remained at the stage of confession had catharsis proved itself a panacea." He also pointed out that the "cathartic confession" frequently contributes to the establishment of a bond with the person to whom the confession is made.[52] It should be noted, though, that at times Jung used the term *confession* much more broadly than in the sense of its traditional association with sin. In some instances, its meaning in his usage was more akin to confiding, with its associations to relief and attachment.

Among the scores and scores of twentieth-century psychotherapy textbooks, it is uncommon to find any mention of confession, let alone any serious consideration of it. In the 1940s, though, Maurice Levine (1902–1971) discussed "confession and ventilation" at some length in a volume intended to guide the general physician in the use of psychotherapeutic methods.[53] He referred to "the method of confession and ventilation" as consisting "essentially of permitting the patient to talk freely, or of persuading the patient to talk freely, of his intimate or personal problems, to discuss some of the things about which he has been feeling ashamed or about which he has been feeling guilty."[54] Levine was clearly aware of the traditional connection between confession and sin and was advocating a means by which a patient might unburden himself and resolve a sense of guilty sinfulness. But his use of the term also included ministering to a patient's need to confide in a confidant. And he included the term *ventilation,* which was coming into common usage in that era to refer to speaking freely, to "getting something off one's chest" in order to achieve a sense of unburdening and relief — and, perhaps further, to clarify and resolve worrisome issues; to ease anxieties or relieve a sense of tension; to put fears to rest; or to feel less isolated and alone in the world. A further indication of the breadth of meaning in Levine's use of "the method of confession and ventilation" was his comment that some people called it "the method of catharsis or psychocatharsis."

Another well-known psychotherapy textbook that discussed confession and ventilation was Lewis R. Wolberg's *Technique of Psychotherapy.*[55] He began by saying, " 'Confession,' 'talking things out,' and 'getting things off one's chest,' in relation to a friend or a professional person, such as a physician, minister or teacher, are common methods of relieving emotional tension. Beneficial effects are due to the release of pent-up feelings and emotions and the subjection of inner painful elements to objective reappraisal." Like Levine, Wolberg saw such activities also as "emotional catharsis." And he concluded by stating that "confession and ventilation are ingredients of all psychotherapies and therefore need not be regarded as a special system."

In his textbook *Theory of Psychoanalytic Technique,* Karl Menninger (1893–1990) discusses the place of confession in psychoanalysis in a way that touches on the traditional sin/guilt motif but goes beyond that in ways akin to the above references to catharsis, confiding, and relief. He refers to psychoanalysis as an "extraordinary situation"

> in which one person is permitted to say whatever comes to mind to another person without suffering punitive consequences for having done so. The patient enters into the contract, as a rule, with misgivings, usually with considerable fear. But, at the same time, he welcomes the opportunity to talk about himself and to discharge a certain pressure of confession. In the early days of analysis the confession relief was spoken of figuratively as "catharsis" and the expression still persists in psychiatry. . . . [The] pressure of an accumulation of unspoken emotionally charged ideas could be released by encouragement in a properly protected opportunity.
>
> . . . The pressure of talk in a two-party situation sometimes seems to stem largely from a sense of guilt and a wish to confess, but at other times it represents a compelling need to establish contact with someone who will "understand." . . . This tendency to relieve "pressure" verbally is a familiar phenomenon, whatever its full explanation, and facilitates the *beginning* of an analysis.
>
> Sooner or later, however, the confessions and confidings of which the early flow of communications consists begin to include material which the patient had not been aware of any need to confess. . . . He finds himself telling tales out of school and admitting things which he had previously denied—perhaps even to himself.[56]

These three examples serve well to illustrate the place of confession in the psychotherapies during the past fifty years or so. Though it was commonly recognized in discussions as a factor in psychotherapy, these were three of the very few instances in which it was mentioned in textbooks. When it was mentioned, the tradition of guilt and sin was usually alluded to, but not always. That is to say, the connection to the tradition of religious confession was not forgotten, but it was rarely given much attention in psychotherapeutic writings. It is very likely that the increasingly strong concern that psychotherapists should be nonjudgmental was significant in this limited reference to confession. The trend was toward emphasizing the aspects of emotional catharsis in confession and in confiding in a trusted person who would not be judgmental. For all the decreased mention of confession, though, Wolberg was not alone in suggesting that confession was omnipresent in psychological healing; and his comment was remarkably similar to the views of many authorities on cross-cultural healing.

This survey of the place of confession over the centuries, and across cultures in more recent times, makes it clear just how common a practice it has been. Sin or wrongdoing has created inner burdens and interpersonal strains for the sinner in a wide variety of social contexts. Whether it has led to the burdensome harboring of a guilty or shameful secret, the resentment of the sinner's fellows for their knowledge of the "offenses" committed, or some uncertain state between these extremes, the sinner's sense of alienation and inner distress has been a mode of suffering, variously viewed as a symptom, a disease, or a disorder of some other sort. Conceived of in whatever way, the act of confessing has brought a significant measure of relief. It may be no more than an unfettered revelation to a trusted friend of the troubled person's guilts and fears. If received by the listener in relatively nonjudgmental fashion, this may provide relief enough, and it may have the further benefit of easing the sufferer's sense of alienation, of rescuing him from his aloneness. As we have seen, though, many cultures have had social functionaries and associated rituals that have provided a well-established context for the confession of sins. Whether the social functionary has been thought of as a human intermediary for a deity or an ancestor or conceived of in modern contexts as a parental surrogate, the authority and wisdom attributed to the listener has commonly enhanced belief in the potential for relief. Further, as frequently forgiveness has been sought and an end to alienation has been hoped for, this attributed authority has usually been perceived as an assurance that these goals were possible. And if forgiveness has been forthcoming, the wisdom attributed to the healer has brought a deeper meaning and a more far-reaching effect from that forgiveness. The assigning of penance, in whatever form, has often seemed like the price of forgiveness or the squaring of a debt for sinners—and has returned to them some sense of control over their own fate. The perceived authority and wisdom of the social functionary has allowed this assigning of penance and has added to its meaning. The inner relief has frequently been accompanied by a sense of reconciliation, whether with the deity, the ancestor, or the sinner's fellows.

Much has been wondered about the readiness of people to confess, whether guilty of the alleged sins or not, particularly in modern times with the advent of so-called brainwashing and the induced confessions of political and military prisoners. As indicated earlier, the traditional explanations of the psychology of confession have usually involved some combination of a relief from the burden of feelings of guilt and an undoing of a sense of alienation from a deity or from the sinner's fellow humans. But the guilty feelings have further entailed a fear of retaliation or the loss of love, and confession has served to ward off such dire fates; the sense of alienation has reflected the sense of having lost love or connectedness. Relating these ideas to parental roots in childhood times is probably not merely speculative, and these roots are also suggested by the long tradition of the priest as "father-confessor." These powerful undercurrents would seem to account for the far-reaching effects of unconfessed wrongdoings and guilty secrets, for their role in severe inner distress and outright illness.

Against this background, medical practitioners — physicians ancient and modern, psychological healers in a variety of forms — have wittingly or unwittingly used these forces in seeking cure or relief for sufferers who come to them for help. Whether the healer's mode of operation has been kindly and benevolent or forceful and authoritarian, the undercurrents in the sufferers have probably been quite similar. Interestingly, many of the historically established rituals for confession, although not medical in nature, have employed a medical metaphor in describing their confessional practices, such as the reference to the priest-confessor as "a physician of souls."

In the realm of social psychology, James W. Pennebaker has argued that catharsis was an inherent aspect of health-promoting confessions. And this investigator has also emphasized that, in such contexts, the confronting of trauma was often crucially associated with the cathartic element in achieving a gainful experience through confession, and that the insight gained was a significant factor.[57]

Finally, the context of a confession has frequently provided the opportunity for confiding — the telling of burdensome matters not associated with sin and guilt but, rather, with anxiety, worry, fear, or grief. This element has sometimes been mentioned in discussions of confession, but has often gone unmentioned. In more recent times, in reference to confession in this or that psychotherapeutic approach, it is clear that the term *confession* has come to be used rather loosely, in a way that includes both confessings and confidings. Occasionally, confession and confiding have each been explicitly identified as elements in a psychotherapeutic process. And in some instances, too, confiding alone has been mentioned. To quote Carl Jung, "One can easily see what it means to the patient when he can confide his experience to an understanding and sympathetic doctor. . . . No longer does he stand alone in his battle with these elemental powers, but some one whom he trusts reaches out a hand, lending him moral strength to combat the tyranny of uncontrolled emotion. In this way the integrative powers of his conscious mind are reinforced.[58]

PART FOUR

Bringing Comfort

8

Consolation and Comfort

Consolation — "the act of consoling, cheering, or comforting . . . allevia-tion of sorrow or mental distress"[1] — would seem to be one of the oldest among the modes of psychological healing. With its verb, *to console,* defined as "to comfort in mental distress or depression; to alleviate the sorrow of (any one); 'to free from the sense of misery,' " we are discussing a rich tradition of ministering to troubled persons. Distress in response to misfortune has been part of the human story since time immemorial. And one's fellows' inclination to respond to that distress with some effort to comfort or console seems to be a natural one, almost as old as the distress itself. Not that such a response has always been forthcoming when someone has been in distress, and perhaps it is too sanguine a view of human nature to think it so natural, but common it has surely been.

Another useful perspective on what consolation is can be obtained from the following early twentieth-century source. Although the context happens to have been one in which Christian consolation was being defined and its history briefly traced, the description fairly represents the phenomenology of a useful consolatory experience.

> In its fullest, and especially in its religious, sense, there is the consciousness of a person whose presence, words, or acts are the source of the feeling of

comfort, and constitute the consoling element. . . . The personal (or quasi-personal) source is always implied. The immediate effect upon the will is that of solace or soothing, restraint from agonizing or neurotic effort, and the inhibition of excited acts. The subconscious effect is that of a tonic, and the will is braced thereby for healthful exercise. Whilst the consciousness of a personal presence and influence is the dominant feature in religious consolation, there is always, in the background at least, the presentation of something that produces pain, distress, or anxiety. Probably in most cases the cause of the painful feeling is at first the focus of attention but the process of consolation forces it into the background as the comfort is being experienced. The consciousness of personal help and support is the positive element in the case, whilst the negative is the sense of relief and mitigation.[2]

Today we may tend to associate an act of consolation with a direct and personal communication from a would-be consoler to a bereaved or otherwise distressed person, sometimes in written form but often in spoken form. And, while we readily think of family members or good friends as carrying out such actions, we also think of consolation as an aspect of the activities of pastors, physicians, psychotherapists, and other professionals whose role includes comforting, soothing, or easing the burdensome lot of suffering persons. Historically, relatively little evidence has survived of the spontaneous acts of consolation offered in direct and personal terms, verbally, by persons close to sufferers. We have, though, rather more evidence of the activities of professional consolers who were called upon to comfort distressed persons, particularly the bereaved, in such direct ways. And we have still more in the way of consolatory literature (letters, treatises, and so on) written either as very personal acts of consolation or as formal consolations to comfort persons not well known to the authors, not to mention manuals and handbooks for the guidance of the professional consoler. Further, many of these written sources were used later to serve audiences beyond those for whom they were originally written. Often enough, written consolations became the basis for spoken consolations, and spoken consolations became recorded as written consolations.

Consolation in Classical Antiquity

Evolving out of the natural human needs mentioned above, and the natural responses to them, writings of a consoling nature appeared in a variety of places in the literature of ancient Greece.

The dead were commemorated in threnodies, which were designed also to console the bereaved, and a great vogue was enjoyed by a *threnos* of Pindar, in which the ideas of the Orphic eschatology were drawn upon for consolation, and which is made use of in the pseudo-Platonic dialogue *Axiochos*. In Athens it was customary, probably after the Persian wars, to engage a rhetor to deliver a funeral oration — like that, e.g., which Thucydides puts into the mouth of Pericles — regarding those who had fallen in battle; and it was usual at the close to address the relatives in consoling terms. . . . Philosophy likewise had at an early stage wrought out certain consolatory lines of thought.[3]

Out of these traditions emerged the formal consolatory piece, the *consolatio*. Themes of comfort and consolation were developed into a set repertoire of arguments that were offered to the troubled in the form of simple letters or philosophical treatises. These *consolationes* were addressed to those suffering as a result of various misfortunes, mainly the loss of loved ones through death, sometimes exile, and occasionally other misfortunes.

> Of the stock arguments (*solacia*), one group is applicable to the afflicted person, the other to the cause of the affliction. Among the former the commonest thoughts are: Fortune is all-powerful — one should foresee her strokes (praemeditatio); has a loved one died? — remember that all men are mortal; the essential thing is to have lived not long but virtuously; time heals all ills; yet a wise man would seek healing not from time but from reason, by himself putting an end to his grief; the lost one was only "lent" — be grateful for having possessed him. As to death, the cause of the affliction, it is the end of all ills: the one who is lamented does not suffer; the gods have sheltered him from the trials of this world. To these *loci communes* consolers sometimes add eulogy of the dead, and almost always of men courageous in bearing misfortune.[4]

The role of the consoler came to be a recognized one, and such a person was often turned to at times of death or disaster, at times of grief and distress. The philosopher as consoler was a crucial constituent of the philosopher as physician of the soul. Antiphon the Sophist (fifth century B.C.) was known for having "founded an art to cure griefs, analogous to that one which among physicians serves as a basis for the treatment of diseases; . . . informing himself of the causes he unburdened and consoled the patients."[5]

The need for consolation in times of bereavement not only brought forth this tradition of comforting remarks from the philosophers; the rhetoricians too became active contributors, although often sacrificing spontaneity in their development of detailed rules for consolation. In general, a tendency developed toward presenting the consolatory messages in a somewhat intellectualized manner, featuring reason as the supreme consoler. And another form of rigidity entered the scene with the contributions of the early Stoics. Taking a sternly disapproving view of the passions as they did, they held that grief and sorrow were particularly reprehensible affects and should be eliminated. Sorrow was not natural and profited neither the mourner nor the dead, and the sorrowing of the bereaved should be firmly checked by reason.

The philosophers of antiquity who undertook to console had a range of themes available to them that presented no conflict with any of the various doctrinal positions. Whatever their philosophical position — Epicurean, Platonist, Stoic, or Neo-Pythagorean — these consolers had ready access to time-tested, all-purpose arguments, for example, that death was no evil, that death came to all and so was no injustice to the particular person, that death was a deliverance from the hardships of life on earth, that life was a loan that eventually had to be repaid.[6] *But* issues related to the propriety or impropriety of grief and mourning brought differences of opinion and practice. The following series of questions gives some perspective on these matters. "What is the nature of grief? Is it an involuntary or voluntary emotion? Natural or unnatural? Is mourning an expression of concern for the deceased or for the mourner himself? Is compassion a sign of an individual's strength or weakness? His wisdom or foolishness? Is it the duty of one who has learned his philosophy well to control or extinguish his sentiments? Can one speak of 'appropriate' grief? Can a person who has dedicated himself to pursuit of the good, and that alone, be affected by those events over which the general run of mankind laments?"[7]

The reaction against the sterner, more rigorous position in these arguments is particularly associated with Crantor of Soli (ca. 335 to ca. 275 B.C.), a philosopher of the Old Academy whose lost work *On Grief* had been written for a friend whose children had died. This work came to serve as a standard, influencing many contributors to the consolatory literature, such as Marcus Tullius Cicero (106–43 B.C.), who drew on it for his own *Consolatio,* composed to comfort himself on the death of his daughter Tullia, and who gave considerable indication of its nature in his *Tusculan Disputations.* The extensive influence of this composition seems to have been related to its treatment of "sorrow not as a reprehensible emotion — in the manner of the Stoics — but rather as a natural impulse, requiring only to be kept in bounds."[8] Both Cicero and Plutarch cited Crantor in a favorable manner for his objection to the Stoic ideal of emotional indifference or insensibility. Cicero quoted him as follows: "I do not in the least agree with those who are so loud in their praise of that sort of insensibility which neither can nor ought to exist. Let me escape illness: should I be ill, let me have the capacity for feeling I previously possessed. . . . For this state of apathy is not attained except at the cost of brutishness in the soul and callousness in the body."[9] And Plutarch said the following in the context of agreeing with these views of Crantor: "The pain and pang felt at the death of a son has in itself good cause to awaken grief, which is only natural, and over it we have no control. For I, for my part, cannot concur with those who extol that harsh and callous indifference, which is both impossible and unprofitable. For this will rob us of the kindly feeling which comes from mutual affection and which above all else we must conserve."[10]

Commonly cited in tracing the consolatory tradition that evolved from the work of Crantor and others are Cicero's lost *Consolatio* mentioned earlier and portions of his *Tusculan Disputations,* in each of which he drew from Crantor's work with appreciation;[11] several of Lucius Annaeus Seneca's (ca. 4 B.C. to A.D. 65) *Epistulae Morales* and two of his *Consolationes,* those known as *Ad Marciam* and *Ad Polybium;*[12] and, again with an appreciative acknowledgment to Crantor, two of the essays in Plutarch's (ca. A.D.46–120) *Moralia, Consolatio ad Apollonium* and *Consolatio ad Uxorem,* the latter written to his wife on learning of the death of their two-year-old daughter, Timoxena.[13] In keeping with Crantor's views, the trend in these writings was toward viewing grief and sorrow as quite natural but needing to be kept in bounds. Although less harsh than was characteristic of the Stoics, Cicero followed in the tradition that conceived of the passions as disorders of the soul and of persons distressed by them as being distinctly unwise. He subscribed to the view that philosophy was the medicine for such souls, and that wise men or philosophers should serve as physicians of the soul by employing the wisdom of philosophy to heal them. The philosopher was to enlist the bereaved person's reason through consolatory counsel in an effort to do away with, or at least subdue, the grief and sorrow, as was advised for other affects. Adopting a modified Stoic orientation, Seneca urged a modest sorrow, rather than an absence thereof, in one of his *Epistulae* on bereavement and grief; but he turned to vigorous admonitions against grief in another. His *Ad Marciam* displays a degree of Stoic harshness, and yet a tender and comforting tone as well. Although manifesting a kindlier tone than was typically Stoic, Seneca did use the standard consolatory rationalizations in his *Consolationes:* "All men must die; there is no need to grieve on our own account or that of the dead; time will ease the sorrow, but let reason do it first."[14] In the *Consolatio ad Apollonium,* while striving for "the mitigation of grief" and an end to the mourning process, Ps.-Plutarch appreciated the naturalness of grief in the face of loss. He thought that there was a time for sorrowing and a time to console in an effort to bring the grief to an end; and he allowed that consolation might be offered prematurely. He was opposed to any Stoic extremes, but he took the view that "sensible is he who keeps within appropriate bounds" and offers the admonition that "reason therefore requires that men of understanding would be neither indifferent in such calamities nor extravagantly affected."[15] In this spirit, Ps.-Plutarch then gave attention to the various traditional consolatory themes and provided an extensive anthology of extracts from the literature of consolation. In Plutarch's *Consolatio ad Uxorem,* the themes were much the same, but the tone and manner were much more personal, reflecting both his relationship to the person being comforted and the fact that he shared in the loss.[16]

The trend toward a greater acceptance of the sufferer's sorrow and distress brought a more humane and empathic tone to the literature of consolation and to the work of the consoler. Interwoven with this trend, instances in which the consoler was personally acquainted with the bereaved seem to have occasioned greater flexibility and spontaneity; these consolations were more personal and more affectively tinged. A certain tension developed between a carefully prescribed form for the *consolatio* and the tendency for a consoler to evince individualized, empathic acceptance of the sufferer's distress. Further, the range of problems which a consolation might address broadened somewhat. While bereavement continued to be the primary concern for which *consolationes* were designed, they were also employed in efforts to ease a variety of illnesses and ailments, to mitigate or cure dejection and despair, and to cope with the fear of death.

Christian Consolation

The tendencies toward a greater acceptance of the sufferer's distress and toward a more individualized response were developed further by early Christian consolers who, "while resorting to pagan arguments, were enabled to renew the genre by the stress laid upon feeling and by the character of their inspiration, which was at once biblical, ethical, and mystic."[17] Although retaining much of both the form and the substance of its classical origins, the Christian *consolatio* evolved toward adding religious counsel, in the service of comfort, encouragement, and support that would help see the bereaved person through a difficult time. Comforters emphasized the treasured memories of the dead person, assured the bereaved person that the two would be together again in the hereafter, reawakened the sufferer's awareness of belonging to the hopeful living, and offered the promise of a life after death. That a period of grief was normal, and probably necessary, before consolation was appropriate or potentially helpful, though not a new idea, came increasingly to be an accepted view. Already apparent in the classical consolatory literature, the tendency to offer comforting appreciations of the person's grief continued. The emphasis shifted from admonishing the sufferer to cease being distressed toward providing relief from distress. Although bringing comfort to the bereaved was, and remained, central to consolation in the Christian tradition, it should be noted that both devotional and homiletical literature indicate several other circumstances in which the administration of consolation was thought to be called for: physical or mental limitations, pain, or distress; anxiety, perplexity, and care; depression and spiritual desolation; difficulty in Christian work, opposition and persecution; death and the fear of death.[18]

In the early Christian consolatory literature that has survived, we find a number of notable contributors from the fourth century. The Cappadocian Fathers — Basil of Caesarea (329–379), his brother Gregory of Nyssa (ca. 330 to ca. 395), and his good friend Gregory of Nazianzus (ca. 329–389) — left extensive consolatory materials, among which many letters and a sermon by Basil are of particular note.[19] Basil employed most of the classical themes, recasting them in Christian form. Biblical quotations and allusions replaced classical quotations, and Biblical personages replaced classical figures. Appreciation of the naturalness of grief came to be illustrated by Jesus' tears at the tomb of Lazarus. The bereaved were soothed and comforted in Christian terms; encouragement was offered; and the afflicted were exhorted to bear up and not grieve inordinately. Also, it became common to give practical counsel to the bereaved about worthy duties that could distract them from their grief, for example, advising a widow to devote herself to the raising of her children as a significant diversion from her sorrow. Basil hesitated to write to the bereaved when the grief was fresh, and he regretted that he was not there to convey his sympathy in person. Although he was trained as a rhetorician and employed familiar rhetorical devices, his consolations demonstrate significant tenderness and variety.[20]

Another early Church Father who had been originally trained as a rhetorician and who made important contributions to the literature of consolation was John Chrysostom (ca. 347–407). Chrysostom had experienced significant personal grief, and the theme of consolation came to permeate his writings, whether treatises, homilies, or letters especially directed to comforting the grief-stricken. "As long as the sore of despondency remains," he advocated applying to it "the medication of consolation."[21] Of special interest, and notably unusual, is the fact that he asked his correspondents to let him know how helpful his consolatory efforts had been.[22] He explains in his "Letter to a Young Widow"[23] that he had "abstained from troubling [her] when [her] sorrow was at its height" and allowed her "to take [her] fill of mourning. . . . For whilst the tempest is still severe, and a full gale of sorrow is blowing, he who exhorts another to desist from grief would only provoke him to increased lamentations and having incurred his hatred would add fuel to the flame by such speeches besides being regarded himself as an unkind and foolish person."[24] He argued that her late husband had gone to another and better life with God, that she was still united with him through her love for him, that she would one day be reunited with him forever, that meanwhile she might find comfort in memories and visions of him, and that she was fortunate to have been with him when he died.

Jerome (ca. 348–420) was another of the early Christian Fathers whose consolatory writings are of some note. He manifested a sincere sympathy, standing "apart from Christian writers of consolation by a show of grief which sometimes apparently cannot be surmounted. His tenderness is expressed in every page of his letters, for he feels deeply with those whom he loves, and he admits that sentiment has a part even in the grief of Christians."[25] In general, by this time Christian writers had "developed the consolatory genre at the expense of the traditional form; in ideas of consolation they stressed new elements, especially the idea of the resurrection." Further, they emphasized "the sweetness of life" and "the life well lived" rather than life's miseries.[26] The idea of the resurrection and of a life beyond death served to mitigate the sorrow of loss and brought hope.

Another Christian leader of this same era who gave considerable attention to consolation was Augustine (354–430). Trained as a rhetor, he was familiar with the Latin philosophers noted for their consolatory writings, particularly Cicero, and with his Latin Christian predecessors.[27] Sharing "the universal need of all men for consolation at the death of their loved ones," Augustine left a rich array of data on loss and grief and on the importance of consolation to the bereaved. Apparently already drawn to sadness in literature and the theater as a youth, in his *Confessions* he told of his own experiences with personal loss prior to his conversion and vividly portrayed his own grief-stricken distress. He was consoled by a family friend on the death of his father, and the passage of time and the consolation of friends gradually eased his grief over the loss of a very close friend. He contrasted these experiences with those after his conversion, including the death of his mother, when he had come to rely on "God as a Consoler." He noted that "it was as a result of his own experience and also of the aid given him by his faith that he was able later to define the qualities of the true consoler, to outline the duties of consolation to others, and to be a consoler himself." In him one finds "the synthesis of the consoled and the consoler."[28] Augustine

> had pondered the words of Scripture which urge the Christian to "weep with those who weep." In his compassion the consoler must feel the sorrow of another, yet he must also be free from all painful emotion when he assists those in need of consolation. "His acts should be characterized by tranquillity

of mind, for he acts not from the stimulus of painful feeling, but from motives of benevolence." Thus Augustine does not set aside the words of Scripture, but qualifies the compassion of the consoler, who by first grieving with the one in distress can then refresh him with consolatory words.[29]

Further, defining the consoling of others as crucial among the tasks of a priest, he imposed this task on his fellow bishops and priests. In addition to the by then familiar themes in consoling the bereaved, Augustine particularly emphasized God as a consoler, Christ as having suffered in order to console by example, and the Holy Spirit as sent to be a comforter. Also, he found a medical metaphor particularly apt, likening God to a doctor, "healing the pain of grief by the promise of another life and by His words recorded in Scripture."[30]

A particularly influential contribution to the literature of consolation was left by Boethius (ca. 480–524), a Roman government leader who, rather than writing to help others or himself to cope with bereavement, wrote *The Consolation of Philosophy* in his prison cell to console himself in the face of disgrace, loss of his worldly goods, exile, and, ultimately, execution.[31] Although there is no certain evidence of it in his *Consolation,* Boethius is now thought to have probably been a Christian. Whatever the case may have been, this work certainly came to be most influential in the Christian tradition, for both consolers and the bereaved, and for others in distress. One of the most translated of works, for many centuries Boethius' *Consolation* provided solace to others, was referred to with respect and appreciation, and served as a model. Interweaving prose and poetry in a dialogue with Philosophy, whom he visualized as a majestic woman in whom he "recognized the face of my physician,"[32] Boethius recounted the details of his distressing situation and vividly portrayed his despair. In a dialogue with the troubled Boethius, Philosophy embarked on some standard rhetorical strategies of consolation, mixing religious overtones into her philosophical argument. She approached the curing of her patient's sickness gradually, leading eventually from gentle persuasion to a more rigorous medicine in the form of philosophical dialectic. "The condition of Fortune's victim is described as a sickness, a disease of the mind leading to anxiety, lethargy, and despair. Philosophy is the physician whose medicines of rational, and therefore human, judgment can restore his soul to health."[33] Through this frank and searching self-exploration Boethius renewed hope for himself and found peace of mind.

Consolation was clearly an element in Christian pastoral care in the period following the early Church Fathers, Augustine, and Boethius; but the "cure of souls" of medieval Christianity tended to emphasize more the confession of sins, penance, and forgiveness, along with the celebration of the Mass and the provision of extreme unction at death. These elements of Christian practice served to provide spiritual guidance and comfort in an evolving system of sacraments. While priests and pastors consoled the bereaved, consolation and comfort were more often brought to the spiritually distressed through the various forms of sacramental healing.[34]

As to physicians, in the Christian era they, too, incorporated consolation and comfort as aspects of caring for their patients. Drawing on the compassion and sympathy that were urged as a crucial factor in an optimal healer-sufferer relationship, they comforted those who were grief-stricken, those who were in pain, those who were burdened by chronic illness, and those who were faced with death. Such efforts to console or comfort those who suffered in these ways were commonly undertaken by the priest or pastor, yet they also tended to become part of the physicianly role. The consolatory activities of the priest were frequently discussed in terms of a medical metaphor, and the priest conceived of himself as engaged in healing activities. And the humane outlines of how a physician should behave included being compassionate and sympathetic, the very root of bringing comfort to a sufferer. Still, though, bringing consolation and comfort to a sufferer continued to be associated more with the role of the priest.

The genre of consolatory writings gradually evolved; eleventh- and twelfth-century monastic literature including letters, treatises, and sermons in response to loss through death. Then, in the twelfth and thirteenth centuries came the "cultivation of the consolatory and remedial realm and the development of moral thought which begins to re-emerge largely under the influence of the revival of rhetoric and classical culture." In tracing these developments, George W. McClure identifies and discusses a series of notable examples of consolatory works which reflect the continuing influence of Cicero, Seneca, and, in several instances, both the form and the substance of Boethius' *Consolation*.[35] Among the humanistic scholars of the late twelfth century was Peter of Blois, cleric and author of a considerable number of consolatory letters, who associated friendship with the duty to be compassionate and to console, and who framed the notion of consolation "in terms of healing, remedial cures."[36] In the second quarter of the thirteenth century, the status of consolation as a remedial practice was nicely illustrated by Albertano da Brescia. Himself a jurist, Albertano wrote his treatise "for his son who was practicing 'in arte cyrurgiae,'" in order to complement the son's medical knowledge. He opened this work by saying: "There are many who are afflicted and depressed in such adversities and tribulation that, because they do not have consolation and counsel in themselves (because of mental perturbation) nor expect it from others, they grow sad so that they go from bad to worse.'"[37]

Consolation and Renaissance Humanism

Even if one discounts the hyperbole that has allowed him to be termed the first modern man and the first humanist, Petrarch—Francesco Petrarca (1304–1374)—was a crucially important figure in the emergence of Renaissance humanism. In addition to his famed poetry and other literary efforts, he made a significant contribution to the realm of consolatory and therapeutic wisdom. In fact, his "interest in tranquillity and consolation is a fundamental part of his vision of a humanistic revival of ancient moral thought."[38] Particularly relevant are Petrarch's self-care and self-analysis in the *Secretum* and his care of others in his letters and in his *De remediis utriusque fortunae*. Most important in his consolatory works was "his development of the therapeutic potential of philosophy and rhetoric." Drawing particularly on Cicero and Seneca, Petrarch "carefully formulates the theory of a healing eloquence, a therapeutic rhetoric which heals the ills of the mind and counters the assaults of *Fortuna*. The development of this craft is one of the central aspects of Petrarch's vision of himself as a *medicus animorum* [doctor of souls]."[39]

In his *Secret, or the Soul's Conflict with Passion*, Petrarch presented an extended account of his personal difficulties and concerns, for he viewed himself as "the victim of a terrible plague of the soul—melancholy; which the moderns call *accidie*, but which in old days used to be called *aegritudo*."[40] This work was organized in the form of a dialogue between Augustinus (St. Augustine) and Franciscus (Petrarch), with Augustinus drawing from Franciscus the distressing details of his condition, and advising, admonishing, exhorting, and consoling him. The dialogue simulated a three-day sequence in which a spiritual adviser guides a sufferer toward tranquillity of soul or peace of mind. In this process Augustinus serves as a spiritual physician, but the character also draws increasingly on the tradition of philosophical consoler, as developed by Plato, Cicero, and Seneca, to bring comfort to Franciscus in the form of secular consolation. Petrarch developed a self-consolation in the guise of a dialogue, which displays a significant kinship to Boethius' *Consolation*.

In his letters, Petrarch in a number of instances consoled people "on bereavement, exile, sickness, absence of friends, fear of death, aging, misfortune." In these contexts, he fashioned "a hybrid humanist-Christian type of consolation, drawing on traditional classical arguments as well as on Christian belief."[41]

Finally, from his concern with his own *accidie-aegritudo* in his *Secret*, Petrarch shifted to concern with the *miseria-tristitia* of others in his *De remediis*, where he definitively emerged as a consoler and *medicus* for those others. In this manual of psychological remedies, he argued against the "windy and sterile disputations" which he associated with scholastic philosophy and in favor of "the true philosophy . . . which in 'certain modest steps leads toward health,' " the true philosophy being the humanism of classical authors such as Cicero.[42] Seeking to aid the troubled in "achieving tranquillity" and "conquering the emotions," he developed a healing craft that was "identified with friendship" and involved a healing rhetoric or eloquence.[43] In Book II of this work, with a significant indebtedness to Cicero and Seneca, Petrarch attended to a wide range of consolatory themes in some detail, including many associated with bereavement and with the problems of a person's own death. In dialogue form, *Reason* contended frequently with *Sorrow* and sometimes with *Fear,* did most of the talking, and provided a scheme of advice and consolation for a long list of misfortunes.[44] Contrasting Book I, with its attention to happiness and joy, to Book II, with its emphasis on sorrow and fear, Charles Trinkaus described "Petrarch as a good rhetorician," who "consoles according to circumstances and disciplines according to necessity, delivering praise and blame."[45]

"As a 'theoretical' consoler of death in the *De remediis,* as an 'applied' consoler in the letters, and as one seeking to meet his own death tranquilly, Petrarch fully presents a rational, consolatory response to the crisis of death."[46] And he made substantial contributions to the development of the role of "the eloquent, healing *medicus*" and to the discipline of rhetor as healer. "As the voice of 'Ratio' in the *De remediis* and as a consoling rhetor in his letters," he "richly develops the technical craft of the humanist *medicus animorum.*[47]

As had many others, Petrarch argued for the significance of reason and its crucial role in leading the sufferer away from the distressing emotions that were plaguing him. The goal was to have reason triumph over the passions, subdue the passions, or do away with the passions. In a sense, consolatory efforts were antidotes to the troubling passions. In a way of thinking introduced by the Stoics, particularly Seneca, a continual conflict existed between reason and the passions (and desires). Reason's striving to prevail was a striving for virtue; the failure of reason to prevail resulted in sin.

Many of Augustinus' consoling comments in the *Secret* have the tidy, rationalized nature sometimes associated with traditional rhetoric and criticized as sterile. Such communications may have been comforting to some, or even to many, but the modern reader might easily find them rather empty, somewhat cold comfort. On the other hand, though, Petrarch strongly identified his healing craft with friendship. To put it in the terms of modern psychological healing, technique alone was not thought to be sufficient. The relationship of healer and sufferer was of critical importance. Further, Petrarch also argued that personal experience with sadness and distress played a significant role in a person's becoming an effective consoler.

Petrarch took up themes and practices that had a long tradition in rhetoric — the art of persuasion and the use of eloquence for healing purposes. And the realm of consolation was a significant one for the application of this healing eloquence. In his "medicaments of words (*medicamenta verborum*)" he drew heavily on the classical philosophers for their consolatory *topoi* and for their style with the healing potential of its rhetoric. In contrast, he was critical of the scholasticism of many medieval philosophers, whom he viewed as rather sterile, mostly form and relatively little substance. But these influences did not produce a pagan consoler. His roots were also Christian, heavily influenced by such as Augustine. He crafted his own interweaving of classical and Christian threads to produce a richly humanistic approach to psychological healing in general and consolation in particular. McClure refers to these trends as "the notion of psychotherapeutic eloquence which, in both antiquity and the Renaissance, can be seen as one of the principal contributions of humanism to the psychological tradition."[48]

Starting from this context, Petrarch looked at contemporary physicans' use of healing eloquence with a rather jaundiced eye. While he appears to have resented deeply physicians' incursions into his own humanistic domain, and while he scoffed at their social and intellectual pretensions, he also clearly had a low estimate of physicians and their practice of their profession.[49] Regarding mental healing and the therapeutic use of words, he stated the following in a letter to a medical acquaintance: "No-one calls a doctor seeking eloquence, but health; necessary for this are herbs not words, scents not style, physic not rhetorical arguments; yours is the care of bodies, leave the care of minds to the true philosophers and orators."[50]

In a letter to another physician, he complained about his own experiences as a patient, commenting that he had "received instead of remedies 'promises and consoling words as if I needed a consoler and moral Philosopher instead of a doctor.'" For Petrarch, words were intended "to cure, heal, and move the mind"; they belonged "to the consoler, moral philosopher, and orator." All this seems to imply that the doctors of his day used "a consolatory type of eloquence." Petrarch would allow them a certain use of words to reassure, to comfort, and to give hope; and such uses of comforting language were clearly an aspect of medical endeavors in that era. But he felt strongly that they should otherwise stay within their limits, attending to their "medical craft," which he conceived of as "mechanical and mute by nature."[51] Petrarch wrote, "The only words appropriate for the doctor's care of the sick are those which encourage the patient to be of good mind to be cured by the medicine if possible."[52]

In a response to Petrarch's criticisms of physicians' use of eloquence, Coluccio Salutati (1331–1406), another prominent Italian humanist, argued in support of a place for healing rhetoric in the doctors' ministrations. He thought that physicians with such skills should certainly use them in the interest of healing the sick. While Petrarch's healing eloquence was "built essentially on ancient moral philosophy," Salutati emphasized more "the aesthetic, affective, natural aspects of eloquence."[53] Though both he and Petrarch formulated "a theory of verbal psychotherapy for the sick. . . . Salutati's theory of medical eloquence for the sick emphasizes the psychoaffective character of eloquence and argues the doctor's possible natural facility in it. Petrarch's healing 'eloquence' as he administers it in his *De remediis* is a highly philosophical, psychointellective craft."[54]

Salutati was himself a consoler of some consequence. In his letters, he indicated his sense of the role of a consoler, the nature of his own practice as consoler, and his personal experience of grief and consolation. For him, letter writing in general was rooted in friendship, and consoling a friend in sadness was a natural part of being a friend.[55] He thought that it was the friendship rather than the rhetoric that accomplished the consoling and the healing; and he argued for the healing power of the consoler rather than that of the consolation. Further, he defined the true nature of the consoler "as one who gives solace both to himself and to another" out of "his own sympathetic grief. For him, the shared experience of grief and solace is essential to true consolation. . . . The consoler's empathy alone is therapeutic. The silent co-sufferer, without words but with compassion alone, can alleviate grief."[56] The true consoler empathically experienced the sufferer's grief and then consoled both the distressed other person *and* himself. Also, Salutati made the point that "efforts of consolation labor in vain" in the face of "the clattering of the passions."[57] The passions needed to be calmed somewhat before consolatory efforts could be effective.

Salutati had drawn extensively on the consolatory traditions of Cicero and Seneca and on the patristic forms of Jerome and Augustine and had been influenced by Petrarch. He had developed a view of consolation rooted in friendship (consolatory efforts being cardinal among the duties of friendship). Then, under the influence of his own bereavements — the loss of first his wife, then his son — his personal grief brought theological themes into play, and a certain dissatisfaction with classical consolation emerged.[58]

Another figure of significant influence in the Renaissance development of consolation was Marsilio Ficino (1433–1499), the crucial contributor to Renaissance Neoplatonism who was trained as a physician and who later became a priest. His numerous letters of consolation mark him as an important consoler, a physician of souls who drew upon Socratic-Platonic thought to console the dying and to provide Platonic solace for the bereaved. Of particular interest among his consolatory themes is his urging the bereaved not to search for the dead person outside themselves, but to "look into one's own soul, where the soul of the departed can be found ever present."[59]

Beyond these notable contributors, numerous other humanists made significant contributions to this flowering of consolatory writings in the fourteenth and fifteenth centuries. These writings appeared in the form of letters, treatises, consolatory dialogues, and even an encyclopedic manual of consolation.[60] These various scholars addressed philosophical issues and spiritual concerns; they shaped forms of pastoral care; they developed a somewhat secular psychology; and they practiced forms of psychological healing.

In this context of the humanist revival of classical learning, a series of scholars shaped and reshaped traditional consolation and the cure of souls into integrated forms of psychological healing. Healing words and a therapeutic wisdom were directed toward solace and tranquillity. These Italian physicians of souls were well grounded in philosophy and had been significantly influenced by Plato, Aristotle, Cicero, and the Stoics, but the approaches they evolved had a considerable admixture of Christianity. From both Petrarch's criticisms and Salutati's supportive contributions, it is clear that physicians, too, sought to console, comfort, and otherwise bring a psychological therapeutic wisdom to bear; but the typical *medicus animorum* of the era was more likely to be a humanist philosopher, a religious functionary, or both. Grief, sorrow, fear, and despair were the commonest forms of psychological distress. And they were commonly "treated" by means that were humanistic, religiously informed, and phrased as a medical metaphor. Physicians certainly served many a sufferer in similar fashion, but such psychological healing was not primarily identified with their roles. The rhetor's persuasion and the consoler's moral therapeutics were integrated into confessional moments in order to help sufferers cope with sorrow and despair. The humanistic psychological healer aided the sufferer in dealing with bereavement and illness, in coping with many other forms of loss and misfortune, and in facing the process of dying and the imminence of death. That more than mere reason was involved in such psychological healing came to be well recognized; affects were taken into account; and some humanistic therapeutists argued that friendship played a crucial role in this healing.

The sixteenth-century physician, mathematician, and scientist Girolamo Cardano (1501–1576) has been depicted as "perhaps the most important and prolific High Renaissance Italian figure in the tradition of consolatory and therapeutic literature." His *De consolatione* (1542) had "an important role in spawning the early modern popularity of consolatory thought." Influenced by Cicero, Cardano went beyond Cicero's emphasis on bereavement to develop consolations for a wide range of human misfortunes, while still giving special attention to the fear of one's own death and the grief of bereavement. The second of the three books in this work was devoted to these last two themes, and it integrated them into one consolatory work. And he made particular use of the theme of immortality in a number of his consolations for death.[61] McClure has pointed out that, along with Petrarch's, Cardano's thought was also particularly influential outside of Italy.

From this rich vein of Italian humanistic contributions to the literature of consolation came many influences that continued through the rest of the sixteenth and the seventeenth centuries, both in Italy and in countries to the north. Editions and translations of many of the classical and patristic consolatory writings appeared. The transalpine world produced its own consolatory literature, drawing on classical, patristic, and medieval sources, and on the Italian humanists. Increasingly, Renaissance consolations were translated into the vernacular, and original works began to appear in individual European languages. And many of these consolatory works were adapted to the literature and practice of pastoral care. Throughout this wide range of consolatory writings, bereavement, death, and the fear of death continued to be the most prominent problems addressed. Attention was also given to problems of illness, and some emphasis was placed on dejection, despair and melancholy.

As to the theologians' ways of dealing with bereavement and death, humanists such as Petrarch and Cardano were rather critical. But those engaged in pastoral care sought to meet such challenges with Christianized versions of humanist "comfort, healing persuasion, and consolation." The pastor shared a "common territorial domain" with the humanist — "namely, the consolation of the distressed, the sad, the fearful, the dying" — and he was not about to abandon it.[62]

Another useful perspective on a crucial aspect of the attitude of the Church toward consolation can be gained from Thomas M. Tentler's extensive study of sin and confession. Instead of the customary emphasis on sorrow and distress, the providing of comfort and relief, and the coping with distressing passions through the activities of Reason or the strengthening of Reason, he connected *consolation* intimately with *discipline* within the traditions of confession, penance, and absolution. Pointing out the element of social control inherent in confession and penance, he commented that "sacramental confession was designed to cause guilt as well as cure guilt." Paired with this discipline was consolation, the bringing of comfort and relief through the cycle of confession, penance, and absolution amounted to a "cure of anxiety." Tentler thus identified "for the institution of forgiveness two social and psychological functions — discipline (or social control) and consolation (or cure of anxiety)."[63] The status and authority of the priest and the strength of the tradition provided "convincing proof that ordained priests truly forgive and effectively console." The process of confession, penance, and absolution brought a sense of being forgiven and of reconciliation with community and with God that was eminently consoling. Despite any tensions between *discipline* and *consolation,* "social control and the cure of anxiety" were "accommodated in one institutional system."[64] Significantly, though, "the emotional center of the sixteenth-century campaign" for reform was "the reformers' denunciation of sacramental confession because it tormented rather than consoled."[65]

Robert Burton and Consolation

Out of this Renaissance background of consolatory activity, Robert Burton developed the "Consolatory Digression" that was positioned so crucially among the healing measures in his *Anatomy of Melancholy.* He offered his own *consolatio* constructed out of "remedies and comfortable speeches" from "our best Orators, Philosophers, Divines, and Fathers of the Church." Though he termed it a "digression," it followed reasonably (and Burton seems to have thought as much himself) on his immediately previous attention to "good counsel, comfortable speeches, persuasion" and "how necessarily they are required to the cure of a discontented or troubled mind."[66] Bearing clear indications of its many debts, this Burtonian consolation contained most of the crucial ingredients from the classical philosophical consolers, their Christian successors, and the humanists that were Burton's more immediate forerunners. Designed as it was to contain "the Remedies of all manner of Discontents," this complex *consolatio* had portions for each of numerous subgroups of misfortunes, just about any misfortune addressed by his consoling predecessors — "Deformity of Body, Sickness, Baseness of Birth, Peculiar Discontents"; "Against Poverty and Want, with such other Adversities"; "Against Servitude, Loss of Liberty, Imprisonment, Banishment"; "Against Sorrow for Death of Friends or otherwise, vain Fear, etc."; "Against Envy, Livor, Emulation, Hatred, Ambition, Self-love, and all other Affections"; "Against Repulse, Abuses, Injuries, Contempts, Disgraces, Contumelies, Slanders, Scoffs, etc."; and "Against Melancholy itself."[67]

Burton first took up the theme that nothing can ever be all good fortune and success for anyone. "Consider the like calamities of other men; thou wilt then bear thine own the better. Be content and rest satisfied, for thou art well in respect of others; be thankful for that thou hast, that God hath done for thee."[68] He then argued the notion that various trials and tribulations are sent to test and strengthen a person; Burton maintained that those who suffered inordinately on earth could look to comfort and pleasant times in heaven; and he advocated trust in God as a way to a sense of support and comfort.

For the various "discontents and grievances" that might "wound the soul of man" and lead to melancholy, whether they affected "body, mind, or fortune," Burton would prescribe "good counsel and persuasion" as antidotes, that the person might be consoled and relieved of his distress.[69] If we are possessed of particular physical liabilities, we may well have compensatory assets; if sick or diseased, it may prove to be for the good of our souls, "a little sickness . . . will correct and amend us."[70] And so he went on to demonstrate how many apparently fortunate human states were not really so great or enviable, and how many apparently unfortunate states had much to be said for them after all.

Consolation was offered to the grief-stricken to the effect that their dead loved one was better off. They were advised that grief, among other passions, should be experienced in moderation. They were reminded that all of us must eventually die; and comfort was offered through the belief in life hereafter. A rationalization was provided for nearly every form of loss of someone close and dear. Diversions in thought and action were suggested to turn the sorrowing person's mind away from preoccupation with the loss.[71]

Much in Burton's consolatory efforts was already familiar. Among the many different influences were frequent reflections of the thought of Cicero, Seneca, Boethius, and Cardano; and Christian consolatory commonplaces were well represented. Further, there seems to have been an element of self-consolation in Burton's efforts, and that too had been true of several of his prominent predecessors. As with so many before him, the explicit emphasis was on reason as crucial. Consolation aimed to provide suitable rationalizations so that reason might be aided in its struggle with the passions and reassert its ascendancy over them. At times it was suggested that reason was the supreme consoler. In modern terms, one might say that a cognitive therapeutic approach was emphasized. And yet affective themes were also prominent. Raising the hope of those who were discouraged or even felt hopeless was of central importance. The frequently cheerful tone and the many encouraging passages for the dejected were inherent aspects of Burton's comfort and counsel. It is fair to say that an affectively tinged comfort and reasoned counsel were intertwined in the interest of consoling the sorrowing sufferer. Further, in some contrast to indications that reason was considered the supreme consoler, one finds in Burton frequent hints of the Christian theme of God as the supreme consoler, although appeals might be made to reason in order to persuade the sorrowful person to accept that view.

The Sixteenth, Seventeenth, and Eighteenth Centuries

In Burton's extended attention to consolation in the psychological healing of melancholia, we have consolatory offerings with clear lines of inheritance from classical, patristic, and humanist predecessors. But moreover, we also have a particularly interesting extension of the keen English-language interest in consolatory writings that had emerged in the sixteenth century. And, still further, we have a window onto the significant place of consolation in the duties and activities of many clergymen in the late sixteenth and seventeenth centuries.

In his "Tudor Books of Consolation," Beach Langston identifies seventy-one consolatory works published in English between 1478 and 1600, even after excluding those written specially to comfort the bereaved. After studying these volumes carefully, he has grouped them into three main categories, according to the consolatory traditions upon which they drew to comfort their readers — Christian, pagan (or classical), and Christian-and-pagan. Using the term *rationalize* in the sense of "to render conformable to reason; to explain on a rational basis," Langston illustrates how the authors of these books used various rationalizations to strengthen and comfort their readers "against the attacks of fear, grief, pain, loss of worldly good, and death itself." Their purpose was "to rationalize the universe; to render it, in the writer's and reader's minds, conformable to reason; to explain the universe in accordance with some just and reasonable pattern; to make the outrageous deeds of fate, fortune, and death seem somehow right." A variety of rhetorical devices were used to persuade sufferers "that they lived in a world rational and somehow good." In the interest of consolation, most of these authors were striving to "justify the ways of God to man," while still endeavoring to conform to observable facts, or at least what was accepted as such in the Christian beliefs of the time. This was aided by the postulation of "another world in which the imperfections of this world would be corrected," as a comfort to those in distress as they faced the trials and tribulations that afflicted them in the here and now. In the tradition of pastoral care, many of the authors were endeavoring "to provide practical help" for those "whose souls and bodies were being tormented."[72]

A large portion of these books was given over to consoling and comforting the reader against the prospect, whether imminent or distant, of death. Some dealt only with consolations for those actually upon their deathbed; some provided consolations against the fear of death for those who were sick; and some offered more general consolations against death, addressed to everyone, both the well and the sick. Although Christians had the consolation of a life hereafter in a better world, the Christian theme of sinfulness was associated with the threat of the alternative of hell and damnation. And so there had been developed the consolatory notion of faith and true contrition as leading to confession and then forgiveness through God's grace.[73]

But Langston finds that another group of books "do not confine themselves to consolations against any one trouble or passion but range over all life's experiences and include even death." The first subgroup here was composed of those which tried "to comfort their readers by urging on them only the comforts of the Christian faith."[74] And these themes were commonly supported with Christianized versions of the classical contempt for worldly things. The works in the second subgroup were not concerned with "the comforts to be obtained from the Christian faith, but with those to be got through natural reason alone."[75] They were editions and translations of classical authors, mainly Cicero, Seneca, Plutarch, and Boethius. The third subgroup included the writings that based "their consolations on both the 'reason' of the Ancients and the faith of St. Paul."[76] Some of the works "used pagan material only for rhetorical ornament," but others "made pagan ideas a vital part of their argument and generally had the highest praise for the Ancients so long as they did not contradict Christian teachings."[77]

These writings and similar publications on the Continent entered a scene in which, for centuries, priests had had the responsibility of providing consolation for their troubled parishioners. They visited the sick to comfort them in their time of suffering. Through confession, penance, and absolution, they brought consolation to those afflicted with the burdens of sinfulness. Deathbed consolations were regularly held to be their duty. And they consoled and comforted members of their flock in other times of distress.

With the Reformation, similar activities became part of the responsibilities of the Protestant clergy. In 1520, Martin Luther's (1483–1546) *Fourteen Comforts for the Weary and Heavy Laden* was published in both Latin and German editions. Originally written as a spiritual consolation for the Elector Frederick the Wise of Saxony (1462–1525) at a time of serious illness, this became a favorite consolatory work over the succeeding centuries.[78] John Calvin (1509–1564) provided numerous letters of consolation to those who were suffering bereavement.[79] And by the end of the century, the Protestant contributions later collected in Langston's "Tudor Books of Consolation" constituted a rising tide of consolatory writings.

Clergymen both in Robert Burton's Anglican tradition and in various other Protestant traditions conceived of consolation as having a significant place among the healing and sustaining activities of seventeenth-century pastoral care.[80] Further, many members of the clergy practiced medicine to one degree or another. "Medical practice was, in fact, a natural extension of the pastor's duty to console his flock in times of sickness."[81] Richard Baxter (1615–1691), the eminent nonconformist divine, brought out, in 1656, an influential handbook on pastoral care, *Gildas Salvianus, or The Reformed Pastor*. Scattered through parts of this work were explicit and implicit references to the significance of consolation. As Baxter stated it at one juncture, "Another part of our work is to comfort the disconsolate, and to settle the peace of our people's souls, and that on sure and lasting grounds. To which end, the quality of the complainants, and the course of their lives, had need to be known; for all people must not have the like consolations that have the like complaints."[82] Also, we find in a collection of Baxter's writings on the care and cure of melancholy persistent indications that consolation had a place among the healing and comforting measures that he advocated. Interestingly, while advising that help be sought from a clergyman more "judicious in his Preaching and Praying, than passionate," Baxter added, "except when he urgeth the Gospel Doctrines of Consolation, and then the more fervent the better."[83] Although Baxter's consoler would thus function in contradistinction to consolers in the earlier tradition, in which the appeal was to the sufferer's reason, that person's consolatory efforts would be in the spirit of the more recent Puritan tradition, in which imaginative appeals were commonly made to the emotions of the listeners and the readers. Also in keeping with this newer tradition, Baxter's writings were heavily scriptural in their references and adornments, in contrast to Burton's "Consolatory Digression," which reflected classical, patristic, and humanist influences. And Baxter expressed himself in a rich Christian idiom that had emerged in the late sixteenth and seventeenth centuries as Puritan preaching and writing flowered.

Akin to *The Reformed Pastor* was *The Country Parson*, written in 1632 but published only in 1652. Its author, George Herbert (1593–1633), a poet and churchman who had long had a connection with Cambridge, identified this work of guidance for a clergyman as falling within the genre of the "Pastorall," that is to say, "a book relating to the cure of souls."[84] In the chapter "The Parson Comforting," Herbert stated that "the Country Parson, when any of his cure is sick, or afflicted with losse of friend, or estate, or any ways distressed," should "afford his best comforts, and rather goes to them, then [than] sends for the afflicted.... To this end he hath thoroughly digested all the points of consolation, as having continuall use of them."[85]

Through the late seventeenth and the eighteenth centuries, the sustaining functions of the clergy continued to include a significant role for consolation and comfort. The Roman Catholic way in the cure of souls had assigned a more significant place to confession, penance, and absolution than the Protestant way, but the long tradition of providing comfort to one's parishioners in times of misfortune or distress remained for most clergy a consistent feature of pastoral care. Whether Catholic of Protestant, they were concerned with bringing solace to the bereaved, sustaining those who faced misfortunes, visiting the sick, and comforting the dying.

Consolation and the Care of the Insane

With the creation of institutions for the insane, an important additional context emerged in which consolation was provided for sufferers. It has become traditional to discuss these institutional settings in terms of their harsh conditions and inhumane practices, with particular emphasis on the themes of confinement and control; and this orientation has not lacked significant evidence to justify it. But, as illustrated by the situation in France, this perspective has resulted in a rather incomplete picture. Well before Philippe Pinel (1745–1826) developed his *moral treatment* for the insane at the end of the eighteenth century, there were glimmerings of a more humane approach — hints of traditional modes of psychological healing at work. Roman Catholic nursing orders in France were already serving the insane in a tradition rooted in pastoral care. And consolation and comfort were crucial in the context of these more humane undertakings.

Christian consolatory literature had long placed special emphasis on ministering to the sick, and so the Christian nursing orders that devoted themselves to the insane were the carriers of a rich tradition of caring and consoling. Their efforts reflected those of religious sick-nurses in general, whose ministerings might be seen as the origin of what French physicians came to term *moral medicine*. Prototypical of these were the Augustinian nursing sisters of the Hôtel-Dieu in Paris. The Hôtel-Dieu had long been "a shelter of charity and consolation which accepted all men, sick or hungry, in accord with the Christian ideal of hospitality." Their consoling ministry entailed "what today would be recognized as the psychotherapeutic component of healing." These sisters knew how " 'to console despair, to temper chagrin, to calm anxiety . . . constantly at bedside talking, consoling.' "[86] For orders such as these, "nursing was a conscious imitation of the life and works of Christ whose charitable qualities the nurses were exhorted to practice." To "the three customary vows of poverty, chastity and obedience," these nursing sisters added "a fourth for the care of the sick."[87] The eminent surgeon Pierre-Joseph Desault (1738–1795), who introduced a surgery school and clinic into the Hôtel-Dieu on the eve of the Revolution, was in some conflict with the sisters around the implementation of new regulations for the management of the hospital. But he charged his students to care for and console the sick in ways rather similar to those urged on the Augustinian nuns by their religious constitution.[88]

Further, a number of Catholic orders undertook important commitments to the care of the insane in particular. Prominent among these were the Brothers of Saint-Jean-de-Dieu, also known as the Brothers of Charity, or the Charitans. This order had its roots in the work of Juan Ciudad (1495–1550), who, in Granada in the early sixteenth century, "dedicated himself to the care of the insane, inspired the new order, and eventually earned sainthood as 'John of God.' "[89] This order prospered in Italy, and was brought to France in 1601 by Marie de Medici of Florence. During the eighteenth century, the motherhouse in Paris, the famous Charité Hospital, came to be very highly regarded. And at this Paris Charité, the brothers trained the nursing personnel for a large network of such houses, or *charités*, in France and its colonies, a number of the houses being devoted to the care of the insane. As was the case in other Catholic orders, novices "were taught to serve the sick as if they were serving Christ: with selfless devotion, gentle kindness, patience, attention to all the details of the patient's physical and spiritual well-being."[90] Also, "the Franciscan monks, or Bon-Fils, the Cordeliers, and the Brothers of the Christian Schools each maintained several *maisons d'aliénés* during the Old Regime." And "the Sisters of the Bon-Sauveur of Caen" cared for "prostitutes and female lunatics."[91]

It was against this background that during the late eighteenth century certain French physicians of note paid interesting attention to consolation. Reflecting the tradition of consolation as an aspect of the physician's activities in ministering to the sick, Pierre-Jean-Georges Cabanis urged the importance of consolation and comfort in caring for those who were ill. "Doubtless it is the duty of the physician to afford the sweetest and most soothing consolations to the patient couched on the bed of sickness; it is he alone, who can penetrate farthest into the confidence of infirmity and misfortune, and, therefore, it is he who can pour the most salutary balm into their wounds."[92] Physician, Idéologue, and hospital reformer, Cabanis interwove medical and philosophical traditions in an effort to reform medicine. And he asserted that the clinically adequate physician must be a humanist and psychologist as well as a medically competent practitioner in the narrower sense. "The physician is doubtless unfit for his profession, who has not learned to read in the human heart, as well as to recognise the presence of the febrile state; or, who in treating a diseased body, cannot distinguish, in the features, in the looks, or in the speech, of his patient, the signs of a disordered mind, or of a wounded heart. . . . How can he revive the dying flame of life, in a body drooping, or devoured by anguish, if he knows not what sufferings he must first alleviate, and what idle dreams he must first dispel?"[93]

Pinel was exposed to the views and values of his friend Cabanis, was probably influenced by the consolatory traditions of nursing orders such as the Brothers of Charity, and was keenly concerned about improvement in the therapeutic lot of the insane. Again and again, he alluded to the significance of consolation in the treatment of mad persons. Along with gentleness, patience, and benevolence, comfort and consolation were crucial in the therapeutic approach that Pinel developed and eventually termed moral treatment. In fact, consolation became a central ingredient of moral treatment. In a 1790 account of his treatment of a deeply troubled young monk, Pinel wrote of assuming "a consoling tone to reestablish calm in the timorous spirit of this unfortunate cenobite."[94] In a 1793 essay discussing "the best method to teach practical medicine in a hospital," Pinel devoted a section to "les remèdes moraux," in which he asserted that he had no wish to deprive the sick of "the consolations of religion." Further, when he was a physician in training, many instances at the bedside had convinced him of "the beneficial effect on the sick of consolatory talk appropriate to reassure them about their condition"; and he would recommend such an approach in the training of young physicians.[95] In 1798–1799, in a work on moral treatment that foreshadowed his more famous *Treatise on Insanity* at many points, Pinel, in citing "the art of consolation" first among "the moral means" for the successful treatment of the insane, indicated that he was being guided by principles well known to such ancients as Celsus and Caelius Aurelianus.[96] Emphasizing "gentle words" and "talking with gentleness,"[97] he urged the use of "consoling talk" and the providing of "consoling hope,"[98] and he cited Pussin's capacity to calm furious maniacs with such consolatory efforts.[99]

Thus it was a familiar theme for Pinel by the time he stated in his *Treatise on Insanity* that "the experience of every day attests the value of consolatory language, kind treatment, and the revival of extinguished hope,"[100] and described a case in which the treatment of the patient was "to console him, to sympathise with his misfortunes, and, after having gradually obtained his esteem and confidence, to dwell upon such circumstances as were calculated to cheer his prospects and to encourage his hopes."[101]

Out of materials such as these, and much more that she has assembled, integrated, and discussed with considerable penetration and wisdom, Goldstein, in her *Console and Classify,* traces the evolution of French moral medicine and Pinel's moral treatment out of medicine's past and the influences of its Idéologue reformers, but also, and to a significant extent, out of the caring pastoral practices of the Catholic parish priest and the comforting consolatory practices of eighteenth-century Catholic nursing orders, particularly those which ministered to the insane.[102] She identifies a degree of struggle between the religious and the physicians for authority over the care of patients and for proprietary rights to the realm of consolatory and caring efforts. And she provides evidence that the physicians of the Revolutionary era, and their immediate professional descendants who might be termed psychiatrists, worked vigorously to divest consolation of its "explicit religious content," to secularize consolatory practices. But these "psychiatrists nonetheless referred to this soothing and empathic therapeutic intervention as consolation; and the name's religious connotations advertised more loudly than they had intended the partially religious inspiration for the new professional function they sought to establish at the expense of the clergy."[103]

The Brothers of Charity were of special interest in this context in view of the kindly, gentle features of their approach to caring for the mad and the recurrent emphasis on consolation as a crucial element in their ministerings to these sufferers. They were urged by "the provincial of the order . . . to be 'courteous and gentle' toward the insane residents of their houses, to 'console them,' to 'speak to them with gentleness and have for them all the courtesy, tenderness and compassion that befits their condition' . . . it was specified that the prior see the lunatics '*one after another and separately,* in order to console them, to guide them to better conduct and to assure himself that they are being treated as they ought to be.' . . . Repeated 'consolations' were especially recommended for the melancholics, whose despair aroused apprehension about possible suicidal intent."[104] Further, the parallels between the approach of the Brothers of Charity and that developed by Pinel and Pussin at the end of the century seem to support Goldstein's well-developed argument that moral treatment had at least some of its roots in the consolatory and comforting practices of the brothers.[105]

As moral treatment evolved in France during the early decades of the nineteenth century, consolation continued to be an essential ingredient; and struggles about who should undertake the consolatory efforts, and the other aspects of moral treatment, continued as clerics and physicians argued the case, which arguments often reflected a larger struggle over whose authority was pre-eminent in an institution. Charenton, near Paris, had been one of the *charités* of the Brothers of Charity that had cared for the insane. Closed in Year III (1794–95) by the Jacobins, it was reopened two years later as a secularized institution for the mad, with moral remedies integrated with physical remedies in the treatment program.[106] François-Simonnet de Coulmiers, an ex-cleric, was appointed as the director. In 1803 de Coulmiers urged "the appointment of a priest to aid in the moral treatment at Charenton and in the 'consolation' that it entailed." He noted that mad persons could find "much consolation in spiritual aid dispensed with wisdom. . . . This moral means could even contribute to reestablishing equilibrium in heads disordered by unforeseen calamities or by revolutionary principles."[107]

Similar themes were still being emphasized in the 1820s and 1830s by Xavier Tissot (1780–1864), a leading member of the Brothers of Charity. At one time a patient who had been successfully treated at Charenton, Tissot founded a half-dozen new institutions for the insane, established moral treatment programs in these settings, and functioned as "director of the moral treatment." Regarding the content of moral treatment, Tissot vigorously advocated his own form of "religious-moral treatment" rather than the "moral-philosophical treatment" of the physicians, whom he viewed as being mainly atheists. "What a difference," he wrote, "between the morality of the Gospel and the maxims of the philosophers! between divine consolations and human consolations!" He outlined a treatment program of prayer, religious consolation, religious music, and sometimes confession. He drew upon

> an in-depth knowledge of the techniques of consolation. A chapter of the general manual of sick-nursing he published in 1829 set forth an entire repertory of consolations to be offered to the afflicted under various circumstances and noted that inventiveness at consolation, a therapeutic gift called the "thousand ingenuities for mitigating chagrin," was an inspiration of the Holy Spirit. "Nothing . . . will better prove your charity toward your fellows than vigilance and constant application in consoling the sick." A sympathetic sharing of pain was sometimes recommended: "If you see a patient who is troubled and anxious, tell him how much you are touched by what he is suffering."[108]

The place that consolation had in moral treatment, and came to have in French psychiatry, can be seen from the following comments in 1836 from Scipion Pinel (1795–1859), Philippe Pinel's son and himself an *aliéniste*. "All physicians, no matter how remarkable their abilities may be, are not necessarily suited to the role of medical director of a hospital for the insane. It is a special vocation, requiring special abilities and a special disposition. Such a person is more than a physician, he is a consoler and a father."[109] Or, as Goldstein stated it, "the nature of the moral treatment endowed the *aliéniste* with something of the persona of a secular priest."[110]

The Nineteenth Century

Traditional consolation and comfort having provided some essential ingredients in the mix that was moral treatment, consoling and comforting continued to have a particular place in medical psychological healing during the first half of the nineteenth century. In the second half of the century, though, the asylums gradually drifted toward a system of custodial care. In the process, moral treatment lost its way and was transformed into a rather narrow version of moral management. As the role for comfort and consolation diminished, asylum treatment became more a matter of discipline, control, and routine care.

In an American example of an asylum physician who actively continued with psychological healing efforts into the second half of the century, Thomas Story Kirkbride (1809–1883) at the Pennsylvania Hospital for the Insane urged and persuaded his patients to abandon their problematic beliefs and behaviors and to espouse the thoughts and behaviors of sane persons.[111] His approach was secular in its content, yet it had much in common with a carefully guided journey toward a religious conversion. There is considerable evidence to suggest that Kirkbride actively sought to gain the trust of the patients, strove to encourage them and to induce a hopeful outlook in them, was sympathetic and kind, and was a source of comfort and consolation.[112]

Kirkbride's approach to psychological medicine was very much in the tradition of the moral treatment handed down from Pinel and the Tukes, but in his time he was more the exception than the rule in the countries where such treatment had flourished. Further, by the 1880s, psychological healing had come to be associated more with the nonasylum care of mentally disturbed persons. Some general physicians, the occasional asylum doctor who had gone into private practice, and a gradually increasing number of the neurologists had taken up the practice of psychological healing. As hypnotism and then suggestion took over in the practice and in the language of medical psychological healing, any explicit mention of consolation or comfort became increasingly rare. How much general physicians or physician-psychotherapeutists consoled or comforted in their clinical work is difficult to know. Surely such efforts remained as aspects of their practice at times, but new language fashions had taken over; and we can only occasionally discern implicit evidence of consolation in the writings left to us.

Although acknowledgment of the significance of consolation and comfort in the literature of the emerging psychotherapeutics may have been limited, the value attributed to consolation was indicated by an essay written as a tribute to the memory of Jean-Martin Charcot (1825–1893). In delivering this eulogy, Jules Claretie (1840–1913), a novelist and member of the Académie Française, chose to focus on Charcot's role as a consoler in extolling his qualities, his capacities, and his contributions. In "Charcot, le consolateur," he discussed him as the psychotherapist who wrote "La foi qui guérit" and "dominated his era and consoled it." He became "a great consoler in his way"; he provided consolation in his clinical setting, "amidst the cries and the sorrows." Claretie concluded on a ringing note: "Evil has been contested, Life has been consoled."[113]

With regard to medical care more generally, the traditional concern that compassion and sympathy should be inherent in the physician's role persisted into the nineteenth century, and intermittently they became the focus for lively

debate. That such compassion and sympathy would naturally lead to providing comfort and consolation tended to be taken for granted but was sometimes
explicitly discussed.[114] Physicians served their patients and their patients' families when they were fearful in the face of severe illness, overburdened by
chronic illness, saddened by loss, or faced with the threat of imminent death;
and their sympathetic and comforting responses in those situations were often
inherent aspects of medical care.[115] The complex of trust, sympathy and compassion, encouragement and hope, and comfort and consolation was well
recognized, although it was sometimes overshadowed by the late century's
burgeoning sense of scientific knowledge about medicine.

Another realm in which comfort and consolation had been, and continued
to be, significant was that of pastoral care or the cure of souls. The caring for
and the curing of troubled souls had always included bringing comfort to
sufferers and consoling them as they faced their losses, misfortunes, and other
distressing experiences. In fact, as one authority on consolation stated it,
"There is no subject more frequently referred to in the whole of devotional
literature than consolation."[116]

Sufferers had sought to be comforted, to have their distress eased. In the
framework of a mystical tradition, efforts were made to achieve a sense of
communion with God or oneness with God. Other sufferers sought comfort
and consolation through prayer, again in an effort to experience a sense of
being in touch with God. And others found comfort in being in touch with
priests or pastors who reduced their aloneness and eased their sufferings
through soothing ministrations. From states of desolation and despair to the
sorrow of bereavement and other forms of distress, religion continued to be a
crucial source of consolation in these ways. As was the case with the physician
who brought comfort, it was important that the pastoral medicus animorum
be able to draw on capacities of compassion and sympathy. And these consolatory and comforting efforts characterized religious psychological healing
throughout the nineteenth century.

Consolation in the Twentieth Century

For our century, Walter Bromberg has stated that "the need for psychotherapy has replaced the need for consolation [to] which religion and philosophy contributed, the first in a practical way, the second more abstractly."[117]
Many would challenge this assertion, and from a variety of viewpoints, but it
alludes to some significant issues nonetheless. For one, the human inclination
to seek comfort in times of distress has not lessened — whether grief-stricken in
response to some loss, suffering an acute illness, burdened by a chronic illness,

fear-ridden in the face of one of life's threats, plagued by guilt or shame, or somehow under a cloud from some other type of misfortune. Although the psychotherapies of our century have certainly been enlisted to respond to those seeking comfort when suffering from these various types of distress, our century's religions and their clergy have surely been turned to by large numbers of such sufferers. And physicians in general have continued to minister to the human need for comfort and consolation, whether or not it has occurred to them to conceive of their activities as a form of psychotherapy.

Pastoral care has continued to be characterized by the traditional elements of the cure of souls — healing and restorative efforts, sustaining, providing guidance, and reconciling.[118] But it has also been influenced by the twentieth century's many psychotherapies. Techniques have been borrowed from this or that mode of psychotherapy and integrated into the practices of pastoral care; and counseling has developed into a distinct aspect of pastoral care. Formal training programs for pastoral counselors have frequently come to include elements from psychotherapeutic training. And some pastoral counselors have conceived of themselves as practicing psychotherapy as part of their pastoral care.[119] In the classical realm of bereavement, the role of the pastor as consoler or comforter has often become somewhat obscured by the language of grief counseling or bereavement counseling. Nevertheless, no matter how a particular member of the clergy has conceived of his or her efforts, bringing comfort or consolation to suffering parishioners has remained a crucial aspect of pastoral care.

In the realm of general medical care, during the twentieth century the tensions between medical science and clinical medicine have intensified. Sympathy and compassion in the practitioner continue to be valued, and practitioners generally recognized these ideals in their practice. Concerns that such values not be lost under the influence of the emerging scientific knowledge have found expression in a considerable literature about the importance of "the doctor-patient relationship" and "the patient as a person." As mentioned earlier, a particularly eloquent representative of these views was Francis Weld Peabody of Harvard Medical School, noted for his clinical caring and for his essay "The Care of the Patient."[120] Showing sympathy, being kindly and humane, and bringing comfort to the sick and the suffering — these attitudes were valued and sought after in physicians; and their significance was attested to in expressions of appreciation — or in complaints when doctors fell short of such standards. In the course of an average practice, physicians met their patients when the latter were in the throes of loss and grief, acute illness, or chronic illnesse, in the grip of other crises, or on the verge of death; and they frequently had significant relationships with patients' families. Whether they were reassuring, frankly consolatory, encouraging, or otherwise comforting, physicians intermittently served their patients in a sustaining role. And they were significant participants in the tradition of inducing and sustaining hope.

Yet in the many varieties of psychotherapy that have characterized psychological healing in the twentieth century, very little formal attention has been paid to comfort or consolation, and the terms themselves have been conspicuously absent from the psychotherapeutic literature. This is not to say that psychotherapists have not provided comfort at times of crisis or in the face of bereavement, but for whatever reasons, it has been uncommon for such contributions or interventions to have been included in accounts of what psychotherapists allegedly do.

The psychotherapeutics that emerged in the latter part of the nineteenth century emphasized the roles of hypnosis and suggestion, then catharsis and abreaction, and eventually persuasion. Accounts of evolving practices were not usually accompanied by references to comforting or consoling, nor would they be in the early decades of the twentieth century. But the general medical practice of assuring and reassuring patients about their ailments, their worries, and their fears gradually found its way into the practice of psychotherapy. As they had for the general physician, these efforts served to re-establish confidence, to encourage, and to bolster sufferers in the face of fear. Suggestion seems to have been a crucial element in assurance and reassurance, but it is also clear that such interventions frequently served to bring comfort to sufferers. When suggestions were delivered with an air of authority, their relations to comforting was often not clear; but when they were rooted in a sympathetic attitude and served to engender hope, their comforting qualities were usually quite clear.

By the 1940s, reassurance had become a recognized factor among the psychotherapeutic interventions that might be employed by the general physician;[121] and it was acknowledged as one of the modes of intervention that might be used by a psychotherapist, particularly as an aspect of supportive psychotherapy. Lewis R. Wolberg included reassurance — along with guidance, suggestion, encouragement, and so forth — in his outline of what constituted supportive therapy; but he added that "reassurance is a partner in all psychotherapies, even where there is a purposeful avoidance of pacifying consolations. The very presence of the therapist serves to conciliate the patient, apart from the auxiliary agencies of placebo and suggestion." He took note of reassuring comments when patients had unrealistic doubts about their ability to get well and of the providing of solace when patients were in the grip of irrational fears. But he also observed that "reassurance is least successful when it is directed at basic, ego-syntonic personality difficulties, particularly devaluated self-esteem and its derivatives."[122] Wolberg also underscored the point that reassurance has commonly been provided "through non-verbal behavior, as by maintenance of a calm and objective attitude."[123] Further, listening carefully and respectfully, having a basically hopeful attitude, and not being overwhelmed by the patient's condition or worries have all served to calm and reassure. And it is also important that reassuring comments not be in the form of empty formulae but rather reflect a basically encouraging attitude and be well grounded in realistic information. To sum up, much in the way of comfort has been brought to sufferers under the rubric of reassurance.

Of particular interest among the psychotherapists has been the work of Paul C. Horton, who argued at length for a central place for the providing of solace. Although he did not use the term *consolation* and only briefly mentioned "consoling" in passing, he has written at length about soothing or solacing, and has used terms such as *solacing objects, vehicles for solace,* and *growth-facilitating soothers.* Borrowing from Donald W. Winnicott, Horton has argued that the "transitional objects" and "transitional relatedness" of the child evolve into various adult uses of transitional objects for comforting and soothing purposes; and he includes the psychotherapist and the psychoanalyst as items that can have such a status and serve such a purpose. Although this representation of solace is somewhat different from the traditional understanding of consoling and comforting, there is clearly a kinship.[124]

Consolation and comfort have also been prominent features of psychological healing in the specialized area of medical psychological care devoted to the bereaved or grief-stricken. As we have seen, consoling the bereaved is nothing new, having long been the province of the philosopher, the pastor, or the physician, not to mention the average citizen who was close to a bereaved person. But, in the wake of Erich Lindemann's studies on loss and grief in the early 1940s,[125] there followed a steady stream of bereavement studies, from the work of Colin Murray Parkes to that of Beverley Raphael[126] and beyond; and ministering to the grief-stricken came to be energetically attended to in psychotherapeutic and general medical contexts. Consoling has been a key activity in much of this work, and yet it has been rare for the language of consolation to be used in the relevant writings. In fact, though there is no mistaking that consolation or the bringing of comfort has frequently been advocated and carried out, Raphael has been the exception in explicitly addressing the subject of consolation in her *Anatomy of Bereavement.*[127]

Consoling and the bringing of comfort to a sufferer are just about as old as our species. For all the evidence regarding man's inhumanity to man, the humane inclination to comfort a suffering fellow human is surely the more basic inclination. In fact, often enough, it seems that suffering is a form of need for another person — a need for a relationship with another. Fortunately, there is also this human inclination to respond with consolatory help.

From ancient Greece, we have considerable evidence to indicate that this human tendency developed into a variety of formal types of consolation. While consolation could be and was applied to many different kinds of misfortune, the literature that survives deals most commonly with bereavement and bringing comfort to the grief-stricken. From these roots developed comforting funeral orations, threnodies, consolatory letters, and consolatory treatises. Then came mourners' manuals, prayer manuals, comforting hymns, and guides to spiritual consolation. And other forms of literature came to serve consolatory purposes: poetry, essays, fiction, and biographies.

The ancient rhetor was called upon to provide consolation for those who had suffered loss. The philosopher as physician of the soul provided consolation as an element in the cure of souls. With the emergence of Christianity, the priest and the pastor became physicians of the soul, and a rich religious tradition of the cure of souls developed. The sense that a sufferer was in distress, sorrow, or even despair, and was in a painful state of aloneness, became common themes. Much effort was devoted to easing that sense of distressing aloneness. Prayers were undertaken both to ease the discomfort and to renew a sense of being in touch with God. Pastors also strove to re-establish a sense of connection with fellow humans for the sufferer.

In the realm of sin and confession, humans commonly felt themselves to be alienated from God and from their fellows; and the process of confession, penance, and seeking forgiveness involved the consolatory benefits of being reconciled with one's fellows and one's God. Spiritual consolations developed as means of coping with despair, desolation, and "being under desertion by God."[128] Repeatedly, consolation was directed toward undoing the experience of feeling despairingly alone through renewing a sense of connection with God. In the various mystical traditions, the person strove to achieve consolation through communion with God, through a sense of becoming one with God. Union with God was considered the ultimate consolation.

Visiting the sick and the dying has long been a recognized context for bringing comfort to sufferers who were fearful, sometimes isolated, and often threatened with a sense of death as the ultimate experience of separation and aloneness. Priests and pastors have always considered such ministering to be an inherent aspect of their pastoral care. Physicians have long had a similar opportunity, and they have often served their patients by bringing comfort in such situations. Rooted in the sympathy and compassion thought natural, they have been natural consolers.

After the emergence of the psychological healing known as psychotherapeutics, comfort and consolation tended no longer to be cited as elements in such clinical work. In the many psychotherapies of the twentieth century, too, there has been little explicit mention of them. But bringing comfort in one form or another has not been at all uncommon. In the various forms of supportive psychotherapy, reassurance, encouragement, and other comforting interventions have been explicitly recognized. In those therapies directed particularly toward bereaved persons, consolation and comfort have often been involved. Meeting up with empathic understanding — feeling truly understood — has been a significantly comforting experience for many a patient. And disturbed patients have frequently found the very establishment of a therapeutic relationship to be comforting. In fact, the relationship itself has proved reassuring or comforting in many instances where that issue was never even considered. Further, it would be the rare psychotherapist who has not met moments in which a patient has experienced a fear-ridden crisis or a grievous loss, and who has, however directly or indirectly, consoled or provided comfort in response.

In looking at the many centuries and many forms of psychological healing, it may be fair to conclude with an old French saying:

> Guérir quelquefois,
> Soulager souvent,
> Consoler toujours.

That is to say, "Cure sometimes, help often, To console (or comfort) always."[129]

PART FIVE

Healing and the Principle of Contraries

9

The Use of the Passions

This chapter is concerned with the instrumental use of the passions as agents to bring about the cure or amelioration of a disease. For many centuries this entailed inducing a passion to counter another passion that was thought to be an integral feature of the disease. Two versions of such therapeutic interventions were scattered through the centuries of medical literature and were to become particularly well known during the Renaissance. One was the displacing of the disturbing passion by inducing another passion. The other was the inducing of a passion opposite to the disturbing one in order to restore a balance in the passions of the mind.

To "rectify these passions and perturbations of the mind" was central to the therapeutics of severe mental disorders, according to Robert Burton, who so ably surveyed the Renaissance's clinical wisdom on mental illness. Rectifying the passions was "the chiefest cure," he said.[1] And the inducing of a passion or emotion was an important technique among the ways of achieving this rectification. As Burton put it, the idea was "to force out one nail with another, to drive out one passion with another, or by some contrary passion . . . to expel one fear with another, one grief with another."[2]

Although the precise origins and the course of development of these modes of treatment are difficult to discern through the mists of time, certain relevant patterns of thought can be detected. Ancient medicine's *principle of contraries* was important, and so was the *doctrine of opposites* on which it was based. Philosophical and medical writings on the *passions* constituted another important source of information for understanding these treatment practices. Then there were the *six things non-natural,* a framework for therapeutic considerations that involved the passions and perturbations of the soul.

To turn for a moment to the meaning of terms in the realm of the passions, it is specially helpful to borrow from Leland Rather who wrote about Thomas Wright's (1561–1623) *The Passions of the Minde in Generall* in the following way. The passions, Rather explains, had been commonly defined "as sensual motions of the appetitive faculty due to the imagination of some good or ill thing." Drawing on Augustine, Wright said that "the motions of the soul (*motus animae*) which the Greeks called *pathê* are called by certain Latins, as Cicero in the *Tusculan Disputations,* perturbations (*perturbationes*). Others called them affections (*affectiones*), others affects (*affectus*), and others expressly passions (*passiones*)." According to Rather, "although they are *acts* of the appetitive faculty," for Wright, "they are called passions . . . because when stirring in the mind they *cause* a passion or alteration in the humors of the body. . . . They are called perturbations because they corrupt the judgement and seduce the will, and affections because 'the soule by them, either affecteth some good, or for the affection of some good, detesteth some il(l).' The passions, then, are internal acts or operations of the soul, bordering on immaterial reason on one side and material sense on the other, 'prosecuting some good thing, or flying some ill thing, causing therewithall some alteration in the body.' "[3]

Contraria Contrariis Curantur

Sharing therapeutic prominence with the various evacuative remedies (cathartics, emetics, bloodletting, and so forth) aimed at reducing a pathological humoral excess, the many remedies based on the principle *contraria contrariis curantur* constituted a crucial portion of ancient therapeutics. Such remedies would have properties that were contrary to the properties of the disease. "Contraries are cured by contraries" or "opposites are cures for opposites," or the principle of contraries, is a theme that emerged clearly in the Hippocratic writings in the fifth and fourth centuries B.C. Against the background notion that "creation was made up of 'opposites,'" many scholars during classical antiquity employed schemes of opposite or contrasting qualities, most commonly "four in number — the hot, the cold, the moist and the dry."[4] The "commonest theory" among the physicians of ancient Greece, "derived no doubt from popular beliefs but expressed as a general doctrine in several Hippocratic texts," was that "opposites are a cure for opposites."[5] In

The Nature of Man, it was said that "diseases caused by over-eating are cured by fasting; those caused by starvation are cured by feeding up. Diseases caused by exertion are cured by rest; those caused by indolence are cured by exertion. To put it briefly: the physician should treat disease by the principle of opposition to the cause of the disease according to its form, its seasonal and age incidence, countering tenseness by relaxation and vice versa. This will bring the patient most relief and seems to me to be the principle of healing."[6]

Later, the principle of contraries was to run like a red thread through Galen's therapeutics, accounting for his many efforts to tailor his remedies so that their qualities were opposite to the qualities of the disease whose treatment was under discussion. In *De temperamentis* (On the temperaments), he developed his theory of temperaments in which the qualities were clearly the cardinal factors.[7] Taking the qualities as the basic conceptual links connecting the various categories, he arrived at therapeutic formulations regarding diet, exercise, medications, and so on, that were keyed to the disease and, at the same time, took into account the individual who had it, in terms of temperament, age, occupation, and the like. Regarding the disease, Galen's governing principle was the Hippocratic *contraria contrariis curantur,* for his remedies aimed at cooling the overheated, warming the chilled, and so forth, or employed a particular combination of qualities in a case where a combination of opposite qualities occurred in excess.[8] Regarding the patient, Galen emphasized the importance of taking individuality into account, advising that remedies be varied according to the nature of the patient and on the basis of similarity to that nature. Yet, while the contrariety of remedies was to be modified by some similarity to the nature of the patient, the basic nature of a remedy was still opposite to the unnatural features present in the patient (that is, to the qualities of the disease).[9]

Rather different from the Hippocratic-Galenic frame of reference was the system employed by the Methodists, in which the disease state was characterized as *status laxus* or *status strictus.* Yet, as the views of Soranus (early second century) make clear, that system still called for therapeutic measures opposite in nature to the prevailing state associated with a disease. In Methodist therapeutics, astringent and constricting remedies were indicated in an unduly relaxed state (status laxus), and relaxing remedies in an unduly tense and constricted state (status strictus).[10] Regarding madness in particular, Soranus advocated efforts to induce in the patient emotions opposite to those with which he was burdened in his sickness. The rationale was that "the particular characteristic of a case of mental disturbance must be corrected by emphasizing the opposite quality, so that the mental condition, too, may attain the balanced state of health."[11]

The Passions

From very early on, the passions or perturbations of the soul were often conceived of in a medical frame of reference. Sometimes they were symptoms in a disease, such as fear and sadness in melancholia. Sometimes they were thought of, in ways akin to a modern psychosomatic approach, as playing a role in the pathogenesis of a disease. And sometimes, they were viewed as states that needed to be influenced or changed in order to move away from disease and toward health. It was this view that provided the framework for inducing passions so that a balance might be restored or an unfortunate passion be replaced by a preferable one — *the rectification of the passions* was a significant element in many centuries of psychological healing. From classical antiquity onward, medicine thought of the passions as states of mind that could influence bodily processes, that might cause disease, and that could cure or modify disease.

In many other contexts, though, the passions were aspects of someone's philosophical views on human nature. Such writings frequently took the form of moral tracts in which it was argued that reason would guide people along a reasonable and virtuous path, unless some passion or other interfered and diverted them into unreason, unhappiness, or sin. In these contexts, passions were sometimes thought of as "diseases of the soul." These diseases of the soul did not usually turn up in medical writings among other diseases, but their appearance in philosophical contexts often entailed the use of a medical metaphor, implying that something was seriously amiss and that corrective measures were called for. And just as moral teachings and practices often came to have a treatment-like language and spirit, medical teachings and practices often acquired moral overtones. The dichotomies of virtuous and sinful, rational and irrational, and healthy and unhealthy were often closely associated, one with another; and each of them held a role in considerations of the passions.

For appreciation of the place of the passions in the various early medical and philosophical contexts, some brief attention to a few of the more influential early theories of the passions is warranted, particularly those of Plato, Aristotle, and the Stoics. For Plato, excesses of pain or pleasure amounted to diseases of the soul, in the sense that great distress or joy diminished a person's capacity to reason. The irrational aspects of the soul that were the wellsprings of appetite and of feeling were located in the abdominal region and in the chest, respectively, and were potential threats to or antagonists of the smooth functioning of the rational soul, located in the brain. The passions that derived from these irrational aspects of the soul were given meanings relating to the bodily conditions associated with them and so were associated with physiology and medical thought. And the ethical meanings given to the same passions placed them within philosophers' theories of the passions and provided the grounds for their inclusion in systems of moral consideration. From the lowest part of the soul (below the midriff) stemmed the various desires and appetites; from the spirited part of the soul (in the chest) came the affections or passions. Here we see the roots of the medieval classification of the concupiscible affections (the desires and appetites) and the irascible affections (the passions). Plato regarded the various passions in part as modifications of pleasure and pain, and in part as distinct from them. Joy and hope were categorized as species of pleasure, and grief and fear as species of pain, a scheme which anticipates the fourfold classification of the passions that was to emerge later.[12]

Aristotle enumerated various passions which he conceived of as occupying a category partway between faculties (or predisposing susceptibilities to such affective states) and formed habits (the results of the repeated exercise of said affects). Habits were capacities for behavior that had become fixed as features of character; in a sense, chronic affective tendencies had become established. While not proceeding to the Stoic conclusion that passions should be suppressed, Aristotle did think that they ought to be brought under conscious control. In general, they were states accompanied by pleasure or pain, even thought of as species of pleasure or pain; but they differed from pleasure and pain in that they were more complex, were "motions of the soul" and not mere complements of a function. He conceived of "somatic passions," which seemed to be the pains of want and the pleasures of replenishment of the appetites, and of other passions, other pleasures and pains, which were of the soul. That some passions were defined as pains or perturbations of the soul did not imply that they were not rooted in bodily processes. Some were described as having origins in both a psychological process and the person's physiological processes. Anger, for example, was defined as a propensity toward retaliation and as an ebullition of the blood about the heart.[13]

In contrast to the Aristotelian belief that the passions should be controlled, the Stoics tended to think that they should be done away with. They viewed them as perverted judgments, except in the case of the wise man (who was knowlegeable, calm, not subject to emotional turbulence). The Stoics sought inner peace as the basic good and thought of the passions as disorders of the soul, disturbing to reason and contrary to nature. The passions were now defined as "diseases of the soul analogous to those of the body" and thought to be distinguishable from one another both in their predisposing temperament and in the nature of the disease itself. Nevertheless, the Stoics allowed a class of "good affections," grouped under cheerfulness, discreetness, and a virtuous habit of will; these were "species of quiet emotion befitting the wise" in contrast to the turbulent passions. They also recognized two other categories of emotions: "the natural affections arising from kinship, companionship, etc.," which were viewed favorably; and "the physical pleasures and pains as distinguished from the elation or depression of mind attending them," which were pleasures and pains viewed "as at least necessary." For the Stoics, in addition to the *feeling state,* the passion involved an *impulse* toward or away from an object and a *judgment* about that object. Their scheme of things allowed for four basic passions: (1) appetite or desire, an irrational inclination toward, implying an opinion of good to come; (2) fear, an irrational recoil from, implying an opinion of impending evil that seems intolerable; (3) pleasure or delight or joy, an irrational expansion or elation of mind, implying a recent opinion of present good; and (4) pain or grief or sadness, an irrational contraction or depression of mind, implying a recent opinion of a present evil. Then, under these four fundamental passions, various Stoics grouped lists of individual affections and emotional dispositions.[14] From those times to the end of the seventeenth century, writers tended to follow the Stoics in seeking to reduce, classify, and logically define the passions.[15]

Like Plato and the Aristotelian writers, the Stoics gave more or less explicit recognition to the physiological roots of the affections. Whereas those earlier authors had evoked the humors and the qualities when considering the bodily conditions associated with the passions, the Stoics tended to think of an enervated pneuma, a most subtle material substance, as the bodily concomitant of the troubled states of the soul that were the passions; but some Stoics expressed notions of dispositions of temperament in terms of the humoralists' qualities. And, for the most part, the Stoics followed the tradition that held that the passions had their seat in the heart.

The Six Non-Naturals

Of special relevance for attention to the passions in the history of therapeutics is the scheme of the *six things non-natural* or the six non-naturals. The term *non-naturals* (not innate) was used to refer to a group of acquired factors, usually six in number, the careful management of which was thought to be crucial to health in the sense later referred to as *hygiene,* and any of which could cause disease if imbalance or disproportion obtained. The six non-naturals were usually air, exercise and rest, sleep and wakefulness, food and drink, (imbalanced) excretion and retention of superfluities, and the passions or perturbations of the soul. As Rather put it, the doctrine of the non-naturals "may be stated briefly as follows: *there are six categories of factors that operatively determine health or disease, depending on the circumstances of their use or abuse, to which human beings are unavoidably exposed in the course of daily life.* Management of the regimen of the patient, that is, of his involvement with these six sets of factors, was for centuries the physician's most important task."[16]

Probably having its origins in a set of factors listed by Galen in his *Ars medica,* this scheme became a standard and significant part of later versions of Galenic medicine. The term *non-natural* came into common use only in the wake of Latin translations of Arabic works largely based on Galen,[17] but *non-natural* was used in works on the pulse by Galen,[18] who seemed to imply that both the term and the classification of six non-natural factors antedated him.[19]

The non-naturals continued to receive significant attention in medical works well into the eighteenth century, and eventually concerns about such matters evolved into the precepts of the physical and moral (psychological) hygiene of more recent times. The doctrine, although it ranked alongside the humoral theory as a significant system of thought for the explanation of both health and disease, remained in active use well beyond the demise of the humoral theory. The non-naturals were frequently given careful attention during consideration of the pathogenesis of a disease and in the outlining of therapeutic plans. In particular, the doctrine's category of the passions or perturbations of the soul provided a crucial means by which the passions could be taken into account in explaining a disease and in undertaking its treatment.

Rectifying the Passions

Although Aristotle was not the first to contribute to a theory of the passions, it seems very likely that the roots of the therapeutic approaches under consideration here are to be found in his writings. At least, Aristotle's views are highly relevant to understanding the evolution of "rectifying the passions." In his *Rhetoric,* in the process of considering the tactics of persuasion and the art of playing upon the emotional susceptibilities of a listener, he undertook an extended discussion of the passions or emotions.[20] He defined emotions or passions as "all those feelings that so change men as to affect their judgements, and that are also attended by pain or pleasure. Such are anger, pity, fear and the like, with their opposites." Emphasizing the importance of a careful study of any passion that one wishes to arouse in a person, he proceeded to discuss a series of them in detail, setting them up in pairs of opposites and thus adumbrating the many later lists and classifications of the passions. He paid some attention to how one might produce or dissipate a passion, and to how one passion might be employed to prevent or neutralize another.

During the centuries that followed, down through the Renaissance and even later, numerous lists and classifications of the passions adhered to his practice of grouping them as pairs of opposites. Pairs of contrasting passions became a commonplace in works studying the nature and function of the emotions in human life. The list of basic affections varied in length, though the most common number was four. Most often it was *desire* contrasted with *fear,* and *joy* contrasted with *sorrow.* Deriving from the Stoics' principles, the contrast between pairs of passions became common, one passion supposedly tending toward good and one turning away from evil: for example, pleasure or joy might lead the soul toward a good and pain or sadness might lead the soul away from an evil. Also, one set of passions in such a classification would be related to a present good or evil, and another set to an anticipated or future good or evil. Further, those passions that we might term positive, such as joy and desire, were thought to dilate the heart, and those that we might term negative, such as sadness and fear, were thought to contract or constrict the heart. From these classificatory schemes reflecting the ancient doctrine of opposites, it was only a short step to determining the opposite of a particular troubling passion and so its natural antidote, and from there to attempting to induce that opposite passion in order to replace the unwanted passion with a preferable one, or to return an imbalance in the passions to a state of equilibrium. As with the other factors among the six non-naturals, the passions of the soul might be thought to be in disproportion or imbalance; and so another passion might need to be induced to restore a balance or equilibrium. That is to say, passions might well be thought of as symptoms in a disease, and they might equally well be used or prescribed for therapeutic purposes. With the regimen developed for a patient often considered to be as important as the medications prescribed, and with the passions being among the non-naturals that were the basis for a regimen, the passions were commonly taken into account in therapeutic planning. The theme of rectification was an inherent aspect of the centuries of advice on the regimen, and the term or one of its cognates became familiar in such advice.

Probably the earliest established advocacy of inducing passions as a corrective measure in the medical treatment of a disease that involved troublesome passions is one found in the writings of Soranus. As noted earlier, in the treatment of madness he advised efforts to induce in the patient emotions opposite to those associated with the sickness so that a balanced state of health might be achieved.[21] This was in a context of advocating therapeutic measures that constituted a regimen for the patient, and that would later come to be thought of as attention to the non-naturals.

For all the centrality of the principle of contraries in Galen's therapeutics, just how he applied it to the passions is unclear. With regard to the various mental disorders recognized in his day, it was not uncommon for him to take the passions into account as symptoms—for example, fear and sorrow in melancholia. Yet he does not appear to have directed his therapeutic measures toward the passions themselves. Although his advocacy of the enlivening effects of dramatic poetry and music is suggestive of efforts to counter melancholia's particular passions, there is no clear indication that Galen saw himself as directly opposing a contrary passion to a troublesome one.

Nevertheless, in *On the Passions of the Soul* and in *On the Errors of the Soul*, Galen did advocate measures directly aimed at the passions. In those works he considered the passions themselves to be "disorders" or "diseases" of the soul and to be in need of "treatment." But those various terms essentially reflected the use of a medical metaphor in contexts where Galen was writing as a moral philosopher who favored the eradication of the passions, or at least a careful control of them. The passions were viewed as "errors of the soul" that were in need of correction, and he was reflecting elements of the Stoic tradition. In those particular writings Galen, as a "physician of the soul," was addressing the "diseases of the soul," in the spirit in which those terms were used in the philosophy of ancient Greece and Rome. Still, though, he thought that the passions of the irascible power might be enlisted or aroused in order to counter the passions of the concupiscible power.[22] In the passage in question, he conceived of "an instrumental role" for the passions in the correction of a distressed or disordered state.[23]

Not long after Galen, contraria contrariis curantur and its application to the "treatment" of troublesome passions gradually found their way into still another tradition, namely, the Christian tradition of the "cure of souls." In his studies of medieval handbooks of penance, John T. McNeill identified the frequent application of the principle of contraries in the advice to confessors ("spiritual physicians" or "physicians of the soul") regarding how they should guide and prescribe for their penitents, passions being prominent among the sicknesses of the soul with which they dealt.[24] For example, Finnian (ca. 525–550) wrote, "By contraries . . . let us make haste to cure contraries and to cleanse away the faults from our hearts and introduce virtues in their places." Then he cited wrathfulness, envy, dejection, and greed as states to be prescribed for in this fashion.[25] Such practices have been traced back to John Cassian (ca. 360–435), who had noted that "the cure for other ailments, viz. anger, vexation, and impatience, has been shown to consist in opposing to them their contraries."[26] In fact, "the whole treatment of sins in the works of Cassian seems largely in accord with this precept."[27] Further, McNeill pointed out that contraria contrariis curantur was to be found "in many patristic treatises," and argued that this "was apparently derived by the Fathers, who were fond of medical analogies in the cure of souls, from the teaching of the 'methodist' school of physicians."[28] Associated with Themison of Laodicea (ca. 50 B.C.), the Methodist school and its use of the principle of contraries had become particularly prominent with Soranus of Ephesus in the early second century A.D.

In the centuries that followed the times of Soranus and Galen, the Aristotelian suggestion that one passion might be induced in order to counter another became an accepted notion in the treatment of madness and mental distress. In conditions that involved disturbing passions, it was advised that the attention to a regimen (that is, to the non-naturals) for the patient should include the arousal of passions opposite to the troublesome ones, such as heat-inducing anger for the cold, frightened person or heat-inducing joy for the cold, sad person. In these instances, the anger or the joy promoted the movement of blood and its warmth from the heart out to the cold periphery of the body. Similarly, worry and fear might be induced in the too joyful, too excited, or too angry person, as blood was returned toward the heart and the overheated body was usefully cooled. In his *Liber Regius,* Haly Abbas (tenth century A.D.) addressed such matters in the final chapter ("De anime accidentibus") of book 5, all thirty-eight chapters of which were devoted to the "things not natural." He gave particular attention to anger, joy, worry, sadness, torpor, fear, and shame.[29] And it was not at all unusual in the writings of Islamic physicians to find accounts of stratagems employed to arouse various passions (particularly fear, shock, and shame) with an eye to healing bodily diseases.[30]

Such attention to the passions in developing a treatment plan became increasingly common during the later medieval centuries. The regulation or modification of the passions in the context of an individualized regimen for a patient became a well-recognized practice, as they were attended to along with the other "six things non-natural." By the late thirteenth century, it was thought that "since the passions most certainly affect health, it is the physician's duty to watch carefully for their influence"; and medical thought on the passions included making "use of them in effecting cures."[31] Further, "medical discussions of the passions" came to be one of "the sources of the focus on man's nature usually thought of as characteristic of Renaissance humanism."[32]

By the sixteenth century, references to the passions as potentially instrumental in correcting troubled states of mind were being made both by physicians in their treatment regimes and by moral philosophers in their prescriptions for "diseases of the soul," in ways that suggest a familiar practice. That one passion might be used to drive out another was becoming a commonplace. In the early sixteenth century, Henry Cornelius Agrippa (1486?–1535) noted that "the passions of the soul" could "take away" as well as "bring some diseases of the mind or body."[33] Later in the century, in devising a regimen for a sufferer in the grip of a distressing passion, Timothy Bright (1550?–1615) advised that, where "other perswasion" has not helped, "a vehement passion, of another sort is to be kindeled, that may withdrawe that vaine and foolish sorowe . . . as of anger, or some feare ministred by another occasion, then that which first was authour of this sadnesse." In this way the new passion "rebateth the force of it which gave first occasion, and as one pinne is driven out with another, so the later may expell the former."[34]

At the end of the century, Felix Platter (1536–1614) provided in his medical textbook both a faithful reflection of sixteenth-century practice and, in light of the several editions of the book, an indication of views that remained influential throughout the seventeenth century. In the process of considering the treatment of "Alienation of the Mind," he carefully catalogued "the perturbations or commotions of the mind." Then, after taking note of other possible psychological interventions to heal disturbing passions, he stated, "But principally in some *passions of the mind* it brings a great deal of help, to move *the Affections of the Mind which are contrary to this affect* that troubles, and so to bring them into a contrary passion, seeing they do bring them to a mean, as contraries are wont to be cured by contraries." He then listed a number of passions that might be particularly troublesome and the contrary passions that should be induced as their antidotes or cures.[35]

With the proliferation of Renaissance works on human nature and prescriptions for behavior, systematic attention to the passions became common indeed. Notable among the seventeenth-century treatises that continued the trend was Wright's *The Passions of the Minde in Generall,* mentioned earlier. Where passions were particularly "vehement" or "outragious," a number of means, which Wright took note of, might "mortifie" or "moderate" them. As one approach to a troublesome passion, he mentioned arranging that "some other passion expelleth it."[36] As he also put it, it was a question of turning "the force of thy soule with as much indeavour as thou canst to the contrarie, and with one naile drive out another."[37]

As noted at the beginning of this chapter, Robert Burton referred to the practice of cure through contrary passions, using the same phrasing as Bright and Wright had of forcing one nail out with another. Within his encyclopedic history of melancholia was embedded a lengthy treatise on the passions and perturbations of the mind, in which he acquitted himself as a moral philosopher more Augustinian than Stoic.[38] Then, in his Partition on treatment, again addressing the passions at length, he included the contrary cure among the various modes of rectifying the passions.[39]

Another significant example of the growing number of works on the passions was *A Treatise of the Passions and Faculties of the Soule of Man* by Edward Reynolds (1599–1676), first published in 1640 and reissued several times later in the century. That work provided a particularly felicitous account of the use of the passions in psychological healing and explicitly noted Aristotle's influence on this tradition. In discussing measures that might be taken to alleviate disorders that "darken the serenitie of mans Mind," he wrote,

> This is done, either by *opposing contrary Passions to contrary;* which is *Aristotles* rule, who adviseth, in the bringing of *Passions* from an *extreame* to a *mediocritie,* . . . or else it is done, by *scattering* and *distracting* of them; and that not onely by the power of *Reason,* but sometimes also by a cautelous *admixture of Passions* amongst themselves, thereby interrupting their free current . . . in the Mind, *Passions,* as they mutually *generate,* so they mutually *weaken* each other. . . . in the *Passions* of the *Mind;* when any of them are *excessive,* the way to *remit* them, is by admitting of some further *perturbation* from others, and so *distracting* the *forces* of the former: Whether the *Passions* we *admit,* be *contrarie* . . . or whether they be *Passions* of a *different,* but not of a *repugnant* nature.[40]

And this theme appeared recurrently in medical writings on the treatment of madness during the rest of the seventeenth century and throughout the eighteenth century.

In his *Two Discourses Concerning the Soul of Brutes* in 1672, Thomas Willis (1621–1675) advised that "the affections of the mind being vehement, and stirred up from thence, are either to be appeased, or subdued by others opposite. Wherefore, to desperate Love ought to be applied or shewed indignation and hatred; Sadness is to be opposed with the flatteries of Pleasure, Musick, a desire of vain glory, or also a *pannick* terror. In like manner, as to the rest of the Passions, you must proceed to quiet, or elude them."[41]

The eighteenth-century status of these psychological measures was reflected in the views of Herman Boerhaave (1668–1738), who so widely influenced Western medicine throughout the century. His clinical writings, enhanced by the commentaries of his student and assistant, Gerard Van Swieten (1700–1772), were considered a prime source of clinical wisdom and included attention to the techniques for "rectifying the passions." In his *Aphorisms* in 1708, Boerhaave took note of "exciting the contrary passions" in a way that suggested its accepted status. In outlining remedies for "Diseases . . . from the Excess of the Circulatory Motion," he stated that "some relate to the mind, others to the body," adding that "of the former sort are such as well asswage any great passion by reasoning, by exciting a contrary passion or diverting it."[42] These three familiar psychological strategies were discussed in more detail by Van Swieten, who commented that it was "a circumstance of great advantage to know what affections are opposite to each other." In this context he specially considered fear and anger as opposites that could be used as antidotes to one another, and observed that these two passions produced opposite changes in the body. Further, that "one affection of the mind may be a cure for another" could be "shewn of the other opposite passions."[43] Then, in considering "the melancholy-madness," Boerhaave wrote that "the first indication" in treatment was "to excite the juices of the brain and nerves to motion, to increase them in quantity, and reduce them into an orderly distribution." Among the familiar psychological approaches to bring about this result, he advocated "introducing cautiously passions of the mind that are of an opposite nature to that of the prevailing melancholy."[44] In his *Commentaries,* Van Swieten referred to "how serviceable it may be to allay disorders raised in the body, by exciting opposite passions in the mind," and continued, "Thus sudden fear quells the heating rage of an angry person; and on the contrary, a timorous man is by anger rendered bold, or daring. Whence it appears, that a prudent rouzing of the passions in the mind, that are of a nature contrary to the patient's melancholy, may be highly serviceable to its cure." He then cited two instances of applying this principle with severely disturbed persons.[45]

Whether one looks at these modes of psychological healing through the eyes of Reynolds, the clergyman whose moral treatise addressed the nature of man and the cure of souls, or through the eyes of Boerhaave, the physician whose medical treatise addressed the healing of both mind and body, one readily recognizes the Aristotelian tradition handed down over so many centuries. The familiar references to pairs of opposite passions are there.[46] Comments to the effect that the healer might either arouse a contrary passion to restore a balanced state of mind or employ one passion to disperse another continued to be made. Whether the language was that of too warm passions and too cool passions, or of an excess of circulatory motion and a deficit of circulatory motion, the theme of excited passions versus subdued passions persisted. And in Boerhaave, the notion that the induction of these psychological states was a ready means of influencing bodily states bespoke a "psychosomatic" orientation that was no new thing even then, though Galenic rather than Aristotelian in its roots. The continuing influence of these views and healing modes was to be found throughout the eighteenth century.

In his *Medicinal Dictionary,* an influential medical encyclopedia published in the 1740s, Robert James (1705–1776) was following Boerhaave very closely when among his treatment recommendations for melancholia he advised "inducing cautiously another Disposition, or Affectation of the Mind, opposite to Melancholy."[47]

In 1758, William Battie (1703–1776), in *A Treatise on Madness,* commented that "if . . . any one particular passion seems to engross the man or continues beyond its usual period, in such case the discretion of the Physician must determine how far it may be adviseable or safe to stifle it by a contrary passion. . . . [Also demanding care was] *unwearied attention to any one object, as love, grief, and despair;* any of these affections will sometimes be annihilated by the tumultuous but less dangerous and sooner subsiding passions of anger and joy."[48]

A student, colleague, and successor of Boerhaave distinguished in his own right, Jerome Gaub (1705–1780), in the second of two significant lectures on "the mutual relations of mind and body in health and disease" in 1763, dealt with the mind and the emotions as causative factors in bodily diseases and as potentially curative factors.[49] Gaub reflected a holistic orientation true to a long-standing tradition and little affected by Descartes, and an easy interactionism of a traditional rather than Cartesian nature. In modern terms, he readily took a psychosomatic, as well as a somatopsychic, perspective. In these and other ways he was quite representative of eighteenth-century medical thought. "Gaub regards an emotion first and foremost as a disturbance of the *mind.* The disturbance is then transmitted to the body, where it gives rise to characteristic effects, harmful or beneficial depending on the circumstances."[50] Gaub took up a series of the passions in turn, detailing their potentially deleterious effects on the body and outlining their use as curative measures. He did not focus on the use of one passion to displace another or neutralize a contrary passion, but he wrote with the assumption that opposite passions had opposite bodily effects and thus that the passion to be induced therapeutically was chosen on the basis of the wished-for opposite effects that it was known to produce. And these clinical considerations were taken into account in the treatment of mental disorders as well as physical disorders.

In Gaub's work are indications of an increased complexity in the cure by "contrary passions." From the simpler notion of the troublesome passion as the symptom, or even as the disorder, that needs therapeutic correction, the concept of the contrary cure had grown to include the troublesome bodily effects and bodily diseases that each passion was thought to cause. This expanded notion meant that a set of disturbing bodily effects or a particular bodily disease might be the basis for the therapeutic induction of a passion that would stimulate the opposite bodily effects. In this way the disturbing bodily effects were neutralized and the sufferer was returned to a balanced state or a state of improved health.

In 1768, in a volume devoted to the place of "regimen" or "management" in the gaining and maintaining of good health, Francis de Valangin (1725–1805) nicely illustrated the conceptual context and therapeutic scheme that for so long had been the "home" for attention to disturbing passions. This treatise on "the management of human life" dealt with that familiar array of factors "by Physicians called the Six Non-Naturals." In his section on "the Affections of the Mind," emphasizing the critical importance of the passions in human life, he stated that "they are, in the moral World, what Motion is in the physical World."[51] The too vehement or otherwise troublesome passion, though, required special attention. "Passions of the Mind are not easily cured by Medicines, but by contrary Passions; Anger and Hope remove Fear; Joy removes Sorrow; and Sorrow removes Joy."[52] In summing up this lengthy section, de Valangin indicated just how significant this doctrine "of very antient date" still was when he remarked, "It appears from what we have said of the Affections of the Mind, that contrary Passions produce opposite Effects in the animal Economy; and that one Affection of the Mind is frequently a Cure for another, that the Sympathy of the Body with the Mind is amazing."[53]

The Passions in Nineteenth-Century Healing

Thus, by the late eighteenth century, it had become common indeed to give detailed attention to the passions. The previous two hundred years had produced scores of works on the subject — religious treatises and works of moral philosophy, philosophical writings on the nature of man, and medical discussions of the passions and their role in pathogenesis and treatment. But the therapeutic use of the passions had come to range far beyond merely inducing one passion to neutralize or displace another. Many different diseases — and not just mental disorders — were thought to be amenable to cure or at least amelioration through the induction of the appropriate passion. Some indication of these trends and the keen interest in them was manifested by the Medical Society of London when, in 1786, it proposed the following question as the topic for its essay prize: "What diseases may be mitigated or cured, by exciting particular affections or passions of the mind?" In his prize-winning essay, William Falconer (1744–1824) discussed at length the passions as either stimulants or sedatives in the cure of a variety of diseases, with the principle of contraries as his guide.[54] Monographs such as Clement Joseph Tissot's (1750–1826) *De l'influence des passions* in 1798[55] and a scattering of dissertations for the M.D. degree at the beginning of the nineteenth century attested further to the interest in the topic during that era.[56]

At the same time, an increasingly significant status was being accorded the passions or emotions in the realm of philosophy. In an emerging tradition, it was argued among eighteenth-century German philosophers that emotion or feeling should be viewed as a distinct and separate faculty. In reaction against Lockean sensationalism and the associationism connected with it, a new faculty psychology was being developed. Largely out of their concerns with aesthetics, Johann Georg Sulzer (1720–1779), Moses Mendelssohn (1729–1786), and Johann Nicolaus Tetens (1736–1807) advocated recognition of an importance and a distinct status for feeling that had hitherto been mainly reserved for knowing or understanding.[57] Immanuel Kant (1724–1804) continued the trend, effectively affirmed the new status assigned the emotions, and took matters a step further, establishing in the 1780s a new triadic scheme of faculties: knowing, feeling, willing.[58] Accordingly, it is Kant who has usually been credited with the origin of the modern three-faculty system of understanding-emotion-will or cognition-affection-conation.[59]

Further, though, the changes occurring in affective psychology gradually brought significant changes in "the psychopathology of affectivity." Given that emotion was increasingly recognized as a distinct and separate faculty of the mind, it became conceivable that some mental disorders might reflect a disturbance in that faculty alone. An "affective disorder" was now possible.[60] Although earlier the faculty of imagination and the faculty of reason had each been thought to be the locus of primary damage in certain forms of madness, the influence of John Locke's (1632–1704) sensationalism had moved eighteenth-century opinion more in the direction of the reason or intellect as the essential locus of damage in madness. But, by the end of the century, Philippe Pinel had developed serious reservations on this point. He noted that "paroxysms of madness are generally no more than irascible emotions prolonged beyond their ordinary limits; and the true character of such paroxysms depends, perhaps, more frequently upon the various influences of the passions, than upon any derangement of ideas, or upon any whimsical singularities of the judging faculty."[61] He put forward quite clearly the notion that some disorders might be limited to the realm of the understanding and others to the realm of the passions. "The powers of perception and imagination are frequently disturbed without any excitement of the passions. The functions of the understanding on the other hand, are often perfectly sound, while the man is driven by his passions to acts of turbulence and outrage."[62] And he represented the reservations many had regarding Locke's views, meanwhile reasserting the existence of purely affective disorders. "We may very justly admire the writings of Mr. Locke, without admitting his authority upon subjects not necessarily connected with his enquiries. On resuming at Bicêtre my researches into this disorder [madness], I thought, with the above author, that it was inseparable from delirium [deranged understanding]; and, I was not a little surprized to find many maniacs who at no period gave evidence of any lesion of the understanding, but who were under the dominion of instinctive and abstract fury, as if the affective faculties alone sustained the injury."[63] When he turned to therapeutic considerations, Pinel made it clear that "the art of counteracting the human passions by others of equal or superior force" continued to be a significant mode of treatment. He advocated employing passions to counter passions in various instances of insanity and emphasized that this "doctrine in ethics" was still "an important department of medicine."[64]

Shortly after the appearance of Pinel's *Treatise on Insanity,* his student, Jean-Etienne-Dominique Esquirol (1772–1840), argued for careful attention to the passions in mental disorders and served notice of things to come, with the publication of *Des passions, considérées comme causes, symptômes et moyens curatifs de l'aliénation mentale,* his inaugural thesis which he had successfully presented to l'Ecole de Médecine in Paris.[65] Both his teacher's views and those prevalent during the eighteenth century regarding the passions as cause and cure of mental disorders were reflected in this work. Later, in his *Des maladies mentales,* Esquirol wrote of "the employment of the passions," as an aspect of moral treatment. "We must oppose, and conquer the most obstinate resolutions, inspiring the patient with a passion, stronger than that which controls his reason. . . . Each melancholic should be treated on principles resulting from a thorough acquaintance with the tendency of his mind, his character and habits, in order to subjugate the passion which, controlling his thoughts, maintains his delirium. . . . A sudden, strong, and unexpected emotion, a surprise, fear and terror, have sometimes been successful."[66] Further, in Esquirol's writings, as in Pinel's, there are clear indications that the traditional attention to the passions in the treatment of mental disorders had now become an integral part of their moral treatment.[67]

A contemporary of Esquirol, Johann Christian Heinroth (1773–1843), was closer to Pinel than to Esquirol in his unequivocal assertion that some mental disorders were the result of primary damage in the realm of emotion rather than of the intellect. In addressing the topic of the *idée fixe,* the fixed preoccupation of melancholic patients that so often developed to become the delusional focus of their concerns, he disagreed with the traditional view that it reflected a primary harm to the intellect or understanding. Starting from that premise, he argued that "it is the disposition which is seized by some depressing passion, and then has to follow it, and since this passion then becomes the dominating element, the intellect is forced by the disposition to retain certain ideas and concepts."[68] Against a background that allowed for an "affective disorder," Heinroth recurrently referred to the passions and "the disposition" as crucial elements in a person's becoming mentally ill, and he advocated psychological measures to influence the passions, as a crucial aspect of treatment. He also took note of "the treatment by opposites of the opposite morbid conditions of the psyche, in as far as their affections are *gradual,* for both exaltation or depression."[69]

The trends of the late eighteenth and early nineteenth centuries continued into the later nineteenth century without dramatic changes. Although an emphasis on madness as basically a derangement of the intellect was still predominant, indications recurred that the notion of it as a primary affective disorder had been retained. Both careful attention to emotions as symptoms requiring treatment and the induction of emotions for therapeutic purposes continued to be elements integrated into the treatment endeavors subsumed under the rubric *moral treatment.* Explicit reference to the "contrary passion" technique continued to be relatively infrequent, and yet it continued to be alluded to by implication in works on the place of the passions in healing.[70]

Some important observations on the place of emotions in treatment were made by Ernst von Feuchtersleben (1806–1849) in a work on medical psychology. "Feeling is most frequently acted upon for" purposes of psychological healing, "and, indeed generally, according to the scheme of 'pleasure and displeasure,' especially the individual feelings. . . . Pleasure and displeasure are employed in therapeutical psychagogics as reward and punishment; content should follow quiet behavior, pain, turbulent behavior."[71] He also noted that "in sensitive individuals and in acute cases, where psychical symptoms predominate," the excitement of emotions invariably afforded "a safe and often a decisive aid, in carrying out the psychical cure." He recognized the theme of cure by "contrary passions," adding, "Of course, in sthenic cases of psychical activity, it is preferable to employ depressing emotions; for instance, fear and horror (the latter always with great caution), and in asthenic cases, exciting emotions; as, for instance, enthusiasm. There are many instances of the cure of psycho-physical states by means of emotions."[72]

In his essay on "the remedial influence of mind" in the 1850s, Dendy noted that "it were not difficult to construct . . . an allopathic table of psychological antagonisms — opposing, for instance, the effects of anxiety, or pride, fear, melancholy, envy, hatred, remorse, by devotion, cheerfulness, self-control, piety: *contraria contrariis curantur.*"[73] He then proceeded to illustrate this principle with numerous instances of psychological healing. Also in the 1850s, in contributions to the leading British textbook of psychological medicine, John Charles Bucknill (1817–1897) made the point that both mental disorders and some physical disorders were "susceptible of cure by an opposing emotion."[74]

Somewhat later, Tuke, in his *Influence of the Mind upon the Body,* gave particular attention to the role of the imagination in psychological healing, but he also focused at some length on the role of the emotions. After first presenting a series of chapters illustrating the place of the emotions in influencing "bodily functions, both in exciting their physiological and pathological action,"[75] he systematically reviewed the evidence for "the influence of mental states upon disorders of sensation, motion, and the organic functions," indicating as he went the place of the imagination and of induced emotion in the successful treatment of these bodily disorders.[76] He then continued on in a chapter on "psycho-therapeutics" in which he considered the influence of the physician on the patient in exciting therapeutically useful mental states such as the emotions, and enlarged his scope to include the treatment of nervous affections and mental disorders.[77] The use of the emotions in healing had become a crucial element in the emerging field of psychotherapeutics.

During the last decades of the nineteenth century, it became rare to refer explicitly to the cure by "contrary passions" or to the therapeutic displacement of one emotion by another, although such modes of treatment might be taken into account in implicit fashion, as they were in Tuke's work. It was still acceptable medical wisdom to refer to the stirring up of particular emotions to cure particular bodily diseases, as illustrated in Tuke's work, but explicit references gradually waned in medical writings. Emotions in psychological healing took on new forms in the realm of "psycho-therapeutics" or "suggestive therapeutics." Disturbing emotional states could be eased or removed by suggestion; suggestion could introduce beneficial emotional states; and further, there were those who thought that emotion was a crucial factor in the very process of suggestion.[78] As the various forms of expressive therapy began to find their place among psychotherapeutic endeavors—such as the catharsis or abreaction of Breuer and Freud's early work, and the free association of Freud's later work—it became a question, at first, of "allowing . . . strangulated affect to find a way out through speech,"[79] and later, of the release of repressed or otherwise avoided emotion.[80] The facilitation of "emotional arousal" would eventually come to be a significant feature of a wide range of psychotherapies; and some of them would carry this facilitation to the extreme of "emotional flooding."[81]

In discussing the basic change agents in psychotherapy, Toksoz B. Karasu has concluded that "affective experiencing" has been a crucial factor. This "affective experiencing" has served to set "the emotional stage for receptivity to change." And "some form of affective experiencing appears to be universally applicable, but perhaps largely as a preliminary stage of treatment."[82] In considering affects in psychotherapy, Donald J. Carek reasons that they have a central and critical role in the psychodynamic psychotherapies, and that an affectively tinged caring and helpful therapeutic relationship is vital. After surveying a range of psychotherapeutic techniques, he concludes that they "regularly imply a role of affect in the psychotherapeutic process with a resultant need to address it in psychotherapeutic strategies." In a summary observation, he states that "the one basic psychotherapeutic function to strive for in psychotherapy, the one basic task to assume is the mobilization and mastery of affect. Much else may and does follow but substantial things happen in and out of therapy only with development of a greater capacity to deal with affect and associated emotional issues."[83]

In brief, by the time the twentieth century was under way, treatment by "contrary passions" or the displacement of one emotion by another belonged to the past. And the induction of specific emotions as agents to cure specific disorders had faded from the scene. Nevertheless, the mobilization of affect had become a significant part of the process in a wide variety of psychotherapies. Emotion had come to be thought of as part of the problem in various new and different ways; and, although emotions were no longer seen as therapeutic agents in themselves, dealing with emotions was part of several new therapeutic solutions.

10

The Use of the Imagination

The imagination served for many centuries as a key element in certain modes of psychological healing of insane and otherwise severely troubled persons. Often enough, this role was extended to a broader range of ailments in a way reminiscent of a modern psychosomatic orientation. Considerable evidence indicates that healing images have been commonly used in shamanistic healing practices across a wide range of cultures[1] and in healing endeavors associated with many religious traditions — in Judaism, Christianity, Islam, and Far Eastern religions.[2] And as the background to their place in Western psychological therapeutics, the imagination and its images have a long and complex history as crucial elements in various schemes of faculties, powers, or functions of the soul or mind.

By the fifteenth and sixteenth centuries, the faculty of imagination was part of a well-established system of faculties in Western thought. This system had evolved gradually, with numerous variations, from its roots in classical Greek thought. And the scheme that I am about to outline is composed of the more common variations. The *vegetative faculty* (or soul) accounted for nutrition, growth, and generation, and human beings shared it with all living matter; the *sensitive faculty* (or soul) accounted for sensation, motion, and the emotions, and human beings shared it with other animals. Exclusive to humankind was the *rational faculty* (or soul), composed of "three speciall powers and faculties

. . . the Imagination, Reason and Memorie."[3] This trio of souls or tripartite soul was commonly conceived of as three aspects of a single, undivided soul, and yet the three were often discussed as though they might be quite separate entities. Three of the bodily organs were frequently associated with these three aspects of the soul, as both their locale and the organ that served their purposes: the liver was associated with the vegetative soul, the heart with the sensitive soul, and the brain with the rational soul. The theory of the *pneuma,* or spirit, provided the means whereby these souls conveyed their influences and brought about their effects. From the vegetative soul and the liver, derived the *natural spirits;* from the sensitive soul and the heart, the *vital spirits;* and from the rational soul and the brain, the *animal spirits.*

With roots in ancient notions such as "seeing with the mind" (Empedocles), the "eye of the soul" (Plato), and the "picture in the mind" (Aristotle), the concept of the imagination evolved within the framework of the three faculties or functions of the rational soul: *imagination, reason,* and *memory.*[4] These were Aristotle's faculties of the soul that were "beyond sensation" — the "post-sensationary faculties," as Harry A. Wolfson termed them. It was this triad that Galen took up in the second century as "the leading functions or ruling faculties of the soul." They came to be called the internal senses, the inward senses, the inward wits, or the spiritual senses, as distinct from the external senses or corporeal senses (vision, hearing, smell, taste, touch). The commonest number was three, with the *common sense* sometimes conceived of as a fourth internal sense and sometimes combined with the imagination.[5] And in a scheme of cerebral localization that appears to date back to Nemesius (born A.D. 340), the imagination was thought to be localized in the anterior cell (our lateral ventricles), the reason in the middle cell (our third ventricle), and the memory in the posterior cell (our fourth ventricle).[6] For these internal senses or psychic functions, it was the animal spirits, stored in the ventricles, that served to convey their influences via the nerves.

Regarding imagination, terminological issues arose, such as whether the common practice of using *imagination* and *phantasia* as synonyms was valid, or whether phantasia (fancy) should be restricted to the production of images in the absence of sensory input. Imagination's functions were, at times, restricted to the forming of images in response to the input from the common sense, but, in various other instances, they were thought to include as well the production of images in the absence of sensory input (fantasies, visions, dreams, hallucinations), the retrieval and use of memory-images, and what we might call the activities of the creative imagination. Viewed another way, the products of the imagination might be accurate, mistaken or even deluded, or creatively idiosyncratic. At times, the language and notions used in discussing imagination seemed to suggest that vision was the only sensory modality involved and that all images were visual, but sometimes the point was made that the language of vision served as a metaphor for the images from any of the five senses.

It was within the system of faculties outlined earlier that the imagination served as a factor in the explanation of mental disorders and as a basis for some of the measures used in treating them. The passions were movements of the soul, caused by the imagination's representations of objects or circumstances. The predominant view had the imagination causing distressing emotional states and various other symptoms of mental disorder. And not infrequently, this role in pathogenesis accounted for various physical disorders. Commonly, a disordered imagination was thought to affect the passions, and to have bodily effects, mediated through the body's humors. Further, aberrant states of the imagination might leave a person susceptible to supernatural influences, and so to the fortunate possibility of divine possession or the unfortunate possibility of demonic possession. There were instances enough where the reason was considered to be the faculty that accounted for a mental disorder, and there was a long trail of arguments about whether the reason or the imagination was responsible in some conditions; but more frequently a malfunctioning or diseased imagination was said to have brought on madness or some other form of severe mental distress. And it was not uncommon, when the reason was thought to be involved, for it to be said that it had been misled by the disordered imagination.

It is also worth noting that the imagination was often viewed as playing a crucial role in the age-old struggle between the rational and the irrational. The imagination was sometimes thought to be aligned with the reason or to serve reason in coping with the input from the external senses and in dealing with the passions and the appetites. At other times, it was viewed as more an aspect of the irrational forces in the soul with which the reason had to contend. And at still other times, the imagination was thought to operate on the border between the rational and irrational aspects of the soul — between the reason and the passions and appetites — sometimes as an asset to reason in the reason's handling of its responsibilities and sometimes as a liability.

The Imagination in Healing

It was this same theoretical scheme that came to serve as a rationale for the treatment of disease, particularly mental disorders. The imagination that could cause harm in the form of disease could do good in the form of curing disease. The *power of the imagination* and the *force of the imagination* became common Renaissance terms for a factor with considerable potential for good or ill.[7]

Although it was not new to take note of the imagination as contributing to disease, explicit and serious attention to this faculty as an agent in therapeutic endeavors seems to have emerged only during the sixteenth century. By the end of the century it was readily taken into account. If one brought a significant change of image to the sufferer's imagination, the imagination would then influence the troubled passions toward a cure. The principle of contraries guided the prescription, and so the effort was to induce an opposite sort of image that it might bring about an opposite sort of passion, with a harmonious affective balance as the goal, or at least a less troublesome passion. In the process, this corrective attention was also conceived of as influencing the humors and the spirits in beneficial ways and as relieving the sufferer of the symptoms.

Representative of these views was the thought of Thomas Fienus (1567–1631), professor of medicine at the University of Louvain, in his *De viribus imaginationis* published in 1608. Following Galen in his medical theory and Thomas Aquinas in his "psychology," Fienus left a treatise that prompted Robert Burton in his own review of the literature on "the Force of the Imagination" to refer to him as "worth all of them together."[8] Fienus argued that the imagination had its pathogenic influences, *not* directly, but "by means of the appetite, the emotions and the motions of the humors and spirits." He added that "the emotions are greatly alterative with respect to the body. . . . Through them the imagination is able to transform the body."[9] The emotions, in turn, "produce change by means of the natural movement of the heart and by means of the movement of the humors and the spirits."[10] In short, "the imagination may be the cause of all those diseases that can be excited by the emotions, and these are many."[11] In detailing his views on the curative effects of the imagination, Fienus emphasized the significance of the patient's "stout faith" in the physician and in the prospect of cure, recounted a series of delusions associated with melancholic disorders, commented that the sufferers were "healed . . . solely by the imagination of health," indicated that "a disease . . . of the mind can be dispatched by an induced imagination of another and opposite nature," and made it clear that the imagination had its curative effects only indirectly via its influence on the emotions.[12]

In his *Anatomy of Melancholy* in 1621, Burton provided us with a detailed account of Renaissance approaches to the care and cure of mental disorders, including a review of the era's practices in the realm of psychological healing.[13] He outlined the faculty psychology reviewed above, "the anatomy of the soul," as he put it. He reviewed the arguments regarding which faculty was

harmed in melancholia, concluding that a damaged imagination had the crucial role in the pathogenesis of that disease, and that the reason was often
affected secondarily. He then related a wide array of psychological treatment
measures to the goal of "correcting" the imagination or restoring its normal
function. Persuasion could bring about an improved state of mind for the
sufferer, and such efforts were thought of as undoing the damage to the imagination and rectifying the passions. Confiding in and taking counsel from a
trusted friend or physician were viewed as enabling the troubled person to
correct the distortions of the imagination and so to be freed from distress and
delusions. Guided by the principle of contraries, one could introduce opposite
sorts of images, right the imbalance, and undo the harm to the imagination;
and similarly, one might induce in the sufferer an opposite emotion to counter
a troubling one. Pleasant sights and diverting thoughts could be useful in this
endeavor. Keeping busy and avoiding preoccupations stemming from idleness
could serve to correct the imagination or keep it from going awry.[14] Burton
repeatedly maintained, " 'Tis thy corrupt phantasy, settle thine imagination,
thou art well."[15]

Burton outlined several ways in which the imagination might be actively
enlisted to promote a cure. He noted that the distressing views or delusional
ideas might be put to rest by fulfilling the person's wishes, and that the real
change in the person's circumstances could be conceived of as influencing the
imagination toward different images and thus bringing about a cure.[16] And
here too was the basis for the traditional "pious frauds," or "artificial inventions," as Burton termed them, aimed at dissuading the patient from belief in
the delusions or countering the distress that they were causing.[17] As Burton's
contemporary, William Vaughan (1577–1641), had put it at the beginning of
the century, "The Physician therefore that will cure these spirituall sicknesses,
must invent and devise some spirituall pageant, to fortifie and help the imaginative facultie, which is corrupted and depraved; yea, hee must endevour to
deceive, and imprint another conceit, whether it be wise or foolish, in the
Patients brain, thereby to put out all former phantasies."[18] Whether it was a
realistic satisfaction of the patient's wishes, a persuasion away from a delusional idea, or a relief of distress within the logic of a delusion, a corrective
image of an opposing nature, it was believed, had been presented to the imagination, which in turn served to relieve, reassure, or calm the person, and so
promoted an abatement of symptoms.

Thus the seventeenth century inherited a "psychology" or "anatomy of the
soul" in which the imagination was, indeed, a force to be reckoned with. At
the beginning of the century Pierre Charron (1541–1603) had said that "the
Power of *Imagination* is exceeding great; This is in Effect the very Thing, that

makes all the Noise in the World: Almost all the Clutter and Disturbances we feel, or make, are owing to it." It was the source of "all our Evils, our Confusions and Disorders, our Passions and Troubles."[19] A generation later, rather less ominously but no less respectfully, Burton commented, "Imagination . . . the wonderful effects and power of it . . . as it is eminent in all, so most especially it rageth in melancholy persons, in keeping the species of objects so long, mistaking, amplifying them by continued & strong meditation, until at length it produceth in some parties real effects, causeth this and many other maladies."[20] But, as we have seen through the eyes of Fienus and Burton, the imagination was also credited with a remarkable potential for therapeutic good. The benefits from charms, amulets, and spells were increasingly attributed to the power of the imagination. The healing efforts of cunning men and wise women, the useful effects of magical healing, and much else that we might think of as a kind of placebo therapy came to be understood as the outcome of a shrewd use of the imagination's healing powers.[21] Therapeutic measures directed toward the mind in the interest of healing mind or body were not new, and the psychosomatic orientation that they reflected was no novelty either, but these matters had come to be understood in terms of the influence of the imagination and how the healer might best go about actualizing that potential influence.

C. E. McMahon has studied the role of "the soul's imaginative faculty in the genesis and remission of disease" at some length. She outlines its "pre-Cartesian history" as follows: the theory stated that images of objects of desire or aversion aroused emotions, which in turn affected the humoral balance, digestion, and other vital functions, sometimes culminating in various forms of pathology and sometimes correcting various imbalances with therapeutic benefit. This theory had come to be used in explaining the therapeutic efficacy of "placebos" in forms such as spells, charms, and talismans.[22] Guided by the principle of contraries, physicians used images opposite to those that were troubling the patient in order to correct the damaged imagination and restore a healthful balance. But McMahon concludes this study with the comment that, "when Descartes redefined soul as 'immaterial substance' or 'mind,' imagination's role in the disease process was irrevocably taken from it."[23] She argued that pre-Cartesian views were "holistic or psychosomatic," but that Cartesian dualism did away with the possibility of such an orientation.

This allegedly disruptive break in the history of the imagination in the pathogenesis and treatment of disease fits well with the various twentieth-century indictments of Descartes for crimes against the wholeness of human beings. Yet it is not at all clear that clinical practice in the late seventeenth and eighteenth centuries changed in any way that could be particularly attributed to Descartes. Neither is it clear that the place of the imagination in the theories of pathogenesis or in the rationales for treatment came to bear a Cartesian imprint to any significant degree. These are complex issues, but they have been addressed in a particularly effective manner by Theodore M. Brown.[24] Focusing on the passions, the somatic influence of the imagination, and the effects of the patient's state of mind on the course of his illness, Brown pointed out that "medical theory long before Descartes had established clear precedents for a theoretical appreciation of the interaction of something very much like mind (psyche) with something very much like body (soma)."[25] In modern terms, both psychosomatic and somatopsychic effects were commonly taken into account. One feature of this orientation, as we have seen, was that a disordered imagination was capable of causing a wide variety of ills; and psychological strategies to influence the imagination were frequently used as means toward a cure. Some thought that the imagination affected the body directly, but the more usual view was that it worked its bodily effects through the passions. As Brown has illustrated well, all this changed very little in the wake of Descartes's contributions.

A confirmed iatromechanist like Giorgio Baglivi (1668–1706) acknowledged the significance of Descartes, but went on to say that "it will be allowable in us to skip these knotty Difficulties, that relate but little to the Cure of Diseases." He asserted that "a great part of Diseases either take their Rise from, or are fed by that weight of Care that hangs upon every one's Shoulders" and "that the Passions or Commotions of the Mind act upon the Body, is certain, and apparent from daily Experience." He then noted that "the Writings of Authors are full of Accounts of the Power of Imagination upon the Organs of the Body," that "vain Fear and sickly Imagination" alone could cause disease, and "that some Diseases are really produc'd by the Passions of the Mind and that the Power of the Imagination has a great Influence both in producing and curing them."[26] Friedrich Hoffman (1660–1742), following too in the iatromechanical tradition so influenced by Descartes, wrote as though a psychosomatic orientation was as persuasive as it ever had been,[27] and his influence was significant in the first half of the eighteenth century. A leading pupil of Boerhaave's and one of his successors at the University of Leyden, Jerome Gaub (1705–1780), acknowledging and not disputing Cartesian dualism, readily described various ways in which the immaterial mind influenced the material body.[28] For further perspective on just how little clinical medicine had changed, the following quotation from Leland J. Rather's study of Gaub illustrates the situation well: "Gaub tells us that while the physician is 'mentally able to abstract body from mind and consider it separately in order to be less confused in the marshalling of his ideas,' in practice 'where he deals with man as he is, should he devote all his efforts to the body alone, and take no account of the mind, his curative efforts will pretty often be less than happy,' for 'the reason why a sound body becomes ill or an ailing body recovers may lie in the mind.' "[29] In addition, Rather comments that "on the whole Gaub's contemporaries ascribed as much or more in the way of bodily change to emotions or 'power of the imagination' than would all but the most convinced proponents of the psychological causation of disease today."[30]

Thus the eighteenth century brought relatively little change in the status of these psychological measures aimed at changing the images in patients' imagination or usefully disabusing them of their delusional ideas. As a leading physician stated it in 1750, "Many Diseases arise from a perverted Imagination; and some of them are cured by affecting the Imagination only. It appears almost incredible, what great Effects the Imagination has upon Patients." Peter Shaw (1694–1763), who was physician to George II and George III, editor of Bacon and Boyle, and translator of Hoffman, Stahl, and Boerhaave, went on to say, "Now, if People may be sick by Imagination, Physicians should endeavour to cure by Imagination. And, of such Cures, there have been so many remarkable Instances." He was critical of the too liberal use of elixirs, pills, and powders in his day. He then hastened to add, "I acknowledge the Effects of Medicine, and am satisfied great Cures have been wrought by the Rule of Art," but he maintained that many of the cures apparently achieved by medicines were really "performed by Nature, by Accident, or by Help from the Patient's Imagination." He also emphasized the importance of providing hope rather than discouragement to patients.[31]

Similarly, a wide variety of other eighteenth-century authorities, medical and nonmedical alike, continued to be concerned with the imagination as a force to contend with in the realm of health and disease. From seventeenth-century terms such as a *disorder in the imagination* and a *Hurt or Error of the Imagination* as ways of explaining madness, there evolved eighteenth-century phrasings such as *disordered imagination, diseased imagination,* and *diseases of the imagination.* Well into the eighteenth century, William Battie maintained that "deluded imagination" was "an essential character of Madness" and "precisely discriminates this form from all other animal disorders."[32] And Samuel Johnson (1709–1784) reflected the thought of many of his contemporaries in stating that madness was "occasioned by too much indulgence of the imagination."[33] Further, as Michael V. DePorte has traced so well, discussions of madness in eighteenth-century literature frequently indicated an active fear of imagination and its potential to lead to madness.[34] The association of the imagination with insanity was well established. The imagination continued to be a factor that was taken seriously and that might well be in need of "correcting" in mental disorders.

As was briefly noted earlier on, in the course of coming to be viewed as a force for therapeutic good, the imagination had increasingly been thought to be the real basis for various cures attributed to amulets, charms, incantations, spells, and the like. Although some suggested somewhat dismissively that certain cures were due to "nothing but the imagination," any disrespect was directed more toward the therapeutic measures taken by irregular healers than toward the power of the imagination. In fact, a considerable respect for the influence of the imagination, whether for good or for ill, prevailed. Much as arguments have been made in more recent times for the constructive use of suggestion or the calculated use of the placebo effect in therapeutic endeavors, serious scholars and clinicians of the seventeenth and eighteenth centuries advocated techniques for influencing the imagination, for employing its powerful potential in the interest of the cure or amelioration of disease.

Toward the end of the eighteenth century, the imagination was again argued to be the key factor in some remarkable therapeutic techniques whose advocates explained them quite differently. Franz Anton Mesmer (1734–1815) developed one such treatment approach, influencing troubled patients and freeing them from their illnesses with techniques that later came to be subsumed under the term *hypnosis*.[35] Mesmer attributed his therapeutic successes to *animal magnetism,* by which he meant that a universal, subtle, imponderable fluid (akin to the magnetic and electrical fluids in the era's physical science) was mobilized by the healer in himself, and its influence was then transmitted to the sufferer; various magnetic devices were used to concentrate it and give it direction in the patient. His techniques produced a *crisis* (convulsive movements) in the patient, which Mesmer maintained was evidence of the disease and the means whereby the imbalance in the patient's own subtle fluid was corrected to produce a cure. In Paris, the success of this technique, the spread of its use, and the accompanying notoriety and criticism eventually led, in March and April 1784, to the appointment of two commissions of inquiry by Louis XVI of France for the purpose of studying Mesmer's work and his claims. Later that year, the reports of these commissions concluded that there was no evidence of the alleged magnetic fluid, and, without denying the beneficial effects, they attributed those effects to the workings of the imagination.[36] The more significant of these two reports, prepared by members of the Academie des Sciences, concluded that "the imagination is the true cause of the effects attributed to Magnetism."[37] The commissioners noted that "the history of medicine includes innumerable examples of the power of the imagination and of the emotions of the soul"; they then cited a series of examples of cures obtained by these means.[38] Repeatedly noting a lack of evidence for any such agent as animal magnetism, and referring again and again to the imagination as the therapeutic factor, they reminded the reader that "the imagination of sick persons is often a considerable influence in the cure of their illnesses."[39]

A second such instance involved a treatment approach developed in the 1790s by an American physician, Elisha Perkins (1741–1799). He employed metallic tractors and maintained that stroking the patient's affected parts with them effected a cure. Early therapeutic successes brought favorable publicity, but doubts and criticism from his peers soon led to considerable controversy. In 1799, John Haygarth (1740–1827), an English physician from Bath, undertook a controlled clinical trial of Perkins' metallic tractors, which involved comparing them with a set of wooden tractors painted to resemble them, and he discovered that the therapeutic results were essentially the same. His findings "prove to a degree which has never been suspected, what powerful influence upon diseases is produced by mere Imagination."[40] And he commented on the similarity between Perkins' tractoration and Mesmer's animal magnetism.[41] He viewed his findings as belonging in the same realm as "the influence of the passions upon disorders of the body," so "excellently illustrated by William Falconer," among others.[42] "These trials . . . clearly prove what wonderful effects the passions of hope and faith, excited by mere Imagination, can produce upon diseases." Further, he concluded that "on this principle we may account for the marvellous recoveries frequently ascribed to empirical remedies, which are commonly inert drugs."[43]

The controversies surrounding mesmerism and Perkinism served to bring into focus the already existing interest in and respect for the power of the imagination in the cause and cure of disease. In tandem with the eighteenth-century interest in the passions as causal factors in disease and as therapeutic agents, this interest in the imagination was a crucial aspect of a lively attention to psychic factors in medical healing. In light of the "psychosomatic" orientation manifested by many eighteenth-century physicians, this was hardly a new trend. Still, late in the century enhanced interest in psychological healing was displayed, along with indications that this realm was thought to have been neglected and that many therapeutic procedures deemed questionable might in fact have a validity based on psychic influences. Further, it was increasingly noted that aspects of the physician-patient relationship generally taken for granted were often crucial to a cure and reflected psychological influences at work. Along this line, the royal commission's report on mesmerism drew on the wisdom of the ages to note that faith in the possibility of getting well and the engendering of hope by the healer were often crucial factors in a cure. The commission members viewed such faith as being "the product of the imagination," which served to calm the sufferer and inspire hope in him.[44]

Jan Goldstein has argued convincingly that, as manifested in the care of the mad, these trends were significant in the emergence of the French psychiatric profession in the nineteenth century. She emphasizes the views of Pierre-Jean-Georges Cabanis on the importance of the imagination—"How many men have been killed, or cured, by imagination!"—and suggests, fairly, that they were characteristic for the times. As she said, "Cabanis' point about the reciprocal influence of *le moral* and *le physique* and the special role of the imagination in mediating the relationship between the two was . . . neither a new nor a particularly controversial one." This perspective, however, "had long been relegated to commonsensical, subscientific status in the medical community." But Cabanis now lent it a "legitimacy . . . by anchoring it in a sophisticated medical-philosophical theory about the nature of man." She observed that Cabanis "thus moved a 'medicine of the imagination' from the shadowy periphery to the center of medical orthodoxy."[45] This "medicine of the imagination" included a "concern for the emotional state of the sick individual" and "the precepts of soothing, [of] reassuring, and of sustaining hope." It was also referred to as "moral hygiene" by Cabanis and Philippe Pinel, and it was out of this matrix of "remèdes moraux" that Pinel developed his moral treatment.[46]

With the developing use of moral treatment and the continuing attention to mesmerism and hypnosis, early nineteenth-century therapeutics did not lack for attention to psychological healing. In fact, even some textbooks of materia medica and general therapeutics came to include brief sections on psychological treatment measures. In the 1830s, in his *General Therapeutics*, Robley Dunglison (1798–1869) accorded a place to imagination in general medical treatment. He noted that a variety of objects, materials, and procedures had been used in a way "calculated to produce considerable effect upon the imagination," and so had been, and could be, "productive of advantage in the treatment of disease." After emphasizing the importance of confidence in the physician and in the remedy, he reasoned that imagination and faith could "render inert medicines efficacious."[47] In the 1840s, Jonathan Pereira (1804–1853) introduced similar views into his *Elements of Materia Medica*. He observed that "the influence of the *imagination* on disease has long been known, and is a fruitful source of fallacy in therapeutics. Extraordinary cures have frequently been ascribed to inert and useless means, when, in fact, they were referable to the influence of the imagination."[48]

Then, in 1872, Tuke's book on "the influence of the mind on the body" was said to be "designed to elucidate the action of the imagination." This volume contained a few scattered references to suggestion, but the language of suggestion had not yet permeated discussions of psychological healing as it would by the end of the century. Tuke wrote of emotion "as the cause, or, at least, the antecedent of bodily change," and of imagination as "a complex mental power" that both belonged with "the intellectual powers" and merged "insensibly into emotional states." It was through the imagination that he conceived of the mind as being affected by psychological factors and, in turn, as having its influence upon the body. A change in the nature of the imagination from "a mere idea, image, or conception, to an irresistible conviction" was "the very mental condition which, from a medico-psychological point of view, is the *desideratum,* in undertaking the treatment of diseases admitting of amelioration from the psychical method." Further, "whatever mental or bodily state can be excited through the senses from without, may arise from within, from Imagination proper." Thus, it was through influencing the imagination that the physician employing the psychical method or, to use another term of Tuke's, "psycho-therapeutics" would bring about the mind's healing influence on the body.[49]

By the end of the nineteenth century, though, references to the role of the imagination in either the cause or the cure of disease were becoming relatively infrequent. As the language of suggestion took over in discussions of psychological healing, much that had previously been attributed to the imagination came to be explained in terms of suggestion and autosuggestion. Alfred Binet and Charles Féré (1852–1907), in their extensive review of animal magnetism and hypnosis, wrote about "this medicine for the imagination, which is entitled to the name of suggestive therapeutics." They discoursed at length on "diseases caused by the imagination — that is, produced by a fixed idea." They emphasized that "there are . . . no imaginary diseases, but there are diseases due to the imagination, and accompanied by real functional disturbances." Just as *malades imaginaires* suffered from disorders brought about by pathogenic ideas associated with the imagination, so might they be cured by ideas acting as therapeutic agents and suggestively influencing the imagination for the patients' betterment. Further, looking back in time, these authors argued that the power of suggestion accounted for cures by quacks such as Greatrakes in the seventeenth century, the exorcisms by Gassner in the eighteenth century, Mesmer's cures, and the various faith healings, all of which had previously been attributed to the power of the imagination.[50] A few years earlier, Féré had written about *la médecine d'imagination,* indicating that it was essentially *thérapeutique suggestive* and that *les maladies imaginaires* were really *les maladies par imagination.*[51] Then, in 1901, Alfred T. Schofield (1846–1929) referred briefly to the imagination in therapeutics, and approvingly quoted a

Professor Hughes, as follows: "The imagination is one of the most effective psychical agencies in modifying the conditions of health and disease." But Schofield went on to assert that the imagination that brought about cures might better be termed the unconscious mind.[52]

A notable exception to the trend away from the imagination and its language was the concept, and the associated technique, of *active imagination* developed by Carl G. Jung during the second decade of the twentieth century. This was the outcome of his self-analysis and the associated confrontation with a series of disturbing emotions and images.[53] He made it part of his psychotherapeutic and analytical methods in the years that followed, as did clinicians who worked in his tradition of psychological healing. He conceived of this technique as striving "to translate the emotions into images — that is to say, to find the images which were concealed in the emotions. . . . As a result of my experiment I learned how helpful it can be, from the therapeutic point of view, to find the particular images which lie behind emotions."[54] He referred to active imagination as a "method . . . in the treatment of neurosis, as a means to bring unconscious contents to consciousness";[55] and he described it as "a method (devised by myself) of introspection for observing the stream of interior images. One concentrates one's attention on some impressive but unintelligible dream-image, or on a spontaneous visual impression, and observes the changes taking place in it."[56] He placed this technique alongside free association, dream analysis, and his own word association method as psychotherapeutic techniques, ways of exploring psychological data. He cautioned, though, that the technique was not without its dangers.

As one considers Jung's various references to the technique, and to the imagination more generally, one finds much to suggest that he had returned the imagination to the status of a relatively independent agency, akin to its place in various faculty psychologies of the eighteenth century and earlier. Edward S. Casey included a particularly valuable study of Jung's thought on imagination in the chapter "The Significance of Imaginative Autonomy" in his book *Imagining*. There he traces the concept of active imagination to roots in Jung's earlier notion of "active fantasy," and notes, "Distinguishing between fantasy and imagination as a result of his study of medieval and Renaissance alchemy, he limits fantasy (*Phantasie*) to being 'a subjective figment of the mind' and promotes imagination (*Einbildungskraft*) into 'an image-making, form-giving creative activity.' Active imagination represents a special employment of this creative power."[57] This process not only facilitated insight into the self, "but at the same time into the archetypal constants that subtend the self. For the aim of active imagination is at once personal and extrapersonal; or more exactly, by taking us more deeply into ourselves it brings us into contact with what is more than ourselves. This 'more' refers to archetypes, which lend lasting shape and structure to what would otherwise be a sheer 'chaotic assortment of images.' "[58] Thus, while using the concept of the imagination in a manner reminiscent of the traditional internal sense or faculty, Jung emphasized a particular aspect of that traditional notion, namely, the creative imagination.

More recently, a whole array of psychotherapeutic uses of the imagination has emerged which can be subsumed under the rubric *guided imagery techniques.* In association with a reawakening of interest in the study of imagery, various enterprising clinicians have developed techniques for stimulating imagery (most often visual) or facilitating the emergence of and attention to imagery as a key aspect of their approach to psychological healing. Suggesting or urging that patients exercise their capacity for imagining, some clinicians have employed "images to explore dimly recognized or repressed ideas, feelings, memories, and fantasies." Others have attempted "to transform current attitudes, emotions, and behavioral patterns by the use of image formation."[59] In these therapeutic activities the imagination has been employed with an eye to releasing pent-up distress, recovering and resolving disturbing memories, achieving useful insight, effecting beneficial cognitive or behavioral changes, or otherwise bringing relief from some troubled state. In brief, the clinician arranges to minimize distractions, employs techniques to promote relaxation, and facilitates the patient's attending to mental images, with varying degrees of guidance or direction.

These guided imagery techniques have evolved out of a veritable maze of influences, only a brief sketch of which can be offered here.[60] Jung's *active imagination* seems to have been an influence. An important early line of development came out of J. H. Schultz's *autogenic training,* a form of self-hypnosis and relaxation. Robert Desoille's *rêve éveillé dirigé* (directed daydream) technique was particularly significant, demonstrating a debt to his teacher, Eugène Caslant, and influences reflected in the work of Roger Frétigny and André Virel and that of Roberto Assagioli. In the 1950s came the highly systematized psychotherapeutic approach of Hanscarl Leuner, called guided affective imagery (GAI). Then, while these European trends were evolving, Joseph Wolpe and others working in the behavior modification tradition were introducing imagery techniques into their work in the United States. And, in ways reminiscent of Jung's active imagination, Fritz Perls and others were making considerable use of imagery in Gestalt therapy. This complex and fascinating realm of guided imagery techniques merits its own detailed study, which cannot be undertaken here, but, for our immediate purposes, it is testimony to the persistence of the imagination as an active focus of approaches to psychological healing.

Although in these various guided imagery techniques we find modern extensions of the long history of the imagination as a factor in psychological healing, it is noteworthy how carefully the language of faculty psychology is eschewed and how regularly the emphasis is on the process of imagining or image formation in operational terms. Still, though, the echoes of the past are strong when one learns that a work titled *Imagination and Healing* by one modern authority developed out of "a series of conferences, entitled 'The Power of the Imagination,'"[61] and another modern authority on imagery in healing entitled one of his books *The Power of the Human Imagination*.[62] These terms would have been entirely familiar and would have echoed with real depth of meaning in the sixteenth and seventeenth centuries.

PART SIX

Bringing Influence to Bear

Animal Magnetism, Mesmerism, and Hypnosis

In the 1770s, certain activities of Franz Anton Mesmer initiated the development of a complex of healing activities that came to be known as animal magnetism or mesmerism and that eventually evolved into hypnosis. Swiss born, Mesmer earned doctoral degrees in both philosophy and medicine, the latter in Vienna in 1766, where he then settled and practiced medicine.

Franz Anton Mesmer

During 1773–1774, Mesmer "undertook in my house the treatment of a young lady aged twenty-nine named Oesterline, who for several years had been subject to a convulsive malady, the most troublesome symptoms of which were that the blood rushed to her head and there set up the most cruel toothaches and earaches, followed by delirium, rage, vomiting and swooning."[1] Influenced by efforts in France, Germany, and Britain that used magnets in the treatment of stomach ailments and toothaches, and by his own theories of planetary influences and magnetic effects on animal bodies, he had Fräulein Oesterline ingest an iron preparation and then applied magnets to her stomach and both legs, regularly bringing her temporary relief from her symptoms. Each time, "she felt inside her some painful currents of a subtle material which, after different attempts at taking a direction, made their way towards the lower part and caused all the symptoms of the attack to cease for six hours."[2]

Out of all this, Mesmer constructed his theory of *animal magnetism,* whereby he explained "the periodical changes which we observe in sex, and in a general way those which physicians of all ages and in all countries have observed during illness." According to him, the heavenly bodies "exert a direct action on all parts that constitute animate bodies, particularly the nervous system, by means of an all-penetrating fluid."[3] As the physical sciences of the era employed ideas of subtle, imponderable fluids to account for a variety of natural phenomena, including magnetism and electricity, Mesmer spoke of an analogy between the properties of animal magnetism and "those of the magnet and electricity." He added " 'that all bodies were, like the magnet, capable of communicating this magnetic principle; that this fluid penetrated everything; that it could be stored up and concentrated, like the electric fluid; that it acted at a distance; that animate bodies were divided into two classes, one being susceptible to this magnetism and the other to an opposite quality that suppresses its action.' "[4]

Reasoning that the magnets that he had used with Fräulein Oesterline were themselves "incapable of such action on the nerves," Mesmer argued that the magnets had served as conduits for the animal magnetism from within his own person and had reinforced its effects. From the accumulation of this subtle fluid in his own body, he had influenced the comparable fluid in the patient, and so had brought about the clinical change. After some months of these treatments, Mesmer ultimately effected a stable cure for his patient. He subsequently "undertook the treatment of various disorders" in other patients, "including, among others, a case of hemiplegia due to apoplexy, stoppages, vomiting of blood, frequent colics, a case of paroxysmal sleep with spitting of blood stemming from infancy, and cases of normal ophthalmia."[5]

Over the next several years, Mesmer was repeatedly embroiled in controversies regarding the usefulness of his treatment method and the validity of his cures; meanwhile, he continued to employ his very personal therapeutic approach. Then in 1776, in the course of countering some of his critics, he discontinued the use of both electricity and magnets as not essential to his ability to cure.[6] Eventually, he gave up the conflicts that had become such a part of his life and, in 1778, moved to Paris. There he soon took up clinical activities once again, guided still by his system of animal magnetism.

By this time, Mesmer's technique involved sitting "in front of the patient with his knees touching the patient's knees, pressing the patient's thumbs in his hands, looking fixedly into his eyes, then touching his hypochondria and making passes over his limbs." Frequently the patient experienced peculiar sensations or fell into a crisis or convulsion. In the early 1780s, when Mesmer's clinical practice was becoming ever busier, he introduced a mode of group treatment involving the *baquet*. This was a tublike vessel that he filled with water and placed in the center of the room; around it as many as twenty patients would sit. Holes had been pierced near the edge of the lid that covered the baquet, one for each patient. Into each hole, an iron rod was inserted, bent outwards at right angles and at different heights, so that each rod could be applied to the afflicted part of a particular patient's body. In addition, a rope joined the baquet to one of the patients and then patient to patient, around the whole group. As one observer described it, " 'the most sensible effects are produced on the approach of Mesmer, who is said to convey the fluid by certain motions of his hands or eyes, without touching the person. I have talked with several who have witnessed these effects, who have convulsions occasioned and removed by a movement of the hand.' "[7]

Although Mesmer had abandoned his earlier view that magnetism and electricity were conveyed by his apparatus from healer to patient, his confidence in his own powers grew, and he continued to interpret his own influence as a subtle magnetic fluid (an animal magnetism) within himself that his techniques and apparatus conveyed into the patient, which stimulated profound emotional and physical restlessness, increasing excitement, and, commonly, an eventual crisis or convulsion. Release and relief were usual outcomes; and clinical improvement was frequently alleged, and was often testified to by the sufferers. The rapport between the healer and the sufferer came to be considered an important factor in bringing about successful treatment. Within this interpersonal process, some contemporary observers and many later commentators saw an intense emotional effect conveyed by a particularly influential, charismatic healer in a way that seemed akin to the development and resolution of sexual excitement; and some warned of the danger of sexual misbehavior or possibly love relationships as outcomes of the magnetizer-patient interaction. Whether or not overt sexual themes emerged, strong dependent ties to the healer frequently developed, and thinly disguised sexual attachment seems to have been common.[8]

Mesmer's years in Paris were eventful, fruitful in clinical successes and acclaim, and yet disappointing to him in that he failed to achieve the official recognition and professional respect that he sought and considered to be his due. At a point of considerable frustration for him, in 1782, friends and disciples endeavored to enlist support for his work, raising funds and developing the Société de l'Harmonie, an association whose members shared both the "secret" of his magnetic treatment and its ownership, and who would serve to teach and publicize Mesmer's method. By 1784, the controversies around

Mesmer and his work led Louis XVI to appoint two commissions of inquiry. Investigating the validity of Mesmer's notion of a magnetic fluid rather than the reality of his cures, the commissions concluded that there was no evidence for the existence of such a fluid. Although they did not challenge the fact of his cures, the commission members did maintain that those cures were essentially due to the effects of the imagination.[9] In the wake of this setback, a number of other criticisms were leveled at Mesmer and his work, troubling treatment failures occurred, and conflicts erupted with some of his disciples. Finally, in 1785, Mesmer left Paris and passed into relative obscurity; the further development of magnetic treatment was taken up by others.

The Marquis de Puységur

In 1784, Maxime de Chastenet, Count de Puységur (1755–1848), while serving as second-in-command of his regiment at Bayonne, had occasion to draw upon his familiarity with animal magnetism in order to effect a dramatic cure of a member of his regiment who had suffered "an apoplectic fit." This was followed by the cure of an injured dog and eventually by mesmeric cures of various regimental members and of residents of the town and surrounding countryside. Count de Puységur compiled a careful account of these events, along with notarized attestations to many of the cures,[10] in which account he referred to the royal commission's report and took some pains to protest against what he considered the unfair treatment of Mesmer. Alluding to the commission's conclusion that Mesmer's clinical results were essentially the result of the imagination, he commented, "If it is here that the effects of the imagination are of value, the academie will be forced to agree that the imagination is the most important doctor on earth."[11] And in acknowledging how meaningful it was to find himself so useful, he referred to "a truth" that he had learned from Mesmer: "How powerful is the influence exerted from one man to another, and the mutual need that we have for one another?"[12]

Prominent as one of Mesmer's most loyal disciples and as a reputable magnetizer, and the older brother of Count de Puységur, Armand Marie Jacques de Chastenet, Marquis de Puységur (1751–1825), introduced changes in technique that were to be particularly significant. It was he who developed the notion of "magnetic sleep" and its usefulness in therapeutic endeavors. He termed this state magnetic somnambulism, by analogy with the "natural somnambulism" that could occur during ordinary sleep. It also came to be known as artificial somnambulism and, much later, as the hypnotic trance. In 1784, Puységur undertook the magnetic treatment of Victor Race, a young peasant whose family had long been in the service of the Puységur family, on the family estate in Buzancy near Soissons. Suffering from a respiratory ailment, Race was mesmerized by Puységur and fell into an unusual type of sleep without the convulsive crisis so often associated with magnetic treatment. In this state, he seemed more alert, aware, and intelligent than he usually did; he spoke clearly and answered questions; when asked about his illness, he guided the magnetizer in the diagnosis and treatment of his condition; and on awakening from this state, he was amnesic for the whole experience. Puységur successfully repeated this procedure with Race several times; and he was cured. Puységur soon found that he was able to repeat the experience with other sufferers and relieve them of their ailments. And he came to term this quieter, nonconvulsive trance state the perfect crisis, making considerable use of the capacity of some patients to guide the diagnostic and therapeutic efforts in a constructive manner. Furthermore, these events led to an increasing demand for his treatment services; eventually he developed a collective form of the treatment in which the patients gathered around an old elm tree, duly magnetized by Puységur, in the town square, with ropes attached to the tree and their ends wound around the afflicted parts of the sufferers' bodies. In Race's case, in time he came to confide in Puységur about personal conflicts and then, following Puységur's suggestions, to take steps to resolve these conflicts after being awakened from the trance state.[13]

With the advent of Puységur's work, and its influence on other magnetizers, began an increasing trend away from the convulsive crisis and a lessened emphasis on the idea of a subtle, physical fluid. Along with the newer emphasis on artificial somnambulism, Puységur drew attention to the importance of the rapport between the patient and the magnetizer, and he introduced the view that a key factor was the magnetizer's *will*.[14] In teaching activities in the latter part of the 1780s, he articulated the principles of magnetic healing as he understood them: "The entire doctrine of Animal Magnetism is contained in the two words: *Believe* and *Want*. I *believe* that I have the power to set into action the vital principles of my fellow-men; I *want* to make use of it; and this is all my science and all my means."[15] As some magnetizers followed more the tradition of techniques advocated by Mesmer and others worked more with the simplified technique of Puységur, there emerged certain conflicts and arguments regarding the physicalist explanatory scheme of the former, versus the animistic explanatory scheme of the latter; and in Puységur's references to the magnetizer's will and the rapport with the patient lay indications of an emerging psychological explanation. Interestingly, it was essentially Puységur's technique that came to be known as *mesmerism* in the early nineteenth century.

Other Early French Contributors

Interest in and attention to magnetic healing waned with the beginning of the Revolution in France, but Puységur's renewed activity around 1805 and his newer publications played an important role in a resurgence of mesmeric therapeutics.[16] His views were taken up by numerous early nineteenth-century mesmerists. Particularly significant, though, was Joseph Philippe François Deleuze (1753–1835), a student of Puységur's writings, much like him in temperament, heavily influenced by him in his approach to magnetic healing. He both handed down the traditions of Puységur's work and had a considerable influence on magnetic healing in his own right.

In his *Histoire critique du magnétisme animal* in 1813, Deleuze provided both the definitive history for the time and a valuable outline of the theory and practice of magnetism.[17] Then, in his *Instruction pratique* in 1825, he provided a detailed manual to guide the practitioner of magnetic therapy.[18] He particularly emphasized that magnetism was a method of healing for those who were ill; and he provided careful instruction about arrangements with the patient and conditions that should be established for the treatment setting. In describing at length the manipulations and passes[19] that were to be employed, he emphasized that the details of the procedures were crucial and that the magnetizer should be consistent in their use, and yet noted that they might well vary from magnetizer to magnetizer. He made quite apparent the intimacy of the work and the physical proximity of magnetizer to patient, though noting that he expected witnesses to be present (preferably only one) and cautioning that the passes should be at more of a distance when the magnetizer was a man and the patient a woman. He was convinced of the idea of a magnetic fluid being transmitted by the magnetizer and of fluid within the patient being influenced and redistributed; and he thought of these measures as restoring an equilibrium or re-establishing "the harmony of the system." The patient experienced warmth emanating from the ends of the magnetizer's fingers; he experienced pains in the afflicted parts, which pains then moved, descended, and were eventually drained out of him; his eyes closed; he felt calm, became drowsy, and slept; and he eventually awakened refreshed. Deleuze commented that the patient sometimes entered a somnambulistic state in which he heard the magnetizer and replied, without awakening; but Deleuze did not consider this a common experience. As had Puységur, he thought that the magnetizer's will was a crucial factor; and Deleuze emphasized that the magnetizer should be committed primarily to the good of the patient—that mere curiosity about the phenomena was insufficient.[20] At least four French editions of his *Instruction pratique* were published over a thirty-year period, it appeared in a number of foreign translations, and it influenced many later authors and practitioners.

During the same era as Deleuze, probably as early as 1813, Abbé José Custodi de Faria (1755–1819), a Portuguese priest working in Paris, was critical of the theory of the physical fluid and the notion of rapport, and he argued that magnetization was due less to the magnetizer than to the subject. His technique was a particularly simple one: the patient was seated in a comfortable chair, his attention was fixed on Faria's open and raised hand, and then the magnetizer commanded in a loud voice, "Sleep!"; the patient would usually fall into a magnetic sleep.[21] Though the term *suggestion* was not employed, later generations could see in Faria's descriptions that the patient was suggestible and that the magnetizer influenced the patient by means of suggestion. General François Joseph Noizet (1792–1885) was much influenced by Faria's views, although he clung to the idea that a fluid was the basis for the influence; Noizet, in turn, is thought to have influenced his friend, Alexandre Bertrand (1795–1831), who is generally credited with a crucial role in the emergence of psychological explanations of magnetism, and particularly of suggestion. Noizet's own treatise on the subject was drafted in 1820 but was not published until 1854. In a 1823 publication, Bertrand still accepted the idea of a universal magnetic fluid; but he had abandoned such a notion by the time his second work appeared in 1826. These three men—Faria, Noizet, Bertrand—are frequently grouped together as early influences in the eventual development of the theory of suggestion.[22]

Elliotson, Esdaile, and Braid

In the 1830s and 1840s, three British medical men played important roles in the ongoing evolution of magnetic therapy. John Elliotson (1791–1868) was the first professor of the practice of medicine at the University of London. Influenced by accounts from France of successful surgery during mesmeric trances, he became interested in mesmerism in the 1830s. This led him to conduct major surgical procedures without pain to the patients, when the latter were in a state of magnetic sleep. As he became an increasingly enthusiastic advocate of mesmerism, he encountered intense opposition, and he eventually was forced to resign his university posts. He went on to work at mesmeric endeavors for some years afterwards, publishing an account of his surgical cases under mesmerism, editing a mesmeric journal, and defending mesmerism eloquently when named to deliver the Harveian Oration in 1846.[23]

Especially significant among those who took up surgical procedures on patients in mesmeric trances was James Esdaile (1808–1859), a friend of

Elliotson. In 1845, while in charge of a hospital in India, Esdaile undertook a potentially painful surgical operation after putting the patient into a mesmeric trance, and it was performed without pain to the patient. This led to a long series of successful operations, without pain, on mesmerized patients. In 1846, Esdaile published a book recounting these cases.[24] Again, controversy arose, and a government investigation took place. But the report that followed was a favorable one, and eventually funds were raised and a mesmeric hospital established under Esdaile's leadership. He returned to his native Scotland in 1851, where he pursued his interest in mesmerism. With the advent of chemically induced anesthesia in the 1840s, mesmerism for surgical anesthesia gradually faded from the scene.

Further in the 1840s, James Braid (ca. 1795–1860), another Scotchman, took up an active interest in mesmerism. Braid had trained as a surgeon and practiced for a time in Scotland, before settling in Manchester. Having witnessed a demonstration of mesmerism, he went to some lengths to satisfy himself that it was not a matter of trickery, and then developed his own skills as a magnetist. But he abandoned the various theories of earlier mesmeric and magnetic therapists. In 1842, in an indignant reply to the publication of a clergyman's critical sermon, he published a brief work, *Satanic Agency and Mesmerism Revisited,* in which he defended the clinical practice while introducing a new explanation for mesmeric phenomena and the rudiments of a new terminology. He took note of three types of theorists: (1) those who attribute the phenomena to deception; (2) those who consider them real phenomena, but "produced solely by imagination, sympathy, and imitation"; and (3) "the animal magnetists, or those who believe in some magnetic medium set in motion as the exciting cause." Then he put forward a fourth category of explanation that would accommodate his own views: "solely attributable to a peculiar physiological state of the brain and the spinal cord." He thought in terms of a "continued effort of the [patient's] will, to rivet attention to one idea," which exhausted both the mind and the various muscles involved in maintaining a fixed stare; of the stillness of the body as diminishing "the force and frequency of the heart's action"; and of all this as resulting in "a rapid exhaustion of the sensorium and nervous system." There ensued "a feeling of giddiness, with slight tendency to syncopy, and a feeling of somnolency," following which "the mind slips out of gear." The true nature of the phenomena lay not "in the operator," but "solely in the individuals operated on keeping their mind and eyes rivetted to one idea, and in one fixed position."[25] He cited a series of cases illustrating remarkable therapeutic benefits. And though he saw himself as having confirmed the facts, he disagreed with previously held theories to explain them. He also maintained that no one could be affected by the procedures "unless by voluntary compliance," and thus they could not be "converted to immoral purposes."[26]

In 1843, Braid elaborated and extended these views in *Neurypnology; or, the Rationale of Nervous Sleep* which is commonly credited with marking a turning point in the history of mesmerism and with effecting the emergence of *hypnotism*. Drawing on the Greek roots for "nerve" and "sleep," Braid had come up with *neuro-hypnology;* then, deleting two letters, he coined the word *neurypnology,* by which he meant "the *rationale,* or *doctrine* of *nervous* sleep, which I define to be . . . . 'a peculiar condition of the nervous system, induced by a fixed and abstracted attention of the mental and visual eye, on one object, not of an exciting nature.' " And he added a list of cognate terms from each of which, as he stated, he dropped the prefix *neuro-* for the sake of brevity. These included: *hypnotism,* nervous sleep; *hypnotist,* one who practices neurypnotism; *hypnotize,* to induce nervous sleep; *dehypnotize,* to restore from the state or condition of nervous sleep.[27] These terms were to become very familiar during the latter half of the century.

Braid believed that he had "now entirely separated Hypnotism from Animal Magnetism" and provided "merely a simple, speedy, and certain mode of throwing the nervous system into a new condition, which may be rendered eminently available in the cure of certain disorders." He had developed "a valuable addition to our curative means, which enables us speedily to put an end to many diseases which resist ordinary treatment," but it was not "a universal remedy." He viewed "the eyes being fixed in the most favourable position, and the mind thus riveted to one idea, as the *primary and imperative conditions.*" He described this condition as quickly leading to "the *primary* stage, or that of *excitement,*" and then to "the *ulterior* stage, or state of *torpor,*" the latter being brought about "by merely affording time for the phenomena to develop themselves." He carefully detailed his technique for the reader as a simple, straightforward, natural set of procedures; and he emphasized that "*all* the conditions" must be strictly complied with. He explained his results as stemming from "a derangement of the state of the cerebro-spinal centres, and of the circulation, and respiratory, and muscular systems, induced . . . by a fixed stare, absolute repose of the body, fixed attention, and suppressed respiration, concomitant with that fixity of attention."[28] He cited brief clinical anecdotes, termed experiments, to illustrate or prove his points: that such procedures surely had curative effects, that no sympathetic influence was conveyed from one patient to another when they were connected by ropes or wires, that subjects varied considerably in their susceptibility to hypnotic influence, that charges against him of "materialism" were not valid, and that phrenological concepts could be integrated with his neurohypnotic notions and shown to have validity, among other matters. He repeatedly emphasized the centrality of the subject's role in hypnotic procedures, doing so in a way that quite diminished the role of "rapport." Although his descriptions of his neurohypnotic efforts frequently seem to indicate the very influence of the hypnotist that he would deny, he may fairly be said to have appreciated the potential for autohypnosis. Also, in later work, he observed that he had failed to establish the validity of thought-reading, of clairvoyance, and of the ability of somnambulists to diagnose diseases.

Out of these efforts came the hypnotism of the middle decades of the nineteenth century, often referred to as Braidism. And Braid's views were influential for the work of many later hypnotists, such as Azam, Broca, Charcot, Liébeault, and Bernheim.

In Braid's descriptions of his procedures and in his clinical vignettes, both in his *Neurypnology* and elsewhere, it is apparent that he, too, employed with his patients what would later come to be termed suggestion. But he repeatedly asserted that the hypnotist exercised no influence on the patient; he maintained rather that it was a more or less mechanical procedure that led to phenomena, which had their origins in the patient. There are hints, though, in some of his later work that he was not unaware of the role of suggestion.[29] In fact, Arthur E. Waite (1857–1942), a later editor of *Neurypnology*, asserted that Braid was the "discoverer" of suggestion.[30] Later, of course, the language of suggestion was increasingly introduced to explain the effects of hypnotic procedures.

The Nancy School and the Salpêtrière School

"In the period from 1860 to 1880, magnetism and hypnotism had fallen into such disrepute that a physician working with these methods would irretrievably have compromised his scientific career and lost his medical practice." So said Henri Ellenberger in introducing his account of the Nancy school of hypnotism.[31] Yet it was this very era in which Auguste Ambroise Liébeault began using hypnosis as a country doctor; he came to make it a central feature of his clinical work. After receiving his medical degree in 1850, Liébeault gradually developed a busy medical practice. Already familiar with magnetism from a book he had read as a medical student and from having magnetized some patients at that time, in 1860 he took up the serious study of mesmerism, giving special attention to experiments with Braid's hypnotism by Eugène Azam (1822–1899), a physician in Bordeaux; after that he increasingly employed hypnotic techniques in his treatment endeavors. Moving to Nancy in 1864, he devoted most of the next two years to writing about his experiences with hypnotic work, and in 1866 he published *Du sommeil et des états analogues,* a book which received very little attention at the time.[32] Liébeault concluded that hypnotic sleep was the same as natural sleep, except that the patient was brought to that state by the hypnotist through suggestion and through concentrating attention on the idea of sleep. A significant rapport existed with the hypnotist. Liébeault's method was a particularly simple and direct one: the patient, sitting in an armchair, was directed to think of nothing and to look steadily at the hypnotist. If the eyes did not soon close spontaneously, Liébeault requested the patient to shut them. Then he made such suggestions as, "Your eyelids are getting heavy, your limbs feel numb, you are becoming more and more drowsy." After a minute or two, he placed his hand on the patient's body and suggested the sensation of local warmth. With the patient in a state of hypnotic sleep, the doctor made simple curative suggestions negating the symptoms of the disease and encouraging good habits of health maintenance.[33]

But Liébeault and his work remained more or less unknown, and certainly unsung, until they came to the attention of Hippolyte Bernheim in 1882. Bernheim, established as professor of medicine at the University of Nancy, heard about Liébeault's work and sought out the relatively unknown local physician-hypnotist; overcoming a certain skepticism, Bernheim took pains to learn from him. He soon incorporated hypnotic techniques as essential features of his own therapeutic work; and he introduced Liébeault's methods into the hospital at Nancy. They became associated as friends and professional colleagues, and before long, Liébeault, his methods, and his views had become widely known through Bernheim's advocacy. They continued to work closely together and, along with Henri Etienne Beaunis (1830–1921) and Jules Liégeois (1833–1908), came to be known as the Nancy school of hypnotism. When in 1884 Bernheim published *De la suggestion dans l'état hypnotique et dans l'état de veille,* he emerged as the spokesman for the group. The work was republished with considerable additional material in 1886, and it appeared in English translation in 1888 under the title *Suggestive Therapeutics.*[34] The views reflected in these writings brought Bernheim and the Nancy group into significant disagreement with Charcot and his followers at the Salpêtrière. Bernheim did not agree that hypnotism had an essential relationship to hysteria; instead, he concluded that it was a psychological state in its own right, and one intimately associated with suggestion. Though indicating agreement with Liébeault's view that "suggested sleep differs in no respect from natural sleep," Bernheim went on to say, "To define hypnotism as induced sleep, is to give a too narrow meaning to the word, — to overlook the many phenomena which suggestion can bring about independently of sleep. I define hypnotism

as the induction of a peculiar psychical condition which increases the susceptibility to suggestion. Often, it is true, the sleep that may be induced facilitates
suggestion, but it is not the necessary preliminary. It is suggestion that rules
hypnotism." He described his approach to the actual hypnotizing as follows:
"I begin by saying to the patient that I believe benefit is to be derived from the
use of suggestive therapeutics, that it is possible to cure or to relieve him by
hypnotism; that there is nothing either hurtful or strange about it; that it is an
ordinary sleep or torpor which can be induced in everyone, and that this quiet,
beneficial condition restores the equilibrium of the nervous system." Then,
once the subject was suitably relaxed, Bernheim proceeded with suggestions
that the patient think of nothing but sleep, that the eyelids were heavy, and
eventually that he or she should sleep. He would vary his technique somewhat
with different types of patients: for example, ask them to fix their eyes on his
eyes or on his fingers, or use gestures in the effort to influence, or use a com-
manding tone of voice. And he was prepared to accept that some would not
sleep but that in those cases he might achieve a state of heightened suggestibility without sleep. His approach was clearly a most flexible one; his adaptabil-
ity in response to individual differences is apparent. In some cases, he emphasized that "we must know the patient's character, his particular psychical
condition, in order to make *an impression* upon him." And scattered throughout this work are allusions to the significance of the relationship or rapport
between the hypnotist and the patient. His clinical data indicate that Bernheim
achieved both the heightened suggestibility and clinical improvement with the
vast majority of his patients.[35] Also, it is of interest to note that he particularly
emphasized the role of imagination in suggestive therapeutics.[36]

With the Nancy position made clear, to the effect that hypnotic phenomena
were the result of suggestion, the contrast with Charcot's position was sharply
defined. The Nancy school took the view that hypnotic phenomena were
essentially psychological in nature and that they were not pathological; and
Bernheim's increasingly clear emphasis on suggestion as a cardinal element
was to influence hypnosis in particular and psychotherapeutics in general for
many years afterward. In sharp contrast, Charcot argued that hypnotism consisted of a series of physiologically determined phases in hysterically pre-
disposed individuals and that the phases were induced and terminated by
physical stimuli (for example, a gong, a light, a magnet, various metals, or
physical contact from the hypnotist).

Already established as a highly regarded neurologist, in 1878 Jean-Martin
Charcot (1825–1893) began his investigations of hypnosis, on a service for
which he was responsible at the Salpêtrière, with women patients whom he
had diagnosed as suffering from hysteria. The hypnotic efforts with these

patients led him to posit three "stages" of hypnotism: lethargy, catalepsy, and somnambulism. His view was that the stages occurred in this order, that each stage had its characteristic symptoms, that the stages were always present as features of a developing hypnotic state, and that they were physiologically determined. For him, a hypnotic state was a pathological condition, an artificially created neurosis akin to hysteria. He argued that hypnosis was not the result of suggestion. He also took the view that the person of the hypnotizer was not of any importance. Charcot and those followers who subscribed to these views came to constitute the Salpêtrière school of hypnotism.[37]

Charcot's outline of these views, presented to the Académie des Sciences in 1882 and published the same year, brought both attention and respectability to hypnotism.[38] The result was a significant increase in hypnotic investigations and in the use of hypnotism in therapeutic endeavors. And it may even be that Bernheim's views met with a better reception in 1884 as a consequence. Then, in 1884–1885, Charcot's crucially significant studies of traumatic paralyses were done, which included demonstrations that certain paralytic states could be both induced and removed under hypnosis; these findings further enhanced the renewed interest in hypnotic work.[39]

As already indicated, just as Charcot was bringing his work on hypnotism to the attention of a larger professional audience, Bernheim was discovering Liébeault's work. Very soon their quite different orientations were being defined in sharp opposition to one another; and vigorous criticisms were directed by each group toward the other group's views. Further, the debates were taken up in medical journals and quickly spilled over into literary journals and into the popular press.[40] Hypnotizability came to be viewed under the influence of Charcot as a sign of mental illness, psychological defect, moral weakness, or weak character; the Nancy school, meanwhile, provided support for those who regarded the hypnotic state as merely a temporary state of heightened suggestibility. Also, considerable alarm was stirred up as to whether hypnotized persons might commit immoral or criminal acts and whether such persons might do harm to others or to themselves. At first, Charcot's prestige and his domination of contemporary medical opinion seemed to bode ill for the just-emerging regard for Liébeault's work; but, gradually, Bernheim's espousal of Liébeault's views, and a growing international respect for the Nancy school, influenced professional opinion in the direction of a psychological explanation for hypnotic phenomena and the view that suggestion was of the essence in bringing about hypnotic states.[41]

The 1880s and the early 1890s encompassed both the waxing and the waning of the disputes regarding hypnotism between the Nancy school and the Salpêtrière school. During the same era, the application of hypnosis in healing contexts and the publication of clinical writings on hypnosis — in addition to neurological investigations using hypnosis, public presentations of hypnosis (or "stage hypnosis"), and the use of hypnosis in parapsychological activities — became increasingly frequent. Paradoxically, though, the very schools of thought that had played such a signal role in bringing about the heightened interest in clinical hypnosis also had a significant influence on the diminishing interest in hypnosis and its clinical use as the nineteenth century came to a close.

In the case of Charcot, both unfair and fair-minded critics brought out more and more the serious limitations of the work at the Salpêtrière and the questionable practices surrounding the recurrent use of a small number of career hysterics for the hypnotic investigations there. Further, the Salpêtrière group had never concerned itself much with hypnosis as a mode of treatment, nor were they particularly sanguine about its therapeutic value; and Charcot himself had never hypnotized a patient. With Charcot's death in 1893, investigations of hypnosis ceased at the Salpêtrière.

In the case of the Nancy school, the focus had always been on the applications of hypnosis in the treatment of the sick. First with Liébeault and then with Bernheim, the attention was directed toward either cure or the relief of suffering; and this Nancy point of view had a wide-ranging influence. But, as his work made it increasingly clear that suggestion was the crucial element in the clinical usefulness of hypnosis, Bernheim gradually made less and less use of hypnosis, arguing that the desired therapeutic effects could equally well be obtained by suggestions to patients in the waking state. With suggestion emerging as the key element in a treatment approach previously associated with hypnosis, hypnosis itself came to be seen as merely a means of establishing a heightened degree of suggestibility. Suggestion might be undertaken with patients in the waking state or in a hypnotic state; as applied in the waking state, suggestion came to be termed psychotherapeutics. In this way, the Nancy influence, which had so enhanced the status of clinical hypnosis, eventually came to diminish the place of hypnosis in the world of clinical endeavors.

For the while, though, clinical hypnosis flourished. Report after report came out regarding successful hypnotic cures, and clinical texts proliferated. In 1888, Max Dessoir (1867–1947), a German psychologist, published *Bibliographie des modernen Hypnotismus,* containing 801 recent titles by some five hundred authors on hypnotism and animal magnetism, and in 1890 a supplement appeared, supplying another 382 titles.[42] The Nancy approach to hypnotism became the prevailing influence in psychological healing, well beyond the confines of Nancy and the borders of France. Numerous authorities who both reflected this influence and extended it had taken the trouble to visit

Nancy and learn directly from Bernheim;[43] for many, the term *Nancy school* thus carried the connotation of this far-flung influence of Liébeault-Bernheim therapeutics.

The work of Auguste Forel (1848–1931) in Switzerland, professor of psychiatry at the University of Zurich and director of the Burghölzli Hospital, did much to spread Bernheim's teaching in Switzerland and subsequently in Germany. Among Forel's significant contributions was his recognition that the personal attitude of the psychotherapist was a critical factor in successful treatment.[44] In Germany, Albert Moll (1862–1939), a psychiatrist, wrote an important book that supplemented Forel's. He introduced hypnotic psychotherapy into Germany and significantly furthered the development of suggestive therapeutics there. He too devoted considerable attention to the place of rapport in hypnosis.[45]

In England, Charles Lloyd Tuckey (1855–1925) and J. Milne Bramwell (1852–1925) were influential practitioners of hypnotism, suggestive therapeutics, and psychotherapeutics; each of these physicians visited Nancy and was profoundly influenced by the work there. In 1889 Tuckey's *Psycho-Therapeutics; or Treatment by Sleep and Suggestion*, appeared. It went through numerous greatly expanded editions, in the course of which its subtitle was changed to *Treatment by Hypnotism and Suggestion*. In this work, he emphasized the influence of the mind on the body and the clinical benefits of hypnotic suggestion on various diseases.[46] Bramwell, in *Hypnotism: Its History, Practice and Theory* (1903), traced the history of mesmerism and hypnotism, particularly emphasized the work of Braid, Liébeault, and Bernheim, and provided useful accounts of how various significant hypnotists went about their work.[47] Though this book was to remain a textbook and standard point of reference for hypnosis, in a new work in 1909 Bramwell indicated that he had come to view hypnosis as essentially a state of increased suggestibility and to see the hypnotic trance as no longer a necessary step in suggestive therapeutics — rather like the conclusion that Bernheim had reached some years earlier.[48] Interestingly, Janet was of the opinion that "treatment by hypnotic suggestion made its way tardily into English-speaking lands, and that this may be the reason why the wave subsided there rather more slowly than elsewhere."[49]

Pierre Janet

Another significant figure in clinical hypnosis from the late 1880s through to the end of the century was Pierre Janet, who, though at the Salpêtrière during the 1890s, was not one of Charcot's disciples and could not be accurately considered a member of the Salpêtrière school; and he could never be classified as a member of the Nancy school. Independent in his views on hypnosis, he practiced a particularly flexible, eclectic version of the psychotherapeutics of the day, with hypnosis as one key technique in his clinical endeavors. An experimental psychologist and physician, he developed his own brand of "psychological analysis and synthesis," with significant elements of deconditioning and reconditioning, advice and counsel, suggestion, and re-education. In many of his psychological investigations and in his therapeutics, he made considerable effective use of hypnosis and hypnotic suggestion, was circumspect in his assessment of their powers, and by the first decade of the twentieth century viewed those who still emphasized clinical hypnosis in their work as being "among the rare authors who are still defending hypnotic suggestion."[50]

After starting out as a young professor of philosophy at Le Havre in the early 1880s, Janet soon began an additional career as a psychological investigator who employed hypnosis in the study of his subjects. After several years of studying a series of hysterical women, he developed from this work his doctoral thesis (later published as *L'automatisme psychologique*), which he successfully defended at the Sorbonne in 1889.[51] That same year he shifted his teaching commitment to Paris and studied medicine there until he received his degree in 1893; he devoted considerable time to clinical investigations of hysteria at the Salpêtrière in the process. Shortly before his death in 1893, Charcot placed Janet in charge of a laboratory of experimental psychology at the Salpêtrière, where Janet continued until 1902, working with many patients in the outpatient department and in his private practice and intensively studying a select few patients over several years. The focus of his clinical research was the neuroses, first hysteria and later neurasthenia; and he continued to make considerable use of hypnosis in both his research and his clinical activities, modes of work that were not always clearly separated. He served the development of psychological healing through his notions of unconscious or subconscious acts, dissociation, and psychological automatisms; and he crucially contributed to the understanding of multiple personalities. As a hypnotist, it is fair to say that he was never really a partisan in the Salpêtrière-Nancy controversies, either as an investigator or as a clinician. His colleagues at the Salpêtrière went in other directions after Charcot's death, apparently rather disapproving of Janet's work; and the Nancy group were critical of his views and practices. He, in turn, found grounds for criticism in both schools of thought.[52]

In his use of hypnosis, a central purpose for Janet came to be the bringing to light of forgotten memories and subconscious fixed ideas that had played a significant role in the development of the patient's symptoms. Bringing these fixed ideas to awareness, working them through, and then undertaking re-educative measures were essential elements of his psychotherapeutics. He particularly stressed the place of rapport in the therapeutic process, noted the tendency for its influence to extend beyond the limits of the hypnotic session, and emphasized the need to control this psychological dependency — or somnambulistic influence, as he termed it — by spacing the sessions.[53]

In 1902, Janet became professor of experimental psychology at the Collège de France. In that decade, he made rather less use of hypnosis, as he developed further his own "psychological analysis" and his own quite flexible and eclectic version of dynamic psychotherapy. "More than a specific psychotherapy," it was, as Ellenberger has suggested, "a general system of psychotherapeutic economics."[54] In his scheme of psychological energy, psychological force, and psychological tension, he classified conditions as hypotonic or hypertonic, and in a way reminiscent of Brunonian notions of a century earlier, his psychotherapeutic efforts were directed toward redistributing psychological energy and increasing or decreasing psychological tension toward normal levels.[55] Janet continued to use hypnosis with hysterical patients, and hypnotic suggestion served as one of the means whereby he could adjust unfortunate levels of psychological tension and achieve a balanced distribution of psychological energy in a patient. But in contrast to the Nancy school's view that hypnosis and suggestion were not abnormal phenomena and that they could be used in the treatment of a wide range of sufferers, he saw them as pathological and particularly associated with hysterics. In general, he came to conceive of hypnosis as a psychotherapeutic fashion that had waxed and waned; and he implied that others who continued to emphasize hypnosis in their clinical work were somewhat outdated in their approach.[56] Still, it remained a meaningful clinical technique for him. In his *Psychological Healing*, he concluded his chapter "History of Suggestion and Hypnotism" by stating, "The decline of hypnotism has no serious meaning. It has been due to accidental causes, to disillusionment and reaction following upon ill-considered enthusiasm. It is merely a temporary incident in the history of induced somnambulism."[57]

Breuer and Freud

Another stream of influence in the realm of clinical hypnotism involved Josef Breuer and Sigmund Freud. Breuer's singular experience in the therapeutic use of hypnotism was to play a particularly significant role in Freud's early work and, indirectly, in the eventual emergence of psychoanalysis. In Vienna of the 1860s and 1870s, as in most of Western Europe, interest in hypnotism was at a low ebb, and a physician who took an interest in it indeed did so at the risk of his reputation. But stirrings of renewed interest in hypnotic phenomena were apparent in the late 1870s, with physicians such as Johann Czermak in

Leipzig and Charles Richet and Charcot in Paris showing the way, although as physiological and neurological investigators rather than as clinicians. These trends created an atmosphere that may have been crucial to Breuer's knowing something about hypnotism, and yet hardly one in which an established and respected physician would readily resort to such a mode of clinical intervention in his day-to-day practice. In Vienna itself, though, indications of renewed interest in hypnotism as a *clinical* activity also manifested themselves, in its use by the neurologist Moritz Benedikt (1835–1920) in severe cases of hysteria.[58]

In 1880–1882, Breuer undertook the treatment of Anna O., a young woman suffering from an array of neurological symptoms. As previously outlined, this treatment came to involve an extensive use of hypnosis and to be termed the talking cure, a version of cathartic therapy.[59]

In November 1882, Breuer first told Freud about Anna O.'s treatment, and the acquaintance between the two men became the context for at least intermittent discussion of her case for some years, culminating in their joint authorship of *Studies on Hysteria* in 1895. In 1885, after three years working in the general hospital in Vienna, Freud was awarded a scholarship abroad from the University of Vienna that allowed him to spend several months (October 1885 through February 1886) in Paris, attending Charcot's lectures and clinics, studying patients at the Salpêtrière, and doing some laboratory work. "When he arrived in Paris, his 'chosen concern' was with the anatomy of the nervous system; when he left, his mind was filled with the problems of hysteria and hypnotism."[60] With Charcot's work prominently in mind, Freud returned to Vienna and entered private practice, concentrating on nervous disorders. At first, he relied on the treatment methods already in common use for nervous disorders — hydrotherapy, electrotherapy, massage, and the Weir Mitchell rest cure. But 1886–1887 was the very period in which hypnotic suggestive therapy reached a peak in Germany and Austria. In this context, and under the influence of Breuer and Charcot, Freud began to use hypnosis in late 1887; by 1888, he had abandoned the use of electrotherapy. Freud not only employed hypnosis in the current fashion of direct hypnotic suggestion but, clearly influenced by Breuer's work, eventually began to induce hypnotic states for the purpose of facilitating cathartic therapy.[61] At the same time, he gradually gave up direct hypnotic suggestion, commenting "In the long run neither the doctor nor the patient can tolerate the contradiction between the decided denial of the ailment in the suggestion and the necessary recognition of it outside of the suggestion."[62]

Whatever the mode of hypnosis, Freud employed it regularly from 1887 to 1892. Though remaining particularly respectful of Charcot's views on many matters, where hypnosis was concerned Freud's work shifted away from Charcot's orientation, "in which there was no place for the therapeutic use of hypnosis."[63] Freud became interested in the work of Liébeault and Bernheim, undertook the translation into German of Bernheim's *De la suggestion* and wrote a preface for it in 1888, visited Nancy to learn from Bernheim in the summer of 1889, and favorably reviewed August Forel's Nancy-influenced *Der Hypnotismus* in 1889. In these contexts, Freud repeatedly took note of Bernheim's view that suggestion "is the basis of the whole of hypnotism" but also evinced concern with the puzzling question, "What in fact *is* this suggestion?"[64] Then, in 1891, he contributed an essay, "Hypnosis," to a medical dictionary, in which he affirmed Bernheim's view as his own opinion. "The true therapeutic value of hypnosis lies in the *suggestions* made during it. These suggestions consist in an energetic denial of the ailments of which the patient has complained, or in an assurance that he can do something, or in a command to perform it."[65]

During the same period, from 1887 to 1892, Freud was making increasing use of Breuer's hypnosis-catharsis method and using direct hypnotic suggestion less and less. Sometime after 1892, he began to use hypnosis less and to develop techniques for producing "the effects of suggestion without the need for putting the patient into a state of hypnosis."[66] In his chapter "The Psychotherapy of Hysteria" in *Studies on Hysteria* (1895), Freud addressed at some length what he judged to be the limitations of working with hypnosis, although he still did not dismiss hypnosis altogether. He sought those other means of obtaining the benefits of catharsis without employing hypnosis, means towards the goal of "bringing clearly to light the memory of the event by which" the symptom had been provoked; by thus evoking the memory, "arousing its accompanying affect"; and finally, through this abreactive process, resolving the symptom.[67] These other techniques were introduced to facilitate cathartic therapy in the waking state. Then, after 1896, he abandoned hypnosis as a therapeutic measure. Much has been made of Freud's discontinuance of hypnosis as a clinical practice. He commented later that he had "despaired of making suggestion powerful and enduring enough to effect permanent cures." And he was particularly concerned that hypnosis masked the patient's resistances, which factors he came to consider crucial in maintaining many illnesses, and important to be understood and resolved in the course of psychotherapeutic work.[68] He also later elaborated on his comments in *Studies on Hysteria* to the effect that he had not been able to hypnotize many of his patients, although it is not clear whether he primarily attributed this to limited hypnotizability or to his own limitations as a hypnotist.[69]

Much later, in his *Autobiographical Study* in 1925, Freud referred to his alteration in "the technique of catharsis" as having "abandoned hypnosis and sought to replace it by some other method, because I was anxious not to be restricted to treating hysteriform conditions." He then went on to say that "increasing experience had also given rise to two grave doubts . . . as to the use of hypnotism even as a means to catharsis."

> The first was that even the most brilliant results were liable to be suddenly wiped away if my personal relation with the patient became disturbed. It was true that they would be re-established if a reconciliation could be effected; but such an occurrence proved that the personal emotional relation between doctor and patient was after all stronger than the whole cathartic process, and it was precisely that factor which escaped every effort at control. And one day I had an experience which showed me in the crudest light what I had long suspected. It related to one of my most acquiescent patients, with whom hypnotism had enabled me to bring about the most marvellous results, and whom I was engaged in relieving of her suffering by tracing back her attacks of pain to their origins. As she woke up on one occasion, she threw arms around my neck. The unexpected entrance of a servant relieved us from a painful discussion, but from that time onwards there was a tacit understanding between us that the hypnotic treatment should be discontinued. I was modest enough not to attribute the event to my own irresistible personal attraction, and I felt that I had now grasped the nature of the mysterious element that was at work behind hypnotism. In order to exclude it, or at all events to isolate it, it was necessary to abandon hypnotism.[70]

Freud did not mention this incident in any other context, and its precise date is unknown; but Léon Chertok and Raymond de Saussure argued plausibly that it must have occurred sometime between 1891 and June 28, 1892. Further, Chertok made a good case for this episode's being at the root of Freud's development of the concept of transference.[71]

Early Twentieth Century

The years following Freud's abandonment of hypnosis were the very years in which overall interest in clinical hypnosis diminished considerably; but it is uncertain just what might be the relation between these two matters. After Charcot's death in 1893, the Salpêtrière rapidly lost its status as a center for hypnotic studies, despite Janet's work, which continued there until 1902. While Bernheim in Nancy continued the active practice of hypnotic suggestion well beyond Charcot's demise, by the late 1880s he was arguing for the frequent effectiveness of suggestion offered in the waking state;[72] and by the first decade of the twentieth century, he had developed more serious reservations about hypnosis. In fact, Janet maintained that by 1901, "Bernheim, the arch-hypnotist, has become a simple moraliser, and is towing in the wake of his whilom pupil Dubois."[73] This was Paul Dubois (1848–1918) who had developed his own system of psychological treatment known as persuasion therapy or moral treatment, among other terms. Originally influenced by Bernheim's suggestive therapeutics, he came to be highly critical of suggestive techniques; he conceived of his own approach as involving "logical persuasion," in contrast to suggestion, which entered "the understanding by the back stairs."[74]

The view that effective suggestive interventions did not require hypnosis as a prelude was the beginning of the end of a golden age for hypnosis. The challenge of the "persuasionists" further diminished the use of hypnosis. To a significant degree, both a loss of interest in hypnosis and reactions against the technique were operative by the first decade of the twentieth century. And it seems that psychoanalytic reservations about and criticisms of hypnosis compounded the situation rather than constituted the primary factor in the lessened use of clinical hypnosis.

The casualties of World War I led to a revival of interest in hypnotic suggestive therapy. As the number of cases of shell shock and other psychological casualties mounted, medical personnel in the armed forces on both sides of the conflict turned to psychological healing measures in an effort to treat the ill. Suggestion and persuasion were in prominent use; various re-educative measures were instituted; and hypnotic techniques were employed, both in an attempt to remove symptoms through direct suggestion and in order to resolve symptoms through the patient's reliving of traumatic experiences. In this latter approach, adopting modified versions of Freud's psychoanalytic views but usually focusing on traumatic experiences from the battlefield rather than sexual conflicts or early childhood experiences, physicians were engaged in a form of brief psychotherapy, in which they induced hypnosis as an expeditious means toward abreactive or cathartic results — not unlike the earlier cathartic therapy of Breuer and Freud. William Brown, for example, terming his approach psycho-catharsis, employed hypnosis to revive traumatic memories and bring about an abreaction of associated affects.[75] J. A. Hadfield (1882–1967) used hypnosis in two ways: (1) to set the stage for direct suggestions that would relieve patients of their symptoms; and (2) to cause patients to regress to the time of their traumatic experience, and then to relive that experience, discharge the related emotions, and reassociate the traumatic experience with the rest of the mind. He coined the term *hypno-analysis* for this second approach.[76] Ernst Simmel employed hypnosis to lift the patient's amnesia, and to allow him to relive the traumatic experience and abreact the associated emotions. He also favored further discussion in the waking state, in the interest of understanding and resolving the underlying conflict and undoing the dissociation.[77]

The renewed interest in clinical hypnosis continued after World War I. It has been suggested both that interest in hypnotic therapy waned once again in the postwar period and that the "new wave of enthusiasm for hypnotherapy . . . persisted to the present day."[78] Certainly, war neuroses became a problem again during World War II, and the clinical need led to another marked increase in the use of clinical hypnosis. But the amount of hypnotherapeutic activity in the interwar years had been far from insignificant. In the 1920s, Brown and Hadfield had continued to advocate the hypnotherapy they had employed during the war. Works such as the second edition of *An Introduction to the Study of Hypnotism* by H. E. Wingfield reflected the continued interest, in its lengthy section on treatment.[79] Henry Yellowlees (1888–1971), in his *A Manual of Psychotherapy* (1923), gave serious attention to hypnosis, to the point of including it among "the methods of psychotherapy." Emphasizing that it did not have "curative value" by itself, he stated that "its great use is to render the process of suggestion more easy and powerful." He also discussed hypnosis as a means to the recovery of repressed traumatic memories, as in the treatment of war neuroses.[80] In 1926, William McDougall (1871–1938), in his *Outline of Abnormal Psychology*, included hypnosis among a range of "psychotherapeutic methods" as a matter of course; in particularly identifying it as a "method of exploration," he noted its role in "the direct relief of symptoms" and referred to it as an "aid to readjustment."[81] And, in Vienna, Paul Schilder (1886–1940) and Otto Kanders were particularly active in the study of hypnosis and its application in psychological healing contexts. After noting that it "may be applied therapeutically in many ways," they emphasized three such applications in particular: (1) "The hypnotically induced sleep is used directly as a healing factor"; (2) "The suggestion given in hypnosis is directed outright against the psychic or physical symptom which is to be eliminated"; and (3) "Forgotten experiences are brought back to memory in hypnosis and are made accessible to the consciousness (cathartic hypnosis)."[82]

Similarly, in the 1930s, for all the alleged diminution in the use of hypnotherapy, a steady stream of useful, and often curative, efforts were made using hypnosis in the treatment of "functional and even organic illnesses." In his survey of the era, Wolberg has detailed an impressive list of such efforts, adding, though, that the majority entailed direct suggestion under hypnosis with the aim of removing symptoms.[83]

With World War II, hypnosis was again called upon in brief therapeutic undertakings to help deal with the new waves of war neuroses.[84] Both direct hypnotic suggestion and hypnosis to facilitate abreaction were employed. It should be noted, though, that narcoanalysis and narcosynthesis were also frequently used, with the same two purposes.

This new wave of clinical hypnotic activity was reflected in the work of Margaret Brenman and Merton Gill (1914–1994) at the Menninger Clinic, both late in World War II and in the immediate postwar years.[85] Others, influenced by the wartime resurgence of hypnotherapeutics, carried this trend into the late 1940s and 1950s. For example, Lewis Wolberg in New York made particularly significant contributions. Jerome Schneck brought together a group of useful contributions in *Hypnosis in Modern Medicine*. And Milton Erickson (1901–1980) continued a long-standing involvement in hypnotherapeutic work. Begun in the 1920s, his contributions were sustained through the 1930s, during the World War II years, and for several decades after the war.[86]

Hypnosis in Recent Times

In the later decades of the twentieth century, hypnosis has continued to be the subject of various controversies. Further, alongside those who have made judicious use of and reasonable claims for hypnotic techniques in psychological healing, some practitioners have been overly dramatic in their hypnotic practices and in their advocacy of hypnosis or have made exaggerated claims for the usefulness of such techniques. Even as some have been cautious about when and how to use hypnosis, others have, because of inexperience, been uneasy about using it at all or have dismissed it out of hand as dangerous.

Some among the various controversies regarding hypnosis have been put to rest as the myths on which they were based have been revealed as lacking substance.[87] First, much has continued to be made of the dangers allegedly inherent in hypnotic practices. By now, though, it is abundantly clear that the dangers alleged are not inherent in the practices; rather, they are the same dangers that might exist with inexperienced, incompetent, or immoral practitioners of any form of psychological healing. Second, it has been frequently argued that "symptom removal using hypnosis may be dangerous to a patient, or may result in symptom substitution," but sufficient evidence has accumulated to suggest that "symptom relief may facilitate rather than hamper the development of insight, the therapeutic alliance, and mastery in other areas." And symptom substitution does not necessarily occur, specially when hypnosis is used noncoercively. A third issue has been whether the hypnotic trance state was a form of sleep. It is now clear that the hypnotic state is "not sleep but a form of intense, focused alertness. Electroencephalogram (EEG) criteria make it clear that the brain is experiencing a form of resting arousal, and the electrophysiology of sleep is absent."[88]

Another issue of importance is the nature of the hypnotist-patient relationship. From the early nineteenth century onward, considerable interest has been shown in the *rapport* between the hypnotist-healer and the patient. At first, this term was used to mean that they were "in communication," that a peculiar state had been induced which allowed the hypnotist to exert an influence on the patient. A shift took place from the notion of a subtle, magnetic fluid mediating this influence to the idea of "the vital principle" and eventually to the view that it was a psychological influence that was communicated. For a while, the "will" of the hypnotist was said to be the crucial factor in the influencing of the patient. Ultimately, the term *rapport* came to mean a harmonious relationship or accord between the hypnotist and the patient. At the same time, though, themes of the patient's dependency and the hypnotist's control became significant, sometimes as explanations of the hypnotic process and sometimes as the focus for concerns and reservations about hypnosis. The more easily a patient responded to the hypnotist's induction procedures and suggestions and the more authoritarian the manner of the hypnotist, the more the themes of dependency and control were emphasized as matters of interest and concern. More recently, it has become clear that "expectations of control and dependency are bound to emerge and must be dealt with metaphorically, if not directly."[89]

Recent investigations have re-emphasized the long-standing view that hypnotic states are natural, rather than pathological, events. David Spiegel and Herbert Spiegel, modern authorities on hypnosis, point out that the hypnotic state is essentially "a form of attentive, receptive focal concentration with a sense of parallel awareness and a constriction in peripheral awareness," and that hypnotizability is a stable and measurable trait, with about two-thirds of an average psychiatric outpatient population being hypnotizable and one-third being highly hypnotizable. Further, Spiegel and Spiegel argue that "the person inducing hypnosis is not projecting anything onto subjects or controlling them, but is showing them how to discover and use their own hypnotic capacities. . . . This approach eliminates the pressure often experienced by therapists to prove themselves by succeeding in hypnotizing the patients, and it also avoids scapegoating the patients for resistance if they are not hypnotized. Although motivation on the part of the patient and the clinician's ability to establish an atmosphere of clinical respect and trust are important, they are necessary but not sufficient conditions for the utilization of hypnosis. The patient's hypnotic capacity is foremost."[90] And so, as Spiegel and Spiegel indicate, the therapist can invite patients to learn about these capacities and apply them in the service of an agreed-upon goal. The argument here is for a noncoercive approach in which the therapist seeks to enlist the patient as a collaborator in a clinical enterprise that is intended to benefit the patient — an approach that would be optimal for most, if not all, psychotherapeutic endeavors.

Regarding the process of induction, procedures have been simplified, the time taken for induction has been shortened, and the process has generally been demystified over the past few decades. The time needed to induce a trance state in a hypnotizable patient can be very brief indeed.

Though hypnosis has little place as a psychotherapeutic practice in and of itself, it has a distinct potential as an adjunctive technique in a variety of psychotherapeutic contexts, whether supportive, re-educative, or psychodynamically oriented. Among the ways in which it can serve as an adjunct to a larger psychotherapeutic endeavor are achieving relaxation and reduction of anxiety and tension; direct suggestion to induce disappearance of symptoms; direct suggestion concerning disappearance of attitudes underlying symptoms; easing of resistances; recovering of repressed memories; and abreaction of traumatic experiences. Further, various combinations of these adjunctive uses have been employed in conjunction with psychoanalytic techniques, to give new meaning to the term *hypnoanalysis*.

12

Suggestion

As noted in the chapter on mesmerism and hypnotism, the language we associate with healing through suggestion did not emerge until the latter part of the nineteenth century. In the wake of Bernheim's *suggestive therapeutics* in the 1880s, suggestion became a recognized element in psychological healing and has continued as such ever since. To some degree, though, this is misleading, as suggestive influences in healing long antedated the mesmerism and hypnotism out of which suggestion seemed to emerge.

The history of healing is replete with ways in which, directly or indirectly, healers have suggested to sufferers that ingesting a particular substance or following a particular procedure would lead to relief or cure. Reassuring words and comforting phrases have, often enough, had suggestive effects that caused sufferers to feel diminished concern about their ailments and even to recover their health. A manner, a gesture, or some other nonverbal message on a healer's part has frequently contributed an effective suggestion that all is well or soon will be. And quite directly, suggestions have at times successfully convinced sufferers that they were no longer ill, but were now well.

The very social context in which a physician or other healer has been sought out for help has commonly included the expectation that healers provide relief or cure; and so, merely by functioning in their role, healers have offered the promise that relief or recovery might well be forthcoming. The very yearning for relief and the state of needing and hoping for a healer's help heighten the sufferer's suggestibility, and quite frequently this has set the stage for useful gains by a patient in response to suggestive elements in a healer's words and actions.

Suggestion is defined as "the action of prompting one to a particular action or course of action; the putting into the mind of an idea, an object of thought, a plan, or the like." And *suggestibility* is used to indicate the susceptibility of a person to suggestion.[1] The *Psychiatric Dictionary* defines *suggestion* as "the process of influencing an individual so that he shows uncritical acceptance of an idea, belief, or other cognitive process. This acceptance is typically expressed as an attitude of belief and/or some action preparatory to carrying out the idea. Some would differentiate between heterosuggestion (when the source of the idea is someone outside the individual) and autosuggestion (when the source of the idea is the individual himself . . .)."[2] And English and English define it in their *Dictionary of Psychological and Psychoanalytical Terms* as "1. the process by which one person, without argument, command, or coercion, directly induces another to act in a given way or to accept a certain belief, opinion, or plan of action. 2. the verbal or other communication by means of which one person induces such action in another." They also add the comment, "There is often an implication that suggestion is devious and designed to circumvent critical consideration."[3] Although this last meaning is not in keeping with the usual practice of therapeutic suggestion, it does reflect an aspect of some of the nonclinical meanings of *suggestion*.[4]

Suggestion and Healing in Earlier Times

Healers' suggestions and the suggestibility of sufferers have long been among the elements that might be usefully present in a healing context. From the healing sleep in the temples of Isis and Serapis in ancient Egypt to the temple sleep in the Aesculapian temples of ancient Greece to the incubation practices associated with Christian churches and their saints, the atmosphere and the beliefs in those settings are generally regarded as having been eminently suggestive in nature.[5] In various combinations, incantations and religious rituals prepared the sufferers suggestively for the possibility of healing; dream interpretation and other divinatory activities further enhanced the expectations of healing help; and the hopes and suggestibility of the sufferers, along with the manner of the priest-healers and their faith in their own procedures, influenced many along suggestively determined paths to improvement or cure. Amulets, talismans, and charms were sought and provided, for their purported curative effects or for preventive purposes, and suggestion played a critical role in their usefulness.[6] And various other magical practices — such as incantations, the casting of spells, and "the king's touch" — have long been used in healing and have come to be recognized as having suggestion at the heart of their successes.[7] Faith healing in a variety of forms — through holy relics, healing shrines, individual healers, and prayerful efforts — has been another reflection of suggestive influences.[8] And it has been argued that many of the healing miracles of Jesus involved suggestion.[9]

Suggestion and Faith

It has long been argued that suggestion is the cardinal element in faith healing and healing miracles. And faith and suggestion have been considered in conjunction ever since suggestive therapeutics came into prominence in the late nineteenth century.

Faith has been defined as "confidence, reliance, trust (in the ability, goodness, etc., of a person; in the efficacy or worth of a thing; or in the truth of a statement or doctrine)";[10] and as "confident belief in the truth, value, or trustworthiness of a person, an idea, or a thing."[11]

In the process of discussing healing and faith, the clergyman-psychologist Leslie D. Weatherhead (1893–1976) concludes that suggestion is a crucial ingredient of faith.[12] Equally concerned with religion and healing, another clergyman-psychologist, Elwood Worcester (1862–1940), said, "In therapeutic practice the action of suggestion rests largely upon faith."[13] Still another clergyman-psychologist, Samuel McComb (1864–1938), in studying "faith and its therapeutic power," concluded that faith had been "an indispensable factor" in a wide variety of healing approaches, both religious and secular. He then added, "What indeed is psychotherapy at bottom but an elaborate system of suggestion, and what would suggestion avail were it not met with trust and faith on the part of the sufferer?"[14]

For the physician and anthropologist W. H. R. Rivers (1864–1922), faith and suggestion were two distinct phenomena that were intimately interrelated in healing; he referred to them as two "processes inextricably interwoven with the employment of therapeutic measures from the earliest stages of medicine down to the present."[15] He commented that "both faith and suggestion are of the greatest importance in psycho-therapeutics"; that faith in the healer and his therapeutic measures had been crucial throughout the history of medicine; and that "the influence of faith and suggestion pervades the whole system of treatment of the sick."[16] And, in a detailed and carefully objective study of faith healing, the British psychiatrist Louis Rose stated that suggestion "is a recognized psychological mechanism and many of the more thoughtful [faith] healers admit that it must play a part in their apparent successes."[17]

At the turn of the twentieth century, a leading voice in general medicine, William Osler, made the following comments on faith and suggestion in healing: "A . . . noteworthy feature in modern treatment has been a return to psychical methods of cure, in which *faith in something is suggested* to the patient. After all, faith is the great lever of life. . . . Faith in us, faith in our drugs and methods, is the great stock in trade of the profession. . . . It is the *aurum potabile,* the touchstone of success in medicine. . . . Faith in the gods or in the saints cures one, faith in little pills another, hypnotic suggestion a third, faith in a plain common doctor a fourth."[18]

Suggestion and Disease

The power of suggestion and the risks of suggestibility have long been recognized in another way, namely, as factors in causing disease. Someone may intentionally or unknowingly make comments that have the suggestive effect of causing another person to become ill; and various objects may deliberately be used to have such an effect or may inadvertently have such an effect.

In 1612, the English physician John Cotta (?1575–1650) wrote about "what fancie and imagination are able to do" in the way of causing all sorts of troublesome symptoms. Cautioning that one should not be too ready to attribute various casualties and illnesses to the devil and wicked men, he outlined the following "historie" to illustrate just how powerful "the juglings of the imaginarie" could be.

> Anno 1607, a Parsons wife of Northamptonshire, dwelling within three miles of the towne, came unto a Physition, complaining of a tumor in one of her breasts. He demanded her among many other things concerning the Sciatica, which he conjectured to vexe her. She denied any acquaintance or notion thereof in all her former life. The same night (being returned home) sodainly about midnight the Sciatica seized painfully and grievously upon her. Some few daies after, it happened another of her neighbours came also unto the same Physition, whom (beside the disease which she her selfe made knowne) he guessed to be troubled with the crampe, and cursorily questioned her thereof. She never before sensibly knowing any such paine, after her returne also that night suffered thereby exceeding torment.[19]

Cotta went on to note that, "It is an easie matter for any impression to worke it selfe into the imagination of a vaine mind."[20]

In the course of reviewing "the force of imagination," Robert Burton, who was a contemporary of Cotta's, cited numerous instances where the imagination was said to have caused a wide variety of symptoms and ailments, the clear indication being that suggestion, as it would later be termed, was at work: "Men, if they see but another man tremble, giddy, or sick of some fearful disease, their apprehension and fear is so strong in this kind that they will have the same disease. Or if by some soothsayer, wise man, fortune-teller, or physician they be told they shall have such a disease, they will so seriously apprehend it that they will instantly labour of it." And he included cases of the imagination's alleged power to mark a fetus with birth defects as a result of the mother's fantasies.[21] This possibility continued to be cited as a worrisome matter in medical folklore during the seventeenth and eighteenth centuries. In his study of Richard Napier's practice between 1597 and 1634, Michael Mac-Donald has noted similar results from the influence of suggestion.[22]

Suggestion and Imagination

Although it was not new to take note of the imagination as a factor contributing to disease, explicit and serious attention to this faculty as an agent in therapeutic endeavors emerged only during the sixteenth century; by the end of the century, though, it was readily taken into account. If a person brought a significant change of image to the sufferer's imagination, the imagination would then influence the troubled passions toward a cure. The principle of contraries guided the prescription, and so the effort was to induce an opposite sort of image, that it might bring about an opposite passion, the goal being a harmonious affective balance or at least a less troublesome passion. In the process, the corrective attention was also conceived of as influencing the humors and the spirits in beneficial ways and as relieving the sufferer of the symptoms.[23] Prominent among those who have left us accounts of this role for the imagination were Thomas Fienus and Robert Burton, each of whom was born in late in the sixteenth century and published a particularly relevant work in the early seventeenth century. Both these authors credited the imagination with a significant potential for causing and curing sickness.[24]

Further, the useful effects of magic in healing, the use of charms and amulets, the contributions of wise women and cunning men, and much else came to be attributed to the healing power of the imagination.[25]

Through the seventeenth century and well into the eighteenth century, medical and nonmedical authorities alike continued to be concerned with imagination as a force to be contended with in both health and disease. The word *imagination* had come to be used in the same way that *suggestion* came to be used in more recent times. Much as arguments have been made in the twentieth century for the constructive use of suggestion or the calculated use of the placebo effect in therapeutic endeavors, during the seventeenth and eighteenth centuries serious scholars and clinicians advocated techniques for influencing the imagination in the interest of the cure or amelioration of disease and suffering.

As was indicated in Chapter 11, in the late eighteenth century the royal commissions named by Louis XVI of France to assess Mesmer's work concluded that any beneficial effects of magnetic healing were due to the workings of the imagination. Then, in the second and third decades of the nineteenth century, several magnetizers introduced psychological explanations of animal magnetism that eventually developed into the theory of suggestion. Gradually the role of imagination in explanations of the cause and cure of disease led to the assigning of a similar role to suggestion.[26]

With the work of James Braid around mid-century, this transformation gradually became explicit, and the term *suggestion* entered discussions of hypnotism. Even though he expressed concern that the attribution of hypnotic phenomena to the imagination tended to be used to discredit or dismiss them, Braid acknowledged that "imagination can either kill or cure"; and he equated "suggestions" leading to ill health or improved health with "the power of the imagination."[27] In his later work, it seems clear the he had a sense of the role of suggestion, and the language of suggestion crept into some of his writings.[28] In 1853 he stated,

> By our various modes of suggestion, through influencing the mind by audible language, spoken within the hearing of the patient, or by definite physical impressions, we fix certain ideas, strongly and involuntarily in the mind of the patient, which thereby act as stimulants, or as sedatives, according to the purport of the expectant ideas, and the direction of the current of thought in the mind of the patient, either drawing it to, or withdrawing it from, particular organs or functions; which results are effected in ordinary practice, by prescribing such medicines as experience has proved stimulate or irritate these organs.[29]

In these regards, A. E. Waite has reasoned that Braid was "the discoverer, so to speak, of suggestion," but that he "by no means fully realised the possibilities of suggestion of the unconscious kind."[30]

Suggestive Therapeutics

In the decades after Braid's time, the concept of imagination continued to be mentioned, though less and less frequently, in explanations of how healers might influence patients toward cure or relief of symptoms. At the same time, the mention of suggestion in such contexts gradually increased. In 1872 Tuke still placed considerable emphasis on the role of imagination in "the influence of the mind upon the body in health and disease"; and it was through the imagination that he conceived of the mind as being affected by psychological factors and, in turn, as having its influence on the body. But Tuke's book contained a few scattered references to *suggestion,* alluding to "mental impressions made on the patient" as "the phenomena of suggestion, or suggestive phenomena."[31] Still, though, the language of suggestion had not yet permeated the discussion of psychological healing in the way that it soon would. Tuke also introduced the term *psycho-therapeutics* for the "General Influence of the Physician upon the Patient in Exciting those Mental States which act beneficially upon the Body in Disease";[32] and that term soon came to be equated with *suggestive therapeutics.*

By the 1880s, much that had previously been attributed to the imagination was coming to be explained in terms of suggestion and autosuggestion. In 1887, in their extensive review of animal magnetism and hypnosis, Alfred Binet and Charles Féré wrote about "this medicine for the imagination, which is entitled to the name of suggestive therapeutics." Looking back in time, these authors argued that the power of suggestion accounted for a variety of cures, some notable and some notorious, which had been attributed to the imagination.[33] Féré had previously written about *la médecine d'imagination,* indicating that it was essentially *thérapeutique suggestive.*[34]

But central to the emergence of suggestive therapeutics was the work of Liébeault and Bernheim in developing hypnotic therapeutics at Nancy.[35] In 1884 Bernheim's *De la suggestion dans l'état hypnotique* appeared, the revised second edition of which was translated in 1888 as *Suggestive Therapeutics.*[36] He defined hypnosis as "the induction of a peculiar psychical condition which increases the susceptibility to suggestion." The hypnotic sleep may facilitate suggestion, but it was not a necessary preliminary. "It is suggestion that rules hypnotism."[37] And it is of interest to note that he particularly emphasized the role of imagination in suggestive therapeutics.[38]

Bernheim's flexible technique allowed him to bring about a state of heightened suggestibility, whether or not the patient could be hypnotized.[39] As a result, he gradually employed hypnotism less and less, and he eventually argued that the same results could be achieved through suggestion to patients in the waking state. Thus hypnotism came to be regarded as a state of heightened suggestibility that had been achieved by suggestion in the first place.

In 1891, in *Hypnotisme, suggestion, psychothérapie; études nouvelles,*[40] Bernheim unequivocally dissociated himself from Liébeault's view that hypnosis was the equivalent of sleep. Rather, he thought that "the sleep-like quality of hypnosis" was "entirely suggested"; and he concluded that the hypnotic state should be regarded as an adjunct to suggestive psychotherapy. "For Bernheim, suggestion was an inescapable part of the doctor-patient relationship. Whether a physician realized it or not, all of his actions conveyed suggestions to his patient. Psychotherapy, as he defined it, was the intentional application of suggestion, in all its various forms, toward a therapeutic goal. . . . In *New Studies,* we see the seasoned wisdom of a clinician who realized that a placebo could be as powerful a therapeutic agent as a "real" drug."[41] In these lectures (given in 1890), Bernheim chronicled a long series of miraculous cures attributed to faith and divine intervention, magical cures, cures through influencing the imagination, early magnetic cures, and late mesmeric cures.[42] He saw this long history of "superstitious medicine" as having crucially involved the unwitting use of suggestion. He concluded that "we have reason to say that everything is in suggestion."[43] He then added some two hundred pages of "Clinical Observations."

Significantly influenced by Bernheim, suggestive practices and the language of suggestion held a prominent place in psychological healing from 1890 to World War I. While cathartic therapy, persuasion, and the growing influence of psychoanalysis were each part of the psychotherapeutic scene, hypnotic therapy and suggestive therapeutics were the more common practices. There were books and journal articles on "suggestion," "suggestive therapy," "suggestion and hypnosis," "suggestion and mental healing," and "psychotherapeutics or suggestion."[44] And journals such as *Suggestive Therapeutics* and *Suggestion* discussed the subject. Hypnosis was commonly viewed as essentially a means of enhancing suggestion. *Suggestion* and *psychotherapy*" (or *psycho-therapeutics*) were frequently used as synonyms.

Further, many other volumes dealing with psychotherapeutics did not make suggestion a central theme and yet devoted considerable attention to the subject—for example, Francis X. Dercum (1856–1931) in his *Rest, Mental Therapeutics, Suggestion* and James J. Walsh (1865–1942) in his *Psychotherapy.*[45] Still other works included at least a chapter on suggestion, or on suggestion and hypnotism—for example, Hügo Munsterberg (1863–1916) in his *Psychotherapy.*[46]

During the same period in which suggestive practices were so prominent, considerable attention was given to persuasion, and it too became a significant feature of psychotherapeutic endeavors.[47] Around the turn of the twentieth century, even as suggestive therapy was in the ascendancy, objections were emerging to suggestion during a patient's waking state, as they already had to hypnotic suggestion. But despite the persuasionists' assertions to the contrary, many critics saw suggestion as the essential element in persuasion therapy, although sometimes suggestion was conceived of as only an oblique form of persuasion. At the very least, they were usually considered to be closely allied. In the next few decades, suggestion and persuasion were each discussed repeatedly in the psychotherapeutic literature, sometimes in conjunction with criticism of one or both and sometimes with an indication that one or the other (or both) was a preferred technique. It was not uncommon for them to be presented as two distinct yet related psychotherapeutic techniques, and to be compared and contrasted in a chapter or section on "suggestion and persuasion."

During the first decade of the century still another trend began to emerge in suggestive therapeutics, namely, *autosuggestion*. Emile Coué (1857–1926), an apothecary, had acted to develop his interest in psychological healing and had studied with Liébeault and Bernheim. After beginning with hypnotic suggestion, he soon became particularly adept in the use of nonhypnotic suggestion; he eventually concluded that autosuggestion was the basis for many suggestive effects. He emphasized that the imagination, rather than the will, was the crucial agency in autosuggestion. In 1910 he started a free clinic for suggestive therapy in Nancy, and out of his efforts the "new Nancy school" emerged. Being especially effective in inducing suggestive effects, Coué turned to promoting the idea that most of the same effects could be achieved by teaching autosuggestion to both those who suffered and those who sought self-improvement in a general educational sense. His famous phrase "Every day, in every way, I am getting better and better," was to be repeated regularly, he advised; and this is a fair reflection of the inspirational and exhortative overtones of his autosuggestive method. After World War I, Coué traveled and lectured widely, and in the 1920s his views and practices became well known and particularly influential in Britain and the United States, where their influence was aided significantly by the writings of Charles Baudouin (1893–1963), Coué's disciple and tireless supporter.[48]

Another keen student of suggestion, the physician and psychologist William Brown, is of particular significance here. His contributions convey a sense of the omnipresence of suggestion in the psychological healing of his era; and as previously noted, they give some indication of the growing significance of psychoanalytically influenced efforts, albeit he was not a psychoanalyst and had his reservations about Freud's views. Like others before him, he first concerned himself with hypnosis, only to later modify considerably his opinion of its usefulness and accord a place to suggestion offered to patients in the waking state. With the advent of World War I, he became one of a key group of psychologically minded medical officers who were heavily involved in, and central to, the British efforts to cope with the huge numbers of battle casualties termed nerve cases, and later sufferers from shell shock. Brown's experience with several thousand of these "psycho-neuroses of war" included lengthy service in a casualty-clearing station behind the lines in France, and in specialty hospitals (such as Craiglockhart War Hospital, near Edinburgh) back in Britain toward the end of the war and afterward.

In many acute cases, Brown found that "the method of *rational persuasion* sufficed to produce a cure if preceded by a thorough physical examination and supported by the arousal of feelings of confidence and enthusiastic expectation of a favourable result"; and he recognized an element of suggestion in such treatment efforts.[49]

In cases "showing extensive amnesia, involving dissociation of intensely emotional psychic states"—hysteria caused by shell shock—he employed *light hypnosis* to restore lost memories and free "the patient from subconscious emotional obsession."[50] He then proceeded to bring about a "working off" or release of repressed emotion, much in the manner of Breuer and Freud's cathartic therapy, recovering repressed memories and undoing dissociation in the process. He termed this procedure "psycho-catharsis or abreaction." He recognized a role for suggestion in the process of hypnosis, and he employed suggestion in facilitating the abreaction. This was followed by efforts toward the reintegration of the dissociated experiences—"re-association or psycho-synthesis"—which was associated with stabilizing the relief from the distress and the physical symptoms.[51]

With patients seen at late stages of their illness, Brown noted an attendant fixation of symptoms, accompanied by a distorted view of the illness on the patient's part, "linked up by numerous bonds of association with earlier emotional incidents of his life equally misunderstood by him."[52] Here he advocated "mental analysis" or "autognosis" (self-knowledge), which he conceived of as "closely akin to re-association."[53]

In summing up, Brown commented that suggestion was "of the utmost importance, since it is a determining condition of the effective working" of psychocatharsis, psychosynthesis, and autognosis. He also argued that suggestion is a crucial element in the role of transference in psychoanalysis.[54] He indicated that suggestion had a distinct role in his clinical work after the war: "One very rarely has occasion to employ it [hypnosis] in civilian practice. Here waking suggestion, persuasion and mental analysis suffice."[55]

After the publication of his *Psychology and Psychotherapy* in 1921, Brown followed up, in 1922, with his *Suggestion and Mental Analysis*. This "Outline of the Theory and Practice of Mind Cure" was organized around the view that there were "two distinct and, in the main, mutually exclusive forms of theory and practice in the field of psycho-therapy, viz. suggestion and auto-suggestion on the one hand, and mental analysis (including the special Freudian system of psycho-analysis) on the other."[56]

To the significance of suggestion put forward in his previous book, Brown now took note of autosuggestion, including particular attention to the work of Emile Coué. He defined "auto-suggestion or self-suggestion . . . in relation to the subconscious" and emphasized the importance of emotion in its operation. "The subconscious responds to suggestion, that is, to affirmations made with belief or conviction. . . . In the case of a good or useful auto-suggestion the emotion should be that of enthusiasm and confident expectation (akin to, if not identical with, faith)." He then noted that "bad auto-suggestions occur involuntarily with all of us from time to time. The emotion which has special power in reinforcing them is the emotion of fear." Further, these bad autosuggestions "tend especially to exaggerate and to prolong ill-health of mind and body," and, often enough, they are the cause of ill health.[57]

Suggestion was also a central factor in Brown's various references to relaxation as an aspect of his approach to psychological healing. This is evident in the careful advice and urging that were part of his attempts to promote a relaxed state during hypnotic efforts. He did much the same in preparing a patient for suggestive therapy. And this emphasis is evident again in his advocacy of quiet sessions devoted primarily to relaxation on a couch. In later writings, he elaborated somewhat on this aspect of his practices, taking note of Edmund Jacobson's (1888–1983) work on "progressive relaxation" in the process.[58] One of Brown's approaches became "suggestion treatment, with progressive relaxation." After twenty-five years of experience, in summing up what he considered the factors of value in psychotherapy, Brown listed the following: "psycho-catharsis and reassociation of the mind, relieving repressions and recalling lost memories by the method of 'free associations,' autognosis, auto-suggestion, progressive relaxation, and the personal influence of the physician."[59]

Another influential British psychiatrist and psychotherapist between the two world wars was Henry Yellowlees (1888–1971), medical superintendent at the York Retreat and later senior consultant in psychiatry at St. Thomas's in London. As so many others did in that era, he dealt with suggestion and persuasion together in his writings. He introduced suggestion as follows: "Suggestion has been defined as 'a process of communication resulting in the acceptance with conviction of the communicated proposition in the absence of logically adequate grounds for its acceptance' (McDougall). It is one of the most important methods of psychotherapy, and, indeed, may be called the most important from the general practitioner's point of view. . . . Suggestibility is a normal characteristic, and varies only in extent in each of us."[60] Much like William Brown, he considered two main categories of psychotherapeutic activity: those related to suggestion and those which were psychoanalytically oriented. He went on to outline various factors which were significant in affecting suggestibility, mentioned the "new Nancy school" and the emphasis by many on the role of auto-suggestion, underlined the role of placebos as an application of suggestion in therapeutics, and took note of the "remedial power of suggestion" in various practices commonly employed by both healers and average citizens.[61] He defined persuasion as "suggestion plus appeal to the patient's common sense."[62] Apparently drawing on the work of Ernest Jones (1879–1958), he mentioned the view that suggestion "really includes two distinct processes": verbal suggestion and affective suggestion. He described the latter as "a *rapport* which depends upon transference," and stated that psychoanalysts held that it was "the essence of suggestion."[63] Finally, in summing up the place of suggestion, Yellowlees said, "In suggestion we have probably the most powerful and readily available single weapon known to medicine. No occasion is too trivial for its use, and it is hard to reach the limit of its possibilities."[64]

While the views and practices of Brown and Yellowlees were representative of many during the interwar years, approaches based primarily on suggestion were gradually losing favor, and psychoanalysis was gradually becoming more influential. Still, suggestion retained a recognized place in psychological healing and continued to be strongly advocated by a few; and it was taken for granted by others, included in a range of techniques that they discussed. At times suggestion was taken into account in considering the placebo effect, and it was recognized by many as an unavoidable aspect of psychotherapeutic endeavors. For the most part, its position had shifted to that of one approach among several, if not one among many. Although psychoanalysts continued to take pains to differentiate suggestive methods from psychoanalytic methods, most recognized that it would be extremely difficult to eliminate suggestive influences altogether — practitioners emphasized the need to be aware of such influences, to attempt to limit them, and to endeavor to analyze them where they could not be avoided. Analysts strove to avoid direct suggestion, but many recognized the considerable potential for indirect suggestive influence in the psychoanalytic situation[65] — for example, the unspoken suggestive implications that there may be explanations and understandings beyond the obvious or beyond the patient's current awareness, that the patient has merit or is not a bad person in the face of his or her convictions to the contrary, that there is hope when the patient is discouraged, or that difficult, complex dilemmas can be understood and resolved. Further, the subtle suggestive effect was always in operation when the psychoanalyst responded to one association rather than another or focused on one issue rather than another.

Reasonably representative of the 1930s was the perspective on suggestion reflected in *Psychotherapy in Medical Practice* (1942) by Maurice Levine (1902–1971). A particularly influential teacher of psychiatry and psychotherapy, Levine had concerned himself with educating general physicians, social workers, psychologists, and laypersons. His book reflected this work and went through innumerable printings and several translations. Levine discussed a wide variety of "methods for the general practitioner" and pointed out when and how a physician might enhance his psychotherapeutic helpfulness to patients.[66] Among these, he included suggestion therapy, noting that it was often facilitated by the patient's endowing the physician with considerable authority and personal influence, well beyond those derived from his actual training and experience. After emphasizing the common tendency for human beings to be suggestible, Levine commented,

> In certain acute conditions the patient can be helped over a difficult situation, or can be helped to get rid of some disturbing symptoms, by authoritative commands, by persuasive suggestions, by impressive treatment, or by the use of placebos which the patient expects to cure him. In less acute conditions, feelings of anxiety may be lessened, feelings of depression may decrease, and certain hysterical symptoms may disappear, when the physician gives some sort of explanation or some sort of treatment, with the strong suggestion that it will have a curative effect. Physicians occasionally use tricks to help bring about this suggestive effect. For example, they may cause an hysterically paralyzed muscle to move by an electric shock, not only as a way of demonstrating to the patient that the muscle is still functioning and in good condition, but also as a strong suggestion that the patient will then be able to move the muscle. In certain acute situations, *e.g.*, in the war neuroses, suggestion therapy may be distinctly and definitely valuable.[67]

Even while indicating the usefulness of suggestion therapy, Levine also discussed some of the objections to such approaches. First, he commented, "an element of trickery" was involved. By "not appealing to the intelligence of his patient," the physician was "working with his antilogical tendencies"; he was "not appealing to the maturity of his patient, but to certain neurotic or infantile attitudes." This was reminiscent of the criticisms of suggestive therapeutics raised by the persuasionists around the turn of the century; and in various forms such comments had been made repeatedly ever since. Second, suggestion was "not an etiologic method of therapy." It was "merely an attempt to cause the disappearance of a symptom," and thus the symptom or an equivalent was likely to recur. He then contrasted it with insight-oriented therapy and with environmental manipulation, both of which were thought to eliminate the cause. Third, the effects of suggestion therapy were "likely to be quite temporary," and it was not likely to be so effective when it was repeated.

Fourth, the patient might well realize that "the physician has been untruthful, in a sense, to him," and so lose confidence in him and perhaps in doctors in general. Each of these objections was familiar and had been frequently raised against suggestion therapy. Levine summed up by commenting, "In general one would say that suggestion therapy may be used when other methods of psychotherapy are either unavailable or unsuccessful, that it may be used in certain emergency situations, and that in the use of suggestion therapy the physician should adhere as much as possible to the truth."[68]

By the end of the interwar years, hypnosis and suggestive techniques in general had, to a significant extent, given way to psychotherapeutic approaches influenced by psychoanalytic methods. In 1940, though, anticipating the prospect of war neuroses to come, a group of British authors attempted to prepare "the present military medical officers" by reviewing their own World War I experience with "large numbers of so-called 'shell-shock' cases fresh from the line or in hospitals abroad and at home."[69] Suggestion had been central in much of the work they reviewed: direct suggestion associated with hypnosis, and both indirect and direct suggestion without hypnosis. J. A. Hadfield authored a chapter, "Treatment by Suggestion and Hypno-Analysis," in which he discussed in some detail suggestion to patients in both the waking and the hypnotic state, as well as hypnoanalysis, this being an amalgamation of hypnotic-cathartic experiences and methods akin to those of psychoanalysis.[70]

As World War II unfolded, the expected wave of psychological casualties occurred in response to the stress of war; and as in World War I, they led to a renewed interest in brief psychotherapeutic techniques associated with suggestion and hypnosis. Suggestion was prevalent, both in association with cathartic or abreactive techniques and as a technique aimed directly at the elimination of symptoms. Catharsis or abreaction was mediated through the induction of a hypnotic state and at times through the use of pharmacological agents to achieve a narcotized state viewed as an equivalent to the state of hypnotic trance.[71] Some important accounts of these treatment efforts make no explicit mention of suggestion, and yet the role of suggestion is often implied. For example, Roy R. Grinker (1900–1993) and John P. Spiegel (1911–1991) reported in detail on psychotherapeutic work with "war neuroses," including cathartic therapy with hypnosis and with narcotic agents, persuasion, and a range of supportive measures. Whether the agent was hypnosis or sodium pentothal, suggestion was employed to promote free expression by the patient, to re-create the traumatic experience in fantasy and so promote a reliving of it, and to overcome resistances to remembering and reliving. Further, suggestion was used to encourage, to provide reassurance, and to enhance other supportive interventions — that is, suggestion was used again and again to further the action of numerous other psychotherapeutic measures.[72] Other World War II medical officers strongly favored hypnosis in the service of catharsis and abreaction and were explicit about the key role for suggestion in the treatment process.

In an extensive report, John G. Watkins provided another account of hypnotherapy with "war neuroses," this time for patients whose persistent symptoms had necessitated their return to a military hospital in the United States. The treatment efforts involved direct suggestion to modify or eliminate symptoms, both during the trance and through posthypnotic suggestions. But Watkins added the caution that "direct suggestion should not be considered as a method of curing an illness."[73] Instead, Watkins advocated the view that such direct suggestions should lead to uncovering traumatic conflicts and working through them with the development of insight. He also commented on the usefulness of suggestion in altering attitudes and in encouraging a positive, cooperative approach to treatment.

Suggestion and Psychoanalysis

During the years in which suggestive therapeutics flourished, psychoanalysis gradually came into prominence as a mode of psychological healing, and psychoanalysts eventually began to express reservations regarding the place of suggestion in psychotherapeutics. As noted in Chapter 11, in the late 1880s Freud had taken up the use of hypnosis in these therapeutics, and hypnotic suggestion had become part of his clinical endeavors.[74] In 1889 he completed a translation of Bernheim's *De la suggestion* into German and visited Bernheim in Nancy. In the preface he wrote for this translation, he emphasized the significance of Bernheim's view that hypnotism was essentially suggestion, but he stopped short of dismissing Charcot's views in favor of Bernheim's. He also expressed his concern that the term *suggestion* was being used rather loosely to refer to too broad a range of phenomena.[75] And he argued that Bernheim, to a large extent, worked with indirect suggestions rather than direct suggestions — that is, that it was "a question . . . not so much of suggestions as of stimulation to *autosuggestions*."[76] As to his own use of suggestion, by the time *Studies on Hysteria* was published in 1895, Freud had essentially abandoned hypnosis and was using direct suggestion with patients in the waking state, in the service of his cathartic therapy.[77] Then, less than ten years later, he made it clear that he had long ago "renounced suggestion" as well as hypnosis; and he took some pains to differentiate "this cathartic or analytic method of psychotherapy" from "hypnotic treatment by suggestion" or any other form of suggestive therapeutics.[78]

Subsequent to these comments, Freud and other psychoanalysts recurrently emphasized how different their treatment approach was from the suggestive therapies; and they vigorously objected to criticism that maintained that successful psychoanalytic treatment was "brought about merely by suggestion."[79] At times, it became rather a point of pride that they did not "alloy the pure gold of analysis" with "the copper of direct suggestion."[80]

Nevertheless, Freud acknowledged certain limited ways in which suggestion still had a relevance for psychoanalysis. On several occasions, he made a brief reference to the use of suggestion in overcoming resistances: "The patient has to accomplish it [that is, overcoming resistances] and the doctor makes this possible for him with the help of suggestion operating in an *educative* sense."[81] He emphasized that the analyst did not use "his personal influence, the factor of 'suggestion,' to suppress the symptoms of the illness, as happens with *hypnotic* suggestion." Rather, in contrast to other psychotherapeutic procedures, he used it "as a motive force to induce the patient to overcome his resistances."[82] Moreover, "psycho-analytic procedure differs from all methods making use of suggestion, persuasion, etc., in that it does not seek to suppress by means of authority any mental phenomenon that may occur in the patient. ... In psycho-analysis the suggestive influence which is inevitably exercised by the physician is diverted on to the task assigned to the patient of overcoming his resistances, that is, of carrying forward the curative process."[83]

Freud also thought of suggestion as retaining a place in psychoanalysis in still another way, namely, as being related to transference. In 1909–1910 a connection between suggestion and transference had been put forward by Sandor Ferenczi and by Ernest Jones. Ferenczi had argued that "the capacity to be hypnotised and influenced by suggestion depends on the possibility of transference taking place."[84] Jones stated that "the phenomena of suggestion in the neuroses are seen to constitute only one variety of a group of processes to which Freud has given the name of Transference." And he added, "The term suggestion covers two processes, 'verbal suggestion' and 'affective suggestion,' of which the latter is the more primary, and is necessary for the action of the former. Affective suggestion is a *rapport,* which depends on the transference (Übertragung) of certain positive affective processes in the unconscious region of the subject's mind."[85] A few years later, referring to Bernheim as "basing his theory of hypnotic phenomena on the thesis that everyone is in some way 'suggestible,' " Freud commented: "His suggestibility was nothing other than the tendency to transference, ... In our technique we have abandoned hypnosis only to rediscover suggestion in the shape of transference."[86] Freud made related comments in two other contexts. Transference was "the same dynamic factor which the hypnotists have named 'suggestibility,' which is the agent of hypnotic *rapport* and whose incalculable behavior led to difficulties with the cathartic method as well."[87] Transference "coincides with the force which has been named 'suggestion.'"[88]

Still, though, Freud continued to emphasize the differentiation of psychoanalysis from the suggestive therapies. As he stated it, the recurrent resolving of the transference "is the fundamental distinction between analytic and purely suggestive therapy," and it is that work that "frees the results of analysis from the suspicion of being successes due to suggestion. In every other kind of suggestive treatment the transference is carefully preserved and left untouched; in analysis it is itself subjected to treatment and is dissected in all the shapes in which it appears."[89]

Suggestion and the Placebo Effect

Still another way in which suggestion has had a place in healing over the centuries has been as a factor in the placebo effect; thus the history of the placebo constitutes a chapter in the history of suggestion. A leading student of placebos and the placebo effect, Arthur K. Shapiro, has defined these terms as follows:

> A *placebo* is defined as any therapy, or that component of any therapy, that is deliberately used for its nonspecific, psychologic, or psychophysiologic effect, or that is used for its presumed specific effect on a patient, symptom, or illness, but which, unknown to patient and therapist, is without specific activity for the condition being treated.
>
> A *placebo*, when used as a control in experimental studies, is defined as a substance or procedure that is without specific activity for the condition being evaluated.
>
> The *placebo effect* is defined as the nonspecific, psychologic, or psychophysiologic effect produced by placebos.[90]

The word *placebo* is borrowed from Latin and means "I shall please." In addition to centuries of use with this meaning, *placebo* also came to convey implications of sycophancy, servility, and flattery. Then, by the late eighteenth century, it began to appear in some medical dictionaries with the definition "a commonplace method or medicine," and in others with the meaning "any medicine adopted more to please than to benefit the patient."[91]

The use of *placebo* with anything like our modern meanings only came much later. In 1894 a medical dictionary defined it as "a make-believe medicine." And, by the middle of the twentieth century, it was being defined as the use in treatment of substances that were "inert" or "inactive."[92] It is only in quite recent times that the definitions have downplayed the notion of humoring the patient and the idea that the substances employed were necessarily inactive, as in the following from the *Psychiatric Dictionary* (1960):

> Any medication used to relieve symptoms, not by reason of specific pharmacologic action but solely by reinforcing the patient's favorable expectancies from treatment. Although a placebo may be an inert substance, as used in present-day research placebos more commonly contain active substances that at least in part mimic the side-effects of the specific therapeutic agent with which the placebo is being compared. Placebo effects include all those psychologic and psychophysiologic benefits and undesirable reactions which reflect the patient's expectations; they depend upon the diminution or augmentation of apprehension produced by the symbolism of medication or by the symbolic implications of the physician's behavior and attitudes.[93]

Yet, as Shapiro pointed out, this definition still did not include any reference to psychological treatment interventions, such as appeared in his own definition a few years later.

Although the modern use of the term and an awareness of how frequently the placebo effect is a factor in treatment have a relatively short history, it has frequently been argued that placebos have been at the heart of therapeutics during most of medicine's history. In fact, Shapiro goes so far as to say that the "history of medical treatment until relatively recently is the history of the placebo effect."[94] But with so much in the history of successful therapeutics retrospectively attributed to the unknowing use of placebos, it is well to be reminded that, however unaware most healers may have been, the knowing use of placebos dates back a very long way. For example, in the Hippocratic writings (fifth and fourth centuries B.C.), the physician was advised, "If the ear aches, wrap wool around your fingers, pour on warm oil, then put the wool in the palm of the hand and put it over the ear so that something will seem to him to come out. Then throw it in the fire. A deception."[95] And, for another example, in the first century A.D., Seneca (4 B.C.–A.D. 65) commented that, with some sufferers, a physician "should dupe by a sugared dose in order to make a quicker and a better cure by using deceptive remedies."[96] And in the *Physical Ligatures* of Qusṭā ibn Lūqā (ca. 830–910), the placebo effect and suggestion were given a significant place in therapeutics. Qusṭā was a physician who both translated from the Greek into Arabic and wrote many medical works of his own. His *Physical Ligatures* was "a learned, 'high medicine' text on the empirical use of magic," in which he made the point, "on no less authority than Plato," that "the mere belief in the efficiency of a remedy will indeed help in a cure"; and numerous manuscripts and early modern printings suggest that his work was widely read in the West. Qusṭā maintained that "a benefit of some drugs in some circumstances is the effect that they have on the mind, provided patients believe them to be remedies." Most of his prescriptions involved "the power of persuasion or suggestion"; and he clearly recognized the placebo effect when he said that "the action of a medicine may be no more than the effect the suggestion has on the mind."[97]

Just how much suggestion is at work in the use of placebos and how much suggestibility affects the experiencing of the placebo effect have been matters of some dispute. It has been argued that suggestion is an essential factor in placebo therapy, whether deliberate, when a healer knowingly prescribes a placebo, or unintentional, when a clinician employs a therapeutic agent that lacks the potential that he believes it to possess; and the sufferer's suggestibility is an important factor in either case.[98] Others have simply equated placebo therapy with suggestive therapy.[99]

Shapiro has pointed out that experimentation has not shown a significant correlation between patients' suggestibility and the placebo effect; but as he also has pointed out, most of the tests of suggestibility have involved "an experimenter rather than a therapist, a subject rather than a patient, and a laboratory rather than a clinical setting," and so these tests may well have little relevance for the placebo effect in clinical contexts.[100] Also, though he wants to claim an important place in past healings for unrecognized placebo effects, Shapiro clearly recognizes that the similar claims for unrecognized suggestion effects have merit. In fact, many remarkable healings of the past that had been attributed to magic, to miracles, to faith, or to imagination, in the nineteenth and early twentieth centuries came to be considered the results of suggestion; and more recently these same healings have been attributed to the placebo effect.[101] Saying that suggestive effects are nothing but placebo effects, or vice versa, seems an acknowledgment that these two phenomena overlap one another or have an important connection with one another. At the very least, the suggestion of help is usually an element in the use of a placebo. Further, among the factors that Shapiro views as significant in the placebo effect are faith, hopeful expectations, the healer's manner and attitude, and the doctor-patient relationship,[102] all of which have been considered significant for successful suggestion in healing contexts.

Attitudes Toward Suggestion Since World War II

The wartime clinical activities cited above continued into the postwar era, first with war veterans and soon as aspects of a postwar boom in psychological therapies. The renewed respect for the therapeutic potential of hypnosis was reflected in the significant role allotted hypnotherapy and in an increasing use of hypnoanalysis, in an increasingly wide range of clinical applications in many Western countries. Suggestion was an ever-present feature of these clinical endeavors, although explicit recognition of its role was often rather limited. Direct suggestion was used to induce and facilitate hypnosis, to facilitate cathartic or abreactive experiences, and to effect the disappearance of symptoms or underlying attitudes in the hypnotic state or through post-hypnotic suggestion. Cautions were usually proffered, though, against direct suggestion to effect merely the removal of symptoms or attitudes without the patient's remembering and in some degree working through the under-lying conflict.

At the same time, suggestion in the waking state continued to be an aspect of treatment in many other psychotherapeutic endeavors of the era, although its inclusion was frequently not made explicit in the relevant psychotherapeutic writings. To what extent direct suggestions were so employed is very difficult to determine; and yet, if for no other ostensible purpose than to facilitate the preferred techniques of a given psychotherapeutic approach, direct suggestions were surely made. And direct suggestions were often used for their diversionary effect — to distract from pain, anxiety, worry, and so on — or in the service of reassurance. As to indirect suggestions, subtle implications were common enough, however witting or unwitting. The tradition of physical interventions that served psychological healing through indirect suggestion — such as faradization and magnets — was alive and well, although with more modern implements, particularly in general medicine. Placebo therapy gradually developed into a world of its own. Indirect suggestion was there raised to the level of an advanced art, though the role of suggestion has often been denied by placebo authorities, just as it has been by many a psychotherapist.

In the 1950s a particularly thoughtful, quite comprehensive, and still relevant survey was made of the place of suggestion in the psychotherapies. Edward Bibring identified five "therapeutic principles" or "groups of basic techniques": suggestive, abreactive, manipulative, clarifying, and interpretive. He used the word *techniques* to refer to "any purposive, more or less typi-fied, verbal or non-verbal behavior on the part of the therapist which in-tends to affect the patient in the direction of the (intermediary or final) goals of treatment." And he thought of them as "applicable to all methods of psychotherapy independent of their respective ideologies or theoretical sys-tems."[103] Bibring then outlined the ways in which suggestion could play a role in psychotherapy.

> The psychiatric meaning of the term refers to the induction of ideas, impulses, emotions, actions, etc., in brief, various mental processes by the therapist (an

individual in authoritative position) in the patient (an individual in dependent position) independent of, or to the exclusion of, the latter's rational or critical (realistic) thinking.

In psychotherapy, suggestion — frequently combined with hypnosis — is purposefully employed in a technical as well as in a curative sense. The technical employment of suggestion aims at the promotion of the treatment process in its various aspects. Technical suggestion may be predominantly formal (for example, to induce the patient generally to fantasy or to dream, whatever fantasy or dream it may be) or predominantly content suggestion (for example, to dream about specific topics or to remember specific events). Curative suggestion aims at that direct change which is characteristic of induction of beliefs, be it a negative belief (denial: making symptoms or attitudes "disappear"), or a positive one (inducing desirable attitudes, etc.). In modern psychotherapy, therapeutic suggestion, in the stricter sense, seems less frequently applied, as compared with the employment of technical suggestion. Suggestion is frequently used in the service of other therapeutic agents. On the basis of a more or less intimate knowledge of the personality, suggestion is purposefully employed, with or without hypnosis, in numerous ways such as to facilitate emotional expression, to help the patient face reality, to overcome or to circumvent resistance, to produce recollections, fantasies and dreams or imaginary or symbolic conflicts, to tolerate anxiety or depression, to encourage the finding of new solutions, even to gain "insight."[104]

Even though since the 1950s explicit discussion of suggestion in psychological healing has become less common, and briefer when it has occurred, its significance does not appear to have changed appreciably. Although its importance has been remarked on less, vigorous reminders of that importance have occasionally been voiced.[105] Bibring's perspective has frequently been cited. Interesting changes have taken place, too, in the pattern of recognition of suggestion's role.

Studies of psychological healing in so-called primitive cultures have frequently reaffirmed the opinion that suggestion is a crucial element in "folk psychiatry."[106] Prince stated flatly, "Suggestion is the most important element in all primitive psychotherapies."[107] In a survey of Judeo-Christian faith healing, Calestro concluded that "suggestion is the most potent factor in the three-thousand-year tradition of faith healing"; and he added, "Throughout the long history of mental healing, suggestion has been an effective therapeutic factor."[108] Suggestion has also continued to be recognized as an important element in psychological healing, through its crucial role in placebo therapy, as increasing attention has been devoted to the placebo effect. As one author put it, suggestion is "the motor behind the placebo effect."[109]

In recent years, hypnosis has gradually come to occupy a less prominent place than it did in the 1940s and 1950s, but it has continued to be employed by many; and suggestion has remained a cardinal element in such clinical work.[110] Beyond hypnosis, suggestion has continued to be thought of as an unavoidable element in psychological healing contexts, its role varying according to the proclivities of the individual sufferer; the circumstances of the sufferer's psychological distress; the status, reputation, personality and manner of the healer; and the nature of the suggestions employed by the healer. As Wolberg stated it, suggestion "is an aspect of every helping situation"; and "suggestion plays a part in every psychotherapeutic relationship even though the therapist seeks to avoid it." Under the rubric of "prestige suggestion," he specially emphasized the significance of the status and manner of the healer in many uses of therapeutic suggestion, commenting, "Among the oldest of techniques is prestige suggestion which is still employed extensively throughout the world by witch doctors, religious healers, and even professional psychotherapists."[111]

In this environment of a decreased explicit recognition of its place in the psychotherapies, it was frequently noted that suggestion was crucial in the various brief or short-term psychotherapeutic approaches, on which growing emphasis was being placed. The impact of World War II and its clinical practices, the resultant development of mental hygiene clinics for veterans, the emergence of public-sector mental health clinics, and the advent of insurance coverage of psychotherapy and the attendant concerns about costs all contributed to a groundswell of such undertakings.[112] Affected by the pressure of time limits and the trends toward focusing on particular problems, short-term therapy often involved greater apparent activity on the therapist's part, rather more directiveness than had been common in the various psychodynamic psychotherapies, and an increased role for suggestion, which in the circumstances also tended to be explicitly acknowledged more often.

Another psychotherapeutic realm in which the place of suggestion has come to be more readily acknowledged is supportive psychotherapy. Suggestion often plays a crucial role in advising, counseling, encouraging, exhorting, or otherwise actively interceding in a patient's life.[113]

To sum up, it is clear that suggestion has been an element in psychological healing over many, many centuries. Although the language of suggestion, as we know it, only emerged in the nineteenth century,[114] the unwitting use of suggestion in healing would seem to have always been with us. In the therapeutic application of charms, spells, and amulets, in the use of magic in healing, and in the various forms of faith healing, suggestion was at work. And the knowing use of suggestive influences in healing was common long before the nineteenth century, albeit without the language of suggestion: as examples, in the history of influencing the sufferer's imagination in the interest of healing, and in the time-honored traditions of placebo therapy.

With the emergence of mesmerism, we have clearer indications of what would become the recognized role of suggestion in healing. In the work of Puységur, we see the beginning recognition of the suggestive influence of the healer on the will of the sufferer — through instructions, advice, and suggestions — in the bringing about of the mesmeric state, in the healing influences on the sufferer during that state, and in the use of post-somnambulistic suggestions. In the early nineteenth-century work of Faria, Noizet, and Bertrand, such efforts became increasingly focused, and in Bertrand's case, notions about imagination and expectant attention were invoked to explain the healing effects. Around the mid-century, Braid introduced the language of suggestion; and hypnotic suggestion and posthypnotic suggestion gradually became common terms. By the end of the century, suggestive therapeutics was flourishing, and suggestion had come to be considered the cardinal element in the healing effects of hypnosis; autosuggestion soon became a matter of keen interest.

As we have seen, acknowledgment of the role of suggestion in psychological healing has come and gone. Denied at one moment, acknowledged but guarded against the next, given pride of place in a treatment approach, or asserted to be omnipresent in healing, suggestion has been assigned various forms of recognition in different psychotherapies. Still, suggestion, whether wittingly or unwittingly employed, has continued to be a factor in most, if not all, forms of psychological healing.

13

Persuasion

Persuasion is another element in psychological healing that has a long and significant history. With the emergence of the "persuasionists" as significant among the psychotherapeutists of the late nineteenth and early twentieth centuries, it has seemed to some that persuasion was primarily a mode of psychological treatment that had arisen as a challenge to the "suggestionists" of the day. But persuasion as a method long antedated the mesmerists, the hypnotists, and those who practiced suggestive therapeutics. Like suggestion, persuasion was far from a latter-day addition to psychological healing.

And what is persuasion in the first place? The *Oxford English Dictionary* defines it as "the action, or an act, of persuading or seeking to persuade; the presenting of inducements or winning arguments; the addressing of reasonings, appeals, or entreaties to a person in order to induce him to do or believe something."[1] English and English add a point of significance in their definition when they include "by an appeal to both feeling and intellect."[2] Hinsie and Campbell say that "persuasion is a method of carrying conviction that aims to prompt the acceptance of a point of view." Of special relevance is their statement, "While almost universal in application, *persuasion* has not gained distinction as a clear-cut form of psychotherapy. It is perhaps a part of all types of psychotherapy, achieving merit as an adjunct."[3] Under the classical term, *rhetoric,* it has had an extremely complex history — a hallowed practice at times and a dubious endeavor at others. To gain some perspective on persuasion, we must have some understanding of the long tradition that is *rhetoric*.

Interestingly, in a brief, but suggestive, study, Erling Eng has raised the hypothesis that rhetoric as the art of persuasion is an ancestor of modern psychotherapy.[4] He hastens to add, "Of course, the rhetorical understanding reclaimed in modern psychotherapy is a new and different mode, one enriched by other modern and related developments." Noting that this was the heyday of the "persuading sleep" of mesmerism, he also makes the provocative suggestion that there may be some connection between "the demise of the rhetorical tradition" in the early nineteenth century and the emergence of the term *psychiatry* in that same era.[5]

Persuasion in Ancient Greece

From careful study of the Homeric epic, Laín Entralgo has shown that significant among the therapeutic uses of the word in ancient Greece was the "persuasive and strengthening conversation with the patient." The use of "pleasant speech" and "beguiling speech" to the end of beneficially influencing the psychological state of the sufferer was clearly recognized and practiced. The psychological basis of the "efficacy of the word" received "the name of 'persuasion' (*peithô*)." *Peithô* (Persuasion) came to be "the goddess of the persuasive efficacy of the word." Eventually, though, rationalizing and secularizing trends transformed this persuasion that once had been divine into something merely important. "The persuasive power of the human word upon the mind of the listener" was illustrated in the Homeric writings, where it was enlisted to cheer up sufferers and divert them from pain. In contrast to incantations and supplications in which the words were addressed to the gods in the interest of healing, persuasive words were addressed directly to sufferers with an eye to influencing their minds and, in turn, affecting their passions and bodily functions. The persuasive word was "pacifying, gentle, beautiful, enchanting, and only very firm and keen minds can resist the power of its enchantment." Vigorous and persuasive words were "the key to interhuman relations." The stirring and modifying of the other person's emotions by the persuader were recognized as significant elements in persuasion. The persuasive word had "the power to take away fear, banish pain, inspire happiness and increase compassion." And so emerged the discipline of rhetoric and the vocation of rhetorician, commonly associated with the Sophist Gorgias (ca. 483–376 B.C.), who thought that the persuasive word acted on the soul as medicines did on the body and who considered rhetoric a means to persuade a sufferer to accept medical care. In the work of Antiphon (fifth century B.C.)

were further indications of the nature of curative persuasion. He believed that the painful could be eliminated, and that a definite technique was available for doing so, which involved "informing himself of the causes of the affliction and speaking to the patient accordingly. Verbal persuasion, acting according to the causes, succeeds in eliminating pain from the mind: the thought and the word of the curative rhetorician, his *logos*, set in order and rationalize the psychic and physical life of the sufferer."[6]

Rhetoric

"Since the time of Greek antiquity, the definition of 'rhetoric' has changed from century to century as the idea of 'rhetoric' has been expanded to cover the whole of the art, or contracted to include only a part. . . . But whatever the particular definition, the term has been applied to the use of language (or of special kinds of language) for the moving, pleasing, or persuading of readers or auditors to specific judgments, decisions, or actions."[7] More often than not, the goal of this art has been persuading, rather than convincing someone strictly as a result of logical argument.

Of particular significance in the history of rhetoric was Aristotle's *Rhetoric*, in which he defined it as "the faculty of observing in any given case the available means of persuasion."[8] "The technical study of rhetoric is concerned with the modes of persuasion," with persuasion being "a sort of demonstration."[9] He stated that three modes of persuasion were available to a speaker. "The first depends on the personal character of the speaker." It is important that the speaker develop a favorable impression of his own character for his auditors, that he inspire confidence and trust: "His character may almost be called the most effective means of persuasion he possesses."[10] "The second [depends] on putting the audience into a certain frame of mind." Here he was referring to influencing the emotions of the hearers. The speaker needed "to understand the emotions — that is, to know what they are, their nature, their causes and the way in which they are excited." He went on in considerable detail about how various emotions might be stimulated, modified, or countered; and he emphasized the importance of knowing the state of mind associated with each emotion, the sort of people that provoked each emotion, and the grounds for a person's emotional reaction. In coming to understand such matters, a speaker became equipped to persuade the hearers through influencing their emotions.[11] "Thirdly, persuasion is effected through the speech itself when we have proved a truth or an apparent truth by means of the persuasive arguments suitable to the case in question."[12] Further on, the sort of person who should be employing the techniques of persuasion is described: "The man who is to be in command of them must, it is clear, be able to reason logically, to understand human characters and excellences, and to understand the emotions."[13]

Subsequent works on rhetoric varied a great deal in their focus, sometimes emphasizing more the preparation, training, and character of the rhetorician, sometimes attending more to the nature of the arguments to be used or the style thought preferable, and sometimes approaching in degree Aristotle's attention to the nature of the auditors or readers and their susceptibility to influence. Further, attention to matters rhetorical was at times diffused through the concerns and practices of a wide variety of disciplines and at other times was focused more on a discrete set of practices as a distinct field of endeavor. And while rhetorical skills and accomplishments in the art of persuasion were respected for the most part, at times rhetoric was not held in such high regard, when it represented "an undesirable hiding of meaning," a questionable level of integrity in a rhetorician, or a way of influencing a person against his best interests.[14]

During the Romantic period, a reaction against rhetoric took place, and the discipline suffered a significant loss of influence and change in status. Then, in more recent times, the terms *rhetoric* and *rhetorical* have often been used to criticize someone's mode of communication, and the art of persuasion has all too often been associated with features similar to those cited by its earlier critics. In an interesting contrast to these trends, it has been argued that the newer rhetoric (since the eighteenth century) has embraced communication and understanding as its goals, and that this development has stood in significant contrast to the coercive persuasion said to have characterized classical rhetoric; but other authorities have strongly disagreed.[15] Whatever the case may have been in these various controversies, it seems that the art of persuasion has long been viewed with some ambivalence. On the one hand, persuaders with integrity have been highly regarded for their skilled use of sound techniques in the interests of their auditors or readers. On the other hand, critics of the art of persuasion have questioned the integrity of persuaders, the soundness of their technique, and the usefulness to auditors or readers of the persuader's efforts. According to another set of criteria, the argument has been whether rhetoric served truth and justice or whether it served deception.

Persuasion, the Passions, and the Imagination

Of particular significance in considering persuasion as an aspect of psychological healing are some interesting trends that seem very likely to have been connected with one another. As pointed out by Brian Vickers, a modern authority on rhetoric, an "increasing stress on persuasion via the passions" became evident between 1540 and 1640.[16] "In the sixteenth, and even more in the seventeenth century, rhetoricians took seriously the perennial claim of rhetoric to sway the passions, and embarked on ever more detailed analyses of psychology and emotion under the power of language." And "this concern with the passions continued until the end of the eighteenth century."[17] As we have seen in previous chapters, attention to the passions, and to the imagination, flourished in the same centuries, in the interest of curing sufferers of various ailments; and surely that was more than coincidence.[18] Ways of influencing the passions, and the imagination, as means of changing particular states of distress or disease became recognized modes of therapeutic endeavor. References to rhetoric were not explicit in medical writings on these topics, but the implication that some communicative mode (language) was entailed in techniques for changing passions or imagery was always quite clear. As Vickers put it, "The power to move the imagination is an essential criterion for the working of rhetoric."[19] He linked rhetoric to painting and music as "expressive, communicative systems. They are linked, further, by their common interest in representing, and appealing to, the passions and the imagination."[20]

Some interesting comments on rhetoric by Francis Bacon (1561–1626) are especially relevant here. He stated that "rhetoric is subservient to the imagination, as Logic is to the understanding; and the duty and office of Rhetoric, if it be deeply looked into, is no other than to apply and recommend the dictates of reason to imagination, in order to excite the appetite and will."[21] He went on to say that "the end of rhetoric is to fill the imagination with observations and images, to second reason, and not to oppress it."[22] Still maintaining that the subject of rhetoric was "Imaginative or Insinuative Reason,"[23] he argued that the "persuasions and insinuations" of rhetoric served to "win the imagination" away from siding with the passions or affections, and so to "contract a confederacy between the reason and imagination against them." Here we see the significance of the art of persuasion in influencing the imagination and, through that influence, in constructively managing the passions.[24]

Not long after Bacon's comments, Robert Burton discussed at length the importance of attention to the passions and the imagination in therapeutics, and indicated that persuasion was an element of some significance in healing. In his encyclopedic attention to melancholia, he advised that, if a sufferer could not satisfactorily manage his own distress, his friends or his physician ought "by counsel, comfort, or persuasion, by fair or foul means to alienate his mind, by some artificial invention, or some contrary persuasion" from the matters that distressed him. He cited Galen as having noted that "many . . . have been cured by good counsel and persuasion alone." Those who might help such sufferers were advised: "By all means, therefore, fair promises, good words, gentle persuasions are to be used, not to be too rigorous at first, or to insult over them, not to deride, neglect, or contemn, but rather . . . to pity, and by all plausible means to seek to reduce them." Nevertheless, where such measures failed, he would countenance efforts "to threaten and chide."[25]

Further, Burton gave serious attention to two other, long-established techniques of psychological healing in which persuasion was central. First, therapeutic ruses or "artificial inventions" were often recommended to relieve a patient of his delusions through correcting his imagination; and Burton cited a series of oft-repeated accounts of such deceptions calculated to cure patients of their delusions.[26] Second, persuasion again enters in as a basic element in Burton's extensive attention to the traditional *consolatio,* whereby the healer was to enlist the sufferer's reason through consolatory counsel in an effort to dissuade him from his troubling passions and distressing thoughts.[27]

During the remainder of the seventeenth century and throughout the eighteenth century, sustained interest was accorded to both the imagination and the passions, both in the form of general concerns about the nature of man and in therapeutic attention to various forms of distress and disease. Although the term itself was infrequently used in such contexts, persuasion continued to be significant in psychological healing through its role in techniques for influencing the imagination and rectifying the passions.[28] In fact, the definitions of persuasion and its cognates had come to include references to influencing the passions. In his *Dictionary* (1755), Samuel Johnson included, in his definition of *persuasion,* "the act of gaining or attempting the passions" and in his definition of *persuasive,* "having influence on the passions"; he defined *persuasiveness* as "influence on the passions"; and in defining *to persuade,* he commented that "*persuasion* seems rather applicable to the passions, and *argument* to the reason."[29] In the developing "management" of the insane in the eighteenth century and in the "moral treatment" that evolved out of it around the end of the century, persuasion was consistently an implied, though unstated, element.[30]

The place of persuasion in this era's psychological therapeutics has been studied by Eric T. Carlson and Meribeth M. Simpson.[31] In addressing the question of "how persuasive techniques (both rational and 'moral' or emotional) were utilized" in the clinical activities of that era, these authors focus particularly on the work of Benjamin Rush (1745–1813). In so doing they concern themselves with what assumptions Rush and his contemporaries held "about the kinds of intellectual and emotional processes that should be manipulated by the physician."[32] Rush set forth three stages of the illness in severe mental disorders, such as mania. In the first or more severe stage, the physician "should acquiesce in the patient's ideas," thereby gaining the patient's confidence and having a calming effect. The second stage was associated with general improvement, or with a less severe disorder in the first place, and "diversionary tactics" were preferred "in order to distract him from thinking about his deluded ideas." The third stage began when the patient was close to recovery, and "at this point it was safe to contradict, reason with, and even ridicule the patient" in the interest of promoting further improvement. Milder disorders could be treated with later-stage techniques sooner or even from the start.[33] Carlson and Simpson, on the assumption that "only in the third stage was reasoning an important part of persuasion," categorize the persuasive efforts of the earlier stages as "emotional persuasion," in contrast to the "rational persuasion" which could be used later. Among these techniques for the earlier stages were the therapeutic ruses or "pious frauds" referred to earlier, the technique of "contrary passions," and the displacement of one emotion by another.[34] The techniques for the earlier or more severe stages involved the manipulation of sensation and emotion but were replaced by a more intellectual approach in the recuperative stages of illness. Still, efforts to influence the emotions were often used in the later stages. Carlson and Simpson take special note of the keen interest of late eighteenth-century physicians "in the manipulation of 'the passions' in curing mental illness." And they add, "although we have been focusing on the use of emotional persuasion in the therapy of incorrect thought, emotions were also used by Rush and the psychiatrists of his era in changing undesirable passions and in modifying behavior." Some contemporaries "were so convinced of the importance of emotions in therapy that they were led to question the value of rational persuasion entirely."[35] This tendency to associate persuasion so intimately with the influencing of the passions was nicely brought out by George Campbell (1719–1796), important among the New Rhetoricians of the era, when he stated in 1776 that "there is no persuasion without moving them [the passions]."[36] That is to say, moving or influencing the passions was an essential factor in persuasion.

In these modes of psychological therapeutics Rush was reflecting trends in the treatment of mentally disturbed persons that had been developed by Philippe Pinel and others toward the end of the eighteenth century. Along with "consolatory language, kind treatment, and the revival of extinguished hope," Pinel had incorporated the emphasis of his era on the therapeutic use of the passions.[37] In fact, the very word *moral*, as used in Pinel's *moral treatment*, not only indicated a psychological approach to treatment but meant that attention to the passions was a key ingredient.[38] In advocating the "innocent ruses" or "pious frauds" so often cited in earlier accounts of the treatment of melancholics' delusions, he indicated that each should be developed individually for the problems and peculiarities of the particular patient.[39] Attention to a disordered imagination was thought to be crucial in these endeavors. These theatrical deceptions for the patient's own good entailed "dexterous" or "innocent strategems" whereby violent patients were calmed by adroit maneuvers that involved agreeing with them to gain their confidence and then diverting them from their disturbing preoccupations.[40] Examination of these three approaches as outlined by Pinel makes it clear that moral or emotional persuasion was a significant, albeit implicit, element in his moral treatment, as it was for others who were part of this newer tradition of psychological healing.

Ruses, Stratagems, and Pious Frauds

Quite distinct from persuasion rooted in the history of rhetorical traditions was the long-standing practice, noted in many medical writings, of various ruses used to persuade insane persons of the lack of validity of their delusions or to influence them to abandon those beliefs. As indicated in previous chapters, some of the accounts of these ruses have relevance in other contexts, but they are also instances of another mode of persuasion. Faced with the relative uselessness of rational argument and persuasion in many cases, physicians developed various tricks or ruses to persuade the sufferers away from their delusions and toward recovery. In some instances, ruses served to persuade patients by demonstrating the absurdity of their delusions. In other instances, patients were persuaded by deceptions carried out within the logic of the delusions. In either type of case, the sufferers were relieved of their delusions and were calmed or reassured, after which they often experienced an abatement of other symptoms. Variously termed cunning stratagems, innocent ruses, artificial inventions, or pious frauds, these efforts began to be described in medical texts at least as early as the first century A.D.

Celsus' brief reference to such practices (ca. 30) is an early example. He commented that some insane persons "need to have empty fears relieved, as was done for a wealthy man in dread of starvation, to whom pretended legacies were from time to time announced."[41] Another early example of such therapeutic ruses was outlined by Galen, although in this case it was not being used to counter a delusion. Galen told of a slave who had sickened with worry at being short some funds in the accounts that he managed for his master. After informing the master that there was nothing physically wrong with the slave, Galen enlisted his cooperation. The master then informed his slave that he would be transferring the management of the funds to another slave; and this was done in such a way as to indicate that the slave would not be called upon to account for the shortage. He soon recovered.[42]

In the second century, Rufus of Ephesus (fl. 98–117) and Galen developed the tradition of citing a series of quite fanciful delusions as aspects of melancholia. The lists of delusions were often rather colorful; it became a common practice to cite a selection of the quite familiar and most striking ones in medical authors' accounts of melancholia; and yet some recognition would be paid to just how individual, and thus nearly endless in their variation, these delusions might be.

With the writings of Alexander of Tralles (525–605), the discussion of the treatment of melancholia included mention of a series of these delusions *along with* the clever and persuasive stratagems used to rid the sufferers of their strange beliefs. These stratagems, too, were handed down, repeated by many a later medical writer, possibly for their strange and almost entertaining effect.

Alexander noted that many melancholics had been cured through a careful attention to the nature of their derangements, with an eye to understanding their psychological origins and developing psychological strategies to influence them toward recovery. Of the cases he cited, one patient was disabused of the delusion that he had been beheaded for having been a tyrant by having a lead cap suddenly placed on his head. A second patient was reassured in the framework of her delusion that she had swallowed a snake, by being made to vomit and seeing a snake that had been surreptitiously placed in the vomitus. Alexander recommended that, except in chronic cases, all manner of contrivances should be tried in an endeavor to cure the various fantastic ideas, especially where there seemed to be an established cause for them in the patient's mind.[43]

As such accounts of therapeutic ruses entered more and more medical writings on the treatment of the insane, the first few in the series tended to be familiar accounts that had been cited by numerous predecessors, and the last one or two might be of more recent vintage, even from the author's own experience. Sometimes the familiar anecdotes were credited to historical predecessors; sometimes they were merely listed as though they might have been from the author's own experience. The lists of familiar examples eventually took on an almost folkloric character.

A representative version of this tradition was left to us by André du Laurens (1560?–1609) in his *A Discourse . . . of Melancholike Diseases*, in 1599. Claiming to write "to the end I may somewhat delight the reader," he listed "some examples such as have had the most fantasticall and foolish imaginations of all others" from "the Greeke, Arabian, and Latine writers," and proposed to "adde some such as I have seene with mine owne eyes." Attributing the account to Aetius, he mentioned the man who was convinced that he had been beheaded "for his tyrannous dealings" and who was "freed from his false imagination" by having an iron cap placed on his head. He cited Alexander of

Tralles as the source for the case of the woman who thought she had swallowed a serpent and was cured by a ruse that appeared to her to demonstrate that she had vomited the snake up. Du Laurens went on to say,

> I have read that a young scholler being in his studie, was taken with a strange imagination: for he imagined that his nose was so great and so long, as that he durst not stirre out of his place, lest he should dash it against something: and the more he was dealt with and disswaded, so much the more did he confirme himselfe in his opinion. In the end a Phisition having taken a great peece of flesh, and holding it in his hand secretly, assured him that hee would heale him by and by, and that he must needes take away this great nose: and so upon the suddaine pinching his nose a little, and cutting the peece of flesh which he had, he made him beleeve that his great nose was cut away.

The chronicler further noted:

> The pleasantest dotage that ever I read, was of one *Sienois* a Gentleman, who had resolved with himselfe not to pisse, but to dye rather, and that because he imagined, that when he first pissed, all his towne would be drowned. The Phisitions shewing him, that all his bodie, and ten thousand moe such as his, were not able to containe so much as might drowne the least house in the towne, could not change his minde from this foolish imagination. In the end they seeing his obstinacie, and in what danger he put his life, found out a pleasant invention. They caused the next house to be set on fire, & all the bells in the town to ring, they perswaded diverse servants to crie, to the fire, to the fire, & therewithall send of those of the best account in the town, to crave helpe, and shew the Gentleman that here is but one way to save the towne, and that it was, that he should pisse quicklie and quench the fire. Then this sillie melancholike man which abstained from pissing for feare of loosing his towne, taking it for graunted, that it was now in great hazard, pissed and emptied his bladder of all that was in it, and was himselfe by that meanes preserved.[44]

In each of these last two cases, there are clear indications of a background of failed effort to persuade the sufferer through reasonable argument, followed by resort to a ruse or stratagem as an alternative form of persuasion.

About two decades later Robert Burton provided a particularly rich account of such cases, taken from both ancient and more recent sources, and all carefully attributed to earlier authors. In discussing various ways of helping those suffering from melancholia, he commented: "Sometimes again by some feigned lie, strange news, witty device, artificial invention, it is not amiss to deceive them. As they hate those, saith Alexander, that neglect or deride, so they will give ear to such as will sooth them up. If they say they have swallowed frogs, or a snake, by all means grant it, and tell them you can easily cure

it, 'tis an ordinary thing." He then retold the story about the delusion of headlessness and the lead cap, which he attributed to "Philodotus the Physician." He quoted Alexander's account of curing the woman who thought that she had swallowed a snake. He narrated Du Lauren's story of the urinary fireman and followed it with that of the cure of the man with the delusionally large nose. And he continued, "Forestus had a melancholy Patient, who thought he was dead; he put a fellow in a chest, like a dead man, by his bed's side, and made him rear himself a little, and eat: the melancholy man asked the counterfeit, whether dead men used to eat meat? he told him yea; whereupon he did eat likewise and was cured. Lemnius hath many such instances, and Jovianus Pontanus of the like. . . . I read a multitude of examples of melancholy men cured by such artificial inventions."[45] In Burton's work, and in that of Du Laurens and others around this time, the tendency was to attribute such delusions to a damaged imagination and to include "artificial inventions" or therapeutic ruses among the ways in which the imagination could be "corrected." That is to say, the physician could introduce images to the patient that would persuade him away from the false or pathological images of his delusion. And it was not uncommon to interweave this form of therapeutic thinking with references to "rectifying the passions" as well.

From the Renaissance through the end of the eighteenth century, these various ruses or therapeutic deceptions were chronicled again and again in medical works, most often as a series of anecdotes to illustrate ways in which melancholic patients had been cured of their delusions and to suggest how a physician might proceed with similar cases.

The Greco-Roman medical tradition had been the source for the many Latin accounts of these artificial inventions, but it also had provided many of the examples for a similar series of Arabic accounts during the Islamic Middle Ages. In citing some of them, J. Christoph Bürgel associated the lead helmet case with Rufus of Ephesus and the snake-delusion case with Galen; and he traced references to these and similar cases in Arabic medical literature. Ishāq ibn 'Imrān (ca. 900) apparently used the lead-helmet ruse successfully. Avicenna's successful treatment of a man who thought that he was a cow, refused to eat, and wished to be slaughtered is mentioned; and this case came to be included in later lists of successful therapeutic ruses. Ibn Malkā was cited regarding a man's delusion that he carried a precious vase on his head and constantly feared knocking it down; working within the logic of the patient's delusion, this physician was able to persuade the patient away from his delusion. This case appeared in a collection of physicians' biographies by Ibn abī Uṣaibi'a, who also mentioned having written a book on such approaches to the treatment of delusions, though this volume has apparently not survived.[46]

The medical views on these matters, at the beginning of the eighteenth century, are fairly represented by the following comments by Michael Ettmüller (1644–1683): "The remote Cause must be taken off either by moral Perswasions, or deceiving the Person with some cunning Stratagem, so as to bring off the melancolic Fantasy. . . . When the melancolic Fancy is deeply lodg'd within 'em, they ought to be undeceiv'd by the means of some Stratagem or Trick."[47]

These practices continued to be mentioned and advocated during the eighteenth century. And late in the century, a representative account of them was included in Diderot's *Encyclopédie,* in a lengthy entry on melancholia and its treatment.[48] In that context, most of the storied delusions and their therapeutic ruses were described. This account emphasized that one must first cure the mind, and then deal with bodily symptoms. Accordingly, the physician must gain the confidence of the patient, enter into and accommodate himself to the patient's delusion, promise him a cure, and then persuade him out of his delusion with some quite "singular" remedy. There followed a series of these delusions and their cures — the belief that some animal was in the patient's body (giving him a vigorous purgative to eliminate the animal, the physician produced a relevant animal as though it had come out in the patient's stool); the belief that the animal was in the patient's head (an incision could be made in the skin and an animal produced through some sleight of hand); the patient's belief that his bones were all as soft as wax (a ruse convinced him that this was no longer the case); the story of the patient who would not urinate (a fire was set for him to douse); the patient's belief that his legs were made of glass (being hit on the legs provoked him to such action that he was persuaded otherwise); and the delusion of being headless (the patient was convinced that this was not the case through the wearing of a lead cap).[49]

Meanwhile, the term *pious frauds* had come into use. The *Oxford English Dictionary* defines *pious fraud* as "a deception practised for the furtherance of what is considered a good object; *esp.* for the advancement of religion."[50] Similar uses of the term seem to have emerged in various writings about religion in the sixteenth and seventeenth centuries, though not without a hint of disapproval regarding such practices. In 1712, in an essay titled "On the Pleasures of the Imagination," Joseph Addison (1672–1719) referred to "pious frauds" having been carried out "to amuse mankind, and frighten them into a sense of their duty."[51] Later, in the 1760s, Voltaire (1694–1778) discussed pious frauds in an entry in his *Philosophical Dictionary;* it was entitled "Frauds," with the subtitle "Should Pious Frauds Be Practiced on the Common People?"[52] "Frauds" is a clever dialogical argument on the theme of the subtitle. It tends to come down on the side of the argument that "we should never deceive anyone," after arguing against the contrasting view that "the people need to be deceived . . . for their own good" and that "the common people" cannot be taught "the truth without sustaining it with fables."[53] "For their own good" implied that pious frauds were used in the interest of promoting and sustaining faith and moral behavior; and that the "common people" would be better off as a result.

In the latter part of the eighteenth century, *pious frauds* was borrowed from these contexts and applied by some physicians to the artificial inventions, ruses, or stratagems recommended for the treatment of the delusions of the insane. William Cullen (1710–1790) apparently used the term in this way.[54] And John Haslam (1764–1844) used the term in the 1790s, commenting that "it is certainly allowable to try the effect of certain deceptions, contrived to make strong impressions on the senses, by means of *unexpected, unusual, striking,* or apparently *supernatural* agents." He indicated that pious frauds were appropriate for those insane persons with a single delusion and a circumscribed derangement.[55]

At the beginning of the nineteenth century, these therapeutic ruses still seem to have had some place. Among a group of interventions that he cited, Pinel wrote of the case of a man who lived in fear that he was to be executed for disloyalty to the government and who, in the 1790s, had been transferred to the Bicêtre hospital where Pinel had charge of his case. At first, Pinel had successfully treated him in the spirit of the moral treatment program that he developed there, setting him up in his trade as a tailor. When he relapsed, Pinel — by then having moved to the Salpêtrière hospital — arranged with Pussin, the governor at the Bicêtre, to set up a simulated trial for the patient in which he was found innocent, and this melancholic man then recovered. Unfortunately, as Pinel reports, the man relapsed later in response to the "imprudent disclosure of the above well intended plot."[56] The implication was apparently that, for their beneficial effects to be sustained, such ruses should not be disclosed to the patient. Pinel's English translator used the term "innocent stratagem" for such interventions; Pinel's term had been "innocente ruse."[57]

During that same decade, though, we find indications of doubt about the usefulness of these therapeutic strategies. John Ferriar (1761–1815) had grave reservations about such efforts "to surprise them into rationality by stratagem." He commented, "I never knew such endeavours answer any good purpose. The stories current in books, of wonderful cures thus produced, are, like most other good stories, incapable of serving more than once."[58]

Nevertheless, such treatment strategies continued to be advocated by many at the beginning of the nineteenth century. Benjamin Rush (1745–1813), for example, cited a significant sample of therapeutic ruses, some being the familiar ones, some being from contemporary authorities such as Cox and Pinel, and some being from his own experience.[59] But gradually, the traditional series of cases ceased to be cited. The oft-repeated stories, and their accompanying clever therapeutic ruses, faded from medical texts. Some troubled themselves to maintain, as Ferriar had, that these ruses were not likely to be effective; and others argued that physicians should not employ trickery, as they should not be deceiving their patients. Still, though, this did not do away with the use of placebos.

By mid-nineteenth century, John C. Bucknill's and Daniel Hack Tuke's well-known textbook, *A Manual of Psychological Medicine*, summed up the matter as follows:

> Systematic works on insanity generally contain examples of the cure of delusions by artifice. Prichard, who has quoted several from Esquirol and Guislain, avows that he has had "no opportunity of making similar experiments," adding, "which, however, I shall certainly attempt whenever it may be in my power, though without sanguine hopes of success." We have less hope than Prichard; for we should not think it worth while even to try the effect of legerdemain upon mental disease. We have seen so many painful instances of objective reality failing to influence delusion in the smallest degree, that we have not the slightest faith in the effect of trick. . . . [here they expressed grave reservations about several of the familiar anecdotes]We are sorry to be able to yield but very imperfect belief to the accounts of the cure of delusions by legerdemain. The modern examples are so uncommonly like the old ones, that it is impossible to resist the suspicion that they have been copied from them.[60]

For the most part, though, medical authors no longer made any reference to such treatment strategies.

From Moral Treatment to Persuasion Therapy

With the further development and continuing use of moral treatment during the first half of the nineteenth century, it is clear that persuasion continued to be a crucial aspect of such therapeutic endeavors. So, too, it is fair to say that persuasion was at work in the influences exerted through the suggestive therapeutics that came to the fore in the last decades of the century. At the same time, explicit references to persuasion as a mode of treatment, or even as an element in psychological healing, were rare for most of the nineteenth century. Around the turn of the twentieth century, though, persuasion became an explicit feature of psychological healing once again.

This change had its roots in a groundswell of objection to hypnosis and suggestion. In varying ways it was argued that hypnosis was disrespectful to patients and undermined their dignity, and that suggestion obtained its results through getting around their judgment by surreptitious means. Prominent in this trend was Paul Dubois, the Swiss physician who had earlier been influenced by Hippolyte Bernheim's suggestive therapeutics and had used those methods for a time. Shifting his emphasis to persuasion, Dubois developed his own system of psychological treatment that was variously referred to as rational therapeutics, rational psychotherapy, moral treatment, moral orthopedics, re-education, and persuasion therapy. In contrast to suggestion, which he thought of as entering "the understanding by the back stairs," he favored persuasion, which for him meant "logical persuasion" that "knocks at the front door."[61] Although both suggestion and persuasion "inculcate ideas," suggestion "is addressed to blind faith" and persuasion "appeals to clear, logical reason."[62] After outlining the innumerable hazards of human suggestibility and the unfortunate results of suggestion, Dubois devoted much of his *Psychic Treatment of Nervous Disorders* to discussing clinical conditions and detailing the nature and the merits of his psychotherapy based on logical persuasion. He would review the patient's habits of a lifetime, explore the meaning of his symptoms, develop an explanation as to how they had come about, teach the patient that he had exaggerated the significance of his ailments and needed to correct this distorted perspective, outline how his difficulties could be overcome, and reason with him so that he could accept the physician's views and proceed to change himself.[63] In this process, Dubois thought of his treatment as appealing to the patient's intellect, making him *"master of himself"* through *"the education of the will,* or, more exactly, *of the reason."*[64] In addition to the elements of his work that he particularly emphasized, others seem quite important when one studies his writings. Among these were the high confidence of the psychotherapist and the forcefulness of his approach, both of which have been characteristic of many successful persuaders. Then, too, he emphasized the doctor-patient relationship, including being a friend to the patient and being truly sympathetic.

Although somewhat less rigorous in his opposition, Joseph Jules Déjerine (1849–1917) followed Dubois in his criticism of both hypnotic suggestion and direct suggestion. Later the chief of psychiatry at the Salpêtrière in Paris, Déjerine had earlier worked under Dubois at Berne, and, like Dubois, he favored a form of persuasion therapy. As he put it, "The conversational attitude, the familiar manner of talking things over, the heart-to-heart discussion, where the physician must exert his good sense and feelings, and the patient be willing to be confidential, — this is what is meant by psychotherapy by persuasion." In contrast to direct suggestions, which he viewed as "restricting the personality," Déjerine argued that persuasion permitted "the personality to develop" and liberated it from the unfortunate attitudes that plagued it.[65] In large measure his approach followed the mode of treatment outlined by Dubois, but there were important differences. As had Dubois, he emphasized the re-education of reason, but, in some contrast to Dubois, in explaining psychoneuroses, Déjerine stressed emotion rather than a weakened will, appealed more to emotion in his persuasive techniques, and aimed at freeing the person from the bad effects of his emotions.

> Reasoning by itself is indifferent. . . . But the moment an emotional element appears the personality of the subject whose mentality one is seeking to modify, is moved and affected by it. . . . From my point of view, psychotherapy depends wholly and exclusively upon the beneficial influence of one person on another. . . . They are only cured when they come to believe in you. . . . Between reasoning, and the acceptance of this reasoning by the patient, there is, I repeat, an element, on the importance of which I cannot insist too strongly; it is sentiment or feeling. It is feeling which creates the atmosphere of confidence without which, I hold, no psychotherapy is possible, that is to say, unless reasoning produces effective action there is no *"persuasion."*[66]

It is of special note that he added, "persuasion can only be applied to individuals whose mental mechanism is virtually sane."[67]

The "suggestionists" had challenged the hypnotists by maintaining that the same useful results could be obtained by suggestion alone, without any need to induce a hypnotic state. The "persuasionists," in turn, challenged the suggestionists, alleging that suggestion ignored the patient's intellect and reason and influenced the patient surreptitiously. In persuasion therapy, as employed by Dubois, it was said that the appeal was strictly to the patients' reason, that they were to be convinced by "logical persuasion." But, then, other persuasionists, such as Déjerine, argued that Dubois's appeal was too much to the intellect, that the emotions were being ignored and needed to be taken into account. And so a revised approach to persuasion was developed which took into account both the intellect and the emotions.

In the context of Dubois' persuasion therapy, education was intermittently an explicit theme — "education of the will, or, more exactly, of the reason," as he stated it.[68] That is to say, the influencing or persuading of a patient toward a healthier outlook and healthier behavior was essentially an educational effort, *or* educational efforts often constituted the way in which a healer strove to persuade a sufferer toward better health. The theme of education as a crucial element in psychological healing was hardly new. Often implicit in earlier healing efforts, it was quite explicit in "the psychical mode of treatment" employed by Ernst von Feuchtersleben (1806–1849) in the "therapeutics" outlined in *The Principles of Medical Psychology* in the 1840s.[69] Later, Pierre Janet, in his *Psychological Healing,* organized a great many data under the rubric "Education and Reeducation,"[70] and the term *re-education* periodically found its way into twentieth-century discussions of psychotherapy. Among the numerous treatment efforts that Janet included under re-education were modes of retraining of patients afflicted with such neurological problems as paralyses and other motor disorders; the training of retarded children; and corrective attention to tics and stammering. He also included various mental disorders — hysterical ailments, phobias, obsessions, and cases of neurasthenia — as appropriate for re-education. But, while it is fair to consider some of these efforts as applications of persuasion, many of them would be more appropriately thought of as instances of conditioning and reconditioning.

Another medical psychologist who emphasized education or re-education as a central theme in his psychotherapeutics was Morton Prince (1854–1929), a contemporary of Janet and rather similar in orientation. This American neurologist and psychopathologist viewed education and therapeutic suggestion as key elements in psychological healing.[71] Early experience with Weir Mitchell's rest cure had brought him to the conclusion that the crucial factors in success with that approach were "largely moral and educational."[72] By the end of the last decade of the nineteenth century, he had developed what he termed the Educational Treatment as the essence of his psychotherapeutics.[73] The education of the patient was central, though echoes of persuasion were apparent at times and of reconditioning at other times.

Persuasion After Dubois and Déjerine

In the decades that followed the work of Dubois and Déjerine, both suggestion and persuasion were mentioned often enough in writings on psychotherapy. As noted in the previous chapter, they were frequently viewed as closely allied, and most often the opinion was that a significant amount of suggestion was inherent in persuasion. Sometimes, though, it was argued that suggestion was merely an oblique form of persuasion. As one authority stated it, "Persuasion is suggestion plus appeal to the patient's common sense. . . . In the former the physician may be said to 'put his cards on the table,' much more than in the latter."[74]

At times, psychotherapists took some pains to avoid techniques and interventions that entailed persuasion, just as some tended to do regarding suggestive techniques. Often, too, a particular psychotherapist, or members of a particular school of psychotherapy, would maintain that persuasion was not a part of his, or their, approach to psychotherapy. Such an assertion sometimes came across as a point of pride, and sometimes it even took on a tone of high morality that such a "sin" was being avoided. Concerns about the propriety of employing persuasion were often an issue. Was it appropriate or ethical to use it at all? If it might be used, how far should a healer go in using it? If it was used, what was proper and what was not? For all these concerns, though, it crept into the work of many psychotherapists, in spite of their denials or in spite of their efforts to avoid it. The giving of advice in order to influence a patient toward certain behaviors, efforts at re-education, exhortations and efforts to inspire, encouragements and reassurances, had long been part of the efforts of physicians. And they were surely resorted to by most psychotherapists at some time or other, however much or however little they might be part of their usual practice, and however much or however little they might be willing to admit it.

In more recent times, in ways that seem to have evolved out of the approaches of Dubois and Déjerine, persuasion has become a recognized aspect of psychotherapy, without being the sum total of any psychotherapeutic approach. In 1942, Maurice Levine, a thoughtful and respected authority, presented persuasion in much the same manner as Déjerine, in particular, and he grouped it with re-education under the heading, "persuasion and reeducation."[75]

Fifty years after the appearance of Dubois's key volume, Lewis Wolberg gave significant attention to persuasion in his massive textbook *The Technique of Psychotherapy*. He included persuasion within the larger context of *supportive psychotherapy* as the generic term. First, he considered it in conjunction with coercion as "authoritative measures which are calculated to bring to bear on the patient rewards or punishments in order to stimulate him toward certain actions." Here he included threats, prohibitions, exhortations, reproaches, and authoritative firmness. He took note of the use of such techniques with some dependent personalities, in instances of "acting-out," in emergency situations, and in cases of uncontrolled emotionality where other methods fail. But he added that "it is rare that a good therapeutic effect will be forthcoming with the use of such authoritative procedures," and that "if they are ever used, [they] should be employed only as temporary emergency measures."[76] He then took up persuasion as a primary psychotherapeutic approach, describing it as follows:

> Persuasion is a technique based upon the belief that the patient has within himself the power to modify his pathologic emotional processes by force of sheer will or by the utilization of "common sense." In persuasive therapy, appeals are made to the patient's reason and intelligence, in order to convince him to abandon neurotic aims and symptoms, and to help him gain self-respect. He is enlightened as to the false nature of his own concepts regarding his illness, as well as the bad mental habits he has formed. By presenting him

with all the facts in his case, he is shown that there is no reason for him to be ill. He is urged to ignore his symptoms by assuming a stoical attitude, by cultivating a new philosophy of life aimed at facing his weaknesses, and by adopting an attitude of self-tolerance. An attempt is made to bring him into harmony with his environment, and to induce him to think of the welfare of others.

A number of psychotherapists, in utilizing persuasion, attempt to indoctrinate their patients with their own particular philosophies of life. The therapist establishes a directive relationship with his patient who seeks the therapist's approval on the basis that the therapeutic authority must know what is best for him. . . . The majority of popular books on mental therapy are modified forms of persuasion.[77]

Although the first of these paragraphs quoted above is very much in the spirit of Dubois, Wolberg proceeded to give a faithful outline of Dubois's persuasion therapy, and to mention briefly Déjerine's modified version of Dubois' work.[78] Wolberg then went on to say,

Modern persuasive methods draw largely, for their inspiration, on the works of Dubois and Déjerine. Stress is laid on cultivation of the proper mental attitude toward life, on the facing of adversity, and on the accepting of environmental difficulties and the tolerance of self-limitations one is unable to change. There is an accenting of the patient's assets and expansion of his positive personality qualities. The patient is taught to control overemotionality, to live with anxiety, to accept and tolerate deprivation, frustration and tension, acquiring proper controls for them. The dynamic basis of many persuasive cures lies in the reinforcing of repression of symptoms by appealing . . . to values significant for the patient, by building up "in the patient a desire to get well," by emphasizing his responsibility to get well, and by helping him to "have a better opinion of himself."[79]

Writing in further discussion of persuasion about "persuasive suggestions," Wolberg made it clear that he viewed persuasion as employing suggestions. He then said that these suggestions "tend toward a redirection of goals, an overcoming of physical suffering and disease, a dissipation of the 'worry habit,' 'thought control' and 'emotion control,' a correcting of tension and fear, and a facing of adversity."[80]

In the expanded second edition of his *Technique of Psychotherapy,* Wolberg reconfigures what he has to say about re-education into a lengthy section on re-educative therapy.[81] He includes some clear applications of persuasion, but he also explicitly recognizes many of his examples as instances of conditioning and counterconditioning. He further views some aspects of the insight-oriented psychotherapies as re-educative in nature.

One author, Patrick J. Mahony, who takes special pains to consider Freud's psychoanalytic endeavors in the light of rhetoric and persuasion, comments that it was "the Greek rhetorical tradition . . . that anticipated psychoanalysis as a logotherapy."[82] He states that "Freud, unwittingly or not, grafted some of Aristotelian dialectic and the catharsis of the *Poetics* onto the *Rhetoric* and thereby created a new persuasive experience in Western history."[83] In summing up, he observes that "first, Freud mapped out the psychomachia, the battle of persuasion raging within the individual himself"; and "second, Freud systematized a new type of persuasion, psychoanalytical therapy."[84] Regarding the place of persuasion in psychotherapy, Mahony goes so far as to suggest that "the ordinary therapist has unwittingly produced rhetoric in a manner similar to Molière's Monsieur Jourdain who, unawares, spoke prose."[85]

Another recent author, Gene M. Abroms, in addressing the question of persuasion in psychotherapy, cites the adroit arguments of such authorities as Jerome D. Frank and Jay Haley who insist that "successful practitioners of nondirective or analytic therapies use techniques of control and persuasion no less than avowedly directive therapists, and it is these techniques which are primarily responsible for therapeutic change."[86] Although sympathetic to the psychoanalytic arguments that the crucial therapeutic factors were the acquisition of insight, the renouncing of maladaptive goals, and the affirming of more mature, constructive goals, Abroms is able to conclude that "persuasion plays an important role in promoting therapeutic change."[87] Nevertheless, he rejects "the claim that it is the sole or primary agent . . . on methodological grounds because it fails to account for individual differences in persuasibility and for the process of incorporating and generalizing new attitudes and behaviors." He maintains that " 'healing through persuasion' says no more than that therapy is an interpersonal process."[88]

More recently, increasing attention has been paid to the role of rhetoric in discussions of psychotherapy. Susan R. Glaser, among others, has studied this issue with care and in detail.[89] Robert Spillane has explored rhetoric in studying "philosophical antecedents of psychotherapeutic ethics."[90] And Frank has developed his thesis regarding the significance of persuasion in psychotherapy to place increasing emphasis on the role of rhetoric.[91]

In addition to these various indications that persuasion may be much more an aspect of modern psychotherapy than many psychotherapists have been willing to admit, persuasion might be said to be at work in other, more subtle ways in psychotherapy. No matter what theories psychotherapists might subscribe to or what set of techniques they might favor, in some way or other, directly or indirectly, knowingly or unwittingly, they usually enlist patients to join them in working within a particular framework. However subtle it may be, some measure of influence or persuasion is at work in this process. Then, as the work of psychotherapy unfolds, it may fairly be said that the psychotherapist often endeavors to persuade or influence the patient in the direction of improvement, better health, or cure. But having taken note of these matters, one can say still more about persuasion in psychotherapy. The patient, too, is usually engaged in efforts to influence or persuade in the psychotherapeutic setting—to persuade the psychotherapist to view him or her favorably and to be kind, and not to judge too harshly—to mention just a few of the possible goals that may be sought through the patient's persuasive efforts.

When one considers the modern psychodynamic psychotherapies, the concept of transference entails another, rather oblique, form of persuasive effort. Transference refers to the inclination of the patient to view the psychotherapist in distorted ways reflecting a projection onto the therapist of attributes associated with significant figures in the patient's past. The patient is not only inclined to misperceive the psychotherapist in such ways, though, but is also inclined unconsciously to influence the psychotherapist toward fitting the misperception or subtly to "persuade" him or her to change in the direction of making the perception an accurate one. Such "persuasion" has led to many a transference-countertransference dilemma. And in many other instances, it has only been the experience, skill, and sensitivity of the psychotherapist that has prevented such "persuasive" efforts on the part of the patient from being successful, and thus disastrous to the treatment enterprise. In fact, it might be said that the concept of transference, and its analysis in treatment, are crucially useful countermeasures to deal with these potentially harmful "persuasions." Further, the lessons learned from investigating and understanding such efforts at persuasion have been, often enough, among the most valuable gains in a psychotherapeutic endeavor.

14

Conditioning and Reward or Punishment

"Learning is the process by which an activity originates or is changed through reacting to an encountered situation, provided that the characteristics of the change in activity cannot be explained on the basis of native response tendencies, maturation, or temporary states of the organism (e.g., fatigue, drugs, etc.)."[1] Among the many theories of learning, one of the most prominent — and widely used as a basis for therapeutic techniques — has been that based on conditioning principles. In addition to its prominent place in animal studies on learning, conditioning is a particularly significant mode of human learning and an integral factor in the acquisition of the habits and the behaviors present in any particular human.[2]

The term *conditioning* as used in some modern approaches to psychological healing — which are subsumed under rubrics such as *conditioning therapies* or *behavior therapies* — is a basic element in the techniques of those modes of treatment and is defined as follows: "According to *learning theory*, the means by which behavior is changed. Conditioning, which takes the form of either *classical* or *operant conditioning*, involves establishing new stimulus-response sequences through a form of environmental manipulation."[3] The application of this term to these practices is derived from the verb *to condition*, in the sense of "to bring to a desired state or condition." In the wake of Pavlov's conditioning experiments with dogs, the meaning of the verb was developed further to include "to teach or accustom (a person or animal) to adopt certain habits, attitudes, standards, etc.; to establish a conditioned reflex or response in."[4] And the general background for these meanings is the long tradition of using *to condition* to mean "to subject to conditions or limitations," often broadly interpreted as environmental manipulation, on the assumption that the environment is a determining factor in thinking and behavior.

Further, a central theme in psychology has been *learning*. That which has been learned has been commonly referred to as a *habit*. Habit has been defined in psychology as "a mental function whose repeated performance results in progressively better accommodation, and is accompanied by a feeling of familiarity and increased facility." *Habituation* refers to "becoming accommodated or habituated with respect to the performance of a given function."[5] A habit is an acquired function, as distinct from those innate functions that have been variously termed faculties, needs, instincts, basic drives, or basic reflex responses. And habituation is the process of developing a habit: as in training programs for animals or humans, child-rearing, conditioning experiments, behavior modification, conditioning therapies, etc. The stimulus-response viewpoint includes the development of habits or skills, as types of *response*. Thus, conditioning is a mode of learning that leads to behaviors (or responses) referred to as habits.

Earlier Instances of "Conditioning"

As Leo Postman, an experimental psychologist, has stated it, our "educational, social, and legal practices" are replete with instances in which rewards and punishments serve as "effective and reliable tools for the modification of behavior." And "philosophical discussions of rewards and punishments as regulators of human conduct have a long and time-honored history."[6] The evidence from past centuries suggests that physicians have called on a good number of practices akin to conditioning, although of course not necessarily employing the language associated with such activities today or the systematic approach that would satisfy the modern behaviorist. But this evidence is only rarely to be found in contexts that we would denominate as healing, in general, or as psychological healing, in particular.

A case in point is the realm of *child-rearing*. Within the scattered indications left to us, child-rearing does seem to have included training measures, educational approaches, and forms of discipline that involved what we would today term "conditioning." Whether carefully calculated or less systematically employed, various schemes of rewards and punishments have long served to mold or change behaviors in directions considered desirable by those involved in rearing and educating children.[7]

In educational approaches in particular, in the early 1800s a program was introduced that would today be referred to as the application of operant conditioning techniques in the classroom.[8] Joseph Lancaster (1778–1838) developed an inexpensive method of educating large numbers of poor children in England.

> Referred to as the "monitorial system," his method utilized students as monitors who performed many of the tasks normally undertaken by a teacher. . . . Student monitors were responsible for teaching and evaluating small groups of individuals in a somewhat regimented fashion. An incentive system was also used in a manner that closely resembles current applications of positive reinforcement in educational settings. Lancaster devised a token economy in which students earned tangible reinforcers for academic performance and deportment. . . . The system spread quickly in the 1800s, and was implemented in many countries throughout the world.[9]

Discipline through rewards and punishments was a key factor in this program, in which forms of social punishment proved more effective than corporal punishment.

Another sphere in which there have been centuries of attention to the molding and shaping of behavior — and indications that something like conditioned responses were striven for and developed — has been that of the *training of animals*. Long before the training of Pavlov's dogs and psychologists' white rats came to serve the study of learning and led to the conditioned response and behaviorism, human efforts to train animals involved "an appreciation of the reactions of a particular species to varied environmental conditions, and the providing or withholding of those conditions." Paul Mountjoy and others have drawn attention to this realm through a careful study of the history of the training of falcons.[10] And Solomon Diamond, in attending to the history of "the learned act," has briefly cited instances in the training of horses, dogs, and camels.[11]

Another instance involving the modification of behavior in animals was described by Kenelm Digby (1603–1665). In discussing how "the Antipathy of beasts towards one an other, may be taken away by assuefaction," Digby observed, "Any aversion of the fantasy may be mastered not only by a more powerfull agent upon the present sense, but also by assuefaction, and by bringing into the fantasy with pleasing circumstances that object which before was displeasing and affrightfull to it: as we see that all sortes of beastes or birdes, if they be taken yong may be tamed and will live quietly together. Dogges that are used to hunt and kill deere, will live frendly with one that is bred with them; and that fawne which otherwise would have been affraide of them, by such education groweth confident and playeth boldely with them."[12]

Earlier Versions of "Conditioning" in Psychological Healing

In contrast to some of the basic elements in the traditions of psychological healing — for example, consolation and confession — conditioning only seldom makes an appearance in the literature before the twentieth century, and we find only limited evidence of anything akin to conditioning as an explicit feature of efforts to ameliorate or cure mental illnesses, psychological disorders, or, for that matter, other forms of human ailments. As with the emerging focus on interpretation associated with the development of psychoanalysis, conditioning was conceived of and developed in a context that belongs mainly to the twentieth century — namely, conditioned reflex experimentation and behaviorism.

Nevertheless, in scattered examples over many centuries, one can identify a few instances in which the treatment measures employed or advocated were very similar to modern conditioning therapies. For example, in discussing patients who were inordinately fearful, Robert Burton advised that they be treated as follows: "As an horse that starts at a drum or trumpet, and will not endure the shooting of a piece, may be so manned by art, and animated, that he can not only endure, but is much more generous at the hearing of such things, much more courageous than before, and much delighteth in it: they must not be reformed abruptly, but by all art and insinuation, made to such companies, aspects, objects, they could not formerly away with. Many at first cannot endure the sight of a green wound, a sick man, which afterwards become good chirurgeons, bold empiricks."[13] Burton was here using *to man* with the meaning "to make tame or tractable," as the term was commonly used in the training of falcons and other hawks. Also, the passage illustrates that there is nothing new in using practices established with animals as the models for conditioning humans.

Probably more common, but not so clearly delineated, have been the instances where techniques based on reward and punishment have been used to change the behaviors and symptoms of the insane and other mentally disturbed persons. As with other forms of deviant behavior, systems of deterrence or inducing sanctions can be identified here and there in accounts of how mentally troubled individuals were persuaded or otherwise influenced to modify or reshape their behavior. Hints of such treatment approaches are rather more easily detected in the management programs for institutionalized insane persons in the eighteenth century and in the moral treatment of the nineteenth century.

An instance from this latter context is to be found in the work of François Leuret (1797–1851) who, toward the middle of the nineteenth century, employed conditioning techniques in his *traitement moral*. A leading figure among the former students of Esquirol, Leuret became chief physician of one of the services at the Bicêtre. He subscribed to primarily psychogenic notions in his view of mental disorders and developed a systematic theory of moral treatment; and his treatment approach involved coercive actions. Mark A. Stewart has noted that one of Leuret's case reports recounted a treatment program in which the technique was akin to Wolpe's modern techniques used to achieve reciprocal inhibition.[14] The patient—Thierry, a thirty-year-old wine merchant—was admitted to the Bicêtre in 1843, with a history of obsessional thoughts that had so worsened that he was no longer able to work. Leuret devised a treatment plan in which the patient received reading assignments of songs that he was to learn and recite or sing for Leuret the next day. His allotments of food were determined by his degree of compliance and success. As the "counterconditioning" program proceeded, his performance became increasingly successful, and his obsessional thoughts gradually disappeared. While some of the tasks—with their elements of reward or punishment—assigned to patients in the various moral treatment programs in the early nineteenth century might well be similarly interpreted as conditioning, it was rare for a treatment regime to be so precisely designed and carried out.[15]

The Emergence of Conditioning in the Twentieth Century

Conditioning, as we in the twentieth century have come to think of it, has its proximal roots in the classical conditioning experiments of Ivan P. Pavlov (1849–1936), the connectionism of Edward L. Thorndike (1874–1944), John B. Watson's (1878–1958) behaviorism, and the operant conditioning experiments of B. F. Skinner (1904–1990).

Classical conditioning refers to

> the complex of organismic processes involved in the experimental procedure, or the procedure itself, wherein two stimuli are presented in close temporal proximity. One of them has a reflex or previously acquired connection with a certain response, whereas the other is not an adequate stimulus to the response in question. Consequent upon such paired presentation of the two stimuli, usually many times repeated, the second stimulus acquires the poten-

tiality of evoking a response very like the response provoked by the other stimulus. The first-mentioned stimulus is called the *unconditioned stimulus* (US), the second-mentioned is the *conditioned stimulus* (CS). The original response is the *unconditioned response* (UR), the newly acquired response for the CS is the *conditioned response* (CR).[16]

This formulation reflects the work of Pavlov, the Russian physiologist whose extensive research with dogs made critical contributions to the understanding of digestion and was the basis for his receiving the Nobel Prize in 1904.[17] From this work he coined a term that was first, and apparently more accurately, translated as *conditional reflex;* but, by common consent, it led to the English terms *conditioned reflex* and *conditioned response.*[18] In Pavlov's work, the concept of association was taken from the traditional context of its application to thoughts and ideas and applied to efforts to deal with learned behaviors — digestive secretions and muscle movements — in objective and quantitative fashion. For Pavlov, conditioning was essentially association by contiguity. As a result, a type of associative learning, or an instance of habit formation, was becoming known as *conditioning.*

Vladimir M. Bekhterev (1857–1927) was also a Russian physiologist, but with a more direct interest in psychology; and he did somewhat similar work to that of Pavlov, but on motor conditioning responses. He, too, drew on the associationist tradition, but he conceived of these responses as reflex in nature and referred to them as *association-reflexes.* After the translations of his work in 1913, he became an important influence in the emerging behaviorism, but it was Pavlov's terms and concepts that became the more commonly used.[19]

Thorndike, with his *connectionism,* was another important contributor to the understanding of learning and, ultimately, to conditioning. The "connection" in connectionism was the one developed between stimulus and response. In "an experimental study of the associative processes in animals" (1898), he

created a kind of experimental associationism. He departed, however, from the classical tradition in several ways. First of all, he chose to study animals, primarily cats and chickens, rather than man. . . . Second, he spoke of the association between sensation and impulse — the conscious concomitant of action — rather than the association between ideas. Third, his experiments convinced him that a sensation and an impulse are most likely to become associated when the animal is satisfied by the consequences of its action, a principle that Thorndike later (1911) named the Law of Effect, because the effect of the action was thought to work retroactively to stamp in the association that led to it. Although animal trainers must have long known the value of rewards, Thorndike's Law of Effect was a genuine modification in the classical principle of association by contiguity. Finally, Thorndike suggested that an association may not require any ideational process in the animal. This suggestion of his was tentative and limited to animals, but it was opposed to the view of classical associationism, and the behaviorists who followed Thorndike extended it boldly.[20]

In the service of this research, Thorndike developed a "puzzle box" from which the animals would learn to escape in order to obtain food as a reward. It was out of this work that an understanding of associational connections was gradually transformed into the behaviorist's conditioned bond between stimulus and response. Thorndike systematically investigated the role of rewards and punishments in learning, and in his connectionism he laid the groundwork for what became instrumental or operant conditioning.

Another important factor in the developing status of the concept of conditioning was John B. Watson's work.[21] As a graduate student at the University of Chicago at the turn of the century, Watson was soon disenchanted by the philosophical aspects of psychology and by the introspective methods of Wundtian experimental psychology. He devoted his efforts to animal research, rapidly emerged as a highly regarded experimental psychologist, and moved to a professorship at Johns Hopkins University in 1908. Expressions of his views at Yale University in 1908 and at Columbia University in 1912 led to the publication of his behaviorist manifesto in 1913, "Psychology as the Behaviorist Views It."[22] Further influenced by acquaintance with the writings of Bekhterev and of Pavlov, Watson advocated the use of conditioning as a basic investigative method for his own work and for that of others. Along with two major books,[23] these efforts brought about the establishment of *behaviorism* as a particularly influential framework in psychology — as a context for many investigative efforts, as a creed for many psychologists, and as a contributor to the language that came to be used in the conditioning or behavior therapies.

Operant conditioning (or instrumental conditioning) refers to

> the complex of organismic processes involved in the experimental procedure (or the procedure itself) wherein a stimulus, having evoked a response that brings into view a rewarding stimulus, thereafter is more likely to evoke that response; or alternatively, the complex of processes or the experimental procedure wherein the stimulus, having evoked a response that prevents or removes a noxious or punishing stimulus, thereafter is more likely to evoke that response. The response that brings the rewarding stimulus or that prevents or removes the punishing stimulus is called the conditioned response, and the stimulus that evokes the CR is called the conditioned stimulus. The stimulus called forth by the conditioned response is called the unconditioned stimulus or the reinforcement.[24]

This formulation reflects the work that B. F. Skinner began at Harvard University in the 1930s and carried out largely with white rats. A white rat that had been deprived of food was placed in a laboratory apparatus that came to be known as the Skinner box, and its exploratory efforts eventually led it to press a bar that produced a food pellet. As satisfaction strengthened the associative linkage, recurrent experiences of the same nature brought reinforcement, and the animal rapidly learned a behavior through operant conditioning.[25]

Working with an emphasis on behavior rather than the physiological processes that might be involved, and studying the organism as a whole, Skinner minimized the role of theory and strove to establish empirical relationships.[26] His operant conditioning reinforced or increased the frequency of desired responses; punished or decreased the frequency of responses not desired; extinguished some responses by discontinuing reinforcers; and exerted stimulus control, by which was meant the reinforcement of a response in the presence of one stimulus and not in the presence of another stimulus.[27] Whereas in classical conditioning a new stimulus-response sequence was established, in operant conditioning an already functioning sequence is strengthened or weakened according to the nature of the reinforcement. Skinner had developed a method for studying a whole new range of learned behaviors.

Others, certainly, were significant contributors to behaviorist psychology — for example, Karl Lashley (1890–1958), Edwin R. Guthrie (1886–1959), and Clark L. Hull (1884–1952)[28] — but it is largely the streams of influence outlined above that have found their way down to recent decades as factors in shaping the conditioning therapies.

Twentieth-Century Conditioning Therapies

Although "behavior change strategies have most likely been employed throughout history . . . [and], in fact, historical precedents can be found for most current behavior therapy techniques, such as exposure, contingency management, aversion therapy, relaxation training, and systematic desensitization,"[29] the conditioning therapies (or behavior therapies) developed into a distinct field of endeavor only in the twentieth century. Out of Pavlov's and Bekhterev's experimental work on conditioned reflexes, and under the influence of Thorndike's contributions and Watson's vigorous advocacy of behaviorism, in the 1920s and 1930s a gradual accumulation of clinical applications for conditioning techniques emerged — although most of these endeavors were undertaken as experimental investigations rather than clinical trials. And Skinner's work on operant conditioning eventually led to numerous further applications of conditioning in clinical work.

The conditioning therapies have also been referred to as conditioned reflex therapy, learning theory psychotherapy, and behavior therapy. Notable among those favoring the term *conditioning therapies* has been Joseph Wolpe, a leader in the development of these modern techniques. In fact, Wolpe has not only tended to use *conditioning* in naming this category of therapeutic efforts, but he has alleged that "conditioning is the basis of all psychotherapeutic change." He commented that successful outcomes in most psychotherapeutic endeavors "usually depend on a process that often occurs inadvertently in all kinds of psychotherapeutic interviews, and that this process is a mode of conditioning — conditioned inhibition based on reciprocal inhibition."[30] While other behaviorally oriented therapists have joined him in thus challenging the views held by other psychotherapists, most of them would prefer to refer to their field of endeavor as behavior therapy or the behavior therapies, as Wolpe came to do himself.

Regarding terminology, in tracing the evolution and differentiation within behavior therapy, Daniel B. Fishman and Cyril M. Franks have said:

> The term *behavior therapy* seems to have been introduced more or less independently by three widely separated groups of researchers: by Skinner, Solomon, and Lindsley in the United States in a status report, to refer to their application of operant conditioning of a plunger-pulling response to bring about social interactions in hospitalized psychotic patients; by Lazarus in South Africa, to refer to Wolpe's application of his "reciprocal inhibition" technique to neurotic patients; and by Eysenck's Maudsley group in England to describe their "new look" at clinical intervention, in which behavior therapy is defined simply as the application of modern learning theory to the understanding and treatment of behavioral and behaviorally related disorders.[31]

As to a definition, behavior therapy has been said to be "the systematic application of principles derived from behavior or learning theory and the experimental work in those areas to the rational modification of abnormal or undesirable behavior."[32] Eysenck would reserve the term *behavior therapy* for the practices of "therapists who explicitly employ behaviour to change habits rooted in the nervous system," and apply the term *psychotherapy* to "what the mind-therapists do." But Wolpe argued that, "despite its etymology 'psychotherapy' should continue to designate the whole field . . . ; and behaviour therapy should be seen as the class of psychotherapeutic practices in which behaviour is deployed in a manner designed directly to bring about change in specific habits."[33]

While *conditioning therapies* and *behavior therapies* have often been used as roughly equivalent terms, many behavioral therapists would point out that behavior therapy includes techniques other than those based on one form or another of conditioning. Still, considering conditioning practices enables us to gain a representative view of how modes of learning may be deliberately or inadvertently employed in psychological healing.

Among the earliest signs of the emergence of modern behavior therapy were clinical applications of conditioning directly associated with Watson's work.[34] Most behaviorist accounts of this history cite the 1920 study by Watson and Rosalie Rayner (1898–1935), in which a conditioned fear reaction regarding white rats and similar objects was induced in "Little Albert," age eleven months, through the use of a Pavlovian conditioning program.[35] These investigators then proposed several conditioning interventions as treatment for this problem, but because Albert left the hospital, they were never able to implement their suggested treatment measures. In 1924, Watson's student, Mary Cover Jones published, on the basis of therapeutic interventions derived from suggestions made by Watson and Rayner, two reports on the use of conditioning in the elimination of various phobias in young children.[36]

During the rest of the 1920s, extensive further experimentation was carried out with conditioning, but little in the way of direct clinical application. In the 1930s the work of Clark L. Hull[37] at Yale University and B. F. Skinner[38] at Harvard University, though not involving clinical efforts, eventually came to influence the clinical work of others in a behavioral direction. Hull's work was reflected in efforts such as the Mowrers' treatment program for enuresis in children[39] and later became an influence in the investigations and clinical efforts of Joseph Wolpe.[40] Skinner's work led to operant conditioning programs such as those with psychotic patients by Ogden R. Lindsley and B. F. Skinner[41] and by Charles B. Ferster and Marian K. DeMyer.[42] In the 1940s Andrew Salter contributed to the slowly increasing stream of clinical applications of conditioning, his work culminating in 1949 in his *Conditioned Reflex Therapy,* influenced by Pavlov's research and Hull's views.[43]

Echoing the eighteenth century's "management" of disturbed patients and the nineteenth century's moral treatment, the milieu therapy programs of the 1940s, 1950s, and 1960s were structured to facilitate favorable behaviors and discourage unfavorable behaviors—in the interest of clinical improvement. Many of those programs were neither structured nor carried out with a conditioning paradigm in mind, yet it was often clear at the time, and certainly in retrospect, that themes of conditioning, reconditioning, and counterconditioning were basic to such clinical undertakings. Reward (or approval) and punishment (or disapproval) were often quite apparent elements; and the social system of the hospital was utilized in the interest of social learning and relearning. Behavior modification was at work. Further, in the 1950s and

1960s, a steady increase took place in the explicit application of Skinner's operant conditioning techniques in training programs for troubled children and in psychiatric hospital settings.[44]

Among such applications were those which came under the rubric of the *token economy* and served groups the size of a hospital ward population and sometimes larger. Although these programs were reminiscent of nineteenth-century educational approaches such as that of Joseph Lancaster mentioned earlier, they derived fairly directly from Skinner-influenced operant-reinforcement research and its clinical applications. In a token economy, clinical staff identified target behaviors and established contingent rewards that could be earned by those behaviors. A token of one sort or another was chosen as the medium of exchange, serving as a reward for the hoped-for behavior and as "currency" that patients could exchange for items or events that they desired. Against a background of careful specification of the responses to be reinforced and the token values associated with each response, patients and clinical staff could work toward an operant conditioning of sought-for behaviors as a clinical goal in the treatment of various mental disorders.[45]

Influenced by the work of Pavlov, by Hull's learning theory, and by Jules M. Masserman's work on experimental neuroses in cats,[46] the psychiatrist Joseph Wolpe induced neurotic disorders in cats and then undertook treatment of those disorders. By the 1950s he was actively developing clinical approaches based on conditioning, deconditioning, and counterconditioning;[47] and his colleague Arnold A. Lazarus applied the term *behavior therapy* to these practices.[48] Wolpe would undertake to condition a new response that was incompatible with the neurotic response (or maladaptive conditioned response) and so to move the neurotic response in the direction of extinction — a process that he termed reciprocal inhibition.[49] Out of this work came the technique known as systematic desensitization: various responses, such as muscular relaxation and assertive responses, were developed in the patient in response to anxiety-provoking situations of gradually increasing intensity, and these conditioned responses served to inhibit the anxiety. This technique and variations on it became particularly significant in behavior therapy.[50]

Also in the 1950s, at the Maudsley Hospital in London, Hans J. Eysenck and M. B. Shapiro began both research and clinical efforts in which conditioning principles were central; and these two men, their colleagues, and their students set in motion another stream of influence in the emerging realm of behavior therapy.[51] Their efforts were significantly influenced by the work of "Pavlov and Hull, who originated the main tenets of modern learning theory" and that of "Watson, who was among the first to see the usefulness of the conditioning paradigm for the explanation of neurotic disorders."[52] Eysenck argued that neurotic disorders were acquired on the basis of classical conditioning, and many of his investigations either led him to that conclusion or were designed to test that hypothesis. His view was that neurotic disorders could be grouped into (1) those with "deficient conditioned reactions" in which the behavior therapist would supplement the situation with the addition of desirable conditioned reactions; (2) those with "surplus conditioned reactions" in which the therapist would counter the surplus reactions with the introduction of other, desirable conditioned reactions.[53] That is to say, cures would be achieved through extinguishing maladaptive conditioned responses and establishing desirable conditioned responses.

Even though the present study has focused on psychological healing in which learning through the influence of conditioning and reward and punishment can be identified—that is, on clinical work explained in terms of stimulus-response theories—the existence of another major family of learning theories, namely, the cognitive theories of learning, must be recognized.[54] In contrast with those who favor stimulus-response theories, investigators or therapists who subscribe to a cognitive learning perspective favor the view that learning involves the acquisition of cognitive structures rather than the acquisition of habits and that insight rather than trial and error is involved in problem solving. That is to say, the cognitive learning perspective takes into account the acquisition of insight and understanding.[55] And it should be added that although some of the clinical work explained by cognitive learning theories may be satisfactorily explained by a conditioning theory, some features of such work cannot be satisfactorily dealt with in that manner.

The "long past, but short history" of conditioning has included many efforts to train or educate humans and various other animals. Various modes of persuasion toward behaving differently have been employed, with overt or covert themes of reward or punishment.

Against this background, and in the more recent past of formal conditioning efforts of a clinical and paraclinical nature, the behavior therapy of the last fifty years has developed into a relatively distinct category of psychological healing. Conditioning emerged out of extensive attention to stimulus-response learning, and with interweavings of reward and punishment, as a primary principle for clinical theory and practice, in which two types predominated: classical or respondent conditioning (from Pavlov's work), and operant or instrumental conditioning (from Skinner's work). Wolpe's systematic desensitization is derived from the respondent tradition, with (positive) counterconditioning in the interest of replacing problematic behaviors with more desirable behaviors. Aversive conditioning also belongs to the Pavlovian tradition and is a form of negative counterconditioning. In operant conditioning, the efforts to change or reshape behavior entail influencing the patient through the consequences of the behavior (rather than influencing through stimuli delivered with the behavior to be reshaped); reinforcement is brought about by rewards or punishments that occur as a result of the behavior that is to be changed, and it too can be positive or negative.

In some of these various techniques, the element of reward or punishment is apparent, and sometimes quite explicit. In others, the role of reward or punishment is much more subtle and may even be denied by those who employ the techniques. In some of these more subtle situations, it is more a matter of approval or disapproval than of reward or punishment. It should be noted, though, that considerable evidence has accumulated to the effect that learning in conjunction with reward is much more effective than learning in conjunction with punishment (or disapproval). Nevertheless, a case can be made for conditioning through reward (or approval) or through merely a lack of reward (or a lack of approval). To sum up, some form of reward or approval has a significant place in a remarkably high percentage of these techniques; and negative factors — whether punishment, disapproval, or merely lack of reward or approval — have a place in some.

Some therapists have been partial to psychoanalytic or psychodynamic approaches to psychological healing but have discerned elements in such treatment approaches that either were akin to the learning theory techniques employed in the conditioning therapies or could be explained in terms of learning theory. Early examples of this viewpoint are found in the work of the American psychiatrist and psychoanalyst, Edward J. Kempf (1885–1971), in the second decade of this century. Interwoven with Kempf's psychoanalytic views were explanations of psychopathology as "conditioned reflex activities," and he cited Bekhterev, Watson, and Lashley as sources of such views. In discussing his treatment efforts, Kempf suggested that a deconditioning process was at work, while at the same time couching matters in psychodynamic terms.[56]

Decades later, the psychiatrist and psychoanalyst Franz Alexander (1891–1964) would comment that, in such clinical approaches, "particularly the principle of reward and punishment and also the influence of repetitive experiences can be clearly recognized." In referring to reward and punishment, he clearly was including experiences of approval and disapproval, and the sense of reward or satisfaction associated with the relief of tension on coming to understand something, on resolving a dilemma or conflict, or on achieving mastery in regard to a problem or task. And Alexander alludes to the role of repetitive experiences in the patient's unlearning old patterns of thought and behavior and learning new ones. He observes that "this complex process of relearning follows the same principles as the more simple relearning process hitherto studied by experimental psychologists." He takes the position that both connectionist and Gestalt theories of learning were probably valid; and so he argues that both learning through trial and error with conditioning influences and learning aided by cognitive processes take place. That is to say, the relearning "contains cognitive elements as well as learning from actual interpersonal experiences which occur during the therapeutic interaction." As he sums it up, the "common basis in all learning," including useful psycho-therapeutic experiences, is "the forging of a connection between three variables: a specific motivating impulse, a specific behavioral response, and a gratifying experience which is the reward."[57]

Another psychiatrist and psychoanalyst, Judd Marmor, put forward the idea that psychoanalytic therapy itself is a learning procedure.[58] And he considered, at length, the relevance of learning theory for understanding the clinical work of psychoanalysts and psychotherapists. "The fundamental problem with which we are faced in psychoanalytic therapy is that of how we can enable or cause the patient to give up certain acquired patterns of thought, feeling, or behavior in favor of others which are considered more 'mature,' 'adaptive,' 'productive' or 'self-realizing.' The learning theorist, if he is a member of the stimulus-response school, structures this as an effort to teach the patient new habit patterns; or, if he belongs to the cognitive school, as an effort to teach the patient new patterns of perception and new cognitive 'insights.' "[59] In the view of the learning theorist, the concept of conditioning plays a major role in any such explanations. According to learning theory investigators, "What seems to be going on in the working-through process [in psychoanalysis] is a kind of conditioned-learning, in which the therapist's overt or covert approval and disapproval — expressed in his nonverbal reactions as well as in his verbal confrontations, and in what he interprets as neurotic or healthy — act as reward-punishment cues or conditioning stimuli."[60] In summing up, Marmor concludes that, without suggesting that conditioning is the be-all and end-all of psychotherapeutic work, "a subtle conditioning procedure usually takes place, in varying degrees."[61]

Some years later, Marmor reported on several studies of the psychothera-peutic process in the work of experienced therapists of different theoret-ical and technical persuasions. Among the eight categories or elements that seemed common to these various clinical approaches, he identified "*operant conditioning* of the patient toward more adaptive patterns of behavior by means of explicit or implicit approval-disapproval cues, and by a correc-tive emotional relationship with the therapist."[62] Parenthetically, it is worth noting that the behavior therapists who were studied made as much use of interpretive statements — as well as suggestion, tension discharge, and other elements not usually said to be aspects of behavior therapy — as did the psychodynamic psychotherapists.

Other scholars have similarly examined various psychotherapies with an eye to identifying a short list of basic factors in such clinical endeavors. Saul Rosenzweig included social reconditioning in his list.[63] And Allen Bergin and Hans Strupp included counterconditioning and reward and punishment in theirs.[64]

PART SEVEN

Cognitive Themes

15

Explanation and Interpretation

Among the meanings of *interpretation* in the English language two definitional traditions are of particular importance for our purposes: one relating to explanation or the act of explaining, and the other to translation or the act of translating. Further, interpretation is the act of offering meaning, signification, or understanding — or the meaning, signification, or understanding offered — whether to another or to oneself.

Among twentieth-century psychotherapists, interpretation has involved the description, explanation, or formulation of the meaning or significance of a patient's communications, usually by the psychotherapist, but often enough by the patient. It has included the explanation of what is obscure and unclear — the perception of less obvious meanings or understandings, and their translation into forms meaningful or useful for the patient. And its significance in psychological healing has been predicated on the considerable usefulness attributed to psychological insight or self-understanding. This intimate association of insight and interpretation has been particularly characteristic of psychoanalysis, and interpretation has been accorded the status of the primary intervention by the majority of psychoanalysts. In these contexts, the meaning of interpretation has usually been that of explanation.

But this activity called interpretation was, of course, nothing new. The desire to know and to understand has long appeared to be a fundamental inclination for humankind. From the young child who asks "Why?" to the average inquiring adult, human beings have always been inclined to search for explanations and to try to understand. As Aristotle stated it, "All men by nature desire to know."[1] In expanding on Aristotle's theme, Jonathan Lear took note of the innate curiosity that is to be observed in humans from earliest childhood but then added, "But curiosity is not, I believe, the best way to conceptualize what drives men on. . . . We cannot simply observe phenomena: we want to know *why* they occur." He further remarks, "We are after more than knowledge, we are after understanding." Restated yet another way, "Understanding, for its part, is man's capacity to grasp how things really are, not just how they immediately present themselves."[2]

Interpretation has been of the essence in the efforts of philosophers ever since such efforts first began; and philosophers long ago developed this inclination into an essential professional activity. They have surveyed human experience in the light of available knowledge, in an effort to determine what is significant in that experience and to give meaning to the living of human life. Interpretation has been a central element in these philosophic endeavors, through which philosophers have striven to explain human behavior, human experience, the natural world, and the wisdom of past thinkers — to themselves and to others. In fact, some have suggested that philosophy *is* the interpretation of such matters.

Further, the multiplicity of interpretations that have been put forward by philosophers — and by the many and varied practitioners of other disciplines dealing with human knowledge — have not been independent of the interpreters who proffered them. The systems of values, beliefs, and assumptions (whether underlying or explicit) held by the interpreters have crucially shaped the nature of their interpretations. In fact, the values, beliefs, theories, and bits of wisdom based on the accumulated experience of human beings might be said to have been used as "instruments" of interpretation and to have been of an interpretive nature themselves. Interpretations and explanations have reflected the developmental background (culture, education, and other aspects of personal experience) and personal assumptions of the interpreter. Further, it is unlikely that the very observations that an interpreter considers in striving to understand and to make an interpretation could ever be purely objective data. Interpretation of some sort is commonly embedded in the very perceptions being considered.

Whether an interpretation is put forward with certainty or tentativeness, it can be viewed as a hypothesis developed in an effort to explain a body of data. Even in the realms of science and religion, where many have been very certain of their interpretations, an interpretation can be no more than a hypothesis that may be met with efforts to verify or disprove it.

Interpretation in the History of Medicine

From the beginnings of medical time, healers have observed, questioned, listened, gathered data, and, in an effort to understand and to provide understanding to others, have formulated hypotheses that have been offered to sufferers and their kin as interpretations or explanations. The very act of formulating a concept of disease constituted an explanation. It began a mode of explaining the nature of sick persons, of giving meaning to their states and their experiences, and of evaluating and interpreting what had come about when persons became ill.[3] Interpretation has always been an inherent element in constructing a diagnosis, too. However crude or however refined the conceptual scheme being used, diagnosis has involved interpretation. In the reasonings that have attempted to trace the process whereby signs and symptoms occurred, developed, and interacted to constitute a particular disorder or disease, arrival at a diagnosis has clearly rested on interpretive thought, some of which has often been conveyed to the sufferer in the form of explanation. Again, determinations of etiology and theories of pathogenesis have been inherently interpretive in nature. Throughout history, when the doctor offered prognostic comments, it was usually after further interpretation, whether or not that was made explicit to the sufferer. And in the rationale for the decisions and procedures of treatment, too, implicit, and sometimes explicit, interpretations were embedded.

In his review of primitive medicine, Henry Sigerist (1891–1957) commented, "All medical actions . . . are determined by the views held of the nature and causes of disease."[4] In fact, therapeutic activity in any culture — whether that culture is deemed primitive or advanced — has tended to be causal rather than symptomatic. The discerning of meaning, of how and why, has usually been a part of the healer's activity; and bringing some form of understanding to the situation has been a natural aspect of comforting, caring for, and curing the sick, whether the interpretation has only guided the healer's ministrations or has constituted an explicit element in those ministrations.

As the centuries of medical history unfolded, so too did theories of disease. Among the ways in which such theories have been categorized, the dichotomy of supernatural explanations versus natural explanations has proved to be of abiding relevance up through the present day. And the details of each theory have provided a system of thought that has guided healers' explanations of disorders, their diagnoses, their prognoses, and their treatment interventions. Whether, in primitive cultures, the explanations have been in terms of breach of a taboo, intrusion of foreign bodies or of spirits, loss of or possession of the sufferer's soul, or the machinations of some witch, interpretations relying on supernatural factors have served both sufferers and healers in countless attempts to ameliorate or cure a sickness. Other cultures, including our own, have made considerable use, in dealing with disease, of explanations based on divine or diabolical interventions. Sinfulness and divine punishment constituted a particularly familiar variant. As to naturalistic explanations, the physicians of classical Greece and Rome frequently invoked the theory of humors and related disequilibria, and the methodists' scheme of tense, astringent states and relaxed, atonic states. Interpretations of disease that relied on the humoral theory continued to be have currency for many centuries thereafter. Then, in the seventeenth century, chemical explanations came to exercise considerable influence; and in the eighteenth century, mechanical explanations came to the fore. In the nineteenth century, the germ theory of disease revolutionized interpretations of disease.

As theories of disease have evolved, healers have gathered observations regarding sick persons, and have used this or that theory to find meaning and to guide them in caring for and endeavoring to cure the sick. The process of explaining or interpreting observations helped healers make their way in the various clinical dilemmas that confronted them — interpretations brought order to uncertainty in both the personal and professional realm, calmed and reassured sufferers and those around them, and guided healers' diagnostic, prognostic, and therapeutic efforts. And with the burgeoning technologies of the last two centuries — stethoscope, microscope, laboratory assessments, radiography, and so on — the increasing observational data have called for a steadily increasing amount of interpretive activity.

Despite the omnipresence of interpretation and explanation, explicit discussion of such activities has been minimal until relatively recent times. Physicians — and healers of every stripe — developed their theories (or subscribed to existing theories) in order to cope with the many illnesses and to follow their vocation. Schemes of explanation have waxed and waned — some long lasting, some short lived — providing meaning for both healers and sufferers, meeting the need for understanding, serving as the basis for diagnostic and prognostic formulations, and guiding therapeutic practices. And these theoretical systems have often been compared with one another, one almost always being deemed better or preferable to another, or it being argued that one has the "truth" and the other has not. Rarely have the common features in these various explanatory schemes been commented on — such as the desire to know and understand, the search for meaning in the experience of being ill, and the other ways in which *different* interpretive systems have served *similar* purposes for healers and sufferers. It is only in our own century that this more objective perspective has developed in any meaningful way.

Interpretation and Psychological Healing

Explanations and interpretations have served healers and sufferers dealing with *mental disorders*, as in the case of other diseases and disorders. Whether the disorders were conceived of in a religious tradition as spiritual ailments calling for spiritual remedies or in a philosophical tradition as states of "unwisdom" or forms of mental distress calling for a wise counselor's guidance, or in a medical tradition as diseases of the head or psychological illnesses calling for medical remedies, healers of all descriptions applied the interpretations and explanations provided by their theories in their search for understanding of the sufferers' sicknesses and for guidance in their healing ministrations. But in contrast to such other modes of intervention as confession or consolation, interpretations and explanations tended not to be viewed explicitly as elements of the healing endeavor. Instead, they were taken for granted as aspects of an approach that provided understanding and guidance to healers and sufferers adopting the approach. Interpretations were an implicit element in efforts to ameliorate a disorder, acquire wisdom, achieve peace of mind, obtain comfort, become contented, or be cured.

It is only in quite recent times that the providing of an interpretation has come to be viewed as an explicit element in healing, or as in itself constituting an agency in a healing process. It was only as psychoanalysis (and approaches influenced by psychoanalysis) developed that interpretations and explanations came to be regarded as critical factors in the healing process — and then it was in conjunction with their role in promoting insight and self-understanding.

Interpretation and Psychoanalysis

Although interpretation has come to be viewed as the cardinal form of intervention on the part of the psychoanalyst, that was not always the case. A brief recapitulation allows us to see just how gradually explanations and interpretations acquired their central position in Sigmund Freud's psychoanalytic treatment process. Influenced by Josef Breuer's experience with Anna O., Freud's prepsychoanalytic efforts had been directed toward the patient's recovering the memory of a traumatic event, re-experiencing the associated affect, and realizing the connection between these matters and the symptoms.

To facilitate the process, Freud employed first hypnotic suggestion and later waking suggestion to prompt this remembering and reliving; and in keeping with the notion that neurotic symptoms were associated with "strangulated" or "dammed-up" affects, the intention was to help the patient achieve a catharsis, along with the abreaction of the affects in question. By the mid-1890s, Freud had gradually shifted to primarily persuasive efforts to get the patient to talk freely in the waking state, in the interest of such remembering and reliving. Then he came to the realization that a patient often actively resisted such urgings to engage in free association; Freud made efforts to identify such resistances and to explain them to the patient, as a step toward eliminating them, so that the clinical work might proceed. In these explanations, we have the beginnings of psychoanalytic interpretations and the rudiments of the emerging practice of psychoanalysis.

Toward the end of the 1890s, Freud's increasing attention to dreams led him and others to propose interpretations of the latent content of dreams. These early interpretive efforts included indicating to the patients the nature of their wishes, drives, and aims, and the conflicts associated with them. During this time, Freud was coming to grips with another type of obstacle to the progress of the treatment, namely, transference manifestations; and in dealing with these as both an interference and a source of useful information, he made contributions toward the understanding of transference themes — patterns of attitude and inclination that patients carried with them from the past and tended to activate in their relationships, including the treatment relationship. In summary, insight or self-understanding was beginning to be viewed as crucial to clinical improvement in psychoanalysis, and interpretation was emerging as the essential technique in acquiring this insight.

Parenthetically, it should be noted that the word *interpretation* was slow to assume the prominent place that it eventually acquired in psychoanalysis. In English, the verb *to interpret* is defined as "to expound the meaning of (something abstruse or mysterious); to render (words, writings, an author, etc.) clear or explicit; to elucidate; to explain." Less common than it once was, but still considered appropriate, is the meaning "to translate." In more recent times (from the late nineteenth century onward), *to interpret* has been used to mean "to bring out the meaning of (a dramatic or musical composition, a landscape, etc.) by artistic representation or performance." As to the noun *interpretation*, all the activities alluded to by the verb could lead to an interpretation; but the commonest meanings have tended to be "explanation," "translation," or "rendering." Regarding the noun *interpreter*, its meanings have included "one who interprets or explains," or translates; and, earlier, "an official or professional expounder of laws, texts, mysteries, etc."[5]

As Rudolf Ekstein has pointed out, two German words, *Deutung* and *Interpretation,* are translated as "interpretation" in English. *Deutung* has most of the meanings just noted and is frequently employed "in religious or superstitious contexts, for example, for prophecies or for fortune telling." And a "*Deuter* may be a *gypsy* who *reads the future* in the palm of a person or an *oracle priestess* or a *seer* who foretells the future, attempts to predict the future from signs, such as symbols in manifest dream content—as is true for the interpretation of dreams as found in the Old Testament or in the writings of antiquity." As to the German word *Interpretation,* it "may also be used in philosophical, religious, or artistic context. It refers frequently to the *attempt to give meaning* to something and is burdened by certain philosophical notions which state an *essential* difference between the sciences which *explain* (erklaerende Wissenschaften) and the sciences which merely *understand* (verstehende Wissenschaften)."[6] Rather than *Interpretation* or *Erklaeren* (explanation), Freud chose the word *Deutung* for the psychoanalytic activities and understandings that English-speaking psychoanalysts later translated as *interpretation.* James Dimon has suggested that Freud was thus avoiding the philosophical debate regarding the alleged differences between *explanation* in the natural sciences (*Naturwissenschaften*) and *interpretation* in the human sciences (*Geisteswissenschaften*).[7]

Freud brought *Deutung* to prominence in psychoanalytic literature with the appearance in 1899 of *Die Traumdeutung* (*The Interpretation of Dreams*), and English translators of his work have consistently chosen to translate that word as *interpretation.* He began this famous work with the following statement: "In the pages that follow I shall bring forward proof that there is a psychological technique which makes it possible to interpret dreams, and that, if that procedure is employed, every dream reveals itself as a psychical structure which has a meaning and which can be inserted at an assignable point in the mental activities of waking life."[8] At the beginning of his chapter "The Method of Interpreting Dreams," he discussed the topic further.

> The aim which I have set before myself is to show that dreams are capable of being interpreted. . . . My presumption that dreams can be interpreted at once puts me in opposition to the ruling theory of dreams . . . for "interpreting" a dream implies assigning a "meaning" to it—that is, replacing it by something which fits into the chain of our mental acts as a link having a validity and importance equal to the rest. As we have seen, the scientific theories of dreams leave no room for any problem of interpreting them, since in their view a dream is not a mental act at all, but a somatic process signalizing its occurrence by indications registered in the mental apparatus. Lay opinion has taken a different attitude throughout the ages. . . . Led by some obscure feeling, it

seems to assume that, in spite of everything, every dream has a meaning, though a hidden one, that dreams are designed to take the place of some other process of thought, and that we have only to undo the substitution correctly in order to arrive at this hidden meaning.[9]

As implied here, Freud chose to side with "lay opinion," arguing that "dreams really have a meaning and that a scientific procedure for interpreting them is possible."[10] He proceeded to demonstrate how one might "translate" the manifest contents of a dream into their latent meanings; how the disguising substitutions, by this process of interpretation, could be transformed and the hidden, unconscious meaning of the dream be made manifest or conscious.

In an outline of "psycho-analytic procedure" a few years later, he wrote of having

developed . . . an art of interpretation which takes on the task of, as it were, extracting the pure metal of the repressed thoughts from the ore of the unintentional ideas. This work of interpretation is applied not only to the patient's ideas but also to his dreams, which open up the most direct approach to a knowledge of the unconscious, to his unintentional as well as to his purposeless actions (symptomatic acts) and to the blunders he makes in everyday life (slips of the tongue, bungled actions, and so on). The details of this technique of interpretation or translation have not yet been published by Freud. According to indications he has given, they comprise a number of rules, reached empirically, of how the unconscious material may be reconstructed from the associations, directions on how to know what it means when the patient's ideas come to flow, and experiences of the most important typical resistances that arise in the course of such treatments. A bulky volume called *The Interpretation of Dreams* . . . may be regarded as the forerunner of an initiation into his techniques.[11]

Although "the details of this technique of interpretation" remained to be published, phrases such as *art of interpretation* and *work of interpretation* were gradually becoming familiar ones. As Freud came to terms with the patient's resistances and began to realize the problems (and usefulness) associated with the patient's transference manifestations, he had slowly modified the view of interpretation suggested in *The Interpretation of Dreams* — it needed to be more than simple translation. Not only did dream interpretation call for more than a translator's glossary of the meanings of dream symbols, but attention to the interpretations of resistance and transference called for considerable patience, careful listening and sustained attention, and a sense of tact and timing. All this contributed to a much more complex notion of what was needed in the way of interpretive activity. In the issue of timing, for example, Freud recognized the problem of premature interpretations; he acknowledged the inclination of the analyst to want to put his own understanding of the patient's difficulties into words before the patient was ready to make any significant use of such information; and he realized the limited usefulness of merely intellectual insight. Then, in 1913 in one of his papers on technique, he brought these various matters together in succinct and cogent fashion.[12]

In his writings and lectures up to this time, when he addressed the topic of interpretation, Freud usually focused on dream interpretation; and to the end of his days, the interpretation of dreams provided the language, the examples, and the general context for most of his discussions of interpretation. Throughout the years, he saw *The Interpretation of Dreams* as the crucial turning point in the development of psychoanalysis; and he held the view that dream interpretation was the aspect of clinical practice that crucially characterized the practitioner as a psychoanalyst. But in the writings of other psychoanalysts and in point of practice, clinical interpretations were also directed to other mental contents, "(parapraxes, symptoms, etc.) and, more generally, to whatever part of the speech and behavior of the subject bears the stamp of the defensive conflict."[13]

In 1934, in his classic study of "the therapeutic action of psycho-analysis," James Strachey (1887–1967) reflected this more general application of the term *interpretation* in psychoanalysts' clinical explanations. Clinical interpretation was not limited to dream interpretation, and it was viewed as the cardinal agency for therapeutic gain in the clinical process. Further, Strachey carefully differentiated "mutative interpretations" from the "purely informative 'dictionary' type of interpretation," the mutative being interpretations that have an emotional immediacy and bring about useful change, and the more conventional interpretations being those which merely provide intellectual insight and are thus less likely to promote change. In addition, he emphasized that it was primarily transference interpretations that were mutative. Though he considered "extra-transference interpretations" less effective, he acknowledged that they probably constituted the majority of the interpretations made and that they had their own key role.[14]

Since Strachey's time, interpretation has continued to be viewed, by the majority of psychoanalysts, as the crucial form of intervention in psychoanalysis; but within that consensus have coexisted significant variations and some controversies. How broadly or narrowly, for example, should the term *interpretation* be applied to the range of psychoanalytic interventions? What should be the relative status of transference interpretations and other interpretations given by the analyst? Are interpretation and insight as crucial to therapeutic gain in psychoanalysis as has so often been argued?

Just what is subsumed under the rubric *interpretation* has ranged from the broadly inclusive — most of the analyst's comments and interventions — to the more limited — "those explanations, given to patients by the analyst, which add to their knowledge of themselves."[15] In addressing this issue in 1951, Rudolph Loewenstein (1898–1976) took a position that has become a reasonably representative one. He indicated that the term should not include instructions and explanations regarding psychoanalytic procedure, interventions that serve to create and maintain the analytic situation, questions, silences, and so forth, but should be reserved for the analyst's verbal interventions that produce "those dynamic changes which we call insight."[16] Further, though, many would carefully distinguish confrontation and clarification from interpretation. Some would say that the first two, in their own right, lead to insight, and would consider them "insight-furthering techniques,"[17] grouping them with interpretation as "technical procedures" subsumed under the heading *analyzing*.[18] Others would give them little separate consideration and would categorize them as either aspects of interpretation or interventions that merely pave the way for eventual interpretations.

In their discussions analysts have gone back and forth regarding the status of transference interpretations: some have taken the position that only transference interpretations should be offered by the analyst, others that such interpretations are the only mutative ones; and yet probably the majority of analysts have valued such interpretations while at the same time merely giving them pride of place in the panoply of interpretations. The concerns about the extreme views on this subject have been dealt with particularly well by Harold Blum. Although he took nothing away from the significance of transference interpretations, Blum made a thoughtful case for the significance of "extra-transference interpretations." He observed that "derivatives of unconscious conflict (and their interpretation) are not limited to transference" and that "transference is not the sole source of analytic insight or locus of analytic work." He moreover commented that "the transference (succeeding the dream) became the 'royal road' to clinical interpretation" but in the end concluded that there really is "no royal road to analytic interpretation. The transference is the main road but not the only road to mutative interpretation, and we do not analyze just transference or dreams, we analyze the patient." "Extratransference interpretation has a position and value which is not simply ancillary, preparatory, and supplementary to transference interpretation."[19] In discussing "kinds of interpretation," Karl Menninger (1893–1990) made a somewhat similar point: "For decades there has been a running debate between proponents of *resistance* interpretation, proponents of *transference* interpretation and proponents of *content* interpretation. From our point of view this can be dismissed in a sentence: All these are necessary at different times."[20]

As to the question of how crucial interpretation and insight are to therapeutic gain in psychoanalysis, most analysts have been in agreement that these factors are crucial indeed. But in the late 1940s and the 1950s, Franz Alexander and his concept of the "corrective emotional experience" were seen as challenging this status and as diminishing the significance of interpretation and insight in psychoanalysis.[21] For a while, this issue received considerable attention, but the central place of interpretation and insight was vigorously reaffirmed by many, and the controversy soon subsided. Representative of such reaffirmations was the view of Edward Bibring. Categorizing Alexander's practices as "experiential manipulation," he acknowledged that the psychotherapies might well hold a place for such "influence through experience" but he asserted that "interpretation is the supreme agent in the hierarchy of therapeutic principles characteristic of analysis."[22]

In recent years, increasing attention has been given to the two-person aspects of the psychoanalytic process, in addition to the traditional emphasis on the patient's intrapsychic realm. Particularly influential, and among the more thoughtful expressions of this trend, have been the contributions of Hans W. Loewald (1906–1993).[23] On the premise that the patient becomes an associate or collaborator in the analytic enterprise, and emphasizing elements of empathy and caring on the analyst's part, Loewald developed the view that clinical interpretations occur within an interactional (patient-analyst) field and reflect an interactional process, in addition to serving as reflections of the patient's intrapsychic activity as understood and communicated by the analyst. He portrayed the analyst's function in this process as somewhat analogous to the developmental and educative roles of a good parent.

A successful psychoanalytic interpretation ultimately involves an understanding on the part of both the analyst and the patient of material the meaning of which the patient has previously been unaware. Beginning with the patient's communications to the analyst, the latter gradually develops his or her understanding of what is being revealed, formulates an interpretation, and, guided by issues related to timing and tact, communicates the interpretation to the patient. A hypothesis has been developed and made explicit for consideration by the patient. The patient's reaction, both in the short run and in the longer run, becomes part of a process of confirmation or disconfirmation. "The patient's corrections, amplifications, and other contributions to the analyst's interpretations must be included in what is considered the interpretive process."[24] Thus the patient's role in a clinical interpretation is multifaceted—it includes the original associations and other communications that contributed to the psychoanalyst's understanding *and* the reactions and responses to the interpretation being put into words. An interpretation is a dynamic process involving both analyst and patient.

In summary, it is clear that interpretation has continued to have a place at the heart of psychoanalytic technique, as an intervention that "brings out the latent meaning in what the subject says and does"[25] — that is, it has a crucial role in providing insight to the patient. Or as Greenson stated it, "To interpret means . . . to make conscious the unconscious meaning, sources, history, mode, or cause of a given psychic event."[26] Further, although a clinical interpretation is an explanation, it is not *just* an explanation. As Ekstein put it, "The primary intent of an analytic interpretation is not to explain but to cure."[27] Still, as Stephen Appelbaum has pointed out in a thoughtful review of the status of insight, the danger exists of overemphasizing the role of insight (and interpretation) and, concomitantly, underemphasizing the role of other elements in both psychoanalysis and psychotherapy.[28]

Interpretation and Twentieth-Century Psychotherapy

Among the numerous psychotherapies that have emerged in the twentieth century, many have been significantly influenced by psychoanalysis. And that influence has frequently entailed subscribing to the psychoanalytic emphasis on insight as a crucial factor in achieving therapeutic gain and on interpretation as the crucial form of intervention in the acquiring of that insight. In one way or another, many authorities on these practices have said much the same thing: for example, "The interpretive process is the central therapeutic activity of the therapist."[29]

Nevertheless, certain psychotherapists (including some who can be termed psychodynamically oriented) have made a particular point of challenging the idea that interpretation and insight merit recognition as cardinal factors in psychotherapy. Some have maintained that interpretation is either unnecessary or counterproductive. Others have retained a place for interpretation but have relegated it to a lesser role. Among these critics, a few have argued that other factors are the central or crucial ones — such as the patient-therapist relationship, catharsis and abreaction, and various modes of learning, unlearning, and relearning.

Prominent among those associated with approaches viewed as noninterpretive is Carl Rogers, with his client-centered therapy. Even though he conceived of the psychotherapeutic process as facilitating the emergence of "insight and self-understanding"[30] and thought of insight as contributing significantly toward therapeutic gain, he had serious reservations about interpretation as a means toward that insight. Rogers held the view that the therapist should work to facilitate the increasingly free expression of patients' attitudes, concerns, and feelings, and that in the process, insightful realizations would tend to emerge spontaneously. This process led to patients gradually acquiring new perceptions of themselves and their experiences, and a new understanding of their symptoms and behavior.[31] Rogers allowed some role for interpretations in this process, yet he had grave reservations about reliance on them: he emphasized that patients generally feared interpretations and experienced them as judgmental and threatening.[32] Over the years, Rogers' reservations about interpretation seemed to increase, and he later commented that "interpretation is not relied on as a therapeutic instrument."[33] Nevertheless, many of the empathic comments made by client-centered therapists amount to interpretive statements; and the therapist's choice of topics to address serves to guide the patient toward particular meanings and insights, and thus stem from underlying interpretations. As to Rogers' concerns about the dangers of interpretations, it might be argued that his emphasis on "accurate empathy"[34] could serve as protection against the danger that the patient will feel judged or threatened.

As many have argued, or at least pointed out, learning in some form or other is a significant aspect of the vast majority of psychotherapies. During the last few decades, a good number of studies have employed learning theory to explain the process of treatment in the psychodynamic therapies.[35] And in this same era, another set of clinical approaches, explicitly based on learning theory, has assumed a significant place among the array of psychotherapies. These have come to be grouped together under the rubric *behavior therapy*. In both these trends, notions of learning and of unlearning and relearning have been called on to describe and explain the techniques and the process of various psychotherapeutic endeavors. Into the former category fall efforts to reconcile the modalities of interpretation and insight with explanations based on learning theory. With regard to the latter category, most behavior therapists have had little to say about interpretation as a mode of clinical intervention. Occasionally, it has been dismissed as an intervention that is associated with psychoanalysis but is irrelevant for the practice of behavior therapy. But more often it has merely been ignored. At the same time, Judd Marmor has argued effectively that psychodynamic therapists and behavior therapists have much more in common in their treatment approaches than either is usually prepared to recognize; and that includes clear evidence that behavioral therapists make interpretive interventions. In fact, in one comparative study, "the behavior therapists made virtually as many interpretive statements as did the dynamic psychotherapists!"[36]

Another psychotherapeutic approach usually considered to be noninterpretive is gestalt therapy. Developed by Fritz Perls, formerly a psychoanalyst, gestalt therapy has drawn on such varied sources as psychoanalysis, phenomenology and existentialism, and Gestalt psychology. It emphasizes the here and now, striving to influence the patient toward a lively, emotionally attuned *awareness* of what is going on within the self. To facilitate this process, the therapist focuses on the patient's behavior, nonverbal communications, and bodily indications of tension. Although gestalt therapists question, encourage free expression, suggest, and cajole, in the interest of facilitating awareness, they characteristically decry the use of interpretation. As one gestaltist put it, "Interpreting behavior is contrary to the Gestalt approach."[37] Perls recurrently criticized the use of interpretation by psychoanalysts. His views on the subject are captured well by the following comment: "In working with a dream, I avoid any interpretation. I leave this to the patient since I believe he knows more about himself than I can possibly know."[38] As still another gestalt therapist stated it, "Instead of interpretation, in Gestalt therapy we have explicitation [*sic*]: the request that the patient himself become aware of and express the experience underlying his present-avoiding behavior."[39]

Nevertheless, interpretation has tended to figure in gestalt therapy in several ways. As with other psychotherapies, the underlying assumptions guiding the clinical work have served as hidden interpretations that have had significant effects on the patients and their treatment. Very frequently, in the therapist's efforts to facilitate the patient's awareness, thinly veiled interpretations are made to the patient without being acknowledged as such. Particularly striking are those moments when patients strive to answer their own "*why* questions" — that is, to make interpretive statements — and the gestalt therapist makes active attempts to dissuade them from such efforts; at such times any comments about what the patient is up to are interpretive in nature. Appelbaum has addressed these sorts of issues most thoughtfully.[40] Acknowledging gestalt therapists' arguments against insight and interpretation, he comments, "gestalt therapy will have to stand up and be counted as a highly effective purveyor of insight, however much gestaltists may dislike their method being characterized in this way." However gestaltists have striven to avoid introducing interpretations, interpretations have crept into their work, whether explicitly, implicitly, or incidentally, as the therapists provide guidance, in working toward increased awareness for the patient. He concludes, though, that "a better distinction than insight and interpretation versus no insight and interpretation would be that gestalt therapists are hypersensitive to the invasion of the interpretive process by emotionally isolated cognition, and have designed their techniques accordingly."[41]

In bringing to a close this discussion of twentieth-century psychotherapies, it is worth remarking that over a good many decades now, thoughtful scholars have contrasted various approaches and have raised the question of just what ingredients in the different psychotherapeutic mixes (or recipes) are crucial to bringing about useful effects for patients. Such scholars have frequently included interpretation, in one form or another, as a significant ingredient in most, if not all, psychotherapeutic approaches. Saul Rosenzweig, in a 1936 study, included "psychological interpretations" in his short list of "common factors in diverse methods of psychotherapy." Within the consistency of any particular psychotherapeutic approach, the interpretations served the purpose of change and reintegration.[42] Some years later, Allen Bergin and Hans Strupp reported on extensive studies of numerous psychotherapies; and they too listed interpretation among the crucial elements.[43] As a third example, Judd Marmor undertook a similar type of study; and on his resultant list of basic factors was cognitive learning or cognitive awareness in which the therapist's interpretations assisted the patient in achieving "a better understanding of the basis of his difficulties" and in correcting "various misconceptions which may exist in his mind."[44]

When one examines the modern scene of approaches to psychological healing, *interpretation* seems to be particularly significant among the variety of interventions employed. Even approaches that appear not to include interpretation as one of their basic elements nevertheless draw attention to it by criticizing it or claiming that they avoid it.

As has been noted, interpretation and explanation are rooted in inherently human inclinations — curiosity, the search for the "why?" of situations and events, the endeavor to know and to understand, and the need to explain events and experiences, for oneself and others. These inclinations relating to the search for meaning have characterized human behavior over the millennia.

Consistently, interpretive elements have been embedded in healing efforts or have underlain them as unstated assumptions, yet interpretations and explanations have rarely been considered agents in the healing process, no matter how construed. And this has been true for psychological healing, just as it has been true for somatic healing.

Only with the emergence of psychoanalysis — and the various psychotherapeutic endeavors influenced by psychoanalysis — has interpretation been conceived of as in itself a therapeutic agency in the process of psychological healing. This occurred because of the intimate connection between interpretation and the acquisition of insight or self-understanding. In the beginnings of psychoanalysis, clinicians worked to bring about clinical gains for patients through a complex process of remembering, realizing the implications of the memories, making connections, and coming to understand issues and conflicts that had, for whatever reasons, been kept out of awareness. Insight came to be of particular significance as this clinical approach evolved further. The gradual unfolding of the healer's role in this process brought into focus that person's activities in facilitating the acquisition of insight. And attention to the healer's activities led to the identification of interpretive activity as a crucial contribution to the healing process. Despite the long history of explicit emphasis on the significance of acquiring self-understanding, only with these twentieth-century developments has the role of interpretation or explanation in gaining that understanding become explicit.

Another context with implications for the history of interpretation in twentieth-century psychological healing has been hermeneutics. One group of authors has characterized hermeneutics as "a family of related approaches that have developed as a corrective to scientism—the modern proclivity to view the natural sciences as models for all forms of inquiry."[45] Commonly defined as the art and science of interpretation, hermeneutics derives from traditions dealing with the interpretation of texts (particularly the Bible), which led in the eighteenth century to concerns regarding the nature of understanding and interpretation in general and eventuated in attention to interpretation within the social, historical, and psychological disciplines. In these domains, the contributions of Wilhelm Dilthey (1833–1911) have played a particularly significant role. He emphasized the centrality of interpretation to the human sciences —a method of understanding human experience and activities based on *Verstehen*. By *Verstehen* he meant the projection of oneself into the historical and social events being considered (or into the experiences of another person), and the resulting acquisition of understanding of those events (or that person) through a form of empathic reliving (*Nacherleben*).[46] Out of these beginnings, hermeneutics came to stress that meanings change and that the orientation of any particular interpreter is rooted in his or her particular historical and cultural past. That is to say, the interpreter meets data with some set of preconceptions that then influence how he or she organizes and interprets those data.

Against the background view that "the central curative aspect of psychotherapy rests on our ability to understand the patient and communicate this understanding back to him or her," Richard Chessick has outlined a possible relevance and usefulness for a hermeneutic perspective in psychotherapeutic endeavors—and thus a way of viewing clinical interpretive activities.[47] He cites Hans-Georg Gadamer to the effect that "to have a method is already to have an interpretation." Further, Gadamer notes the presence in the human sciences of "a dialectic or mutual influence between the subject of interpretation and the interpreter, in which, as the horizons of each coparticipate, meaning is generated in that particular dyadic pair at that particular time and place."[48] That is to say, "understanding is dialectical and is a linguistic process that makes interpersonal communication the locus in which meaning is determined. . . . Knowledge is the consequence of a dialectic altering both parties."[49] This statement seems akin to the oft-noted observation of recent years that, in psychotherapy and psychoanalysis, interpretation is a "two-person" process.

As has just been noted, the twin recognitions of the role of sociocultural factors in the development of interpretations and of the "two-person" nature of interpretation in psychotherapeutic contexts may owe something to the influence of hermeneutics. But there are problems with a hermeneutic perspective in the realm of psychological healing. A crucial issue is that the application of hermeneutics to such healing contexts can overlook the very fact that they are *healing* contexts. In the extreme, we have those hermeneuticists who would view the sufferer as analogous to a text and so run the risk of misunderstanding the complex role of the sufferer and the interaction between healer and sufferer. A hermeneutic scheme could moreover place limitations on generalizability from any interpretation, even within the clinical work with a single patient. Associated with that are the risks inherent in extremes of relativism that pass beyond useful understanding. Such a relativistic view of interpretations could leave healers so uncertain about the meaning and the therapeutic potential of what they are doing that the possibility of therapeutic effectiveness could be seriously vitiated. A further danger here might be the tendency toward nihilism or at least serious discouragement — or perhaps it is discouragement that leads to espousal of a hermeneutic perspective.

In view of the emergence of interpretation as an explicit and significant element in so much of twentieth-century psychological healing, and in light of the ferment stirred up by the proponents of a hermeneutic orientation, it seems fair to conclude this chapter by quoting the philosopher Richard J. Bernstein: "the twentieth century might be labeled 'the Age of Interpretation.'"[50]

16

Self-Understanding and Insight

The word *insight* has its roots in the idea of "internal sight," that is, perceiving "with the eyes of the mind or understanding." It originally entailed "the notion of penetrating into things or seeing beneath their surface with the eyes of the understanding." The *Oxford English Dictionary* defines it as follows:

1. Internal sight, mental vision or perception, discernment; in early use sometimes, Understanding, intelligence, wisdom.
2. The fact of penetrating with the eyes of the understanding into the inner character or hidden nature of things; a glimpse or view beneath the surface; the faculty or power of thus seeing.[1]

A very recently published dictionary describes insight as: "1. The capacity to discern the true nature of a situation; penetration. 2. The act or outcome of grasping the inward or hidden nature of things or of perceiving in an intuitive manner."[2]

In twentieth-century psychiatry and psychology, *insight* has included meanings such as: "the process by which the meaning, significance, pattern, or use of an object or situation becomes clear; or the understanding thus gained." But it has particularly come to imply a person's, often a sufferer's, understanding of his or her own condition. It is defined further as "(1) Reasonable understanding and evaluation of one's own mental processes, reactions, abilities; self-knowledge. (2) The greater or less understanding of one's true condition when mentally ill; e.g., the ability to recognize the irrationality of some of one's impulses."[3] And, in many of the twentieth-century psychotherapies, the goal of acquiring insight and the process entailed by the efforts to reach such a goal became central issues. Insight became a basic element in such clinical undertakings, and its acquisition was often viewed as either the cause or the result of clinical improvement. Many other aspects of psychotherapeutic activity were thought to derive their significance from their contribution to the acquisition of insight.

"Know Thyself"

The exhortation to self-understanding — "Know thyself" — was carved on the temple at Delphi in ancient Greece, along with the companion inscription "Nothing too much." And it was associated with the Delphic Oracle, the supreme oracle of Greece in classical times, presided over by the god Apollo.[4] Apollo's functions particularly included music, prophecy, and medicine. "He is often associated with the higher developments of civilization, approving codes of law, inculcating high moral and religious principles, and favouring philosophy (e.g., he was said to be the real father of Plato)."[5] Further, he was reputed to have been the father of Aesculapius, physician, hero, and god of healing.[6]

These two inscriptions on the temple at Delphi — "Know thyself" and "Nothing too much" — reflected themes that were the essence of the highly regarded sophrosyne, a concept that evolved to mean self-knowledge, self-restraint, and moderation. One of the principal types of imagery associated with the word in ancient Greek literature was that "of health, or the healing of disease. This metaphor is implicit in the very word sophrosyne, whose etymology suggests saving the reason or keeping it sound. . . . When the doctrine of the 'goods' of body and soul became a commonplace in Hellenistic philosophy, sophrosyne was regularly defined as health of soul."[7] Eventually, sophrosyne came to be viewed as one of the four cardinal virtues, along with wisdom, justice, and courage.[8]

Sophrosyne was intimately associated with Socrates in Plato's writings, through both his own search for this quality or attribute and his discussions of it. In *Charmides,* the concept was explored by Socrates in almost agonizing detail, and it was defined as self-knowledge by Critias, with reference to the Delphic "Know thyself."[9] In *Phaedrus,* Socrates defined it as self-knowledge and referred to his own quest for such knowledge, with reference to the Delphic saying.[10] And in *Alcibiades I,* Socrates again discussed sophrosyne as self-knowledge and referred to the Delphic Oracle.[11]

In the centuries following Plato's time, *sophrosyne* was often used with more emphasis on self-restraint and moderation but, periodically, with an emphasis on self-knowledge. Cicero (106–43 B.C.) illustrated both aspects of this trend. Both early on and in his later writings, he mentioned the notion of temperance (sophrosyne), with the emphasis on self-restraint and moderation.[12] While this was his more common interpretation of temperance (sophrosyne), he did use it to mean self-knowledge, and those instances were significant. In discussing contemplation of the universe and the secrets of nature, Cicero commented, "To the soul occupied night and day in these meditations there comes the knowledge enjoined by the god at Delphi, that the mind should know its own self and feel its union with the divine mind, the source of the fulness of joy unquenchable."[13] And he emphasized that when "Apollo says, 'Know thyself,'" he does not mean "Know thy body," but, rather, "Know thy soul."[14]

Then, in the course of discussing wisdom as "the mother of all good things," in noting that "love of wisdom" is the source of the term *philosophy,* Cicero remarked, "For she [philosophy] alone has taught us, in addition to all other wisdom, that most difficult of all things — to know ourselves. This precept is so important and significant that the credit for it is given, not to any human being, but to the god of Delphi. For he who knows himself will realize, in the first place, that he has a divine element within him, and will think of his own inner nature as a kind of consecrated image of God; and so he will always act and think in a way worthy of so great a gift of the gods."[15]

From these two instances, one can detect themes that were to become important in later Christian tradition: self-knowledge associated with the search for a sense of union with God; and self-knowledge as the path to a person's realization of "a divine element within him." And for Cicero, they showed how the contemplative life served the pursuit of temperance/sophrosyne, and how the achieving of temperance/sophrosyne brought with it harmony in the soul, *tranquillitas animi,* or what in the twentieth century might be called peace of mind. Decrying the relative inattention (in comparison with the attention to bodily diseases and the art of healing them) to "the sickness of the soul" and the "art of healing for the soul," Cicero discussed this "art of healing" at considerable length. By this "art," he meant philosophy; and through this art, afflicted persons might serve as their "own physicians," and philosophers might serve as "physicians of the soul."[16] Temperance, as one of the cardinal virtues, was an ideal and was considered a goal in efforts to heal the sick soul.

In the centuries immediately after Cicero, the emphasis was more on self-restraint and moderation as the essential meanings of *sophrosyne,* and Cicero's Latin equivalent, *temperantia,* was commonly the term of choice. With both later Stoic and early Christian philosophers, this was the case. Frequently concerned with the cardinal virtues — wisdom, justice, courage, and sophrosyne (temperance) — they emphasized restraint and moderation of the appetites and the passions and harmony in the soul. Increasingly the efforts toward temperance entailed pursuit of the contemplative life, longing for wisdom, ascetic practices, and a search for purity; and these activities were a means toward "assimilation to God" or "imitation of the Divine."

The by then preponderant Greek view that sophrosyne was essentially self-restraint gradually developed into the Christian emphasis on self-control, including its more extreme versions of chastity and purity. Mention of self-knowledge as an aspect of sophrosyne/temperance had become relatively infrequent, but when it did occur, it was associated with striving toward the imitation of God or a sense of union with God.[17] A significant instance is found in the writings of Clement of Alexandria — a Christian scholar probably born in Greece who came to Alexandria around 180, he studied with St. Pantaenus and succeeded him as director of the catechetical school there.

Clement of Alexandria (ca. 150–ca. 215) placed considerable emphasis on self-control in his *Paedagogus,* but he also addressed the importance of self-knowledge as a means to knowing God. Together, self-control and self-knowledge could lead to purification and "assimilation to God." As Clement believed, "To know oneself has always been, so it seems, the greatest of all lessons. For, if anyone knows himself, he will know God; and, in knowing God, he will become like him . . . by performing good deeds and cultivating an independence of as many things as possible."[18] Helen North has suggested that certain passages in Plato's writings had a critical influence on Clement's association of sophrosyne with the imitation of God.[19] Insofar as Clement employed *sophrosyne* to mean that self-control was a significant factor in seeking to be like God, this may well be so. But Plato was referring in these contexts to the aspect of self-control in sophrosyne, whereas in the passage just quoted from the *Paedagogus* Clement was associating another aspect of sophrosyne, self-knowledge, with the imitation of God. In this latter regard, his view seems to be more reminiscent of Cicero's views.

A somewhat similar view of the significance of self-knowledge was expressed by Plotinus (205–270). Variously referred to as "Neoplatonist philosopher and mystic" and "the founder of Neoplatonism," Plotinus was a Greek or perhaps a Hellenized Egyptian. Although he favored the interpretation of sophrosyne that stressed self-control and moderation, he nevertheless gave meaningful consideration to self-knowledge. He viewed contemplation as a means by which a soul could attain union with God, although he identified himself neither with the pagan religion of his time nor with Christianity. Like other philosophers of Roman times, Plotinus attended to the cardinal virtues, with an emphasis on self-control of the appetites and passions and on the notion of purification. In his view, the virtues served the soul in its efforts to escape the material world and ascend toward unity with the Divine Mind. Sophrosyne was "a kind of agreement and harmony of the appetitive [part of the soul] with the rational part." Sophrosyne now took "the form of a turning (or conversion) towards the Divine Mind . . . , for in the Divine Mind itself sophrosyne consists in turning towards itself." Through a process of purification, the soul was enabled "to contemplate the Divine Mind and, by contemplating, to become one with it."[20] In addressing these matters, Plotinus placed some emphasis on the acquisition of self-knowledge. In a complex discussion of "self-knowing," he indicated that the acquiring of self-knowledge — the pursuit of the Delphic "Know thyself" — must entail contemplative efforts to know God, and that knowing God was the path to self-knowledge. For Plotinus, these two "knowings" were essentially inseparable.[21]

Augustine paid particular heed to self-knowledge in several of his writings, beginning with the following prayer from 386: "O God, who art ever the same, let me know myself and thee."[22] Influenced by Platonic thought, by Cicero, and by Plotinus and Neoplatonism, this African-born teacher and philosopher eventually came under the influence of Ambrose, bishop of Milan, and was converted to Christianity in 386. Augustine became a priest and served for many years as bishop of Hippo. His writings were a significant influence on the Christian world of the Middle Ages, and they have continued to be important in Christian thought ever since.

In his considerations of temperance, or sophrosyne, Augustine discussed self-restraint more in the sense of moderation than in regard to the extremes of purity and chastity as had so many of his Christian predecessors; he was seriously concerned as well with the theme of self-knowledge. For him, the acquiring of self-knowledge was a commendable task, something to be sought for and worked at, even if never fully achieved. And he associated self-knowledge with inwardness, a self-exploration in the pursuit of such knowledge — an inner experience that would later come to be termed introspection.[23] As one author has stated it, "The *Confessions* are indeed a large-scale exercise in creating such self-knowledge from the formless chaos of memory, an attempt to penetrate into what Augustine elsewhere calls 'the more obscure depths of the *memoria*' by seeking to disclose to the mind's conscious gaze the truth lying latent and unsuspected within itself."[24] Through such efforts a person could reach a measure of self-knowledge — and achieve that peace of mind that so often has been the goal of psychological healing.

In *De Trinitate,* Augustine argued that the mind must seek to know itself, in order that it may love itself;[25] he discussed at length the mind's search for self-knowledge, and the logic of such an effort;[26] and he considered the purport of the Delphic injunction, "Know thyself," suggesting that it was "that the mind should reflect upon itself, and live in accordance with its nature."[27]

In the sixth century, the philosopher and statesman Boethius (ca. 480–524) conveyed a sense of the significance of self-knowledge in the following passage from *The Consolation of Philosophy,* presented in the form of a dialogue with Philosophy. She (Philosophy) has earlier employed a medical metaphor in considering how she might help Boethius in his distress: "If you expect a physician to help you, you must lay bare your wound."[28] Further along, in her role as a physician of the soul, she says, "I know the cause, or the chief cause, of your sickness. You have forgotten what you are. Now therefore I have found out to the full the manner of your sickness, and how to attempt the restoring of your health. You are overwhelmed by this forgetfulness of yourself." False opinions "breed a dark distraction which confuses the true insight." And Philosophy proposes to help in dissipating "this darkness" so that the troubled Boethius may be restored to self-awareness and peace of mind.[29]

Throughout the Middle Ages, if the maxim "Know thyself" was seldom directly cited in Christian writings, the theme of self-knowledge was a persistent concern. Further, the theme "was given a heightened importance in the writings of the later medieval Mystics." As had Plotinus and certain of the early Christian Fathers, they considered self-knowledge essential to attainment of knowledge of God and to the realization of their yearned-for goal of union with God. For them, the path to that goal was through self-examination and recognition of their faults, and through the ensuing sorrow and confession.[30] Self-knowledge was "a door, the entrance to the most intimate chamber," "a ladder by which the soul may ascend to the heights," "a highway leading to contemplation," and "the haven into which a ship sails through storm and calm." One mystic wrote of self-knowledge as a "large and high mountain" which the soul would strive to ascend; another "resolved to form a 'cell of self-knowledge' within her own heart and dwell therein."[31] In the late Middle Ages, writers repeatedly affirmed the importance of knowing oneself, coming to a knowledge of one's sins, humbling one's spirit, and hunting out the faults to which one was inclined.[32] Union with God was the explicit reason offered for striving toward self-knowledge; the implicit goal was peace of mind.

In the sixteenth and seventeenth centuries, the injunction "know thyself," according to Eliza Wilkins, "again assumed a place of some importance in secular literature; while discussions of the theme of self-knowledge, some of them of considerable length, occur rather frequently in ecclesiastical writings."[33] Noted lay authors in most of the European languages addressed the subject; Richard Baxter's *The Mischiefs of Self-Ignorance and the Benefits of Self-Acquaintance* offers an example of the way religious writers treated the subject of self-knowledge; and, whether in Latin or in the vernacular, the maxim frequently served as the title for a poem or identified a topic within a poem.[34] Within this vast literature, the implications of "Know thyself" varied a good deal. Among secular authors, it was used to mean taking one's own measure, knowing one's place, or forming a true estimate of one's capacities and virtues; or it served as "a warning against pride and vainglory and a general overestimate of one's self"; to know oneself was to be truly humble and moderate, or to know the limits of one's wisdom. In the ecclesiastical literature, "Know thyself" frequently was applied to recognizing one's faults or acknowledging that one was a sinner and should repent. The ancient philosophical implications to knowing one's soul had acquired a strongly Christian coloration; and knowing oneself continued to be considered the essential pathway to knowledge of God. This sense of self-knowledge took on the overtones of the modern term *conversion*.[35] The quest for self-knowledge was given great significance; it was the beginning of virtue and wisdom; and it was difficult to attain. "In the religious writings of these centuries, as of those which had preceded, the beginning of self-knowledge is achieved by prolonged self-examination and reflection."[36]

In the eighteenth century, references to and discussions of self-knowledge were less frequent. In most of these discussions, self-knowledge was considered in ways already familiar: knowing one's measure, knowing one's ability, recognizing one's mortality, knowing the limits of one's wisdom, knowing one's faults, or knowing one's soul.[37] As to how one might gain such self-knowledge, a number of different means were suggested: "looking at our neighbor as into a mirror, or listening to his opinion of us, whether he be friend or foe; the study of philosophy and literature and the pursuit of education in general; adversity; retirement for reflection and other religious observances." These methods were not at all new, but meanwhile a less familiar approach had joined them and would eventually become significant: acquiring self-knowledge through the study of humankind.[38]

From the late eighteenth century to the end of the nineteenth century, both the Delphic injunction and the theme of self-knowledge continued to flourish in Western literature. Most of the familiar implications of "Know thyself" persisted. In addition, though, a newer perspective came into prominence — the search for self-knowledge through one's associations with others — including knowing others, comparing oneself with others, and learning how others perceived one. Given the increasing emphasis on other selves, concerns arose about the social aspects of knowing oneself — a social self-knowledge and a knowledge of one's relations with others — and this was accompanied by ethical implications.[39] And occasionally notice was taken of the self-awareness and self-realization that might be gained from moments of vivid emotion.

During the late nineteenth century and on into the twentieth, a modest but steady inclination persisted to bring up the saying "Know thyself" in philosophical discussions, in essays on the pursuit of knowledge, in considerations of how to be a better or a wiser person, and occasionally in the title of an article, a book, or a poem. As a phrase, it still had a considerable appeal. Cogitations on the theme of self-knowledge or self-understanding seemed to come from a well that would never run dry. A far from exhaustive search of the literature turns up dozens of references to both the maxim and the theme. These trends put one in mind of the not infrequent suggestion that "Know thyself" is at the very heart of philosophy and of the search for knowledge in general. As Samuel Taylor Coleridge (1772–1834) stated it in the early nineteenth century, "The postulate of philosophy and at the same time the test of philosophic capacity, is no other than the heaven-descended KNOW THYSELF!"[40] Or, as the philosopher William Knight (1836–1916) put it early in the twentieth century, "The old Socratic maxim 'know thyself' lies at the very root of all human progress, personal, social, or political. We must know ourselves before we can know anything else adequately. . . . I take the Socratic motto 'know thyself' as the basis of everything else worth knowing."[41]

Of particular interest, though, is the emergence, also in the late nineteenth and the twentieth centuries, of significant attention to the notion that matters outside a person's awareness, yet "within" him or her, in a manner of speaking, may influence the person's frame of mind, mental state, or behavior — that is to say, the idea that gave rise to to the terms *the subconscious, the unconscious, unconscious mental phenomena,* and so on. And acquiring knowledge of that aspect of oneself became a new form of self-knowledge. This trend became closely associated with the development of psychological healing as a distinct endeavor — whether termed psychotherapy, psychoanalysis, or whatever. In this developing field, self-knowledge gradually assumed a crucial role, and *insight* or *psychological insight* became its commonest name. Recognition of the heritage of this new version of self-knowledge is reflected in the observations of the modern scholar Bennett Simon: "the Socratic imperative 'Know thyself' is a root of the notion of understanding as part of the process of healing."[42] And he identified as follows the common thread running through philosophy's long tradition of seeking to know oneself, and the twentieth-century pursuit of self-understanding as critical to psychological healing. "Philosophy . . . can serve as a way to put a man in touch with his true self, and truly help him to know himself. This is the sense in which the Socratic ideal comes closest to ideals held up by various schools of psychoanalysis and psychotherapy — ideals of an integrated awareness of the self, of one's own past, present, and future, and of the relationship between oneself and one's group."[43]

Insight and Psychoanalysis

Whereas the idea of insight or self-knowledge has a long history in psychoanalysis, the term *insight* only entered the language and literature of psychology in more recent decades. Josef Breuer and Sigmund Freud alluded to the concept in 1893, in an article that became the first chapter of *Studies on Hysteria* in 1895. As noted in earlier chapters, these authors had learned that a patient's symptom could be caused to disappear by bringing a disturbing memory into awareness, along with its accompanying affect. Recollection without affect usually produced no result.[44] The physician's efforts were directed toward the patient's recovering the memory of the traumatic experience, re-experiencing the associated affect, and realizing the connection between this experience, with its affect, and the symptoms. That is, the experiential, affective and cognitive elements in the process together led to the disappearance of the symptoms.

Once all three aspects of this process are considered important, the patient's self-knowledge[45] — the *coming to know* and the *knowing* — can be seen to encompass both a cognitive and an emotional awareness. But the patient might show reluctance or resistance to acquiring this self-knowledge, as Freud pointed out at some length in *Studies on Hysteria*.[46] Gradually Freud shifted from primarily persuasive efforts to foster remembering to an appreciation of the significance of the resistances themselves; and so the analytic work intended to lead to the patient's self-knowledge came also to include efforts to bring about an understanding of the resistances. As he noted later, physicians' tendency, once they had come to an understanding of the patient's conflicts and symptoms, was to explain that understanding to the patient, at times in a rather intellectual mode and without due appreciation of the value of the patient's understanding the resistances. For the moment, the analyst might employ suggestion or persuasion, rather than analysis.

In 1913, Freud looked back at these problems as follows.

> Are not the patient's ailments due to his lack of knowledge and understanding and is it not a duty to enlighten him as soon as possible — that is, as soon as

the doctor himself knows the explanations? The answer to this question calls for a short digression on the meaning of knowledge and the mechanism of cure in analysis.

It is true that in the earliest days of analytic technique we took an intellectualist view of the situation. We set a high value on the patient's knowledge of what he had forgotten, and in this we made hardly any distinction between our knowledge of it and his. We thought it a special piece of good luck if we were able to obtain information about the forgotten childhood trauma from other sources . . . as in some cases it was possible to do; and we hastened to convey the information and the proofs of its correctness to the patient, in the certain expectation of thus bringing the neurosis and the treatment to a rapid end. It was a severe disappointment when the expected success was not forthcoming. How could it be that the patient, who now knew about his traumatic experience, nevertheless still behaved as if he knew no more about it than before? Indeed, telling and describing his repressed trauma to him did not even result in any recollection of it coming to mind.

. . . There was no choice but to cease attributing to the fact of knowing, in itself, the importance that had previously been given to it and to place the emphasis on the resistances which had in the past brought about the state of not knowing and which were still ready to defend that state. Conscious knowledge, even if it was not subsequently driven out again, was powerless against those resistances.[47]

This amounted to a combination of "knowing with not knowing." Here we have the seeds of later discussions about intellectual insight versus emotional insight.

In addition to the attention to resistances, Freud's focus gradually shifted from efforts to aid the patients in recovering the affect-laden memories of the repressed traumatic experiences to efforts to aid them in becoming aware of their wishes, drives, and aims, and the conflicts associated with them. The nature of the self-knowledge being sought was changing, but insight was still considered a vital element in treatment.

And this complex of efforts soon came to be accompanied by interpretive endeavors toward understanding the transference themes that tended to emerge in the treatment. These patterns of attitude, inclination, and behavior that patients carried with them from the past, and tended to activate unwittingly in their relationships, were "transferred" to the analyst and thus served as active factors in the treatment process. A type of reliving and re-experiencing occurred in the transference, with emotional concomitants; the analyst's interpretations facilitated the acquisition of an understanding of these attitudes, inclinations, and behaviors; and thus the option to change those which were problematic could be made available to the patients. The self-knowledge thus gained might include an awareness of how patients felt and why they felt that way, of what they did with and to others, of why these behaviors occurred, and of how their inclinations had come to be as they were. The so-called working-through phase of analysis involved consideration and reconsideration of these matters, along with opportunities for the patients to employ the insight gained in the interest of changing problematic aspects of their lives.

While the goals of psychoanalysis were being modified in the ways outlined above, insight or self-understanding continued to be valued as a central element in the work toward clinical improvement—and interpretation came to be considered the crucial technique through which the analyst facilitated acquisition by the patient of this self-knowledge. Samuel Slipp has provided a cogent summary that is relevant here. "Freud believed that psychoanalytic cure came from insight, facilitated by the therapist's interpretations and reconstructions of associative material and dreams, and by the patient's reliving of old conflicts in the transference to the analyst. Insight served as a bridge between the past and the present. It was as if part of the patient were frozen (fixated) in the past and doomed repeatedly to act out the past through behaviors in the present. Cure was possible only after the patient remembered these conflicts and understood the unconscious wishes and fears underlying them."[48] And numerous other authorities on psychoanalysis have emphasized the view that insight, particularly as conveyed through interpretations, is the essential element in psychoanalytic cure. Harold Blum has maintained that "insight propels the psychoanalytic process forward and is a condition, catalyst, and consequence of the psychoanalytic process."[49] Further, "analytic 'cure' is primarily effected through insight and not through empathy, acceptance, tolerance, etc."[50] Lloyd H. Silverman posed the question: "What is the psychological process that brings about change in psychoanalytic treatment?" In answer, he stated, "The consensus among psychoanalysts is that the *main* agent of change is insight, with the qualifications that the insight must be experienced emotionally as well as cognitively and that it must be 'worked through.'"[51]

Interwoven through the decades of psychoanalytic discussion and argument about insight has been a continual emphasis on the significance of emotional insight for the accomplishment of therapeutic gain. It has been repeatedly argued that, without a convincing emotional accompaniment to the self-understanding being acquired, it was merely intellectual insight and had little mutative effect. The problems alluded to by these terms, and the vagaries of their meanings, were discussed at length by Gregory Zilboorg (1891–1959)[52] and subsequently by many others.[53] And a variety of other terms have been used in discussions relevant to these contrasted modes of insight. As mentioned earlier, James Strachey wrote about two types of interpretation—"the purely informative 'dictionary' type of interpretation" and "the mutative interpretation" that is "emotionally 'immediate' " — and thereby implied that two types of insight stood in similar contrast to each other.[54] Jerome Richfield used the terms *descriptive insight* and *ostensive insight* for his pair of contrasted notions, the latter of which referred to those "insights which incorporate actual, conscious experience of their referents."[55] And he cited Bertrand Russell's similar dichotomy of "knowledge by *description*" and "knowledge by *acquaintance*."[56] In discussing these same issues, John R. Reid and Jacob E. Finesinger favored the dichotomous pairing of "neutral insight" and "dynamic insight."[57]

Finally, to extend and deepen our sense of psychoanalysis and the patient's insight — to touch on, however briefly, the efforts of the patient and the psychoanalyst in their striving towards self-knowledge for the patient — I turn to the particularly thoughtful contributions of Hans Loewald (1906–1993). "The patient, who comes to the analyst for help through increased self-understanding, is led to this self-understanding by the understanding he finds in the analyst." Through clarifications and interpretations, "the analyst structures and articulates, or works towards structuring and articulating, the material and the productions offered by the patient. If an interpretation of unconscious meaning is timely, the words by which this meaning is expressed are recognizable to the patient as expressions of what he experiences. They organize for him what was previously less organized and . . . [enable] him to understand, to see, to put into words and to 'handle' what was previously not visible, understandable, speakable, tangible."[58] Loewald was speaking here of what he called "integrative experiences in analysis." He later expanded these comments somewhat, as follows:

> What seems to be of essential importance is insight or self-understanding as conveyed, as mediated by the analyst's empathic understanding, objectively stated in articulate and open language. . . . If defenses do not interfere, it is experienced by patient and analyst alike as authentic responsiveness. This responsiveness *is* an essential element in what we call emotional insight because it frees the patient for nondefensive responses of his own. Interpretations of this kind explicate for the patient what he then discovers to have always known somehow, but in the absence of its recognition and explication by the analyst such knowledge could not be acknowledged and grasped.[59]

To expand just a bit further, in all these efforts the analyst is working to understand the patient — to develop an understanding of the patient that can help the patient acquire crucial insight or self-knowledge in striving toward gainful change.

Several controversies among psychoanalysts have included an element of challenge to the status of insight as an essential factor in psychoanalytic treatment. One of the liveliest of these controversies revolved around Franz Alexander's (1891–1964) concept of the "corrective emotional experience" and some of the technical modifications associated with it. As Alexander saw it, when the analyst was taking pains to be radically (and obviously) different from the patient's transference expectations of him, the patient achieved an emotional readjustment that might or might not have been brought about through interpretation and insight; and if insight was acquired, it might well be the effect rather than the cause of the emotional readjustment.[60] Many of Alexander's psychoanalytic contemporaries saw him as dangerously diminishing the significance of interpretation and insight.

Another controversy in psychoanalysis that has had significant implications for the role of insight is associated with Heinz Kohut's self psychology. Kohut's thoughts on "the nature of the psychoanalytic cure" were discussed in some detail in his posthumous book, *How Does Analysis Cure?* He took note of "the traditionally accepted claims that the acquisition of verbalized knowledge (often referred to as insight) constitutes the essence of the psychoanalytic cure — 'the talking cure.' "[61] While not entirely abandoning a place for interpretation and insight in the achieving of improvement or cure, he accorded "insight a far lesser place in the curative scheme of things than does classical analysis."[62] With "a psychology of the supraordinate self and its developmental struggle for cohesion, with a psychopathology and a therapy based on conceptions of deficit and of restoration rather than of conflict and its resolution,"[63] and out of the complex of the patient's introspection and the analyst's empathy, Kohut derived as the goal of psychoanalysis "the establishment of empathic in-tuneness between self and selfobject on mature adult levels."[64] In summing up, he said, "A successful analysis is one in which the analysand's formerly archaic needs for the responses of archaic selfobjects are superseded by the experience of the availability of empathic resonance, the major constituent of the sense of security in adult life." He added that "broadened insight" might accompany these gains, but that it was "not the essence of cure."[65]

Whether or not the insight acquired leads to useful change has been another factor debated in recent decades. The basic scheme had been this: interpretation is the crucial intervention, and insight is the crucial result of an accurate interpretation. Often unstated, and yet commonly assumed, was the view that insight then led to useful change. When interpretation did not necessarily lead to insight, psychoanalysts concerned themselves with questions regarding the accuracy of an interpretation, the issue of timing and the patient's readiness to receive the interpretation, and the patient's resistance. But then when an interpretation did lead to insight, the insight did not necessarily lead to change for the patient. Concerns at this point revolved around the issue of intellectual insight versus emotional insight. But, when the insight was suitably emotional and convincing to the patient, what was the problem if the insight did not lead to useful change? "Working through" was the aspect of psychoanalytic work that was thought to deal with this not uncommon outcome — that is, the issue would be met and met again in various guises in the analysis, and gradually the obstacles to useful change would be resolved. And then, insight could eventually come to be made use of in action.

Some analysts, though, influenced by such instances of the patient's acquisition of insight without concomitant change, began to turn to notions such as *will* and *action*. Noting that "insight alone is ineffective," in 1956 Allen Wheelis argued that will and its efforts were crucial in making use of insight and moving on to change in one's personality and character, in one's ways of relating to other people, and in other behaviors that had previously been problematic.[66] That is to say, effort of will led to constructive action and so to useful change. Earlier, Wheelis had written on "the place of action in personality change" in a way that led to these later views on the need for a combination of insight and action.[67] And years later, in his book *How People Change,* he touched on insight as follows:

> The most common illusion of patients and, strangely, even of experienced therapists, is that insight produces change; and the most common disappointment of therapy is that it does not. *Insight is instrumental to change, often an essential part of the process, but does not directly achieve it.* . . .
>
> The place of insight is to illumine: to ascertain where one is, how one got there, how now to proceed, and to what end. It is a blueprint, as in building a house, and may be essential, but no one achieves a house by blueprints alone, no matter how accurate or detailed. . . . The sequence is suffering, insight, will, action, change.[68]

Arthur F. Valenstein touched briefly on this theme in 1962, citing Wheelis in the process. "However vital and veritable it may become, there is nothing magical about insight; in and of itself, it is not equivalent to a change in behavior, nor does it *directly* produce the relatively conflict-free readaptation which is the hoped-for outcome of a successful psycho-analysis. For there to be final adaptive change, alterations in behavior, whether subtle or obvious, must somehow come about as a result of modifications of action patterns."[69] Some years later, Valenstein elaborated considerably. After some discussion of "will" and the "will to action and change," he summed up as follows: "Acting and behaving in significantly different ways consequent to the elective use of insight lead to personal and consonant interpersonal change, as the modified or new action patterns are worked through."[70] In short, actualization of the benefits from insight necessitated efforts of the will and concomitant results in action.

Insight and Twentieth-Century Psychotherapy

Much of the history of insight in twentieth-century psychotherapy is a reflection of insight's place in the evolving history of psychoanalysis, as already outlined. In the name of psychoanalytically oriented psychotherapy, dynamic psychotherapy, and related categories, a wide range of approaches to psychological healing have accorded psychological insight a status very similar to that given it by the psychoanalysts. In fact, many of these approaches have been categorized together under the rubric *insight psychotherapy*. A representative opinion from the relevant literature is that expressed by Edward Bibring in 1954. Speaking of "dynamic psychotherapies" as a group, he espoused the commonly held view that insight was a crucial "curative agent"; and again reflecting a common opinion, he identified interpretation as the primary intervention in the gaining of insight, but allowed that clarification could also contribute to that end.[71] Although as Judd Marmor has argued, various of these clinical approaches may have described their version of what constituted insight in rather different terms from one another, each has tended to assign insight an essentially similar role in its particular view of psychological healing.[72]

As previously noted, Franz Alexander had raised questions about insight in psychoanalysis. And he and Thomas French also focused attention on insight in the psychotherapies in ways that were significant in the 1940s and continued to be for years thereafter. For purposes of discussion, they distinguished two general categories of psychotherapy: supportive therapy and insight (or uncovering, or expressive) therapy. "Supportive therapy is used primarily for the purpose of giving support to the patient's ego with no attempt to effect permanent ego change; uncovering or insight therapy is used primarily for the purpose of achieving a permanent change in the ego by developing the patient's insight into his difficulties and increasing the ability of his ego to deal with them, through the emotional experiences in the transference situation. Since both types of approach are present in almost all treatments, however, this distinction is not absolute."[73] They argued that in planning a psychotherapy, "emotional readjustment, not insight" was the goal; that in the second of their psychotherapeutic categories, helping the patient to acquire insight was the "most effective means of bringing about the necessary emotional readjustments"; and that "it is the emotional readjustment which may result from insight that is our real therapeutic goal, and not insight for its own sake."

They then went on to say, "Indeed, not infrequently, the relationship between insight and emotional readjustment is just the opposite from the one we expect in a standard psychoanalysis. In many cases it is not a matter of insight stimulating or forcing the patient to an emotional reorientation, but rather one in which a very considerable preliminary emotional readjustment is necessary before insight is possible at all."[74] Further, they commented that some psychotherapists "tremendously overvalue the therapeutic efficacy of insight."[75] And they cited cases in which "the insight, instead of being the cause of the therapeutic improvement, was one of the important results of a therapeutic improvement made possible by other means."[76]

In subsequent considerations of these views, many psychoanalysts saw the role of insight as having been seriously diminished. Nevertheless, years later, while discussing "the dynamics of psychotherapy in the light of learning theory," Alexander emphasized the place of both emotional and cognitive elements in the "relearning process," indicated that these two elements were "intricately interwoven," noted that the psychoanalytic literature referred to the combination as "emotional insight," and stated that this insight was "the central factor in every learning process including psychoanalytic treatment."[77]

Bibring saw the work of Alexander and French as illustrative of "the shift in emphasis from insight through interpretation to experiential manipulation. It seems to have become a common trend in various methods of dynamic psychotherapies."[78] And this division of psychotherapeutic approaches into insight therapy versus experiential manipulation was taken up by many, particularly psychoanalysts. Also, there was some tendency to divide the psychotherapies into those that focused on acquiring insight through interpretation versus those that emphasized clinical gain through aspects of the doctor-patient relationship, including such as Alexander's "corrective emotional experience," Winnicott's "holding environment," and identification with the psychotherapist. Further still, certain therapists differentiated between psychotherapies that focused on insight and those which focused on affect. All in all, insight had come to be considered far from the only key to psychotherapeutic gain, but it was still accorded a significant place.

Among other twentieth-century psychotherapists who placed some emphasis on insight, a few held views somewhat distinct from these largely psychoanalytic trends. In the 1920s, one such contributor was William Brown, who had had a central role in World War I work with shell-shock victims. Influenced by Freud's work and yet disagreeing with him in many ways, Brown thought that psychotherapy should include efforts toward self-knowledge, and he coined the term *autognosis* (self-knowledge) for "the process whereby the patient gains an ever-deepening insight into the exact nature of his mental condition. It is a complex psychological process in which the patient endeavours to obtain an objective view of his own mind, its past development, present condition, and strivings towards the future, so far as his symptoms are concerned. It is more than a mere intellectualizing of the mind — although this is a very important element — since it stimulates and purifies that power of intuition or direct insight as regards psychological matters which all men possess to a greater or lesser degree." And he particularly maintained that "the autognostic method" should be used with "all forms of psycho-neurosis."[79]

Brown's terminology apparently found little favor with other psychotherapists of his era, but it was taken up by W. H. R. Rivers (1864–1922), a physician, psychologist, and anthropologist who shared many of Brown's views and, like him, had been very involved in clinical work with World War I shell-shock victims. In an essay on psychotherapeutics in the early 1920s, he discussed autognosis at some length and commented that "the process by which the patient learns to understand the real state of his mind and the conditions by which this state has been produced forms a very important therapeutic agency which may be called 'autognosis.' "[80]

More recently, in the 1940s, out of his work in child guidance and counseling, the clinical psychologist Carl R. Rogers developed what came to be known as client-centered therapy. While this approach gradually assumed a place as a form of psychotherapy quite distinct from the various psychoanalytically influenced therapies, Rogers shared with such approaches an emphasis on nondirectiveness and on the value of insight. For him, the psychotherapeutic process facilitates the emergence of "insight and self-understanding" which can lead, in turn, to an acceptance of the self and progress toward "new levels of integration" for the client.[81] From the increasingly free expression of their attitudes, concerns, and feelings, clients gradually acquire new perceptions of themselves and their experiences, a new understanding of the meaning of their symptoms and the patterns of their behavior. Rogers terms these realizations *insight* and *self-understanding* and emphasizes that they are "learnings with deep emotional concomitants, not learnings of intellectual content."[82] Instances of insight gained are steps in a larger process of gradually increasing self-understanding. Despite grave reservations about the use of interpretations, he would allow them some role in the development of insight, but he underscores the importance of timeliness.[83]Rogers' emphasis on the spontaneous nature of the moments of insightful realization is a reflection of his nondirective approach. He states that "insight is an experience which is achieved, not an experience which can be imposed."[84] In summing up, he explains, "It involves the reorganization of the perceptual field. It consists in seeing new relationships. It is the integration of accumulated experience. It signifies a reorientation of the self." New recognitions gradually led to a new way of perceiving oneself.[85] Also, he emphasizes the importance of the psychotherapist's own self-understanding in the efforts to work successfully with the troubled client.[86]

Insight and Clinical Psychiatry

While the various emphases on insight or self-knowledge were evolving in psychoanalysis and psychotherapy, the term *insight* had a distinct and largely separate history in twentieth-century clinical psychiatry. In Hinzie and Shatzky's *Psychiatric Dictionary, insight* was defined as "the patient's knowledge that the symptoms of his illness are recognized as abnormalities or morbid phenomena."[87] This definition reflected usage in psychiatric hospital settings for many years before this dictionary's publication in 1940, and it continued to do so for years thereafter. When a patient suffered from unrealistic fears, strange thoughts, delusions, or hallucinations, psychiatrists were concerned to know whether he thought that he was sick, or even insane. If he thought so, if he was aware that he was mentally ill, he was deemed to have insight; if not, he was said to lack insight. Assessing the patient on this point was one of the elements in the standard clinical examination of psychiatric patients, and it was later a part of a clinical routine, "doing a mental status." As Zilboorg described it in 1950,

> In medical schools, and later in mental hospitals, we were taught . . . that insight is the knowledge that one is mentally ill. The term was and still is frequently used with the descriptive addendum, "insight as to illness." Patients were noted in their case histories as having recovered with or without insight. It was assumed that the patient's normal behavior was clear and known to the patient himself, and the knowledge of what was not normal was sufficient to guide him, or at least a great therapeutic advance. Thus the schizophrenic was considered better off if he said that he knew that all his strange thoughts were "crazy," that the voices he heard were not real voices. The "manic-depressive" patient was considered better off if and when he would "admit to himself" that his moods were abnormal "swings"; he would then, it was averred, be able to recognize the beginning of these swings and take "appropriate measures" — from self-control to consulting a psychiatrist or seeking shelter in a mental hospital.[88]

Some rough-and-ready principles emerged from these concerns about "insight and illness," although none of them could be said to be always valid. It was frequently suggested that frankly psychotic patients lacked insight. A glimmer of insight during a psychotic episode was considered a good prognostic sign. Patients might or might not acquire insight after their recovery, and the prognosis was thought to be more favorable in cases where such insight had been acquired.

The roots of this usage can be found in Emil Kraepelin's (1856–1926) *Psychiatrie* at the turn of the century. In the fifth edition in 1896, he commented that, other than the disappearance of observable symptoms, insight was the most important indication that recovery from insanity had occurred. It was a sign that the patient had recovered his normal perspective on himself and that he knew that he had been mentally ill. Without clear and complete insight regarding his disorder, he could not be considered to be fully recovered. Indications of the development of insight during the course of the illness constituted evidence of a favorable prognosis. From this passage, though, it is not clear just what insight might consist of — beyond the patient's realization that he was or had been mentally ill.[89] And this passage was repeated almost unchanged in subsequent editions of Kraepelin's textbook.

Further, in the sections on specific clinical disorders in his fifth edition appeared a few brief references to the absence of insight or to limited insight. Then, in the sixth edition of *Psychiatrie*, Kraepelin added, here and there, a few more such brief references, again in the discussions of clinical syndromes; and the additions continued in the seventh and eighth editions.[90] In these contexts, insight was not often noted to have been present during an episode of illness; when insight was observed during an illness, the patient tended to be in a depressed state; and some degree of insight was more often found with improvement or recovery.

During the early decades of the twentieth century, these Kraepelinian perspectives gradually came to characterize psychiatrists' clinical accounts, especially when the patient was or had been in a mental hospital.[91] It became commonplace to attend to whether insight was present, absent, or partially present. A determination of the patient's status regarding insight became an aspect of mental examinations, and reports of these examinations usually included some mention of this status. Beginning in the first decade of the century, the widely influential psychiatrist Adolf Meyer (1866–1950) made the assessment of insight a routine part of his determination of "the mental status" or "the mental condition" of each patient: "The patient's judgment concerning himself and the situation and his disease ('insight')."[92] Meyer continued to attend to this topic both as a clinician and as a teacher who had a far-reaching influence in his own setting at Johns Hopkins University, in numerous other centers that were influenced by his pupils, and in the practice of many psychiatrists elsewhere.

That this kind of attention to insight had become widespread was further

attested by statements made by David K. Henderson (1884–1965) and Robert D. Gillespie (1897–1945) in their *Text-Book of Psychiatry*. These two authors, having trained with Meyer at Johns Hopkins, returned to Great Britain and produced the textbook, which was to be one of the most influential in English-speaking psychiatric contexts for many years. First published in 1927, the textbook went through numerous editions over the next several decades, and each edition included the following comments in the chapter "Method of Examination," under the heading "Insight and Judgment." "The questions here relate to the amount of realisation the patient has of his own condition; does he realise that he is ill, that he is mentally ill, that he is in need of treatment in a mental hospital? Does he acknowledge that his ideas have been due to his disordered imagination? Does he show poor judgment regarding the question of discharge, plans for the future, family responsibilities, and ethical standards?"[93] Further along in this same work, in discussing delusions, these authors observed: "*Insight* in the form of the patient's own criticism of the fact of his holding delusional beliefs is a related problem of even more significance. A person who entertains a false belief, but at the same time admits that it might be unjustified, and who may spontaneously talk of it as a delusion, is, as a rule, more amenable to treatment than one whose beliefs admit of no criticism."[94] And brief references to the topic of insight, similar in spirit, became characteristic of many psychiatric texts from the 1920s onward.

The philosopher-psychiatrist Karl Jaspers (1883–1969) discussed insight in "The Patient's Attitude to His Illness," a chapter in his *General Psychopathology*. After addressing such themes as a patient's perplexity and awareness of change in the face of a sudden onset of acute psychosis, and the various opinions that a patient may assume toward his illness (including self-interpretations of a delusional nature) as he strives to understand what is happening to him and somehow to work through his symptoms,[95] Jaspers turned to "the patient's judgment of his illness." In this category, he searchingly examined the various phenomena and problems that psychiatrists had come to consider when evaluating a patient's insight.

> When the judgment is a psychological one the patient makes himself aware of his experience and the manner of it. The ideal of a "correct" attitude to experience is achieved by patients when they "have insight into their illness." ... We will now describe features in patients' attitudes which appear when they turn away from content [of their illnesses] to their own selves and the experience they are having, and ask the reason for what is happening. They are in short passing a judgment on their illness either in its individual aspects or as a whole. We are concerned here with everything that can be collectively called awareness of illness or insight into the illness.

The term *"awareness of illness"* is applied to the patient's attitude when he expresses a feeling of being ill and changed, but there is no extension of this awareness to all his symptoms nor to the illness as a whole. It does not involve any objectively correct estimate of the severity of the illness nor any objectively correct judgment of its particular type. Only when all this is present and there has been a correct judgment of all the symptoms and the illness as a whole according to type and severity, can we speak of *insight,* with the reservation that the judgment can only be expected to reach that degree of accuracy attainable by the average, normal individual who comes from the same cultural background as the patient. . . .

Patients' self-observation is one of the most important sources of knowledge in regard to morbid psychic life; so is their attentiveness to their abnormal experience and the elaboration of their observations in the form of a *psychological judgment* so that they can communicate to us something of their inner life. . . .

. . . In psychosis there is no lasting or complete insight. . . . Individual phenomena may be judged correctly but, apart from that, the innumerable manifestations of the illness are not recognised as such and inversely there are morbid feelings where the content is a false one and is itself a symptom. For instance, a melancholic patient considers she is rotting away physically or a paranoid patient thinks his thought-processes are being interfered with by external machinations. . . . In acute psychoses there are transient states of far-reaching insight. . . . Sometimes at the beginning of a process we find considerable insight, the correction of delusions, the proper assessment of voices, etc., which one might well consider as recovery and a benign psychopathic state, but insight of this sort is quite transient.[96]

As to "attitude to psychosis after recovery," there tends to be "a clear picture of complete insight . . . in patients who recover from deliria, alcoholic hallucinosis or mania." But, in other psychotic conditions, it is more uncertain: insight may not be present or may be rather limited, and at times, apparent insight may not stand up to careful scrutiny. Again, in patients' attitudes to their illness in chronic psychosis, insight is quite uncertain, often more apparent than real. Frequently enough, such patients learn to say what might favorably impress psychiatrists and other people.[97]

In his singularly thoughtful comments, Jaspers frequently conveyed sophisticated phenomenological data, quite beyond most of the routine assessments of insight that psychiatrists were reporting during the years in which the several editions of his *Allgemeine Psychopathologie* were appearing (1913 to 1959).[98] Occasionally, his statements were far-reaching enough that they might subsume insight as it was being considered by psychoanalysts, but most of the time he seems to have been approaching the notion as the general psychiatrist was, albeit in a more penetrating and profound way. Although I can say on the basis of personal experience that I have heard most of what Jaspers says on this subject discussed thoughtfully at one time or another, no one else seems to have brought it together as effectively or presented it as meaningfully in a written context.

The pursuit of insight or self-understanding has a long history as a crucial element in psychological healing. And the ailments against which it has been brought to bear have ranged from unwisdom or ignorance to various errors of the soul, sinful states, forms of psychological distress, and modern syndromes of mental illness. From the Delphic injunction "Know thyself," and Socratic attention to the theme, through many religious and philosophical versions of knowing one's self and on down to the twentieth-century concerns with psychological insight, self-knowledge has repeatedly been emphasized as a goal of value for the individual and an element in achieving an improved or healthier state. It has been represented as a way of guarding against arrogance and hubris and as a path toward valued humility; as a way to acquire wisdom and avoid ignorance; as a way to come to know other things and other people; as the way to come to know God; as the path to knowledge of one's faults and thence to self-improvement; as a means of developing self-respect and self-esteem; and as a means to attain understanding of how one got into difficulties or became ill, and so as a crucial help toward the resolution of difficulties, the recovery from illness, and so forth. Through philosophical writings, theological works, and general literature, and on down to twentieth-century psychoanalytic, psychological, and psychiatric literature, self-understanding has been advised, prized, sought after, and found helpful. And during the past hundred years, the pursuit of self-knowledge has come, more and more, to entail efforts to know things about oneself considered to be "unconscious" or "subconscious," and so particularly difficult to get to know—such as the nature and roots of one's patterns of behavior in relation to others, the origins of one's symptoms, and the sources of one's inclinations, dispositions, predilections, and habits.

Though the twentieth-century verdict is not unanimous, coming to know oneself is still widely regarded as eminently useful in efforts toward psychological healing. Such new knowledge (or recovered "old" knowledge, as the case may be) has been observed to play a crucial role in achieving integrative or reintegrative gains of crucial value to the individual,

Further, it has often been noted that sorrow and suffering serve as aids in the acquisition of self-understanding. They have been the stimuli that have caused many a person to embark on the quest for self-knowledge. And this quest has been an integral aspect of numerous psychological healing endeavors; peace of mind, relief or cure and other forms of personal gain have often been achieved in intimate association with the process of coming to know oneself.

17

Self-Observation and Introspection

Like so many of the elements considered in this work, self-observation is no new thing. Variously referred to as inward perception, looking inward, self-scrutiny, self-examination, self-inspection, introspection, reflection, the activity of the inner sense, and so forth, it has been an activity of humankind for a very long time.

Human beings have long observed the operations of their own minds or inspected the flow of their own mental events, whether in an effort to know more about themselves or for the grander purpose of increasing their knowledge of "mind." The mental activities that came to be known as consciousness — sensations, feelings, thoughts, images, memories, and so on — have always been of interest to human beings, and thoughtful persons have studied consciousness as a way to gain knowledge about themselves and their species. The fruits of self-observation from the minds of wise thinkers have been valued as useful knowledge. A person's inward perceptions have been found useful in the pursuit of self-understanding and, often enough, in the process of psychological healing. And the psychologists of the nineteenth and twentieth centuries developed deep respect for "the introspective method," which was to be followed, however, by negative reactions to conclusions based on that same method.

With regard to psychological healing in particular, the theme of seeking insight or self-understanding[1] makes some degree of self-observation a necessary activity. In order to follow the injunction "know thyself," one must, somehow or other, observe oneself. "Looking within" has served the pursuit of knowledge about humankind in many a philosophical context, and, under the rubric of *introspection,* it served for many years as an important investigative method in psychology; but also, it has been an element in efforts to acquire self-knowledge in the interest of personal healing benefits.

Looking Inward and the Philosophers

Frequently to be noted in histories of philosophy are brief comments to the effect that introspection has been a method employed in the search for and the gaining of knowledge about humankind, particularly regarding the human mind. Historians of psychology have considered it a significant method in the long philosophical prologue to modern psychology.

Robert I. Watson has suggested that "one of the first instances, if not the first, of a systematic use of introspection" was the self-examination inherent in the Socratic "Know thyself"; many have echoed that perception.[2] Certainly, over many centuries, interest in the contents of human consciousness has occasioned the use of self-observation, by whatever name, as a method for observing and studying the nature of those contents. Though the process as such has been little studied until recent times, over the centuries scattered explicit references have been made to self-examination as a means toward self-knowledge or knowledge of mind; and allusions to mental contents have implicitly pointed to self-observation or introspection.

Prominent among the philosophical students of the inner self were Plotinus and Augustine. Plotinus employed this "turning inward" to study the forms of mental activity, in order to understand and teach about transcendental experience; but in the process, he developed some ideas regarding self-consciousness and made a significant contribution to the study of the mind.[3]

Influenced by Neoplatonic thought, most likely through the work of Plotinus, Augustine undertook a searching examination of both his life and his inner experience, with God as "physician of my most intimate self," in an effort to "heal my sicknesses."[4] In the spirit of Plotinus' exhortation to "go into yourself," to "look within the soul and not at external things,"[5] he explored his inner world, his mind. "By the Platonic books I was admonished to return into myself." And so he "entered into my innermost citadel" and searched "with my soul's eye."[6]

In this undertaking Augustine strove "through my inward perception"[7] and through confession to bring forth all he knew and could find out about himself. His *Confessions* amounted to a type of self-analysis. It entailed a systematic effort, through introspection and unsparing frankness with himself, to recover and integrate a lifetime of experiences and memories. He confessed, worked at understanding himself, and strove to correct or improve himself.[8]

Then, later, in Book X of *The Trinity,* titled "The Realization of Self-Knowledge," Augustine discussed at length "the mind's search for knowledge of itself."[9] During this discussion, he raised the question, "What can be the purport of the injunction, Know thyself?" and proceeded to answer it, "I suppose it is that the mind should reflect upon itself, and live in accordance with its nature."[10] As was mentioned in Chapter 16, he associated self-knowledge with an inwardness, a self-exploration in the pursuit of such knowledge, that would later come to be termed introspection.[11]

In the writings of some of the humanist scholars of the Renaissance, particularly those who drew on self-examination as a source of data, introspection again emerged as a significant element in self-understanding and in the understanding of mankind. Petrarch and Michel de Montaigne (1533–1592), in the early and late Renaissance, respectively, were important instances of this trend.[12] Much influenced by that remarkable observer of self St. Augustine, Petrarch paid special attention to the individual human, his soul, and his problems, and this introspectionist bent particularly manifested itself in his *Secretum* and in some of his letters.[13] In the *Secretum,* he employed the form of an imaginary dialogue between Augustine and himself, through which he sought a healing experience for his melancholic illness. This "thorough exploration of the innermost recesses of the human soul"[14] bears some kinship to both the self-examination of a penitent in confession and the inward searching of a modern sufferer in a psychotherapeutic context. In considering Petrarch's letters, Morris Bishop commented, "He had a very unusual taste for introspection; he examined his own behavior with pensive delight. He gives his correspondents — and posterity, his more remote correspondent — the most complete picture in existence of the inner and outer life of a medieval man."[15]

Michel de Montaigne emerged as an introspectionist of consequence in his later essays. Like Socrates — indeed, he has been referred to as the French Socrates — he started from the position that he knew little or nothing, was guided by the Delphic "Know thyself," and employed self-examination in the service of acquiring self-knowledge and, through it, knowledge of humankind. P. Mansell Jones gives him a central position in his book *French Introspectives.* Jones comments:

> Montaigne's interest in the self is therefore an interest in its moral and social *rapports* — never a purely scientific or "psychological" investigation,

> never pure or purposeless introspection. . . . Usually it [this interest] occurs
> in the form of a recommendation of self-examination as a means to self-
> improvement, or as the initial stage in a proper realisation or adaptation of
> the self. There are thus two types of introspection discernible in the *Essays*.
> The one occurs when the author attempts to define (and defend) the *Essays* as
> the expression of the self of the writer; the other, when he applies his judg-
> ment to himself in view of correction or improvement. This type of self-
> examination never reaches the depths of introspection to which the former
> sometimes attains.[16]

As Montaigne stated it in his essay "On Practice": "For many years now the
target of my thoughts has been myself alone; I examine nothing, I study nothing, but me; and if I do study anything else, it is so as to apply it at once to
myself, or more correctly, within myself."[17] In his last essay, "On Experience,"
he remarks: "I study myself more than any other subject. That is my metaphysics; and that is my physics."[18]

During the seventeenth century Robert Boyle (1627–1691), famous for his
contributions to chemistry and physics, commented on the potential usefulness of introspection: "We know but very little of the nature of our own minds,
though, to discover that, we need not rove into, much less wander beyond the
world without us; but only reflectingly take notice of what passes within
ourselves; nor need we anatomical knives, or geographical globes, or optical
telescopes or microscopes, or any other material, or elaborate instruments, to
investigate and detect what we seek for; the human mind being itself the
subject, the object, the faculty, the organ, and the instrument, of the knowledge it should attain."[19] Wise in the ways of scientific investigation and the use
of instruments, Boyle described introspection as an "instrument" for the study
of the human mind.

A significant deepening of the understanding of human consciousness derived from the efforts of John Locke in *An Essay Concerning Human Understanding* (1690). Through the practice of introspection, though not using that
term, Locke searchingly examined the experience of the sensations and other
mental activities. As he stated it, one of the two sources of "the *materials* of
thinking" is "our observation employed . . . about the internal operations of our
minds perceived and reflected on by ourselves." This activity he named reflection, and he stated further that "the ideas it affords being such only as the mind
gets by reflecting on its own operations within itself." In contrast to sensation
and the external senses, which he viewed as the other source of "the *materials* of
thinking," he also referred to this second source as internal sense.[20]

Regarding the English term *introspection,* it seems to have come into use in
the latter part of the seventeenth century. Matthew Hale (1609–1676) had
commented that many things about human nature "are discernible by Observa-

tion, and by no other Observation, so well as by a mans Observation of himself." Further, "We may easily by inspecting and observing our selves, know much concerning our own Souls and the operations of them."[21] Then he used the term *introspection* in the sense that was to become familiar: "The actings of the Mind or Imagination it self, by way of reflection or introspection of themselves, are discernible by Man."[22] By the time Samuel Johnson's *Dictionary* was published (1755), introspection was defined in Hale's exact words.[23]

The terms *introspection* and *reflection* served one philosopher or another to refer to self-observation or looking inward. Although Hale and Johnson seemed to suggest that they were synonyms, not infrequently *introspection* implied self-observation in a relatively narrow sense, while *reflection* had a somewhat wider meaning that included a "turning back on" the mental contents and considering what was observed. But by whatever name and in whatever form, these self-inspection activities continued to play a role in the views of a good number of eighteenth- and nineteenth-century philosophers concerning the mind. Among them were British empiricists and associationists, such as David Hume (1711–1776), David Hartley (1705–1759), James Mill (1773–1836), John Stuart Mill (1806–1873), and Alexander Bain (1818–1903), and the French empiricist and associationist Etienne Bonnot de Condillac (1715–1780).[24] These scholars had little to say about reflection or introspection as topics. Rather, their tendency was to assume the worth of self-inspection and to proceed to use it as an important method of observation for the study of consciousness and as a means of providing the data for their analyses. These very philosophers were forerunners of modern psychology, and their work tends to be given a place in the history of psychology.

Another eighteenth-century philosopher, Thomas Reid (1710–1796) – a leading member of the Scottish School – addressed the issue of introspection quite directly and gave it a central place for purposes of investigating the human mind. He acknowledged that "to attend accurately to the operations of our minds . . . is no easy matter even for the contemplative"; but in introspection or reflection, an "instrument" was available for studying the "anatomy of the mind" – in fact, he was of the opinion that it was "the only instrument by which we can discern the powers of the mind."

> I claim no other merit, than that of having given great attention to the operations of my own mind, and of having expressed, with all the perspicuity I was able, what, I conceive, every man who gives the same attention, will feel and perceive. . . .
>
> . . . All that we know of the body, is owing to anatomical dissection and observation, and it must be by an anatomy of the mind that we can discover its powers and principles. . . .
>
> An anatomist who hath happy opportunities, may have access to examine

with his own eyes, and with equal accuracy, bodies of all different ages, sexes, and conditions; so that what is defective, obscure, preternatural in one, may be discerned clearly, and in its most perfect state in another. But the anatomist of the mind cannot have the same advantage. It is his own mind only that he can examine with any degree of accuracy and distinctness.[25]

While not having much in common with the empiricists and associationists just mentioned, like them Reid valued introspection and like them he left a heritage that became part of the nineteenth century's emerging discipline of psychology.

Self-Examination, Confession, and Pastoral Care

The theme of self-examination has been manifested in religious writings over many centuries. Notable instances can be found in the Old Testament: "Let us search and try our ways, and turn again to the Lord";[26] and in the New Testament: "Examine yourselves, whether ye be in the faith; prove your own selves."[27] In another New Testament context, self-examination is urged (or possibly demanded) as a prelude to participation in the sacrament known as the Eucharist, or Holy Communion: "But let a man examine himself, and so let him eat of *that* bread, and drink of *that* cup."[28]

In scattered contexts over the succeeding centuries, self-examination was frequently mentioned. As already noted, a prominent example was Augustine's sustained examination of his inner experience in his *Confessions*. He examined his inner life with unsparing frankness in the interest of self-healing; he left a record that became part of the history of confession. Manuals for confessors and other forms of instruction or advice have dealt with confession, with regard sometimes to the self-examination that the penitent should have made in preparing for confession and sometimes to the confessor's duty to instruct penitents about preparing themselves. In these contexts the issue is either a faithful and searching reflection on what sins the penitent might have committed or the achieving of an appropriate degree of contrition about those sins, or both.[29] Though the idea of self-examination as a preparation for confession was hardly new by the time of the Council of Trent (1545–1563), only at that point does it seem to have been laid down as an absolute requirement. In a decree dealing with confession and penance, it was stated that "all the mortal sins, of which, after a diligent examination of themselves, they are conscious, must needs be by penitents enumerated in confession, even though those sins be most hidden, and committed only against the two last precepts of the decalogue. . . . After each has examined himself diligently, and searched all the folds and recesses of his conscience, he [shall] confess those sins by which he shall remember that he has mortally offended his Lord and God."[30] This particular decree, and the other decrees and canons issuing from the Council of Trent, reflected the efforts of the Roman Catholic Church to reaffirm and strengthen its traditions and practices in the face of growing Protestant disaffection; and confession was a particular issue in it. This self-examination was frequently referred to in subsequent manuals for confessors and guides for penitents.[31]

As just noted, self-examination was intimately associated with confession and penance — that is, it was part of a system of belief and action that was a crucial constituent of the realm referred to as "the cure of souls." Confession was commonly conceived of as a practice that served a healing purpose; and penance was frequently referred to as medicine for sin or medicine for the soul. Penitents were thought of as "morally diseased"; sins were viewed as "symptoms of disease"; and confessors were referred to as physicians of the soul.[32] Self-examination was urged as a crucial step toward the penitent's recognition of sin which, in turn, was the beginning of healing. Spiritual health had been lost through sin, and so the goal of the process was the recovery of that health. Although this language tradition reflected, at least initially, the use of a medical metaphor in discussing certain forms of mental distress, the sense of a metaphor gradually gave way to a literal usage. Sin-laden states of mind came to be regarded as serious illnesses; and ministering to those types of distress came to be a form of psychological healing. Caring for and endeavoring to heal the "sin-sick soul" was the work of the Church's physicians of the soul. Confession and penance constituted only one aspect of a pastor's healing efforts; "the cure of souls" became recognized as the province of churches in general. The practices derived from the spiritual guidance of a pre-Christian era became the pastoral care of later centuries.[33]

In the wake of the Reformation, self-examination or introspection was attended to in a somewhat different manner in various Protestant Christian settings. Despite the shift away from the Roman Catholic emphasis on and approach to confession, the root issue in the Protestant "cure of souls" still seems to have been to provide "a remedy for sin." In the Church of England, self-examination was still recommended, in conjunction with confession to God and making amends, as a way of ministering to a troubled conscience.[34] But the tendency in the Protestant denominations was more toward self-examination as a crucial means whereby a person could progress in spiritual development. They thought of the cure of souls in terms of spiritual growth through a series of stages. Even if confession in those contexts no longer had the place it had once had, considerable concern was devoted to identifying and dealing with sin. The systems of stages in spiritual development were based on the idea of moving from a state of sinfulness toward a state of salvation or holiness. Pastors were expected to be familiar with the inner life, and so to be able to counsel their parishioners and assist them along their developmental paths; and clergy were urged to examine themselves, in part so that they could be more effective counselors for their parishioners.[35] A significant example of the Protestant emphasis on self-examination can be found in a lengthy discourse on the subject by Jonathan Edwards (1703–1758).[36] In exhaustive fashion, he discussed the ways in which a person might have sinned, how that person should be on the alert against sin, and how self-examination should be pursued in the interest of detecting sinfulness and correcting it.

Another way in which self-examination was urged on Protestants was through recommendations that they should conduct a regular "stock-taking" of their thoughts and actions. This was advised as a daily practice — or weekly, or less frequently but regularly — again in the interest of identifying sins and correcting them; and it was advised in order to cultivate and improve the sinners' souls.

Whether as an aid to confession or as an aid to spiritual development, self-examination involved a searching out and acknowledging of one's sins — the ferreting out of sin was considered to be in the interest of a full and good confession, and thus as a step toward being forgiven and receiving absolution; acknowledgment was considered an important aid to improving the state of one's soul. Both were vital aspects of "the cure of souls."

Introspection and the Psychologists

Nineteenth-century philosophers evinced *both* a continuing interest in introspection in the study of the human mind *and* an increasingly vigorous criticism of this method of psychological investigation. But the latter half of the nineteenth century brought a new emphasis on introspection — and definitions such as the following: "The action of looking within, or into one's own mind; examination or observation of one's own thoughts, feelings, or mental state."[37] The long history of self-observation or looking inward had set the stage for the designation of introspection as a central method for investigation in psychology. After a heyday for introspection, a period of considerable controversy followed.

Beginning around the middle of the nineteenth century, the new experimental psychology began to take shape. Developing out of the tradition of empiricism, with its inherent dualism and its connection with associationism, and significantly influenced by physiologists such as Hermann von Helmholtz (1821–1894) and by Gustav Fechner (1801–1887) and his psychophysics, this new psychology began to differentiate itself from philosophy, and introspection assumed a significant role in the new investigative methods. Wilhelm Wundt (1832–1920), a pioneering experimental psychologist at Leipzig, made crucial contributions to this process, gradually shaping a systematic physiological psychology and establishing one of the earliest experimental laboratories in psychology. He developed introspection as a central means for investigation, in tandem with experimental control of its conditions. He laid down careful rules for the proper use of introspection, and the observers who participated in his various experiments were carefully trained in the use of the method.[38]

Another psychologist who came to prominence in the same era as Wundt was William James (1842–1910). Trained in medicine, a philosopher of significance, and the founder of an early psychological laboratory, James became a leading figure among American psychologists. Both impressed by the new experimental psychology and continuing to be something of a philosophical psychologist, he valued introspection, but the way he applied it was not really consonant with either of these two traditions. James emphasized the significance of states of consciousness, and he gave introspection a key role in those phenomena. In *The Principles of Psychology* (1890), he assigned a central place to introspection, in the following terms:

> *Introspective Observation is what we have to rely on first and foremost and always.* The word introspection need hardly be defined — it means, of course, the looking into our own minds and reporting what we there discover. *Every one agrees that we there discover states of consciousness.* So far as I know, the existence of such states has never been doubted by any critic, however sceptical in other respects he may have been. . . . All people unhesitatingly believe that they feel themselves thinking, and that they distinguish the mental state as an inward activity or passion, from all the objects with which it may cognitively deal. *I regard this belief as the most fundamental of all the postulates of Psychology,* and shall discard all curious inquiries about its certainty as too metaphysical for the scope of this book.[39]

Another experimental psychologist who advocated the systematic use of introspection as an investigative method was Edward B. Titchener (1867–1927), an English student of Wundt, who completed a doctorate under his tutelage and in 1895 went to Cornell University. He became a leader in American psychology and influenced many others toward a systematic use of the introspective method.[40] For both Wundt and Titchener, the basic elements of observation were sensations, feelings, and images; they also examined combinations of those elements, such as perceptions, ideas, and more complex combinations; psychology was viewed as the science of consciousness;

and introspection became the essential method for investigating the contents of consciousness.[41] Again like Wundt, Titchener thought that the observers should be carefully trained to engage in introspection. And Titchener's emphasis on introspection allowed him to state: "Psychology is based upon the introspections of a large number of trained observers."[42]

In the hands of these two men, the age-old practice of introspection as "the contemplation of one's own experience" was developed and sharpened into the means for observing and reporting on "what *mental content* or process is present, and the description thereof in terms of *elements* and attributes."[43] The long tradition of "looking inward" had been developed into a central feature of what came to be called structural psychology.

Edward G. Boring, experimental psychologist and historian of experimental psychology, has commented that "classical introspection . . . went out of style after Titchener's death in 1927 because it had demonstrated no functional use and therefore seemed dull, and also because it was unreliable."[44] But others had questioned introspection's place as a prime investigative method long before that time, and in 1913 John B. Watson, the so-called father of behaviorism, had vigorously challenged its status.[45] Watson and his nascent behaviorism had a strong influence on the changing views of introspection. As he so pointedly stated it, "Psychology as the behaviorist views it is a purely experimental branch of natural science. Its theoretical goal is the prediction and control of behavior. Introspection forms no essential part of its methods, nor is the scientific value of its data dependent upon the readiness with which they lend themselves to interpretation in terms of consciousness."[46] But, as Boring has said,

> Actually the repudiation of dualism by modern experimental psychology led only to the surrender of the word "introspection," not to the abandonment of the method. The general method (not classical introspection) is used without the name (1) in phenomenological description as the Gestalt psychologists use it and as it is employed in the description of experience in perception; (2) in psychophysics where are determined the relations of conscious events, usually of a sensory nature, to magnitudes of the stimulus, especially in the determination of the sensory thresholds and sensory scales; and (3) in the protocols of patients as they describe their consciousness to psychiatrists and psychoanalysts, sometimes in free association on the psychoanalytic couch, sometimes in projective tests, . . . where the subject, for diagnostic purposes, reports the train of thought aroused in him by an equivocal stimulus or situation.[47]

Regarding the various ways in which *introspection* has been, is, or might be employed (in psychology), Peter McKellar has pointed out: "The word introspection does not denote a single method, but a family of methods." Further, it was the classical introspection of Wundt and Titchener that had been so roundly criticized and essentially abandoned, and that mode of introspection was only one member of this "family of methods."[48] McKellar took note of the introspection associated with phenomenalism, as manifested in the work of the Gestaltists and that of the phenomenological philosophers; the way in which Freud and those he influenced employed introspection in their work; and the use of introspection in projective testing techniques.[49] McKellar commented on the kinship between introspection and some instances of biographical data, whether obtained from a subject by a psychologist or other type of interviewer, or whether subject and author were the same person. And he cited Dostoevsky as an instance of an author drawing on introspective sources in his writing.

> The Russian novelist Dostoevsky, whom incidentally Nietzsche assessed as "the only psychologist from whom I had anything to learn," was not a professional psychologist. His writings of life in a Siberian convict settlement provide biographical and introspective data of value to the understanding of desocialisation and regression (*The House of the Dead*). Elsewhere he records the subjective experiences which occur previous to an epileptic attack (*The Idiot*). As Dostoevsky was himself epileptic there is reason to believe he was drawing on his own introspections. Elsewhere (*The Gambler*) he takes the reader into the subjective experiences of an individual struggling with a vice from which he cannot free himself; biographical data again suggest sources in Dostoevsky's own life history. Yet elsewhere the novelist portrays the thoughts and feelings of a hardened criminal (*Letters from the Underworld*), and of an individual who experiences dissociation of personality (*The Brothers Karamazov*).[50]

And McKellar observed that, in one way or another, introspective methods are still used in areas of psychological investigation, such as thought, imagination, perception, emotion, and motivation.[51] As he summed it up, "Investigators who have been curious about human experience and behavior have, in fact, used a *variety of methods* of introspection. . . . Rather than attempt formal definitions it is suggested that it is better to recognize a *family of introspective methods,* together with methods which shade into related techniques of a biographical kind.[52]

Self-Observation and Psychoanalysis

With the development of psychoanalysis around the end of the nineteenth century, Sigmund Freud brought self-observation (*Selbstbeobachtung*) into the very center of a mode of psychological healing. As he learned just how valuable his patients' reports of their mental activities could be for his own understanding of their difficulties and as a basis for his therapeutic interventions, he came to emphasize to the patients the importance of their self-observations and of their communication of those observations to the psycho-analyst. This developed into a practice whereby the patient was to communicate freely to the analyst everything that came to mind, without reservation or editing.

In his *Interpretation of Dreams* (1899), Freud commented:

> I have noticed in my psycho-analytical work that the whole frame of mind of a man who is reflecting is totally different from that of a man who is observing his own psychical processes. In reflection there is one more psychical activity at work than in the most attentive self-observation, and this is shown amongst other things by the tense looks and wrinkled forehead of a person pursuing his reflections as compared with the restful expression of a self-observer. In both cases attention must be concentrated, but the man who is reflecting is also exercising his *critical* faculty; this leads him to reject some of the ideas that occur to him after perceiving them, to cut short others without following the trains of thought which they would open up to him, and to behave in such a way towards still others that they never become conscious at all and are accordingly suppressed before being perceived. The self-observer on the other hand need only take the trouble to suppress his critical faculty. If he succeeds in doing that, innumerable ideas come into his consciousness of which he could otherwise never have got hold.[53]

Freud then discussed at some length the ideas that the patient should "concentrate his attention on his self-observation" and that this self-observation should be "uncritical"; this practice eventually became "the fundamental rule of psycho-analytic technique."[54] Freud continually emphasized the significance of this "state of quiet, unreflecting self-observation" as the means whereby the patient might become fully aware of the contents of his or her consciousness and communicate them to the analyst.[55]

In the years that followed, self-observation continued to hold a central position in clinical psychoanalysis; and psychoanalysts made a point of differentiating the self-observing function from the "experiencing" function—that is, from the experiencing of the sensations, feelings, thoughts, and memories that were being observed. This came to be referred to as a differentiation of the ego into an experiencing ego and an observing ego.

The practice of self-observation was regularly advocated, yet it was relatively uncommon for the term *self-observation* to be used. Occasionally, though, in discussions of the process of psychoanalysis, people talked about self-observation, but they would apply terms such as *introspection* to it instead. And sometimes such discussions would take note of the fact that self-observation, by whatever name, was a factor in the analyst's activity as well as in the patient's.[56]

As the patient's acquisition of insight or self-understanding came to be viewed as a crucial element in the clinical gains brought about through psychoanalysis, the patient's self-observing activity came to be thought of as particularly significant among the factors that facilitated that acquisition of insight. Robert L. Hatcher has carefully considered insight and self-observation in tandem. He describes "the function of self-observation as the observation of any and all contents, characteristics, and activities of the person, and the relationships among these features."[57] In addition to "experiential self-observation" — avoiding, as Freud originally suggested, application of the critical faculty[58] — "reflective self-observation" takes place when the patient attempts to organize and integrate data (whether in response to the analyst's comments or to his own incipient realizations) and move toward insight. "Experiential self-observation is the process which provides the content of the analysis," and reflective self-observation facilitates the movement toward insight or self-understanding.[59]

Heinz Kohut, a psychoanalyst who favored the term *introspection,* argued for the central role of self-observation in the somewhat different language of his self psychology. Pointing out that "our thoughts, wishes, feelings, and fantasies ... cannot be observed by our sensory organs," Kohut commented, "They have no existence in physical space, and yet they are real, and we can observe them as they occur in time: through introspection in ourselves, and through empathy (i.e., vicarious introspection) in others. ... We speak of physical phenomena when the essential ingredient of our observational method includes our senses, we speak of psychological phenomena when the essential ingredient of our observation is introspection and empathy."[60] He further emphasized that "introspection and empathy play ... a role in *all* psychological understanding."[61] And he conceived of introspection and empathy, operating in tandem, as crucial elements in psychoanalytic work. The introspective efforts of the patient, the analyst's own introspective activity, and the analyst empathically serving as a witness to the patient's introspection all reinforced one another.

Introspection and the Psychotherapies

As the psychotherapeutics of the late nineteenth century took shape — incorporating hypnosis, suggestion, and persuasion — self-examination, by whatever name, did not seem to enter into those healing efforts. With Wundt's work in experimental psychology, introspection as an activity and a term was achieving a new significance; but this had no particular connection with therapeutics. Introspection in the popular mind was often considered "morbid" — the sign of a weakness and self-involvement that could easily become pathological; and such a view was not confined to the realm of the popular. Against this backdrop, the use to which Freud would put self-observation in psychoanalysis became pivotal.

Introspection or self-observation, as it became significant in psychoanalytic treatment, gradually began play a key role in many other twentieth-century psychotherapies, particularly those influenced by psychoanalysis — the psychodynamic psychotherapies. Whether the particular clinical approach urged a thoroughgoing unreflective observation of and reporting on a person's mental experiences or whether a reflective consideration of those mental experiences was also a feature of the approach, some form of self-observation was a prime element in those various modes of treatment.

As Watson and his behaviorism entered the scene, the introspectionism of Wundt and Thorndike was vigorously criticized; and psychoanalytic practice, including introspection, also came under attack. As Boring and McKellar have pointed out, many psychologists disowned introspective methods in the wake of the behaviorist campaign; but in the clinical domain some forms of introspection remained crucial. The various types of behavior therapy that developed were versions of psychological healing that did not call on introspection. But a good number of psychotherapeutic approaches continued to rely on self-observation, albeit often with little explicit discussion of its role. And as self-observation was often associated with the pursuit of self-understanding, these treatment approaches came to be categorized by some as the insight-oriented psychotherapies.

In these ways, and by these different names, self-observation has been a significant component in people's efforts to learn about themselves and to apply that learning to good purpose. In a history of introspection, Anna Robeson Burr remarked on "the world's general intellectual disposition to 'look within' ";[62] she took note of its crucial role in the evolution of philosophy, of its place in the history of both confession and religion in general, and of its reflection in many an autobiography. But Burr did not address the role of introspection in psychological healing, except for its function in confession.

Nevertheless, modes of ameliorating a sufferer's distress and healing the disorders of a troubled psyche figure prominently among the useful purposes of introspection. Introspective efforts in the search for wisdom and peace of mind have always been inherent in the contributions of philosophers. In the history of the cure of souls, self-examination has again and again served healing purposes. In the narrowly medical sphere, though, "looking within" was for centuries rarely mentioned. It was only when certain psychological healing trends were ushered in around the beginning of the twentieth century that self-observation emerged clearly as an explicit element in physicians' treatment endeavors. Psychological healers came to advocate self-observation, to indicate its value to a sufferer, and to provide guidance in its practice. And as has been mentioned, those engaged in pastoral care needed to have a clear understanding of "the intricacies of inwardness."[63]

The process of looking inward — whether regarded as a means to identify sin and thus bring relief to the soul or as an instrument to increase self-awareness while eliminating the symptoms of a psychiatric disorder — has been an element in numerous approaches to psychological healing over time. Confessional practices continue to offer an important form of self-examination. And numerous clinical endeavors continue to make significant use of self-observation.

Scholars and healers continue to find some variant of introspective method invaluable — and perhaps unavoidable — in their work.

PART EIGHT

Concluding Considerations

18

Overview and Afterthoughts

Much has been made of the culture-bound nature of certain psychological healing practices, on the grounds that they are not easily transferable
to another cultural setting, not easily understood by healers in another culture, and not easily compared with its healing practices. The same problems
have also been raised in the "cross-cultural" situation of various subcultures
within the same larger society; each subculture's healing practices may well
differ in that they cohere around alternative ethnic customs, religious beliefs, or medical views. Similar difficulties can easily arise if one compares
psychological healing practices over time. Cultural influences have admit-
tedly shaped practices across societies and across the centuries and have produced seemingly very different embodiments of the psychological aspects of
caring and curing, yet the present study suggests that some elements or themes
transcend space and time, and that cultural influences give different "faces"
in different times and places to a group of basic elements. Wax and wane
though they have, certain concepts and the related practices seem to have
survived both changes in name and the fluctuation in their theoretical contexts. Threads of meaning and application have persisted from era to era, from
one framework to another, in a way to suggest that at least a few elements are
fundamental to psychological healing. The evidence leaves one wondering

whether human nature might have some limiting influence on the number and nature of such elements.

Toward an Integrated View

That a variety of healing approaches might share a group of basic elements is not suggested to minimize their differences. The theories and ideologies that support and explain particular psychological healing approaches can vary significantly from one another and thus render any meaningful comparisons apparently impossible; and of course, practitioners have generally tended to exploit these differences to argue for the alleged uniqueness and superiority of their particular approach. Certain rituals are and always have been associated with any particular approach, and they are rationalized in light of its theory and maintained to be absolutely essential to its practice. These theories and rituals are far from unimportant, and in many ways they are crucial. They provide a common ground for the sufferer and the healer where they can communicate with each other and work with a sense of shared values and goals. But just as one can discuss a profound philosophical issue — or the price of bread — in a number of different languages, so can one seek and find relief or cure in a number of different psychological healing approaches with their different theories and rituals.

There is a bedrock to healing that is related to our shared human nature. Symptoms occur and a human being suffers. Doing what comes naturally, the sufferer reaches out for help. The sufferer's approach may vary, depending on the person's past experience with fellow humans in general and potential helpers in particular. No matter how large man's inhumanity to man might seem to loom, I would argue that most people have a fundamental tendency to respond with compassion and some inclination to be helpful. In almost any culture, certain persons have extended and developed this inclination, and so have become recognized as healers. The more severe or complex the sufferer's symptoms are, the more likely that person is to consult someone designated a healer by the culture. Usually the sufferer has a story to tell the healer — what hurts, what is troubling, the nature of the suffering; and the healer listens and provides "witnessed significance"[1] for the sufferer's account. The healer may also inquire, comment, and eventually provide explanation, advice, and a plan of treatment. We see, at this rudimentary level, the basic role played by the talking, the listening, and the healer-sufferer relationship. If this beginning encounter develops into an ongoing treatment relationship, these three elements, in all their complexity, continue to be crucial. I have argued that this is the case for psychological healing, but it is also the case in healing contexts in general. Despite twentieth-century efforts to attend to the importance of the physician-patient relationship, inattention, or attention of a problematic quality, to the significance of these basic elements is responsible for many a problem in modern medicine and other contemporary healing situations.

Although the healer-sufferer relationship has received much more attention as a therapeutic factor in more recent times, it has been a central element in most modes of psychological healing. As has been detailed earlier, themes of trust, sympathy, compassion, and hope have long been held to be significant; and attention to empathy has become a modern concern. As Franz Alexander summed it up, "There is little doubt that much of the therapeutic success of the healing profession, of the medicine man and of the priest as well as of the modern practitioner, has been due to the undefined emotional rapport between physician and patient."[2]

Most of the other elements focused on in this volume have significant connections with this basic model. Consolation seems to have grown out of human experiences with loss and grief, and the natural reaction of others to respond with compassion and efforts to comfort.

The tendency of a human being to need other human beings has served to develop the healing potential of the healer-sufferer relationship in other ways. This context became the natural setting in which sufferers could confide their troubles and ease their sense of burden and distressing aloneness and could confess in a quest for forgiveness, an easing of a sense of guilt, and reconciliation with others. And the opportunity to express themselves often brought cathartic or abreactive relief from emotional burdens.

The relationship has commonly provided a situation in which influence might be brought to bear, with suggestion and persuasion having long histories as cardinal forms of influence in the service of healing. Themes of reward and punishment (approval and disapproval) have come into focus more with the advent of modern behavior therapies, but conditioning practices, too, have a long history in the influencing of people, albeit only recognized in more recent times.

When the focus has been more on irrational factors, special attention has been devoted to modifying the passions or the imagination.

Concerns with rational factors have been manifested in attention to reason and understanding. Accordingly, explanations and interpretations have commonly had a place in healing modes over the centuries. The search for insight and self-understanding has often been emphasized. And self-observation has tended to be an element in those approaches which featured self-understanding. This group of elements has been crucial for many a sufferer in coming to a sense of "knowing" what all the suffering has been about; and "knowing" has offered a way for sufferers to move from suffering helplessness to some sense of mastery and control over their lives.

The Modern Psychotherapeutic Scene

The twentieth century has become the chronological home for an almost infinite array of approaches to psychological healing, yet it is clear from the basic elements reviewed in this volume that all the modern approaches evidence significant indebtedness to the past — both the recent and distant past. In varying combinations, modern modes of psychotherapeutic endeavor have been constructed out of mixes of the basic elements discussed in the preceding chapters, although a claim to uniqueness frequently surfaces. As examples of these combinations or mixes, we will examine: (1) psychoanalysis and psychoanalytically influenced psychotherapies; (2) the behavior therapies; and (3) the so-called humanistic psychotherapies, such as client-centered therapy, existential therapy, and gestalt therapy.

In psychoanalysis, so often referred to as the talking cure, both talking and listening are central elements. The healer-sufferer relationship, too, is central, and the significance of empathy is increasingly noted. Aspects of this relationship are taken into account and dealt with in terms of transference and countertransference. Catharsis or abreaction was a crucial element in the early stages of the development of psychoanalysis; and though its significance has lessened over time, it has continued to be an intermittent aspect of the clinical approach. The evocation of the emotions and the relief derived from freely expressing them are considered an indispensable part of therapy. Confession, while not usually taken note of and not a prominent feature, has continued to play a part, as does confiding. Psychoanalysts have regularly denied that suggestion and persuasion have any place in psychoanalytic endeavors, but at least occasionally they may find their way into this form of clinical work. Consolation is not usually noted to be an element in psychoanalysis, but it would be rare for a psychoanalytic treatment to proceed without some grieving for losses and experiencing of solace. Of course, interpretation and insight are consistently recognized as aspects of psychoanalytic work, and are often said to be the *essential* elements. Self-observation is a cardinal factor. As we have seen, the themes of conditioning, and reward or punishment (approval or disapproval), though subtly present in learning and change in psychoanalysis, are usually far from explicit

As to the psychoanalytically influenced psychotherapies, it is fair to say that their situation is similar to that already described for psychoanalysis. Listening, talking, and the healer-sufferer relationship are all central features. Facilitating the grieving over losses and providing consolation is common enough. In some approaches, catharsis and abreaction may be more emphasized, and the evocation of and free expression of emotions are frequently regarded as significant. Suggestion and persuasion may be more readily allowed into the mix than in psychoanalysis. Confession and confiding commonly have their place. Interpretation and insight are often crucially important, as is self-observation. Conditioning and forms of approval or disapproval are often subtly present. Hypnosis has, of course, been an integral aspect of hypno-analysis and has been an adjunct in some psychodynamic therapies.

In the behavioral therapies, conditioning and reward and punishment practices are central elements. In the more recent past, behavior therapy has increasingly taken account of cognitive factors and shown a tendency to emphasize cognitive restructuring more and conditioning less; but some have argued that this restructuring is still based on versions of conditioning. With its roots in a strict focus on behavior, the early years of behavior therapy did not seem to give much attention to talking and listening, except in acquiring data for the initial behavioral analysis and in providing instructions and receiving reports. But though it is unlikely that this inattention was ever as extreme as a Watsonian behaviorism might seem to imply or as critics have suggested, these two elements and the nature of patient-therapist communication have become much more significant, especially with the increasing emphasis on cognition in behavior therapy. And the healer-sufferer relationship has come to be considered a more important factor in behavior therapy. It has commonly been alleged that behavior therapists minimize or deny the significance of the person and of the relationship in their therapy, but it appears that the basis for such allegations is diminishing, given the increased attention paid to the person of the patient and the more deliberate use of the relationship in treatment. In fact, behavior therapists have increasingly taken to structuring their behavior in the relationship with a view to enhancing treatment in general or reinforcement in particular. Suggestion and persuasion have some place, but neither behaviorists themselves nor their critics have made much of them one way or the other. As to interpretation and insight, most behaviorists have excluded them from behavior therapy by definition; and it has been common for them to decry these two elements as inessential to psychological healing and as characteristic only of the benighted activities of therapists influenced by psychoanalysis. Yet, as Marmor has pointed out, interpretive efforts seem to occur — whether wittingly or unwittingly, whether acknowledged or not — in the clinical activities of many behavior therapists.[3] Catharsis and abreaction, confession, and consolation would seem to have little or no place in these clinical undertakings.

Prominent among the "humanistic" psychotherapies is Carl Rogers' client-centered therapy. Talking and listening are central elements, much as they are in the psychoanalytically influenced therapies. Unfettered communication is actively encouraged; and the therapist provides keenly attentive listening. The healer-sufferer relationship is strongly emphasized—though the term is not employed—as being at the heart of this approach. The triad of conditions considered essential for the therapist to provide gives some indication of the Rogerian view of the optimal version of this relationship: accurate empathy, unconditional positive regard (or nonpossessive warmth), and genuineness. Though not so overtly as in the behavior therapies, a conditioning process is clearly at work. The therapist's person and behavior are employed to condition the patient toward positive self-regard—to an increased sense of self-worth. Early on, Rogers harbored serious reservations about interpretation, and his reservations increased over the years. Still, though, client-centered therapists have tended to engage in veiled interpretive activity in their empathic comments and through the nature and timing of other interventions. As to insight, Rogers conceived of his treatment process as promoting the emergence of insight and self-understanding, and he thought of this as a significant contribution toward therapeutic gain; but he favored the facilitation of the patient's free expression, rather than interpretation, as the means toward such insight. Like the psychoanalytically influenced therapies, client-centered therapy does not include suggestion and persuasion among its usually acknowledged elements; but as with those other approaches, there is some tendency for suggestion and persuasion to find their way into this treatment mode. Catharsis or abreaction and confession can also be factors in Rogerian clinical work, but they appear to be neither emphasized nor denied by therapists of this persuasion.

It is much more difficult to consider the elements or ingredients that combine to constitute existential therapy. It has frequently been noted that it can be misleading to speak of "existential therapy"—that it is perhaps better to think in terms of an existential trend within psychotherapy or an existential dimension within various approaches to psychotherapy or an existential influence that might occasionally or pervasively color the psychotherapy of a particular therapist. It is more an orientation and a set of values that can influence a variety of psychotherapeutic approaches, without in itself constituting a distinct therapeutic method. Out of a background in the writings of Søren Kierkegaard, Edmund Husserl's phenomenology, Karl Jaspers' phenomenological psychopathology, the existential analytics of Martin Heidegger, and the philosophical contributions of Jean-Paul Sartre, existential therapy emerged in Europe during the interwar years in the clinical endeavors of such psychiatrists as

Ludwig Binswanger and Eugène Minkowski. In the post–World War II era, this orientation flourished in Europe and by the 1950s had found its way across the Atlantic to North America, where it was brought to some prominence in the work of Rollo May and James F. T. Bugental, among others.

In addition to the various influences just noted, to some degree existential therapy developed in response to dissatisfaction with elements of psychoanalytic thought that were perceived as reductionistic, mechanistic, and deterministic. And yet existential therapists draw significantly on techniques associated with psychoanalysis and the psychodynamic psychotherapies. The approach is characterized more by a different orientation toward the other person rather than by a different set of techniques. There is much less emphasis on diagnosis or on a search for causal factors in the patient's past. Instead, attention is focused on the patient's current experience, on an explanation of feelings and relationships in the present — or, as some existentialists might put it, the emphasis is on the here and now, on the patient's being in his or her world at this point in time. Techniques are generally adapted to the individual patient, with an emphasis on efforts to understand the patient and on the crucial role of empathy. Concerned with the sufferer's alienation from self and others, and attending to the anxiety experienced in the face of the threats inherent in his or her very existence, the existential therapist undertakes a dialogue with the sufferer in an egalitarian relationship, in the interest of the sufferer's taking responsibility for his or her "being-in-the-world" and becoming able to move toward full encounter and shared experience with others. Talking and listening are as significant as in most other forms of psychological healing. The healer-sufferer relationship is of crucial importance, as it is in many other approaches, but the emphasis is on equality and authenticity, on openness, and on its being mutually influential in the here and now. As one might guess, the themes of transference and countertransference are seldom at the forefront. Interpretation is common enough, but its foci fall within the boundaries already mentioned. Insight is sought, but within these same bounds. Self-observation is called upon, as it is in so many modern psychotherapies. Suggestion and persuasion are not officially recognized elements in this approach, but they nevertheless play a role.

The third approach to be considered in our sample of humanistic psychotherapies is gestalt therapy, which first came into prominence in the 1950s. Although it makes use of concepts from Gestalt psychology, to a significant extent it developed out of psychoanalysis and has an indebtedness to the work of Wilhelm Reich. Frederick S. ("Fritz") Perls, the founder of gestalt therapy, was a psychoanalyst who integrated influences from and reactions against psychoanalysis into an approach with some kinship to existential therapy and

Reich's characterology. Putting emphasis on the here and now, the gestalt therapist functions quite directively and, without ignoring verbal communications, attends carefully to various bodily and behavioral clues from the patient — breathing patterns, evidence of tension, and other nonverbal communications. In the interest of the patients' developing an awareness of what is happening within themselves, the therapist points out these clues, urges them to speak about what the clues mean and to take responsibility for that meaning, and, in the process, commonly evokes related affects in the patients. In this way, various "disowned" or suppressed aspects of the patient become manifest, recognized, and "owned." The use of awareness exercises and other forms of experimentation within a session, along with an emphasis on bodily awareness, the experiencing of affect, and the role of encounter, have all come to characterize gestalt therapy. While talking and listening are far from insignificant in this clinical approach, the emphasis on nonverbal communication and the therapist's careful visual observation give those two cardinal elements a somewhat different status from what is usual in most psychotherapies. As to the healer-sufferer relationship, gestalt therapists affirm that a nonjudgmental acceptance by the therapist is optimal (though they would probably decry this use of "healer-sufferer"); yet many of them, though they may argue to the contrary, actively work to facilitate the possibility of change in the patient. Suggestion and persuasion are quite evidently at work; but it seems that these elements are neither advocated nor discredited or disowned. Catharsis or abreaction and confession are common components, but no special emphasis is placed on them. Gestalt therapists characteristically decry the use of interpretation and downplay the value of insight, yet these factors do figure in this approach.[4] Awareness, which is vigorously emphasized, is closely akin to the acquisition of insight. And even though therapists may make no direct attempt to convey insight, their efforts to expand the patients' awareness often constitute de facto interpretations. "Explaining" remarks are not at all uncommon. Self-examination is a crucial factor. Regarding any undercurrents of conditioning and reward or punishment, they are, as in most psychotherapies, very likely to be present in some fashion, but it is never explicit. As with many other approaches, approval or disapproval seem to play a role, but this is not usually acknowledged by gestalt practitioners.

In addition to these categories of modern psychological healing, supportive psychotherapy merits some brief mention here. As noted in an earlier chapter,[5] the healer-sufferer relationship, listening, and talking — the bedrock of psychological healing — are crucial elements in such clinical work. Varying admixtures of persuasion, suggestion, and conditioning are frequently present in supportive therapy. And any of the other basic elements mentioned in previous chapters may occasionally be a factor.

Afterthoughts

Just as the basic elements enumerated here have served many modes of psychological healing over the centuries and have been crucial constituents in our modern psychotherapies, so they may be found, in varying combinations, in other twentieth-century contexts. For instance, the issues involved in considering the role of the healer-sufferer relationship lie at the root of twentieth-century discussions of humanism and medicine. The literature of medicine has swung back and forth between the significance of technological advances and the need to retain humane influences in the practice of medicine. Concern has repeatedly been voiced that the training of young physicians is overwhelmingly skewed toward our technological advances and seriously deficient with regard to these humane influences. How to balance or integrate the two streams of influence has been a perennial question. And now we have managed care threatening to do more harm to the humane practice of medicine than technology has. How do we protect the care of patients from the dehumanizing dangers posed by these twin demons, technology and managed care?

We can readily see just what a central place the healer-sufferer relationship has in such concerns. Healers can put into practice various combinations of the basic elements which are rooted in that relationship — to provide an attentive, listening ear; to allow confiding, confessional, and cathartic moments; to comfort and console; to evoke and deal with emotions; to arouse and sustain hope; to provide thoughtful suggestion or persuasion; to integrate explanation or interpretation with these other ingredients; to promote self-understanding and the potential for mastering difficult illness-related situations. Though more obliquely than in a purposive psychotherapeutic endeavor, psychological healing nevertheless takes place in general medical contexts as well, where, as elements in healer-sufferer transactions, the factors we have been considering can make the difference between therapeutic success and failure. Their successful use in therapeutic contexts is a reflection of a humane orientation at work in healing. Before anyone gets the mistaken idea that I would suggest that healing is nothing but a matter of employing psychological factors to influence sufferers toward better health, I wish to emphasize that these factors will frequently not be sufficient, but that they will very frequently be necessary.

Another relevant area of modern controversy has been that surrounding the various forms of alternative medicine and holistic medicine. Without discounting what such practitioners do or how they explain what they do, I would again suggest that in one or another combination these basic elements frequently play a crucial role in alternative healing traditions, too. Of course, the healer-sufferer relationship is once again a cardinal ingredient. But wherever such practitioners are therapeutically successful, it is likely that they have made deliberate or intuitive use of at least a few of these basic elements.

But as I bring this volume to a close, I must return to the place of these basic healing elements as the essence of psychological healing and the place of psychological healing within healing in general. For all the evidence that it can be very considerably aided by medicine and procedures, *healing is, at its root, a natural phenomenon.* And psychological healing frequently plays a crucial role in healing, despite the tendency of medicine to lose sight of this fact in our era of technological marvels.

It was not without justification that so many generations of healers attributed much to the healing power of nature. But more frequently, healers have taken credit for what was just happening naturally. Still, though, in functioning in ways that were naturally human and providing some mixture of the basic elements that constitute psychological healing, healers have often been the agents contributing significantly to the furtherance of these natural trends.

Among those with a disposition toward caring and curing, some have brought inclinations and temperaments specially suited to the practice of psychological healing — a respectful and interested way of listening; a readily felt trustworthiness; a compassionate and sympathetic response to those who suffer; a capacity for arousing and sustaining hope; and a calm response to disturbing or frightening clinical states. In more recent times, such natural dispositions have been enhanced and strengthened through training and experience. Whether in earlier times or in our own era, suitably disposed healers have been instrumental in the sustaining and healing of many a sufferer through psychological means.

Combinations of these basic elements of psychological healing — whether deliberately, thoughtfully practiced in a form of skilled psychotherapy or provided indirectly as an invaluable adjunct to general medical care — are the essence of *care of the psyche.* And neglect of the psyche has meant, more often than not, neglect of the sufferer and the sufferer's health.

Notes

Chapter 1: Introduction

1. The term *psychological healing* was used by Eden and Cedar Paul as the English title for their translation of Pierre Janet's *Les médications psychologiques* (Paris: Alcan, 1919) — *Psychological Healing: A Historical and Clinical Study,* 2 vols. (New York: Macmillan, 1925). Henri F. Ellenberger, who wrote so well about Janet in *The Discovery of the Unconscious: The History and Evolution of Dynamic Psychiatry* (New York: Basic Books, 1970), preferred to translate the same book title as *Mental Healing.*

2. James Mark Bedwin (ed.), *Dictionary of Philosophy and Psychology . . . ,* 2 vols. (New York: Macmillan, 1901), 2: 394–95.

3. Ibid.

4. James A. H. Murray et al. (eds.), *A New English Dictionary . . . ,* 13 vols. (Oxford: Clarendon Press, 1888–1933), 7: 1553.

5. Josef Breuer and Sigmund Freud, *Studies on Hysteria* (1895) in *The Standard Edition of the Complete Psychological Works of Sigmund Freud,* trans. and ed. James Strachey, Anna Freud, et al., 24 vols. (London: Hogarth Press, 1955–1974), 2: 282–83.

6. Jerome D. Frank, *Persuasion and Healing: A Comparative Study of Psychotherapy,* rev. ed. (Baltimore, Md.: Johns Hopkins University Press, 1973), 1–3.

7. Hippolyte Bernheim, *Hypnotisme, suggestion, psychothérapie: Etudes nouvelles* (Paris: Octave Doin, 1891). Recently translated by Richard S. Sandor as *Bernheim's New Studies in Hypnotism* (New York: International Universities Press, 1980).

8. Albert Willem van Renterghem and Frederik van Eeden, *Clinique de psychothérapie suggestive fondée à Amsterdam* (Brussels: Manceaux, 1889). A much longer account

was published by these authors in 1894: *Psycho-thérapie: Communications statistiques, observations cliniques nouvelles* . . . (Paris: Sociétés d'Editions Scientifiques, 1894).

9. Frederik van Eeden, "The Theory of Psycho-Therapeutics," *Medical Magazine,* 1895, *1,* 232–57 [232–33].

10. Frederik van Eeden, *Happy Humanity* (Garden City, N.Y.: Doubleday, Page, 1912), p. 68. Better known as a poet, novelist, and playwright, Van Eeden also attended Charcot's lectures in Paris during a stay there as a medical student. Like Van Eeden, Van Renterghem had studied at Nancy.

11. Bernheim (n. 7), *New Studies,* pp. 18, 36.

12. Daniel Hack Tuke (ed.), *Dictionary of Psychological Medicine,* 2 vols. (Philadelphia: Blakiston, Son, 1892), 2: 1034.

13. Hippolyte Bernheim, in Tuke (n. 12), *Dictionary,* 2: 1217.

14. Daniel Hack Tuke, *Illustrations of the Influence of the Mind upon the Body in Health and Disease* (London: Churchill, 1872), pp. 419–54.

15. Frances Power Cobbe, "Faith Healing and Fear Killing," *Contemporary Review,* 1887, *51,* 794–813.

16. C. Lloyd Tuckey, *Psycho-Therapeutics; or Treatment by Sleep and Suggestion* (London: Baillière, Tindall and Cox, 1889).

17. W. C. Dendy, "Psychotherapeia, or the Remedial Influence of Mind," *J. Psychol. Med. & Mental Pathology,* 1853, *6,* 268–74. Dendy was a British surgeon who had originally presented this paper to the Medical Society of London in 1853.

18. Tuke (n. 14), *Influence of the Mind,* p. 381.

19. Van Eeden (n. 9), pp. 233, 235.

20. John T. McNeill, *A History of the Cure of Souls* (New York: Harper Torchbooks, 1965).

21. Pedro Laín Entralgo, *The Therapy of the Word in Classical Antiquity,* trans. L. J. Rather and John M. Sharp (New Haven, Conn.: Yale University Press, 1970).

22. Forest E. Clements, "Primitive Concepts of Disease," *University of California Publications in American Archeology and Ethnology,* 1932, *32* (No. 2), 185–252; Ari Kiev (ed.), *Magic, Faith, and Healing: Studies in Primitive Psychiatry Today* (New York: Free Press, 1964); Ellenberger (n. 1), *The Discovery of the Unconscious,* pp. 4–40; Kenneth M. Calestro, "Psychotherapy, Faith Healing, and Suggestion," *Int. J. Psychiat.,* 1972, *10,* 83–113 [88–93].

23. Janet (n. 1), *Psychological Healing;* George Barton Cutten, *Three Thousand Years of Mental Healing* (New York: Charles Scribner's Sons, 1911); Walter Bromberg, *Man Above Humanity: A History of Psychotherapy* (Philadelphia: Lippincott, 1954); Nigel Walker, *A Short History of Psychotherapy: Its Theory and Practice* (London: Routledge & Kegan Paul, 1957); Jan Ehrenwald (ed.), *The History of Psychotherapy: From Healing Magic to Encounter* (New York: Jason Aronson, 1976); Richard Chessick, *Great Ideas in Psychotherapy* (New York: Jason Aronson, 1977); Ellenberger (n. 1), *The Discovery of the Unconscious;* Dieter Wyss, *Depth Psychology: A Critical History,* trans. Gerald Onn (New York: Norton, 1966); James R. Barclay, *Foundations of Counseling Strategies* (New York: John Wiley & Sons, 1971); Donald K. Freedheim (ed.), *History of Psychotherapy: A Century of Change* (Washington, D.C.: American Psychological Association, 1992.

24. Adam Crabtree, *Animal Magnetism, Early Hypnotism, and Psychical Research, 1766–1925: An Annotated Bibliography* (White Plains, N.Y.: Kraus International Publications, 1988); Crabtree, *From Mesmer to Freud: Magnetic Sleep and the Roots of Psychological Healing* (New Haven, Conn.: Yale University Press, 1993); Alan Gauld, *A History of Hypnotism* (Cambridge: Cambridge University Press, 1992).

25. Ernest Jones, *The Life and Work of Sigmund Freud*, 3 vols. (New York: Basic Books, 1953–1957); Peter Gay, *Freud: A Life for Our Time* (New York: Norton, 1988); Reuben Fine, *A History of Psychoanalysis* (New York: Columbia University Press, 1979); Lawrence Friedman, *The Anatomy of Psychotherapy* (Hillsdale, N.J.: Analytic Press, 1988); Robert S. Wallerstein, *The Talking Cures: The Psychoanalyses and the Psychotherapies* (New Haven, Conn.: Yale University Press, 1995).

26. McNeill (n. 20), *A History of the Cure of Souls;* Charles F. Kemp, *Physicians of the Soul: A History of Pastoral Counseling* (New York: Macmillan, 1947); William A. Clebsch and Charles R. Jaekle, *Pastoral Care in Historical Perspective* (New York: Jason Aronson, 1975); E. Brooks Holifield, *A History of Pastoral Care in America: From Salvation to Self-Realization* (Nashville: Abingdon Press, 1983); W. J. Sheils (ed.), *The Church and Healing* (Oxford: Basil Blackwell, 1982); Ronald L. Numbers and Darrel W. Amundsen (eds.), *Caring and Curing: Health and Medicine in the Western Religious Traditions* (New York: Macmillan, 1986); Lawrence E. Sullivan (ed.), *Healing and Restoring: Health and Medicine in the World's Religious Traditions* (New York: Macmillan, 1989); Leslie D. Weatherhead, *Psychology, Religion, and Healing* (London: Hodder and Stoughton, 1951).

27. Quoted by L. J. Rather in *Mind and Body in Eighteenth Century Medicine: A Study Based on Jerome Gaub's De regimine mentis* (Berkeley: University of California Press, 1965), p. 10. Translated from Pierre Jean George Cabanis, "Coup d'oeil sur les révolutions et sur la réforme de la médecine," in Cabanis, *Oeuvres philosophiques,* 2 vols. (Paris: Presses Universitaires de France, 1956), 2: 247.

28. Ari Kiev (ed.), *Magic, Faith, and Healing: Studies in Primitive Psychiatry Today* (New York: Free Press, 1964); Ellenberger (n. 1), *The Discovery of the Unconscious,* pp. 4–40; Calestro (n. 22); Arthur Kleinman, *Rethinking Psychiatry: From Cultural Category to Personal Experience* (New York: Free Press, 1988), pp. 108–41.

Chapter 2: Psychological Healing in Ancient Greece and Rome

1. Richard D. Chessick, "Socrates: First Psychotherapist," *Amer. J. Psychoanal.,* 1982, 42, 71–83 [76]. Of a different opinion are Bennett Simon, *Mind and Madness in Ancient Greece: The Classical Roots of Modern Psychiatry* (Ithaca, N.Y.: Cornell University Press, 1978); Christopher Gill, "Ancient Psychotherapy," *J. Hist. Ideas,* 1985, 46, 307–25; Luis García Ballester, "Diseases of the Soul (Nosemata tes Psyches) in Galen: The Impossibility of Galenic Psychotherapy," *Clio Medica,* 1974, 9, 35–43.

2. Pedro Laín Entralgo, *The Therapy of the Word in Classical Antiquity,* ed. and trans. L. J. Rather and John M. Sharp (New Haven, Conn.: Yale University Press, 1970), pp. 139–70. I am indebted to this fine study in much of this chapter.

3. Gill (n. 1), p. 310.

4. Simon (n. 1), *Mind and Madness in Ancient Greece,* p. 123.

5. E. R. Dodds, *The Greeks and the Irrational* (Boston: Beacon Press, 1957), pp. 76–80. In Herodotus, Dodds was drawing on bk. 4.79.

6. Ibid., p. 22.

7. Ibid., p. 21. Of course, such practices have hardly been limited to so-called primitive cultures. Derived from a Greek verb meaning "to conjure out," *exorcism* meant "the expulsion of evil spirits from persons or places by incantations, magical rites or other means." Hugh Chisholm et al. (eds.), *The Encyclopaedia Britannica,* 11th ed., 29 vols. (New York: Encyclopaedia Britannica, 1910–1911), 10: 80. *Exorcism* became the common term for such conjurations in Christian contexts.

8. Laín Entralgo (n. 2), *Therapy of the Word,* pp. 22–23.

9. For a crisp outline of the essence of these matters, see N. G. L. Hammond and H. H. Scullard (eds.), *The Oxford Classical Dictionary,* 2nd ed. (Oxford: Clarendon Press, 1970), pp. 129–30, 543–44; for an extensive collection of ancient references, both literary materials and inscriptions, to Aesculapian temple healing and a detailed study thereof: Emma J. Edelstein and Ludwig Edelstein, *Asclepius: A Collection and Interpretation of the Testimonies,* 2 vols. (Baltimore, Md.: Johns Hopkins Press, 1945); for some interesting comments from a particularly thoughtful scholar, Dodds (n. 5), *Greeks and the Irrational,* pp. 110–16; for a survey of incubation from ancient times to modern times: Mary Hamilton, *Incubation, or the Cure of Disease in Pagan Temples and Christian Churches* (London: Henderson et al., 1906); for a detailed account of a lengthy career as a devout Aesculapian temple patient, C. A. Behr, *Aelius Aristides and the Sacred Tales* (Amsterdam: Adolf M. Hakkert, 1968).

10. If one was a believer, the cures were termed *religious,* and, if one was not a believer, they were termed *magical.* The other fellow's views were magical or pagan, whereas one's own views, of course, reflected the true religion. This principle was to be recurrently at work over the centuries in the judgment of amazing or miraculous cures.

11. Ibid., pp. 23–25, 29–30.

12. Ibid., pp. 64–69.

13. Ibid., p. 88.

14. Ibid., pp. 91–97.

15. Ibid., p. 104. Not to be confused with Antiphon the orator, this Antiphon was a Sophist and an interpreter of dreams. It is said that "at Corinth, fitting up a room near the market-place, he wrote on the door that he could cure by words those who were in distress" Plutarch, "Lives of the Ten Orators," trans. Harold North Fowler, in *Plutarch's Moralia,* trans. Frank Cole Babbitt et al., 15 vols. (Cambridge: Harvard University Press, 1949–1976), 10: 342–457 [351]. It is generally thought that this work was *not* by Plutarch.

16. Laín Entralgo (n. 2), *Therapy of the Word,* pp. 120–23, 126.

17. Ibid, p. 163.

18. Ibid., pp. 178–81.

19. For a detailed study of *persuasion,* see Chapter 11.

20. Laín Entralgo (n. 2), *Therapy of the Word,* p. 69.

21. These two elements of psychological healing will each be dealt with in detail in later chapters, catharsis in Chapter 6 and consolation in Chapter 8.

22. Simon (n. 1), *Mind and Madness in Ancient Greece,* p. 180, 182–86.

23. Plato, *Charmides,* in *The Dialogues of Plato,* 2 vols., trans. B. Jowett, intro. Raphael Demos (New York: Random House, 1937), 1: 6 [*Charmides,* 156–57].

24. The Stoic school of thought began with Zeno of Citium (335–263 B.C.). Other significant figures in this tradition were Cleanthes (331–232 B.C.), Chrysippus (ca. 280–207 B.C.), and, later, Seneca (5 B.C.–A.D. 65), Epictetus (ca. 55–ca.135), and Marcus Aurelius (121–180). See Whitney J. Oates (ed.), *The Stoic and Epicurean Philosophers* (New York: Modern Library, 1940); Frederick Copleston, *A History of Philosophy,* 8 vols. (Westminster, Md: Newman Press, 1946–1966), 1: 385–400, 421–25, 428–37; Cicero, *Tusculan Disputations,* trans. J. E. King (Cambridge: Harvard University Press, 1966); Seneca, *Moral Essays,* trans. John W. Basore, 3 vols. (Cambridge: Harvard University Press, 1965–1975); R. S. Peters (ed.), *Brett's History of Psychology* (London: Allen & Unwin, 1962), pp. 146–58; H. M. Gardiner, Ruth Clark Metcalf, and John G. Beebe-Center, *Feeling and Emotion: A History of Theories* (New York: American Book, 1937), pp. 64–80.

25. Peters (n. 23), *Brett's History of Philosophy,* p. 143.

26. Ibid., p. 156. From Diogenes Laërtius on Zeno.

27. Cicero (n. 24), *Tusculan Disputations.* The quotations that follow in the text are drawn mainly from Books III and IV of this work.

28. Ibid., bk. III, iii.

29. Ibid., bk. III, xxxi–xxxiv.

30. Ibid., bk. III, xxv.

31. Ibid., bk. III, xxxiv.

32. Seneca, *Ad Lucilium Epistulae Morales,* trans. Richard M. Gummere, 3 vols. (Cambridge: Harvard University Press, 1967–1971). The following is drawn, mainly, from vol. 3, epistle 95, and partially from vol. 3, epistle 94.

33. Seneca (n. 24), *Moral Essays,* 2: 2–97 [bk. VI].

34. Ibid., 2: 219 [bk. IX, ii. 10].

35. Ibid., 2: 221 [bk. IX, ii. 15].

36. Ibid., 2: 237–39 [bk. IX, ii. 3].

37. Ibid., 2: 239 [bk. IX, ii. 5].

38. Galen, *On the Passions and Errors of the Soul,* trans. Paul W. Harkins, ed. and intro. Walther Riese (Columbus: Ohio State University Press, 1963), pp. 31–33, 44, 48, 52–54, 66.

39. Ibid., pp. 53–54.

40. Ibid., p. 49.

41. Walther Riese viewed these practices as a form of psychotherapy, see his introduction to and interpretation of Galen (n. 38), *Passions and Errors,* pp. 20, 112, 120, 124; Owsei Temkin referred to Galen here as appearing "in the guise of the Stoic psychotherapist," *Galenism: Rise and Decline of a Medical Philosophy* (Ithaca, N.Y.: Cornell University Press, 1973), pp. 38–39; George Sarton said that Galen had offered "psychotherapeutic guidance," *Galen of Pergamon* (Lawrence: University of Kansas Press, 1954), p. 72; Rudolph E. Siegel wrote at some length on "Galen's psychotherapeutical concepts," *Galen on Psychology, Psychopathology, and Function and Diseases of the Nervous System* (Basel: Karger, 1973), pp. 275–78; Henri F. Ellenberger referred to this work as "philosophical psychotherapy," *The Discovery of the Unconscious: The History and*

Evolution of Dynamic Psychiatry (New York: Basic Books, 1970), p. 42. But Ballester was sternly opposed to such views, arguing that a "Galenic psychotherapy" was impossible (n. 1); Laín Entralgo would surely regard Galen's approach as a "therapy of the word" and would probably grant that it had "psychotherapeutic features," but he would very likely maintain that it was not a systematic "verbal psychotherapy" — *Therapy of the Word* (n. 2). Simon would probably view Galen here as "the philosopher as therapist" and physician of the soul, but it is not clear that he would approve of terming this work "psychotherapy" — *Mind and Madness in Ancient Greece* (n. 1); Gill would seem to have taken a position that would not allow these practices to be categorized as psychotherapy (n. l).

42. James A. H. Murray et al. (eds.) *A New English Dictionary . . . ,* 13 vols. (Oxford: Clarendon Press, 1888–1933), 7: 1553; Denis Leigh, C. M. B. Pare, and John Marks (eds.), *A Concise Encyclopaedia of Psychiatry* (Lancaster, England: MTP Press, 1977), p. 305.

43. Martha C. Nussbaum, *The Therapy of Desire: Theory and Practice in Hellenistic Ethics* (Princeton, N.J.: Princeton University Press, 1994). In this very interesting book, Nussbaum has systematically addressed the place of psychological healing in Hellenistic philosophical thought and practice — in the works of the Epicureans, Skeptics, and Stoics. Again, this was a philosophical therapeutics and not a part of medical therapeutics.

44. Caelius Aurelianus, *On Acute and on Chronic Diseases,* ed. and trans. I. E. Drabkin (Chicago: University of Chicago Press, 1950), pp. 543–53.

45. Ibid., pp. 547–49. This element will be dealt with in detail in Chapter 9.

46. Arthur J. Brock, *Greek Medicine: Being Extracts Illustrative of Medical Writers from Hippocrates to Galen* (London: Dent & Sons, 1929), pp. 213–14.

47. This practice will be dealt with in some detail in Chapter 12.

48. Spencer L. Rogers, "Egyptian Psychotherapy," *Ciba Symposia,* 1947, 9, 617–22 [618].

49. Heinrich von Staden, *Herophilus: The Art of Medicine in Early Alexandria* (Cambridge: Cambridge University Press, 1989), p. 8.

50. Kenneth G. Zysk, *Religious Healing in the Veda* (Philadelphia: American Philosophical Society, 1985), pp. 8–9.

51. Ibid., pp. 62–63.

52. K. C. Dube, "Nosology and Therapy of Mental Illness in *Ayurveda,*" *Comparative Medicine East and West,* 1978, 6, 209–28.

53. C. V. Haldipur, "Madness in Ancient India: Concept of Insanity in *Charaka Samhita* (1st Century A.D.)," *Comprehensive Psychiatry,* 1984, 25, 335–44 [338].

Chapter 3: The Healer-Sufferer Relationship

1. G. E. R. Lloyd (ed.), *Hippocratic Writings* (Harmondsworth, England: Penguin Books, 1978), p. 67.

2. Darrel W. Amundsen and Gary B. Ferngren, "Evolution of the Patient-Physician Relationship: Antiquity Through the Renaissance," in Earl E. Shelp (ed.), *The Clinical Encounter: The Moral Fabric of the Patient-Physician Relationship* (Dordrecht: Reidel, 1983), pp. 3–46 [4].

3. Plato, *The Dialogues of Plato*, 2 vols., trans. B. Jowett (New York: Random House, 1937), 1: 31–52 [*Lysis*, 217].

4. Hippocrates, *Precepts*, in *Works of Hippocrates*, 4 vols., trans. and ed. W. H. S. Jones and E. T. Withington (Cambridge: Harvard University Press, 1923–1931), 1:305–33, [319]. The majority of scholars interpret the "love of art" in this Hippocratic passage as implying the physician's "love of art," which joins with his "love of man" to play a crucial role in healing. But Edelstein reasoned quite differently, to the effect that what was being referred to was the patient's "love of the art." He argued that, if such "philanthropy" was present on the physician's part, then "'love of the [medical] art' will be kindled in his patients, a state of mind that greatly contributes to their speedy recovery, especially when they are dangerously sick" — see Ludwig Edelstein, "The Professional Ethics of the Greek Physician," in *Ancient Medicine: Selected Papers of Ludwig Edelstein*, ed. Owsei Temkin and C. Lilian Temkin, trans. C. Lilian Temkin (Baltimore, Md.: Johns Hopkins Press, 1967), pp. 319–48 [321, and n. 4]. Apparently implying previous agreement with Edelstein, Temkin has recently indicated that he can no longer accept Edelstein's interpretation; and he now subscribes to a view that is essentially the same as that of most other scholars. Owsei Temkin, *Hippocrates in a World of Pagans and Christians* (Baltimore, Md.: Johns Hopkins University Press, 1991), p. 31, and n. 88. Amundsen and Ferngren (n. 2) have questioned the use of this passage "as a proof-test for the existence of a philanthropic motive in Greek medicine." They maintain that "the physician here is simply being encouraged to show kindness, in return for which a patient can be expected to exhibit a love of the physician's art." While they share Edelstein's view that the physician's attitude may well engender a favorable reaction in the patient, these authors consider *philanthropia* here to mean "little more than 'kindly or friendly' [sentiments]" (p. 26).

5. Edelstein (n. 4), p. 320.

6. Pedro Laín Entralgo, *Doctor and Patient*, trans. Frances Partridge (London: World University Library/Weidenfeld and Nicolson, 1969), pp. 21–22. This author has argued that friendship (*philia*) was the cornerstone of the doctor-patient relationship in the ancient world (pp. 17–29); and he goes on to reason that, in one form or another, it continued to be a crucial element in the art of healing during subsequent centuries.

7. Ibid., p. 26.

8. Hippocrates, *Decorum*, in *Works* (n. 4), 2: 269–301; Hippocrates, *Physician*, in *Works* (n. 4), 2: 305–13.

9. Hippocrates, *Epidemics I*, in *Works* (n. 4), 1: 147–211 [165].

10. Hippocrates, *Physician*, in *Works* (n. 4), 2: 311–13.

11. Plato (n. 3), *Dialogues*, 1: 604–8, 610–11 [*The Republic* I, 340–42, 346].

12. Ibid., 2: 491 [*Laws* IV, 720].

13. Ibid., 1: 671 [*The Republic* III, 406].

14. Seneca, *Moral Essays*, 3 vols., trans. John W. Basore (Cambridge: Harvard University Press, 1975), 3: 395–97 [*On Benefits*, VI, 16].

15. Celsus, *De medicina*, 3 vols., trans. W.G. Spencer (Cambridge: Harvard University Press, 1935–1938), 1: 41 [Proem. 73].

16. Edelstein (n. 4), p. 338.

17. Ibid.

18. Ibid., p. 345. This passage from Libanius has also been given careful attention by Temkin (n. 4), *Hippocrates,* p. 221. And the full context of the passage has been translated and discussed by Richard M. Ratzan and Gary B. Ferngren, "A Greek Progymnasma on the Physician-Poisoner," *J. Hist. Med. Allied Sci.,* 1993, *48,* 157–70.

19. Edelstein (n. 4), p. 345.

20. Ratzan and Ferngren (n. 18), p. 161.

21. As Temkin has said, "Even if this portrayal is exaggerated, there must be some truth in it, since otherwise the prosecutor could not count on approval"—Temkin (n. 4), *Hippocrates,* p. 221, n. 55.

22. Luke 10:30–37, *Holy Bible.*

23. Laín Entralgo (n. 6), *Doctor and Patient,* pp. 53–57.

24. Temkin (n. 4), *Hippocrates,* pp. 160, 252, 256.

25. Darrel W. Amundsen and Gary B. Ferngren, "Philanthropy in Medicine: Some Historical Perspectives," in Earl E. Shelp (ed.), *Beneficence and Health Care* (Dordrecht: Reidel, 1982), pp. 1–31; Amundsen and Ferngren (n. 2), pp. 3–46.

26. Paul Delatte, *The Rule of St. Benedict: A Commentary,* trans. Justin McCann (London: Burns Oates & Washbourne, 1921), p. 237.

27. Ibid., p. 258.

28. Loren C. MacKinney, "Medical Ethics and Etiquette in the Early Middle Ages: The Persistence of Hippocratic Ideals," *Bull. Hist. Med.,* 1952, *26,* 1–31, p. 4.

29. Cassiodorus Senator, *An Introduction to Divine and Human Readings,* trans. and annotated by Leslie Webber Jones (from *Institutiones Divinarum et Saecularium Litterarum,* ed. R. A. B. Mynors) (New York: Columbia University Press, 1946), p. 135.

30. Laín Entralgo (n. 6), *Doctor and Patient,* pp. 53–100; MacKinney (n. 28); Darrel W. Amundsen, "The Medieval Catholic Tradition," in Ronald L. Numbers and Darrel W. Amundsen (eds.), *Caring and Curing: Health and Medicine in the Western Religious Traditions* (New York: Macmillan, 1986), pp. 65–107; Amundsen and Ferngren (n. 2).

31. Laín Entralgo (n. 6), *Doctor and Patient,* p. 77.

32. James A. H. Murray et al. (eds.), *A New English Dictionary . . . ,* 13 vols. (Oxford: Clarendon Press, 1888–1933), vol. 9, pt. 2. In addition to our more familiar meaning of *sympathy* as an interpersonal notion, the *OED* cites the long-standing use of the term in medicine to denote "a relation between two bodily organs or parts . . . such that disorder, or any condition, of the one induces a corresponding condition in the other." In ancient medicine, this meant a special type of resonance between body organs or parts whereby, when one organ or part was diseased or injured, another might *sympathetically* be likewise affected. Over the centuries, the "communication" that was thought to make this possible was variously attributed to the humors, the nerves, or the blood. Although there is a certain conceptual common ground to these two notions of sympathy, they have served separate purposes and have had rather separate histories; sympathy as a concept in physiology and pathology flourished over many centuries and began to wane in the early 1800s, whereas sympathy as an interpersonal concept has retained its meaning into our own time.

33. Ibid., vol. 2.

34. A. S. Aglen, "Compassion or Pity," in James Hastings et al. (eds.), *A Dictionary of the Bible . . . ,* 5 vols. (New York: Charles Scribner's Sons, 1902–1919), 1: 462.

35. Augustine, *Concerning the City of God Against the Pagans,* ed. and intro. David

Knowles, trans. Henry Bettenson (Harmondsworth, England: Pelican Classics, 1972), p. 349 (Book IX, chap. 5).

36. Paracelsus, *Selected Writings*, ed. and intro. Jolande Jacobi, trans. Norbert Guterman (New York: Pantheon Books, 1951), p. 142.

37. Ibid., pp. 144, 146.

38. D. D. Raphael (ed.) *British Moralists, 1650–1800*, 2 vols. (Oxford: Clarendon Press, 1969), 1: 342–43.

39. Francis Hutcheson, *A System of Moral Philosophy*, 2 vols. [ed.] Francis Hutcheson, M.D. (London: Millar and Longman, 1755), 1: 1–37.

40. Ibid., 1: 19–20.

41. David Hume, *A Treatise of Human Nature*, ed. L. A. Selby-Bigge (Oxford: Clarendon Press, 1964), pp. 316, 318–19.

42. Ibid., pp. 575–76.

43. Ibid., p. 593.

44. Adam Smith, *The Theory of Moral Sentiments*, ed. D. D. Raphael and A. L. Macfie (Oxford: Clarendon Press, 1991), pp. 9–10.

45. Ibid., pp. 10, 43.

46. Ibid., p. 10.

47. Ibid., pp. 11–12.

48. Ibid., pp. 13–15.

49. Ibid., p. 226.

50. Walter Jackson Bate, "The Sympathetic Imagination in Eighteenth-Century English Criticism," *English Literary History*, 1945, *12*, 144–66.

51. Samuel Johnson, *A Dictionary of the English Language* . . . , 2 vols. (London: Knapton, Longman, Hitch and Hawes; Millar, and Dodsley, 1755), vol. 2.

52. James Beattie, *Essays on Poetry and Music, as They Affect the Mind* . . . , 3rd ed. (London: Dilly and Creech, 1779), pp. 181–82.

53. Ibid., p. 159.

54. Norman S. Fiering, "Irresistible Compassion: An Aspect of Eighteenth-Century Sympathy and Humanitarianism," *J. Hist. Ideas*, 1976, *37*, 195–218.

55. Roy Porter, *Mind-Forg'd Manacles: A History of Madness in England from the Restoration to the Regency* (Cambridge: Harvard University Press, 1987), pp. 89–96.

56. John Gregory, *Lectures on the Duties and Qualifications of a Physician* (London: Strahan and Cadell, 1772), pp. 19–21.

57. Ibid., pp. 22–23.

58. Pierre-Jean-Georges Cabanis, *On the Relations between the Physical and Moral Aspects of Man*, 2 vols., trans. Margaret Duggan Saidi, ed. George Mora, intro. Sergio Moravia and George Mora (Baltimore, Md.: Johns Hopkins University Press, 1981) 2: 598. Sophie Condorcet, Cabanis's sister-in-law, translated "Adam Smith's *Theory of Moral Sentiments* and prefaced it with eight rambling *Lectures on Sympathy* . . . dedicated to Cabanis" (Martin S. Staum, *Cabanis: Enlightenment and Medical Philosophy in the French Revolution* [Princeton, N.J.: Princeton University Press, 1980], p. 149).

59. P. J. G. Cabanis, *Sketch of the Revolutions of Medical Science, and Views Relating to Its Reform*, trans. and ed. A. Henderson (London: Johnson, Murray, and Constable, 1806), pp. 385–86.

60. F. A. Mesmer, *Mesmerism:* . . . *Original Scientific and Medical Writings of*

F. A. Mesmer, trans. and comp. George Bloch, intro. E. R. Hilgard (Los Altos, Calif.: William Kaufmann, 1980), pp. 34–35.

61. Ibid., p. 135.

62. Murray et al. (n. 32), *OED*, vol. 9, pt. 2.

63. See n. 32.

64. Lester S. King, *The Road to Medical Enlightenment, 1650–1695* (London: Macdonald/American Elsevier, 1970), pp. 141–45; Leo M. Zimmerman, "Surgery," in Allen G. Debus (ed.), *Medicine in Seventeenth Century England* (Berkeley: University of California Press, 1974), pp. 49–69 [57–61]. The extent to which these matters were related to magical healing can be seen in Keith Thomas's chapter "Magical Healing" in his *Religion and the Decline of Magic: Studies in Popular Beliefs in Sixteenth and Seventeenth Century England* (London: Weidenfeld and Nicolson, 1971) pp. 177–211.

65. Adam Crabtree, *From Mesmer to Freud: Magnetic Sleep and the Roots of Psychological Healing* (New Haven: Yale University Press, 1993), pp. 39–41, 47.

66. Ibid., p. 73.

67. Ibid., pp. 73–74, 95.

68. Ibid., pp. 74–75.

69. Bate (n. 50), pp. 144–45.

70. Horace Mann et al., *First Annual Report of the Trustees of State Lunatic Hospital,* December 1833, in *Reports and Other Documents Relating to the State Lunatic Hospital at Worcester, Mass.* (Boston: Dutton and Wentworth, 1837), pp. 37–44 [41].

71. Arthur Schopenhauer, *On the Basis of Morality,* trans. E. F. J. Payne, intro. Richard Taylor (Indianapolis, Ind.: Bobbs-Merrill, 1965), pp. 65–66.

72. Ibid., pp. 148–49, 162.

73. Ibid., pp. 143–44.

74. Worthington Hooker, *Physician and Patient; or, a Practical View of the Mutual Duties, Relations and Interests of the Medical Profession and the Community* (New York: Baker and Scribner, 1849), pp. 383–84.

75. Ibid., pp. 385–90.

76. For example, Henry Edwin Morrill, "Formation of Medical Character," M.D. thesis, University of Pennsylvania, 1840; W. A. Moody, "The Responsibility and Duty of the Physician," M.D. thesis, University of Nashville, 1851; Thomas J. Beall, "The Physician's Calling," M.D. thesis, University of Pennsylvania, 1858.

77. Martin S. Pernick, *A Calculus of Suffering: Pain, Professionalism, and Anesthesia in Nineteenth-Century America* (New York: Columbia University Press, 1985), pp. 115–20.

78. Ibid., p. 114. Quoted from *The Water-Cure Journal,* January 1860, 29, 3–4, which reprinted "Female Physicians" from the *Philadelphia Bulletin.*

79. William Osler, *Aequanimitas,* 3rd ed. (Philadelphia: Blakiston, 1945), pp. 3–6.

80. William Osler, *The Collected Essays of Sir William Osler,* 3 vols., ed. and intro. John P. McGovern and Charles G. Roland (Birmingham, Ala.: Classics of Medicine Library, 1985), 1: 12. The quotation within a quotation is taken by McGovern and Roland from Wilbur C. Davison's foreword in John P. McGovern and Chester R. Burns, *Humanism in Medicine* (Springfield, Ill.: Charles C Thomas, 1973), p. vii.

81. Regina Markell Morantz-Sanchez, *Sympathy and Science: Women Physicians in American Medicine* (New York/Oxford: Oxford University Press, 1985); Rebecca J. Tan-

nenbaum, "Earnestness, Temperance, Industry: The Definition and Uses of Professional Character Among Nineteenth-Century American Physicians," *J. Hist. Med. Allied Sci.,* 1994, *49,* 251–83 [262–70].

82. Morantz-Sanchez (n. 81), *Sympathy and Science,* pp. 191, 197.

83. Ibid., p. 63.

84. Agnes C. Vietor (ed.), *A Woman's Quest: The Life of Marie E. Zakrzewska, M.D.* (New York: Appleton, 1924), p. 266.

85. Morantz-Sanchez (n. 81), *Sympathy and Science,* pp. 210–11.

86. N. D. Jewson, "The Disappearance of the Sick-Man from Medical Cosmology," *Sociology,* 1976, *10,* 225–40 [229].

87. Ibid., p. 230.

88. Jonathan Lear, *Love and Its Place in Nature: A Philosophical Interpretation of Freudian Psychoanalysis* (New York: Farrar, Straus & Giroux, 1990), p. 5.

89. William Chase Greene, *Moira: Fate, Good, and Evil in Greek Thought* (New York: Harper Torchbooks, 1963), p. 109.

90. Francis Weld Peabody, "The Care of the Patient," in *Doctor and Patient: Papers on the Relationship of the Physician to Men and Institutions* (New York: Macmillan, 1930), pp. 27–57 [56–57]. Emphasis added. This paper was originally published in *J. Amer. Med. Assoc.,* 1927, *88,* 877–82.

91. Peabody (n. 90), pp. 29, 31.

92. Ibid., pp. 47, 49, 54, 57; and Oglesby Paul, *The Caring Physician: The Life of Dr. Francis W. Peabody* (Boston: Francis A. Countway Library of Medicine and Harvard Medical Alumni Association, 1991), chap. 6.

93. Peabody (n. 90), pp. 48, 49.

94. Ibid., pp. 49–50.

95. Josef Breuer and Sigmund Freud, *Studies on Hysteria,* in *The Standard Edition of the Complete Psychological Works of Sigmund Freud,* 24 vols., ed. and trans. James Strachey et al. (London: Hogarth Press, 1955–1974), 2: 3–305 [282–83]. Emphasis added. This set of volumes will henceforth be referred to as *Standard Edition.*

96. Sigmund Freud, "On Beginning the Treatment," in *Standard Edition* (n. 95), 12: 123–44 [139–40].

97. C. G. Jung, "The Therapeutic Value of Abreaction," in *The Collected Works of C. G. Jung,* 20 vols. in 21, ed. Gerhard Adler, Michael Fordham, Herbert Read, and William McGuire, trans. R. F. C. Hull (Princeton, N.J.: Princeton University Press, 1953–1979), 16: 129–38 [132–33].

98. Breuer and Freud, *Studies on Hysteria,* in *Standard Edition* (n. 95), 2: 301–4.

99. Sigmund Freud, "Fragment of an Analysis of a Case of Hysteria," in *Standard Edition* (n. 95), 7: 3–122 [116–20].

100. Sigmund Freud, "Five Lectures on Psycho-Analysis," in *Standard Edition* (n. 95), 11: 3–55 [51–52].

101. Sigmund Freud, "The Dynamics of Transference," in *Standard Edition* (n. 95), 12: 99–108.

102. Sigmund Freud, "Observations on Transference-Love: Further Recommendations on the Technique of Psycho-Analysis III," in *Standard Edition* (n. 95), 12: 159–71.

103. Sigmund Freud, "The Future Prospects of Psycho-Analytic Therapy," in *Standard Edition* (n. 95), 11:141–51 [144–45].

104. Adolph Stern, "On the Counter-Transference in Psychoanalysis," *Psychoanalytic Review,* 1924, *11,* 166–74 [167–68].

105. Paula Heimann, "On Counter-Transference," *Int. J. Psycho-Anal.,* 1950, *31,* 81–84.

106. Ibid. This use of the term is illustrated well in Heimann's paper, a study in which various levels and potentials of the healer-sufferer relationship are effectively delineated. As to the evolution of meanings for the term *countertransference,* these developments have been traced in detail by Douglass W. Orr, "Transference and Countertransference: A Historical Survey," *J. Amer. Psychoanal. Assoc.,* 1954, *2,* 621–70 [646–57]; and by Joseph Sandler, Christopher Dare, and Alex Holder, *The Patient and the Analyst: The Basis of the Psychoanalytic Process* (New York: International Universities Press, 1973), pp. 61–70.

107. Ralph R. Greenson and Milton Wexler, "The Non-Transference Relationship in the Psychoanalytic Situation," *Int. J. Psycho-Anal.,* 1969, *50,* 27–39 [29]. The emergence and development of this concept in psychoanalysis has been outlined in Sandler, Dare, and Holder (n. 106), *The Patient and the Analyst,* pp. 27–36.

108. While this is so, and earlier uses of the term *sympathy* sometimes included the very meaning usually given to *empathy* today, modern authors have often taken some pains to differentiate the two. It has frequently been emphasized that empathy entailed "feeling into" the state of another person, whereas sympathy involved "feeling with" the other person, with the suggestion that the latter, while eminently responsive, was quite unreliable as a clue to the other person's feelings and state of mind. Also, it has not been uncommon for the two terms to be used as synonyms, although this has been more the case in common parlance than in clinical frames of reference. As an example of the comparing and contrasting of these two concepts, see Lauren G. Wispé, "Sympathy and Empathy," in David L. Sills (ed.), *International Encyclopedia of the Social Sciences,* 17 vols. (New York: Macmillan and Free Press, 1968), 15: 441–47 [441].

109. For detail on the historical development of empathy, see Chapter 4.

110. Recent examples of this trend are: Howard Spiro et al. (eds.), *Empathy and the Practice of Medicine: Beyond Pills and the Scalpel* (New Haven: Yale University Press, 1993); Ellen Singer More and Maureen A. Milligan (eds.), *The Empathic Practitioner: Empathy, Gender and Medicine* (New Brunswick, N.J.: Rutgers University Press, 1994).

111. F. L. Cross and E. A. Livingstone (eds.), *The Oxford Dictionary of the Christian Church,* 2nd ed. (Oxford: Oxford University Press, 1974), pp. 665–66.

112. Hebrews, 6:19.

113. Maurice B. Strauss (ed.), *Familiar Medical Quotations* (Boston: Little, Brown, 1968), p. 217.

114. W. A. F. Browne, *What Asylums Were, Are, and Ought to Be . . .* (Edinburgh: Adam and Charles Black, 1837), p. 178; see Samuel T. Coleridge, *Table Talk of Samuel Taylor Coleridge . . . ,* intro. Henry Morley (London: George Routledge and Sons, 1884), p. 174.

115. Hooker (n. 74), *Physician and Patient,* pp. 46, 344–56.

116. Daniel Hack Tuke, *Illustrations of the Influence of the Mind upon the Body in Health and Disease, Designed to Elucidate the Action of the Imagination,* 2nd ed. (Philadelphia: Henry C. Lea's Son, 1884), pp. 46–47, 51–52, 426.

117. Sigmund Freud, "Psychical (or Mental) Treatment," in *Standard Edition* (n. 95), 7: 283–302 [289].

118. James J. Walsh, *Psychotherapy: Including the History of the Use of Mental Influence, Directly and Indirectly, in Healing and the Principles for the Application of Energies Derived from the Mind to the Treatment of Disease* (New York: Appleton, 1912), p. 91.

119. Jerome D. Frank, Lester H. Gliedman, Stanley D. Imber, Anthony R. Stone, and Earl H. Nash, "Patients' Expectancies and Relearning as Factors Determining Improvement in Psychotherapy," *Amer. J. Psychiat.*, 1959, *115*, 961–68 [967].

120. Jerome D. Frank, "The Dynamics of the Psychotherapeutic Relationship: Determinants and Effects of the Therapist's Influence," *Psychiatry*, 1959, *22*, 17–39 [30–39].

121. Jerome D. Frank, "The Role of Hope in Psychotherapy," *Int. J. Psychiat.*, 1968, *5*, 383–95 [383–84].

122. Jerome D. Frank, "Psychotherapy: The Restoration of Morale," *Amer. J. Psychiat.*, 1974, *131*, 271–74 [271].

123. Thomas M. French, *The Integration of Behavior*, 3 vols. (Chicago: University of Chicago Press, 1952–1958), vol. 1.

124. Ibid., 3: 42, 410.

125. Hans W. Loewald, "On the Therapeutic Action of Psycho-Analysis," *Int. J. Psycho-Anal.*, 1960, *41*, 16–33.

126. Maxwell Gitelson, "The Curative Factors in Psycho-Analysis: I. The First Phase of Psycho-Analysis," *Int. J. Psycho-Anal.*, 1962, *43*, 194–205 [198–99].

127. William F. Lynch, *Images of Hope: Imagination as Healer of the Hopeless* (Baltimore, Md.: Helicon Press, 1965), pp. 31–32.

128. Ibid., p. 21.

129. Ezra Stotland, *The Psychology of Hope* (San Francisco: Jossey-Bass, 1969), pp. 1–2.

130. Modern authorities have discussed various groups of such factors, and the relevant literature is vast. For a few significant contributions, see Carl R. Rogers, "The Necessary and Sufficient Conditions of Therapeutic Personality Change," *J. Consult. Psychol.*, 1957, *21*, 95–103; Arthur K. Shapiro, "The Placebo Effect in the History of Medical Treatment: Implications for Psychiatry," *Amer. J. Psychiat.*, 1959, *116*, 298–304; Shapiro, "A Contribution to the History of the Placebo Effect," *Behav. Sci.*, 1960, *5*, 109–35; Jerome D. Frank, *Persuasion and Healing*, 2nd ed. (Baltimore, Md.: Johns Hopkins University Press, 1973); Frank, "Therapeutic Components of Psychotherapy," *J. Nerv. Ment. Dis.*, 1974, *159*, 325–42; Hans H. Strupp and Suzanne W. Hadley, "Specific vs Non-Specific Factors in Psychotherapy: Controlled Study of Outcome," *Arch. Gen. Psychiat.*, 1979, *36*, 1125–36. For useful reviews, see Hans H. Strupp, "Psychotherapy Research and Practice: An Overview," in Sol L. Garfield and Allen E. Bergin (eds.) *Handbook of Psychotherapy and Behavior Change: An Empirical Analysis*, 2nd ed. (New York: John Wiley & Sons, 1978), pp. 3–22; Arthur K. Shapiro and Louis A. Morris, "The Placebo Effect in Medical and Psychological Therapies," in Sol L. Garfield and Allen E. Bergin (eds.), *Handbook of Psychotherapy and Behavior Change: An Empirical Analysis*, 2nd ed. (New York: John Wiley & Sons, 1978), pp. 369–410.

131. Robert Burton, *The Anatomy of Melancholy*, ed. Floyd Dell and Paul Jordan-Smith (New York: Tudor, 1948), p. 223.

132. Laín Entralgo (n. 6), *Doctor and Patient.*

133. Leo Tolstoy, *War and Peace,* trans. Louise and Aylmer Maude (New York: Simon and Schuster, 1942), p. 727 (bk. 9, chap. 16).

134. Michael Balint, *The Doctor, His Patient, and the Illness,* 2nd ed. (London: Pitman Medical, 1968), p. 240.

135. Ibid., pp. 239–51.

136. Ibid., p. 276.

137. Richard J. Baron, "Bridging Clinical Distance: An Empathic Rediscovery of the Known," *J. Med. & Philosophy,* 1981, *6,* 5–23 [21].

138. Carol Matthau, *Among the Porcupines: A Memoir* (New York: Turtle Bay Books, 1992), p. 223.

Chapter 4: The Listening Healer

1. Wendell Johnson, *Your Most Enchanted Listener* (New York: Harper, 1956), p. 20.

2. Frieda Fromm-Reichmann, *Principles of Intensive Psychotherapy* (Chicago: University of Chicago Press, 1950), p. 7.

3. Dietrich Bonhoeffer, *Life Together,* trans. and intro. John W. Doberstein (New York: Harper & Row, 1954), pp. 97–99.

4. Don Ihde, *Listening and Voice: A Phenomenology of Sound* (Athens: Ohio State University Press, 1976), chap. 1.

5. Aristotle, "Metaphysics," in *The Complete Works of Aristotle,* 2 vols., rev. Oxford translation, ed. Jonathan Barnes (Princeton, N.J.: Princeton University Press, 1984), 2: 979b22–80a27.

6. Aristotle, *Sense and Sensibilia,* in *Works* (n. 5), 1: 436b18–37a2, 437a4–6, 437a11.

7. Ibid., 1: 437a4–6.

8. Ibid., 1: 437a11.

9. Aristotle, "On the Soul," in *Works* (n. 5), 1: 435b24–25.

10. R. S. Peters, *Brett's History of Psychology,* edited and abridged (London: Allen & Unwin, 1962), pp. 109–10.

11. Simon Kemp, *Medieval Psychology* (Westport, Conn.: Greenwood Press, 1990), p. 45.

12. Leonardo da Vinci, *Selections from the Notebooks of Leonardo da Vinci,* ed. Irma A. Richter (London: Oxford University Press, 1952), p. 110.

13. Book of Psalms, *Holy Bible, Containing the Old and New Testaments* (London: British and Foreign Bible Society, n.d.), Ps. 102.

14. Ibid., Ps. 130.

15. Ibid., Ps. 141.

16. Ibid., Ps. 142.

17. Paul R. Fleischman, *The Healing Zone: Religious Issues in Psychotherapy* (New York: Paragon House, 1989), pp. 7–8, 14.

18. James A. H. Murray et al. (eds.), *A New English Dictionary . . . ,* 13 vols. (Oxford: Clarendon Press, 1888–1933), 1: 566.

19. William A. Clebsch and Charles R. Jaekle, *Pastoral Care in Historical Perspective* (New York: Jason Aronson, 1975), p. 50.

20. Ibid., pp. 53–54.

21. E. B. Holifield, *A History of Pastoral Care in America: From Salvation to Self-Realization* (Nashville, Tenn.: Abingdon Press, 1983), p. 15.

22. Sander L. Gilman (ed.), *The Face of Madness: Hugh W. Diamond and the Origin of Psychiatric Photography,* intro. Eric T. Carlson (New York: Brunner/Mazel, 1976).

23. Michel Foucault, *The Birth of the Clinic: An Archaeology of Medical Perception,* trans. A. M. Sheridan Smith (New York: Pantheon Books, 1973), p. ix.

24. Josef Breuer and Sigmund Freud, *Studies on Hysteria,* in Sigmund Freud, *The Standard Edition of the Complete Psychological Works of Sigmund Freud,* trans. and ed. James Strachey, Anna Freud, et al., 24 vols. (London: Hogarth Press, 1953–1974), 2: 30, 33–37.

25. Henri F. Ellenberger, "The Story of 'Anna O.': A Critical Review with New Data," *J. Hist. Behav. Sci.,* 1972, *8,* 267–79 [275–76].

26. Sigmund Freud, "Recommendations to Physicians Practising Psycho-Analysis," in *Standard Edition* (n. 24), 12: 111–12.

27. Ibid., 12: 115–16.

28. An effective and representative summary of "How the Analyst Listens," was provided by Ralph R. Greenson in his textbook on psychoanalytic technique, *The Technique and Practice of Psychoanalysis* (New York: International Universities Press, 1967), pp. 100–101.

29. Paul Ricoeur, *Freud and Philosophy: An Essay on Interpretation,* trans. Denis Savage (New Haven, Conn.: Yale University Press, 1970), p. 409.

30. Theodor Reik, *Listening with the Third Ear: The Inner Experience of a Psychoanalyst* (Garden City, N.Y.: Garden City Books, 1951), pp. 144, 146–47.

31. Ibid., p. 150.

32. Charles Edward Gauss, "Empathy," in Philip P. Wiener (ed.), *Dictionary of the History of Ideas,* 5 vols. (New York: Scribner's Sons, 1973–1974), 2: 85–89.

33. Theodor Lipps, "Empathy, Inner Imitation, and Sense-Feelings," trans. Max Schertel and Melvin M. Rader, in Melvin M. Rader (ed.), *A Modern Book of Esthetics: An Anthology* (New York: Henry Holt, 1935), pp. 291–304 [302].

34. Jørgen B. Hunsdahl, "Concerning Einfühlung (Empathy): A Concept Analysis of Its Origin and Early Development," *J. Hist. Behav. Sci.,* 1967, *3,* 180–91.

35. Edward B. Titchener, *Lectures on the Experimental Psychology of the Thought-Processes* (New York: Macmillan, 1926), p. 21.

36. Freud, *Jokes and Their Relation to the Unconscious,* in *Standard Edition* (n. 24), 8: 186, 195–97.

37. Freud, *Delusions and Dreams in Jensen's Gradiva,* in *Standard Edition* (n. 24), 9: 45.

38. Freud, *Group Psychology and the Analysis of the Ego,* in *Standard Edition* (n. 24), 18: 108, 110. Basch has urged a significant correction to the *Standard Edition* translation given here. Rather than that empathy enables us "to take up any attitude at all towards another mental life," he points out, Freud's implication was that "empathy was indispensable when it came to taking a position regarding another person's mental life." Michael Franz Basch, "Empathic Understanding: A Review of the Concept and Some Theoretical Considerations, *J. Am. Psychoanal. Assoc.,* 1983, *31,* 101–26 [103].

39. Theodore Schroeder, "The Psycho-Analytic Method of Observation," *Int. J. Psycho-Anal.*, 1925, *6*, 155–70 [159].

40. Ibid., p. 162.

41. Helene Deutsch, "Occult Processes Occurring During Psychoanalysis," in George Devereux (ed.), *Psychoanalysis and the Occult* (New York: International Universities Press, 1953), pp. 133–46 [136–37].

42. Sandor Ferenczi, "The Elasticity of Psycho-Analytic Technique," in Sandor Ferenczi, *Final Contributions to the Problems and Methods of Psycho-Analysis,* ed. Michael Balint, trans. Eric Mosbacher and others, intro. Clara Thompson (New York: Basic Books, 1955), p. 89.

43. Ibid., p. 90.

44. Ibid., pp. 92, 94.

45. Ibid., p. 96.

46. Ibid., p. 100.

47. There were a few exceptions — e.g., Robert Fliess, "Metapsychology of the Analyst," *Psychoanal. Quart.*, 1942, *11*, 211–27; Robert P. Knight, "Psychotherapy of an Adolescent Catatonic Schizophrenic with Mutism: A Study in Empathy and Establishing Contact," *Psychiatry,* 1946, *9*, 323–39.

48. Robert Fliess, "Countertransference and Counteridentification," *J. Am. Psychoanal. Assoc.*, 1953, *1*, 268–84; Christine Olden, "On Adult Empathy with Children," *Psychoanalytic Study of the Child*, 1953, *8*, 111–26 (New York: International Universities Press, 1953); Olden, "Notes on the Development of Empathy," *Psychoanalytic Study of the Child,* 1958, *13*, 505–18 (New York: International Universities Press, 1958); Heinz Kohut, "Introspection, Empathy, and Psychoanalysis," *J. Am. Psychoanal. Assoc.*, 1959, *7*, 459–83; Roy Schafer, "Generative Empathy in the Treatment Situation," *Psychoanal. Quart.*, 1959, *28*, 342–73; Ralph R. Greenson, "Empathy and Its Vicissitudes," *Int. J. Psycho-Anal.*, 1960, *41*, 418–24.

49. Schafer (n. 48), p. 342.

50. Kohut (n. 48).

51. Greenson (n. 48), p. 418.

52. Charles Horton Cooley, *Sociological Theory and Social Research,* intro. and annot. Robert Cooley Angell (New York: Henry Holt, 1930), p. 290.

53. George H. Mead, *Mind, Self and Society: From the Standpoint of a Social Behaviorist,* ed. and intro. Charles W. Morris (Chicago: University of Chicago Press, 1934), pp. 253–57.

54. Carl R. Rogers, *Client-Centered Therapy: Its Current Practice, Implications, and Theory* (Boston: Houghton Mifflin, 1951), p. 29.

55. Greenson (n. 48), p. 421.

56. Evelyne Schwaber, "Empathy: A Mode of Analytic Listening," *Psychoanal. Inquiry,* 1981, *1*, 357–92; Schwaber, "Narcissism, Self Psychology and the Listening Perspective," *Annual of Psychoanalysis,* 1981, *9*, 115–32 (New York: International Universities Press, 1981); Schwaber, "Particular Perspective on Analytic Listening," *Psychoanalytic Study of the Child,* 1983, *38*, 519–46 (New Haven, Conn.: Yale University Press, 1983).

57. Schwaber (n. 56), "The Listening Perspective," p. 117.

58. Ibid., pp. 117–18.

59. Ibid., pp. 118, 124, 127.

60. Schwaber (n. 56), "Empathy," p. 358.

61. Ibid., p. 389.

62. Richard D. Chessick, *The Technique and Practice of Intensive Psychotherapy* (New York: Jason Aronson, 1974), p. 205.

63. Richard D. Chessick, *The Technique and Practice of Listening in Intensive Psychotherapy* (Northvale, N.J.: Jason Aronson, 1989), p. 21. Chessick's five "listening stances" are: (1) Freud's drive/conflict/defense orientation; (2) the perspective of object relations theory; (3) the phenomenological point of view; (4) Kohut's self psychology viewpoint; and (5) the interactive approach.

64. A representative work, such as that of Aloysius Roeggl, contained a detailed catalogue of sins, admonitions, and remedies, with advice regarding interrogation, *but* not a word about listening. Aloysius Roeggl, *The Confessional,* 6th ed., trans. and adapt. Augustine Wirth (New York: Benziger, 1882).

65. E.g., Gerald Kelly, *The Good Confessor* (New York: Sentinel Press, 1951), pp. 11–12.

66. Quentin Donoghue and Linda Shapiro, *Bless Me, Father, For I Have Sinned: Catholics Speak Out About Confession* (New York: Donald I. Fine, 1984).

67. Kenneth R. Mitchell and Herbert Anderson, *All Our Losses, All Our Griefs: Resources for Pastoral Care* (Philadelphia: Westminster Press, 1983), p. 118.

68. Arthur Kleinman, *The Illness Narratives: Suffering, Healing, and the Human Condition* (New York: Basic Books, 1988), pp. xi–xii.

69. Edward Shorter, *Bedside Manners: The Troubled History of Doctors and Patients* (Harmondsworth: Viking, 1986), pp. 252, 254, 256.

70. Howard M. Spiro, *Doctors, Patients, and Placebos* (New Haven, Conn.: Yale University Press, 1986), pp. 73–74.

71. Attributed to William Osler, but the exact source has not been identified.

Chapter 5: The Talking Cures

1. Plato, *The Dialogues of Plato,* 2 vols., trans. B. Jowett (New York: Random House, 1937), 1: 3–27 [6] [*Charmides,* 157].

2. Helen North, *Sophrosyne: Self-Knowledge and Self-Restraint in Greek Literature* (Ithaca, N.Y.: Cornell University Press, 1966).

3. Pedro Laín Entralgo, *The Therapy of the Word in Classical Antiquity,* trans. L. J. Rather and John M. Sharp (New Haven, Conn.: Yale University Press, 1970), pp. 112, 121.

4. North (n. 2), *Sophrosyne,* p. 153.

5. Laín Entralgo (n. 3), *Therapy of the Word,* chaps. 1 and 2.

6. Ibid., p. 71.

7. Aeschylus, *Prometheus Bound,* trans. David Grene, in *The Complete Greek Tragedies,* 4 vols., ed. David Grene and Richmond Lattimore (Chicago: University of Chicago Press, 1959), 1: 303–51 [325] [*Prometheus Bound,* 379–82].

8. Cicero, *Tusculan Disputations,* trans. J. E. King (Cambridge: Harvard University Press, 1945), bk. III, xxxi.

9. Laín Entralgo (n. 3), *Therapy of the Word,* pp. 87–102.

10. Ibid., p. 91.

11. Ibid., pp. 97–98.

12. Ibid., pp. 108–38.

13. Ibid., p. 123.

14. Ibid., pp. 126–37.

15. Plato (n. 1), *Dialogues,* 2: 491 [*Laws* IV, 720].

16. Rufus of Ephesus, "On the Interrogation of the Patient," in Arthur J. Brock (ed.), *Greek Medicine: Being Extracts Illustrative of Medical Writers from Hippocrates to Galen* (London: Dent & Sons, 1929), pp. 112–24.

17. Ibid., pp. 113–14.

18. Laín Entralgo (n. 3), *Therapy of the Word,* pp. 139–70.

19. For detailed attention to this theme, see Chapter 9.

20. Hippocrates, *Humours,* in *Works of Hippocrates,* 4 vols., trans. and ed. W. H. S. Jones and E. T. Withington (Cambridge: Harvard University Press, 1923–1931), 4: 61–95 [81] [*Humours,* IX].

21. Aristotle, *Rhetoric,* in *The Complete Works of Aristotle.,* 2 vols., ed. Jonathan Barnes (Princeton, N.J.: Princeton University Press, 1984), 2: 1356a3–25, 1377b15–1378a20.

22. Laín Entralgo has reasoned at length on this matter (n. 3), *Therapy of the Word,* pp. 183–229.

23. Caelius Aurelianus, *On Acute Diseases and on Chronic Diseases,* ed. and trans. I. E. Drabkin (Chicago: University of Chicago Press, 1950), p. 551.

24. Donald Lemen Clark, *Rhetoric in Greco-Roman Education* (New York: Columbia University Press, 1957); George A. Kennedy, *The Art of Persuasion in Greece* (Princeton, N.J.: Princeton University Press, 1963); Kennedy, *Greek Rhetoric Under Christian Emperors* (Princeton, N.J.: Princeton University Press, 1983).

25. Richard M. Ratzan and Gary B. Ferngren, "A Greek Progymnasma on the Physician-Poisoner," *J. Hist. Med. Allied Sci.,* 1993, *48,* 157–70.

26. For a more detailed account of this theme, see Chapter 8.

27. Martha C. Nussbaum, *The Therapy of Desire: Theory and Practice in Hellenistic Ethics* (Princeton, N.J.: Princeton University Press, 1994).

28. Ibid., pp. 13–15.

29. Ibid., p. 49.

30. Robert Burton, *The Anatomy of Melancholy,* ed. Floyd Dell and Paul Jordan-Smith (New York: Tudor Publishing, 1948), pp. 471–75.

31. Ibid., p. 476.

32. Ibid., pp. 777–78.

33. Ibid., pp. 491–557.

34. Galen, *On the Passions and Errors of the Soul,* trans. Paul W. Harkins, intro. Walther Riese (Columbus: Ohio State University Press, 1963).

35. Josef Breuer and Sigmund Freud, *Studies on Hysteria,* (1895), in *The Standard Edition of the Complete Psychological Works of Sigmund Freud,* 24 vols., trans. and ed. James Strachey, Anna Freud, et al. (London: Hogarth Press, 1955–1974), 2: 30.

36. Ibid., pp. 33–37.

37. Ibid., p. 56.

38. Ibid., p. 63.

39. Ibid., chaps 1, 4.

40. Ibid., p. 280.

41. Freud, "The Neuro-Psychoses of Defence" (1894), in *Standard Edition* (n. 35), 3: 50.

42. Freud, "Psychical (or Mental) Treatment" (1905), in *Standard Edition* (n. 35), 7: 283, 292. This work has usually been cited as having been published in 1905, but that publication was actually the third edition, with no changes in the text. The first edition was published in 1890. See James Strachey, "Editor's Introduction" to Freud's "Papers on Hypnotism and Suggestion," in *Standard Edition* (n. 35), 1: 63–64.

43. Breuer and Freud, *Studies on Hysteria,* in *Standard Edition* (n. 35), 2: 106–24, 135–81, 255–305. These references are to the cases of Miss Lucy R. and Fräulein Elisabeth von R., and to Freud's chapter "The Psychotherapy of Hysteria."

44. Freud, *Interpretation of Dreams* (1900), in *Standard Edition* (n. 35), vols. 4–5.

45. Ibid., 4: 101.

46. Ibid., 4: 102. In a detailed study of free association, Patrick Mahony mentions several accounts of earlier behaviors that have some kinship to free association, although it is uncertain what their influence on Freud might have been and although they do not address the role of talking in psychological healing. "The Boundaries of Free Association," *Psychoanalysis and Contemporary Thought,* 1979, 2, 151–98 [152–53].

47. Freud, *Introductory Lectures on Psycho-Analysis* (1916–17), in *Standard Edition* (n. 35), vols. 15–16, 15: 17.

48. William Labov and David Fanshel, *Therapeutic Discourse: Psychotherapy as Conversation* (New York: Academic Press, 1977), p. 8.

49. Ibid., p. ix.

50. Ibid., p. 1.

51. Ibid., p. 349.

52. Kathleen Warden Ferrara, *Therapeutic Ways with Words* (New York: Oxford University Press, 1994), pp. 3–5.

53. Ibid., p. 167.

54. Ibid., p. 168.

55. Brian Bird, *Talking with Patients,* 2nd ed. (Philadelphia: Lippincott, 1973), p. 1.

Chapter 6: Catharsis and Abreaction

1. James A. H. Murray et al. (eds.), *A New English Dictionary.*

2. Ibid.

3. Ibid.

4. Sue Walrond-Skinner, *Dictionary of Psychotherapy* (London: Routledge & Kegan Paul, 1986), p. 45.

5. Ibid., p. 2.

6. Horace B. English and Ava Champney English, *A Comprehensive Dictionary of Psychological and Psychoanalytical Terms* (New York: Longmans, Green, 1958), p. 77.

7. Ibid., p. 2.

8. G. B. Kerferd, "Katharsis," in Paul Edwards (ed.), *The Encyclopedia of Philosophy*, 8 vols. (New York: Macmillan Publishing and Free Press, 1967), 4: 326–27.

9. J. H. T. [J. H. Tufts], "Catharsis," in James Mark Baldwin et al. (eds.), *Dictionary of Philosophy and Psychology*, 3 vols. (New York: Macmillan, 1901), 1: 161–62.

10. Ibid., p. 162. By 1931 the number of different interpretations had grown to more than 1,400, and numerous new interpretations have appeared since then. Teddy Brunius, *Inspiration and Katharsis: The Interpretation of Aristotle's The Poetics VI, 1449 b 26.* (Uppsala, Sweden: 1966), p. 9.

11. E. R. Dodds, *The Greeks and the Irrational* (Boston: Beacon Press, 1957), p. 37.

12. Pedro Laín Entralgo, *The Therapy of the Word in Classical Antiquity*, ed. and trans. L. J. Rather and John M. Sharp (New Haven, Conn.: Yale University Press, 1970), p. 41.

13. Ibid., pp. 128–29.

14. Ibid., pp. 131–32.

15. Ibid., pp. 135–37.

16. The passages that have been assiduously studied and argued about by so many scholars over the centuries are *The Poetics*, 6, 1449 b 24–28, and *The Politics*, VIII, 7. Aristotle, *The Complete Works of Aristotle*, 2 vols., ed. Jonathan Barnes (Princeton, N.J.: Princeton University Press, 1984). Laín Entralgo (n. 12), in his *Therapy of the Word*, tended to favor "compassion and fear," but the commonest translation has been "pity and fear," and an occasional translation has been "pity and terror."

17. Laín Entralgo (n. 12), *Therapy of the Word*, pp. 183–239.

18. Emma J. Edelstein and Ludwig Edelstein, *Asclepius: A Collection and Interpretation of the Testimonies*, 2 vols. (Baltimore, Md.: Johns Hopkins Press, 1945), 2: 145–58.

19. Brunius (n. 10), *Inspiration and Katharsis*, pp. 68–79.

20. Teddy Brunius, "Catharsis," in Philip P. Wiener (ed.), *Dictionary of the History of Ideas*, 4 vols. (New York: Charles Scribner's Sons, 1968–1973), 1: 269.

21. Dodds (n. 11), *Greeks and the Irrational*, pp. 76–78.

22. Ibid., p. 37.

23. The modern experimental studies of James W. Pennebaker have strongly supported the notion that catharsis was an inherent aspect of health-promoting confessions. See James W. Pennebaker, "Confession, Inhibition, and Disease," in L. Berkowitz (ed.) *Advances in Experimental Social Psychology*, vol. 22 (New York: Academic Press, 1989).

24. Brunius (n. 20), "Catharsis," p. 267.

25. Franciscus Mercurius Van Helmont, *The Spirit of Disease; or, Diseases from the Spirit: Laid open in some Observations Concerning Man, and his Diseases. Wherein is showed how much the Mind influenceth the Body in causing and curing of Diseases . . .* (London: Sarah Howkins, 1694), pp. 46–47. Cited by Richard Hunter and Ida Macalpine, *Three Hundred Years of Psychiatry, 1535–1860* (London: Oxford University Press, 1963), pp. 256–57.

26. Benjamin Rush, *Medical Inquiries and Observations, upon the Diseases of the Mind* (Philadelphia: Kimber & Richardson, 1812), p. 343. Cited by Eric T. Carlson and Meribeth M. Simpson, "Moral Persuasion as Therapy," in Jules H. Masserman (ed.), *Current Psychiatric Therapies*, vol. 4 (New York: Grune & Stratton, 1964), p. 21.

27. Jakob Bernays, *Grundzüge der verlorenen Abhandlung des Aristoteles über Wirkung der Tragödie* (Breslau: Eduard Trewendt, 1857). Reprinted in *Zwei Abhandlungen über die aristotelische Theorie des Dramas* (Berlin: Wilhelm Hertz, 1880).

28. Laín Entralgo (n. 12), *Therapy of the Word,* pp. 186–89, 200.

29. Josef Breuer and Sigmund Freud, *Studies on Hysteria,* in Sigmund Freud, *The Standard Edition of the Complete Psychological Works of Sigmund Freud,* trans. and ed. James Strachey, Anna Freud, et al., 24 vols. (London: Hogarth Press, 1953–1974), 2: ix–xxxi, 22–28. The French term *absence* was used to refer to a period of apparent unconsciousness, characterized by suspended or merely automatic activity and by amnesia for events during that period.

30. Ibid., p. 35.
31. Ibid., p. 46.
32. Ibid., p. 3.
33. Ibid., p. 6.
34. Ibid., pp. 8–11.
35. Ibid., p. 17.
36. Ibid., pp. 262, 266–67.
37. Ibid., pp. 268–70.
38. Ibid., pp. 283–84, 287.

39. P. M. F. Janet, *L'automatisme psychologique: Essai de psychologie expérimentale* (Paris: Alcan, 1889), pp. 439–40. It is also significant that Janet's cathartic work with Lucie was reported in 1886, "Les actes inconscients et le dédoublement de la personnalité pendant le somnambulisme provoqué," *Revue Philosophique,* 1886, 22, 577–92.

40. Breuer and Freud, *Studies on Hysteria,* in *Standard Edition* (n. 29), 2.

41. Pierre Janet, *Psychological Healing: A Historical and Clinical Study,* 2 vols., trans. Eden and Cedar Paul (New York: Macmillan, 1925) 1: 589–698.

42. Ibid., pp. 601–2.

43. Pierre Janet, *Principles of Psychotherapy,* trans. H. M. and E. R. Guthrie (London: Allen & Unwin, 1925), p. 41.

44. Janet (n. 41), *Psychological Healing,* 1: 681–87.

45. Breuer and Freud, *Studies on Hysteria,* in *Standard Edition* (n. 29), 2: 7, quoting J. R. L. Delboeuf, *Le magnétisme animal* (Paris: Germer Baillière, 1889).

46. Breuer and Freud, *Studies on Hysteria,* in *Standard Edition* (n. 29), 2: 7; Alfred Binet, *Les altérations de la personnalité* (Paris: Germer Baillière, 1892), p. 243.

47. H. Bourru and P. Burot, "Un cas de neurasthénie hystérique avec double personnalité," *First International Congress of Experimental and Therapeutic Hypnotism* (Paris: Doin, 1889), pp. 228–40.

48. L. Chertok, "On the Discovery of the Cathartic Method," *Int. J. Psycho-Anal.,* 1961, 42, 284–87.

49. Ibid., p. 285.

50. Ibid., p. 286. Ellenberger would surely have disagreed with this suggestion of priority. As he pointed out, in 1886 Janet "published the result of his work with the patient Lucie." He goes on to state that this case "is considered the first cathartic cure on record." Henri F. Ellenberger, *The Discovery of the Unconscious: The History and Evolution of Dynamic Psychiatry* (New York: Basic Books, 1970), p. 755. Though this assertion

appears to have been aimed at Breuer and Freud's claim for Breuer's priority (Anna O. was treated in 1880–1882), it would seem also to contradict Chertok's claim for Bourru and Burot, who did their clinical work in 1887 and reported it in 1889. Yet these competing claims must all yield to the data I will cite on Hoek's work, carried out in 1851 and reported in 1868. All this merely adds strength to the view that cathartic notions were "in the air" in this era.

51. Onno van der Hart and Kees van der Velden, "The Hypnotherapy of Dr. Andries Hoek: Uncovering Hypnotherapy Before Janet, Breuer, and Freud," *Am. J. Clin. Hypn.,* 1987, *29,* 264–71. For the original publication of this case, see A. Hoek, *Eenvoudige mededeelingen aangaande de genezing van eene krankzinnige door het levens-magnetismus* ('s Gravenhage: De Gebroeders van Cleef, 1868).

52. Van der Hart and van der Velden (n. 51), p. 265.

53. Ibid., pp. 265–66.

54. Freud, "Sexuality in the Aetiology of the Neuroses," in *Standard Edition* (n. 29), 3: 282.

55. Freud, "Freud's Psycho-Analytic Procedure," in *Standard Edition* (n. 29), 7: 249.

56. Freud, "On Psychotherapy," in *Standard Edition* (n. 29), 7: 259.

57. Freud, *Three Essays on the Theory of Sexuality,* in *Standard Edition* (n. 29), 7: 163.

58. Freud, "A Short Account of Psycho-Analysis," in *Standard Edition* (n. 29), 19: 194.

59. Sandor Ferenczi, "The Principle of Relaxation and Neocatharsis," in Sandor Ferenczi, *Final Contributions to the Problems and Methods of Psycho-Analysis,* ed. Michael Balint, trans. Eric Mosbacher et al., intro. Clara Thompson (New York: Basic Books, 1955), pp. 115–18.

60. Ibid., pp. 118–19.

61. Franz Alexander, "The Problem of Psychoanalytic Technique," in Franz Alexander, *The Scope of Psychoanalysis, 1921–1961: Selected Papers of Franz Alexander* (New York: Basic Books, 1961), p. 228.

62. Ralph R. Greenson, *The Technique and Practice of Psychoanalysis* (New York: International Universities Press, 1967), pp. 48–49.

63. Paul A. Dewald, *The Psychoanalytic Process: A Case Illustration* (New York: Basic Books, 1972), pp. 621–22.

64. William A. Binstock, "Purgation Through Pity and Terror," *Int. J. Psycho-Anal.,* 1973, *54,* 499–504 [504].

65. Bennett Simon, *Mind and Madness in Ancient Greece: The Classical Roots of Modern Psychiatry* (Ithaca, N.Y.: Cornell University Press, 1978), p. 141.

66. Michael P. Nichols and Melvin Zax, *Catharsis in Psychotherapy* (New York: Gardner Press, 1977), p. 1.

67. Martin Stone, "Shellshock and the Psychologists," in W. F. Bynum, Roy Porter, and Michael Shepherd (eds.), *The Anatomy of Madness: Essays in the History of Psychiatry,* 2 vols. (London: Tavistock, 1985), 2: 250–51.

68. Ibid., p. 243.

69. William Brown, "The Revival of Emotional Memories and Its Therapeutic Value (I)," *Brit. J. Psychol., Medical Section,* 1920, *1,* 16–19 [16].

70. Ibid., pp. 16–18.

71. W. McDougall, "The Revival of Emotional Memories and Its Therapeutic Value (III)," *Brit. J. Psychol., Medical Section,* 1920, *1,* 23–29 [25, 28].

72. C. G. Jung, "The Therapeutic Value of Abreaction," in Herbert Read et al. (eds.), *The Collected Works of C. G. Jung,* 20 vols. (Princeton, N.J.: Princeton University Press, 1957–1979), 16: 129–38 [131]. This is a slightly revised version of the original which appeared in *Brit. J. Psychol., Medical Section,* 1921, 2, 13–22.

73. Ernst Simmel, "War Neuroses," in Sandor Lorand (ed.), *Psychoanalysis Today* (New York: International Universities Press, 1944), pp. 227–48.

74. Jose Brunner, "Psychiatry, Psychoanalysis, and Politics During the First World War," *J. Hist. Behav. Sci.,* 1991, 27, 352–65.

75. Simmel (n. 73), p. 227.

76. Ibid., p. 246.

77. E.g., John G. Watkins, *Hypnotherapy of War Neuroses: A Clinical Psychologist's Casebook* (New York: Ronald Press, 1949).

78. E.g., J. S. Horsley, "Narco-Analysis," *J. Ment. Sci.,* 1936, 82, 416–22.

79. E.g., Roy R. Grinker and John P. Spiegel, *Men Under Stress* (Philadelphia: Blakiston, 1945).

80. E.g., H. J. Shorvon and William Sargant, "Excitatory Abreaction: with Special Reference to Its Mechanism and the Use of Ether," *J. Ment. Sci.,* 1947, 93, 709–32.

81. E.g., Anthony Hordern, "The Response of the Neurotic Personality to Abreaction," *J. Ment. Sci.,* 1952, 98, 630–39.

82. E.g., C. H. Rogerson, "Narco-Analysis with Nitrous Oxide," *Brit. Med. J.,* 1944, 1, 811–12.

83. Edward Bibring, "Psychoanalysis and the Dynamic Psychotherapies," *J. Am. Psychoanal. Assoc.,* 1954, 2, 745–70 [745–46].

84. Ibid., pp. 748–49.

85. J. L. Moreno, "Psychodrama," in Silvano Arieti (ed.), *American Handbook of Psychiatry,* 3 vols. (New York: Basic Books, 1959–1966), 2: 1375–96; Moreno, *Psychodrama* (New York: Beacon House, 1946).

86. Binstock (n. 64), p. 503.

87. Wilhelm Reich, *Character-Analysis* (New York: Orgone Institute Press, 1949); Reich, *Selected Writings: An Introduction to Orgonomy* (New York: Farrar, Straus and Cudahy, 1960), pp. 57–186.

88. Alexander Lowen, *Bioenergetics* (New York: Coward, McCann & Geoghegan, 1975).

89. Ibid., p. 45.

90. Frederick Perls, Ralph E. Hefferline, Paul Goodman, *Gestalt Therapy: Excitement and Growth in the Human Personality* (New York: Dell, 1951); Joen Fagan and Irma Lee Shepherd (eds.), *Gestalt Therapy Now: Theory, Techniques, Applications* (New York: Harper Colophon, 1971); Erving Polster and Miriam Polster, *Gestalt Therapy Integrated: Contours of Theory and Practice* (New York: Brunner/Mazel, 1973); Chris Hatcher and Philip Himelstein (eds.), *The Handbook of Gestalt Therapy* (New York: Jason Aronson, 1976).

91. Polster and Polster (n. 90), *Gestalt Therapy Integrated,* p. ix.

92. Arthur Janov, *The Primal Scream: Primal Therapy, the Cure for Neurosis* (New York: Putnam's Sons, 1970).

93. Ibid., p. 385.

94. Joseph T. Coltrera and Nathaniel Ross, "Freud's Psychoanalytic Technique — From

the Beginnings to 1923," in Benjamin B. Wolman (ed.), *Psychoanalytic Techniques: A Handbook for the Practicing Psychoanalyst* (New York: Basic Books, 1967), pp. 23–24.

95. Berkowitz has termed the advocates of such approaches ventilationists. Leonard Berkowitz, "The Case for Bottling Up Rage," *Psychology Today*, 1973, 7, 24–31.

96. Percival M. Symonds, "A Comprehensive Theory of Psychotherapy," *Am. J. Orthopsychiatry*, 1954, 24, 697–712 [699].

97. Ibid., p. 711. This theme can be found as a red thread running through the literature of cathartic therapy over many decades. Freud, in Breuer and Freud, *Studies on Hysteria*, in *Standard Edition* (n. 29), pp. 282–83; Jung (n. 72), p. 132; Simmel (n. 73), p. 244.

98. Frederick H. Lowy, "The Abuse of Abreaction: An Unhappy Legacy of Freud's Cathartic Method," *Can. Psychiat. Assoc. J.*, 1970, 15, 557–65 [562].

99. Nichols and Zax (n. 66), *Catharsis and Psychotherapy*, pp. 1, 210, 217.

100. T. J. Scheff, *Catharsis in Healing, Ritual, and Drama* (Berkeley: University of California Press, 1979), pp. 13–14.

Chapter 7: Confession and Confiding

1. James A. H. Murray et al. (eds.), *A New English Dictionary . . .* , 13 vols. (Oxford: Clarendon Press, 1888–1933), 2: 801.

2. Anna Robeson Burr, *Religious Confession and Confessants: With a Chapter on the History of Introspection* (Boston: Houghton Mifflin, 1914), p. 19.

3. Raffaele Pettazzoni, "Confession of Sins and the Classics," *Harvard Theological Review*, 1937, 30, 1–14 [14].

4. James Hastings (ed.), *Encyclopaedia of Religion and Ethics*, 13 vols. (New York: Charles Scribner's Sons, 1908–1927) 3: 825–26.

5. *Encyclopaedia Britannica*, 11th ed., 29 vols. (New York: Encyclopaedia Britannica, 1910–1911), *see* "Confession."

6. Quentin Donoghue and Linda Shapiro, *Bless Me, Father, For I Have Sinned: Catholics Speak Out About Confession* (New York: Donald I. Fine, 1984), p. 15.

7. Henry Charles Lea, *A History of Auricular Confession and Indulgences in the Latin Church*, 3 vols. (New York: Greenwood Press, 1968), 1: 227–73.

8. H. J. Schroeder, *Disciplinary Decrees of the General Councils: Text, Translation, and Commentary* (St. Louis: Herder, 1937), pp. 236–96.

9. Ibid., pp. 259–63.

10. *Encyclopaedia Britannica*, 14th ed., 24 vols. (Chicago: William Benton, 1956), *see* "Confession."

11. John T. McNeill, "Medicine for Sin as Prescribed in the Penitentials," *Church History*, 1932, 1, 14–26.

12. Galen, "Quod optimus medicus sit quoque philosophus," in Galen, *Opera omnia*, ed. C. G. Kühn, 20 vols. (Leipzig: Cnobloch, 1821–1833), 1: 53–63 [61].

13. Stephen R. Ell, "Concepts of Disease and the Physician in the Early Middle Ages," *Janus*, 1978, 65, 153–65 [156].

14. Stephen D'Irsay, "Patristic Medicine," *Ann. Med. Hist.*, 1927, 9, 364–78.

15. John T. McNeill and Helena M. Gamer, *Medieval Handbooks of Penance . . .* (New

York: Octagon Books, 1979), p. 44. For Cassian, see his *Conferences,* ed. Edgar C. S. Gibson, in *The Nicene and Post-Nicene Fathers,* 2nd series, vol. 11 (Grand Rapids, Mich.: Eerdmans, 1978).

16. McNeill and Gamer (n. 15), *Medieval Handbooks of Penance,* pp. 45–46.

17. Robert Grosseteste, *Templum Dei,* ed. Joseph Goering and F. A. C. Mantello (Toronto: Pontifical Institute of Mediaeval Studies, 1984); E. J. Arnould, *Le manuel des péchés: Etude de littérature religieuse anglo-normande (XIIIe siècle)* (Paris: Librairie Droz, 1940); Robert Mannyng of Brunne, *Handlyng Synne,* ed. Idelle Sullens (Binghamton, N.Y.: Medieval & Renaissance Texts & Studies, 1983).

18. E. J. Arnould (ed.), *Le Livre de Seyntz Medicines, The Unpublished Devotional Treatise of Henry of Lancaster* (Oxford: Blackwell, 1940).

19. E. R. Dodds, *Pagan and Christian in an Age of Anxiety* (Cambridge: Cambridge University Press, 1965), p. 28, n. 2.

20. Pettazzoni (n. 3), pp. 2–3.

21. Ell (n. 13), p. 157.

22. Schroeder (n. 8), *Disciplinary Decrees,* p. 260.

23. McNeill (n. 11); McNeill and Gamer (n. 12), *Medieval Handbooks of Penance.*

24. Schroeder (n. 8), *Disciplinary Decrees,* p. 263.

25. Ibid., pp. 263–64; Lea (n. 7), *History of Auricular Confession,* 1: 262–67.

26. Known also for his *Breviarium Bartholomei,* an extensive compilation from the medical writings considered authoritative in his time, Mirfeld had knitted together numerous selections, both medical and theological, in this chapter from his *Florarium Bartholomei,* otherwise a theological treatise. Percival Horton-Smith Hartley and Harold Richard Aldridge, *Johannes de Mirfeld of St. Bartholomew's, Smithfeld: His Life and Works* (Cambridge: Cambridge University Press, 1936), p. 127.

27. Michael MacDonald, *Mystical Bedlam: Madness, Anxiety, and Healing in Seventeenth-Century England* (Cambridge: Cambridge University Press, 1981); MacDonald "Religion, Social Change, and Psychological Healing in England, 1600–1800," in W. J. Sheils (ed.), *The Church and Healing* (Oxford: Basil Blackwell, 1982).

28. Robert Burton, *The Anatomy of Melancholy,* ed. Floyd Dell and Paul Jordan-Smith (New York: Tudor Publishing, 1948), p. 966 [pt. 3, sec. 4, memb. 2, subs. 6].

29. John Sym, *Lifes Preservative Against Self-Killing . . .* (London: Dawlman and Fawne, 1637), pp. 311–26; a valuable facsimile reprint of this work is available, edited with an introduction by Michael MacDonald (London/New York: Routledge, 1988).

30. Ibid., pp. 316–19.

31. MacDonald (n. 27), *Mystical Bedlam,* p. 177.

32. Henri F. Ellenberger, "The Pathogenic Secret and Its Therapeutics," *J. Hist. Behav. Sci.,* 1966, 2, 29–42.

33. Ibid., p. 29.

34. Raffaele Pettazzoni, *La Confessione dei peccati,* 3 vols. (Bologna: Zanichelli, 1929–1936). The materials on so-called primitive societies are found in vol. 1. This volume has been published in enlarged and revised form as *La confession des péchés,* 2 vols., trans. R. Monnot (Paris: Librairie Ernest Leroux, 1931–1932), with these materials in vol. 1. See also H. S. Darlington, "The Confession of Sins," *Psychoanalytic Rev.,* 1937, 24, 150–64; Weston La Barre, "Confession as Cathartic Therapy in American Indian

Tribes," in Ari Kiev (ed.), *Magic, Faith, and Healing: Studies in Primitive Psychiatry Today* (New York: Free Press, 1964).

35. Pettazzoni has stated that sexual offences were the commonest confessed sins among so-called primitive peoples — "Confession of Sins: An Attempted General Interpretation," in Raffaele Pettazzoni, *Essays on the History of Religions,* trans. H. J. Rose (Leiden: Brill, 1954).

36. Ibid., pp. 53–54.

37. Darlington (n. 34), p. 150.

38. Pettazzoni (n. 35), pp. 49–50.

39. La Barre (n. 34), p. 45.

40. E. Fuller Torrey, *Witchdoctors and Psychiatrists: The Common Roots of Psychotherapy and Its Future* (Northvale, N.J.: Jason Aronson, 1986), p. 88.

41. Ibid., pp. 107–8.

42. Murray et al. (n. 1), *Oxford English Dictionary,* 2: 803.

43. Francis Bacon, *The Essayes: Or Counsels Civill & Morall of Francis Bacon* (New York: Heritage Press, 1944), pp. 86–87.

44. Burton (n. 28), *Anatomy of Melancholy,* pp. 471–72 [pt. 2, sec. 2, memb. 6, subs. 1 and 2].

45. See Chapter 3.

46. Josef Breuer and Sigmund Freud, in *Studies on Hysteria,* in James Strachey, Anna Freud, et al. (eds.), *The Standard Edition of the Complete Psychological Works of Sigmund Freud,* 24 vols. (London: Hogarth Press, 1953–1974), 2: 210–11.

47. Ibid., p. 282.

48. Freud, *The Question of Lay Analysis,* in *Standard Edition* (n. 46), 20: 189.

49. C. G. Jung, "Psychotherapists or the Clergy," in Herbert Read et al. (eds.), *The Collected Works of C. G. Jung,* 20 vols. in 21 (Princeton, N.J.: Princeton University Press, 1957–1979), 11: 344.

50. Jung, "Yoga and the West," *Collected Works* (n. 49), 11: 536.

51. Jung, "Problems of Modern Psychotherapy," *Collected Works* (n. 49), 16: 55.

52. Ibid., pp. 59–60.

53. Maurice Levine, *Psychotherapy in Medical Practice* (New York: Macmillan, 1947), pp. 109–21.

54. Ibid., p. 113.

55. Lewis R. Wolberg, *The Technique of Psychotherapy,* 2nd ed., 2 vols. (New York: Grune & Stratton, 1972), 1: 87–90.

56. Karl Menninger, *Theory of Psychoanalytic Technique* (New York: Basic Books, 1958), pp. 100–101.

57. James W. Pennebaker, "Confession, Inhibition, and Disease," in L. Berkowitz (ed.), *Advances in Experimental Social Psychology,* vol. 22 (New York: Academic Press, 1989).

58. Jung, "The Therapeutic Value of Abreaction," *Collected Works,* (n. 49), 16: 132.

Chapter 8: Consolation and Comfort

1. James A. H. Murray et al. (eds.), *A New English Dictionary . . . ,* 13 vols. (Oxford: Clarendon Press, 1888–1933), 2: 865.

2. J. G. James, "Consolation, Comfort (Christian)," in James Hastings (ed.), *Encyclopaedia of Religion and Ethics,* 13 vols. (New York: Charles Scribner's Sons, 1908–1927), 4: 71–72.

3. W. Kroll, "Consolation (Greek and Roman)," in Hastings (n. 2), *Encyclopaedia,* 4: 73–74.

4. N. G. L. Hammond and H. H. Scullard (eds.), *The Oxford Classical Dictionary,* 2nd ed. (Oxford: Clarendon Press, 1970), p. 279.

5. Pedro Laín Entralgo, *The Therapy of the Word in Classical Antiquity,* ed. and trans. L. J. Rather and John M. Sharp (New Haven, Conn.: Yale University Press, 1970), pp. 97–98. See Pseudo-Plutarch, *Antiphon* in *Vitae Decem Oratorum,* 833 c–d. Plutarch, *Plutarch's Moralia,* trans. Frank Cole Babbitt et al., 15 vols. (Cambridge: Harvard University Press, 1949–1976), 10: 351 (trans. Harold North Fowler). Probably not actually by Plutarch, thus designated Pseudo-Plutarch, or Ps.-Plutarch.

6. Robert C. Gregg, *Consolation Philosophy: Greek and Christian Paideia in Basil and the Two Gregories* (Cambridge, Mass.: Philadelphia Patristic Foundation, 1975), p. 81.

7. Ibid., p. 82.

8. Kroll (n. 3), p. 74.

9. Cicero, *Tusculan Disputations,* trans. J. E. King (Cambridge: Harvard University Press, 1966), III: 6.

10. Plutarch (n. 5), *Plutarch's Moralia,* 2: 111. Both this passage and the previous one from Cicero are drawn upon in an extensive and valuable treatment of the issues involved in "the problem of 'appropriate grief' " by Gregg (n. 6), *Consolation Philosophy,* chap. 3.

11. Cicero (n. 9), *Tusculan Disputations.* Themes of the developing tradition of consolation are particularly to be found in Books I and III.

12. Seneca, *Ad Lucilium Epistulae Morales,* trans. Richard M. Gummere, 3 vols. (Cambridge: Harvard University Press, 1967–1971), 1: epistle 63, and 3: epistle 99; Seneca, *Moral Essays,* trans. John W. Basore, 3 vols. (Cambridge: Harvard University Press, 1965–1975), 2: bks. 6 and 11.

13. Plutarch (n. 5), *Moralia,* 2: 105–211; 7: 575–605.

14. Seneca (n. 12), *Moral Essays,* 2: viii.

15. Plutarch (n. 5), *Moralia,* 2: 113.

16. Ibid., 7: 575–605.

17. Hammond and Scullard (n. 4), *Oxford Classical Dictionary,* p. 279.

18. James (n. 2), pp. 71–73.

19. For the following outline I am indebted to Gregg (n. 6), *Consolation Philosophy.*

20. Sister Mary Melchior Beyenka, *Consolation in Saint Augustine* (Washington, D.C.: Catholic University of America Press, 1950), pp. 18–19.

21. John Chrysostom, "The Homilies on the Statues," trans. W. R. W. Stephens, in *Nicene and Post-Nicene Fathers,* 14 vols., ed. Philip Schaff (New York: Christian Literature, 1886–1889), First Series, 9: 315–489 [381].

22. Beyenka (n. 20), *Consolation,* p. 24.

23. John Chrysostom, "Letter to a Young Widow," in *Nicene and Post-Nicene Fathers* (n. 21), 9: 121–28.

24. Ibid., p. 121.

25. Beyenka (n. 20), *Consolation,* pp. 27–29.

26. Ibid., p. 30.

27. In one of his writings Augustine used *consolatory* as a synonym for *exhortatory,* reflecting perhaps his training in rhetoric, where consolatory speech was classified under exhortatory speech — see Beyenka (n. 20), *Consolation,* p. 70. Certainly, the art of persuasion is apparent in much of the consolatory literature.

28. Ibid., pp. 31–37. Saint Augustine, *Confessions,* trans., intro., and annot. Henry Chadwick (Oxford: Oxford University Press, 1991), bks. III, IV, IX.

29. Beyenka (n. 20), *Consolation,* p. 44.

30. Ibid., pp. 44–45, 50. Here Beyenka draws on numerous instances of these themes scattered through many of Augustine's works. See her pp. 56–57.

31. Boethius, *The Consolation of Philosophy,* trans., ed., and intro. Richard Green (Indianapolis, Ind.: Bobbs-Merrill, 1962); Howard Rollin Patch, *The Tradition of Boethius: A Study of His Importance in Medieval Culture* (New York: Oxford University Press, 1935).

32. Boethius (n. 31), *Consolation,* p. 7.

33. Ibid., p. xxiii. The medical metaphor is not merely the editor's contribution. Such usages are scattered within Boethius' text.

34. John T. McNeill, *A History of the Cure of Souls* (New York: Harper Torchbooks, 1951); Charles Jaekle and William A. Clebsch, *Pastoral Care in Historical Perspective* (New York: Jason Aronson, 1964).

35. George William McClure, Jr., "The Renaissance Vision of Solace and Tranquillity: Consolation and Therapeutic Wisdom in Italian Thought." Ph.D. dissertation, University of Michigan, 1981, pp. 52–76. Here, and in the discussion of consolation in the Renaissance, I am indebted to this valuable study and to its published version, *Sorrow and Consolation in Italian Humanism* (Princeton, N.J.: Princeton University Press, 1991).

36. McClure (n. 35), *Renaissance Vision,* pp. 59–62.

37. Ibid., pp. 73–74. Translated and quoted by McClure from Albertano da Brescia, *Liber consolationis et consilii,* ed. Thor Sundby (London, 1873), p. 1.

38. McClure (n. 35), *Renaissance Vision,* pp. 77–78.

39. Ibid., p. 79.

40. Petrarch, *Petrarch's Secret, or the Soul's Conflict with Passion* . . . , trans. William H. Draper (Westport, Conn.: Hyperion Press, 1978), p. 84. Petrarch outlined the details of his clinical state on pp. 84–106.

41. McClure (n. 35), *Renaissance Vision,* pp. 111–12.

42. Ibid., pp. 122–24.

43. Ibid., pp. 127, 131.

44. Petrarch, *Petrarch's Remedies for Fortune Fair and Foul,* trans. and commentary by Conrad H. Rawski, 5 vols. (Bloomington: Indiana University Press, 1991), vols. 3–4. Thomas Twyne, *Phisicke against Fortune* . . . Written in Latine by Frauncis Petrarch (London: Richard Watkyns, 1579).

45. Charles Trinkaus, *The Poet as Philosopher: Petrarch and the Formation of Renaissance Consciousness* (New Haven, Conn.: Yale University Press, 1979), p. 127.

46. McClure (n. 35), *Renaissance Vision,* p. 157.

47. Ibid., p. 160.

48. Ibid., p. 167.

49. Ibid., pp. 175–93.

50. Ibid., p. 177. Translated and quoted by McClure from Francesco Petrarca, *Rerum senilium libri*, III, 8, in *Opera omnia* (Basel, 1554), p. 861.

51. McClure (n. 35), *Renaissance Vision*, pp. 178–80. Translated and quoted by McClure from Francesco Petrarca, *Rerum senilium libri,* XII, 12, in *Opera omnia* (Basel, 1554), p. 1002.

52. McClure (n. 35), *Renaissance Vision,* p. 698, n. 4. Translated and quoted by McClure from Francesco Petrarca, *Invectivae contra medicum,* in *Opera Latine di Francesco Petrarca,* 2 vols., ed. A. Bufano (Turin, 1975), II, 930.

53. McClure (n. 35), *Renaissance Vision,* p. 203.

54. Ibid., pp. 207–8.

55. Ibid., pp. 211–15.

56. Ibid., pp. 223–25.

57. Salutati, quoted ibid., p. 239.

58. Ibid., pp. 255–67.

59. Ibid., p. 367.

60. Ibid., pp. 399–489.

61. Ibid., pp. 490–92, 500.

62. Ibid., pp. 562–66.

63. Thomas N. Tentler, *Sin and Confession on the Eve of the Reformation* (Princeton, N.J.: Princeton University Press, 1977), pp. xiii, xvi, 12–15.

64. Ibid., pp. 347–49.

65. Ibid., p. 351.

66. Robert Burton, *The Anatomy of Melancholy,* ed. Floyd Dell and Paul Jordan-Smith (New York: Tudor, 1948), p. 491.

67. Ibid., pp. 497–557.

68. Ibid., p. 495.

69. Ibid., p. 497.

70. Ibid., p. 499.

71. Ibid., pp. 532–40.

72. A. D. Beach Langston, "Tudor Books of Consolation." unpublished Ph.D. dissertation, University of North Carolina, Chapel Hill, 1940, pp. vii–x.

73. Ibid., pp. 231–35.

74. Ibid., pp. 241–42.

75. Ibid., p. 289.

76. Ibid., p. 344.

77. Ibid., p. 391.

78. Jaekle and Clebsch (n. 34), *Pastoral Care,* pp. 209–23.

79. Ibid., pp. 224–32; McNeill (n. 34), *Cure of Souls,* pp. 203–5.

80. Michael MacDonald, "Religion, Social Change, and Psychological Healing in England, 1600–1800," in W. J. Sheils (ed.), *The Church and Healing* (Oxford: Basil Blackwell, 1982), pp. 101–25; MacDonald, *Mystical Bedlam: Madness, Anxiety, and Healing in Seventeenth-Century England* (Cambridge: Cambridge University Press, 1981), pp. 172–231; McNeill (n. 34), *Cure of Souls;* Jaekle and Clebsch (n. 34), *Pastoral Care.*

81. MacDonald (n. 80), *Mystical Bedlam,* pp. 222–23.

82. Richard Baxter, *Gildas Salvianus: The Reformed Pastor,* ed. and intro. John T. Wilkinson (London: Epworth Press, 1939), p. 81.

83. Samuel Clifford, *The Signs and Causes of Melancholy . . . Collected out of the Works of Mr. Richard Baxter . . .* (London: Cruttenden and Cox, 1716), p. 123.

84. George Herbert, *A Priest to the Temple, or, the Country Parson,* in *The Works of George Herbert,* ed. F. E. Hutchinson (Oxford: Clarendon Press, 1970), pp. 224, 556.

85. Ibid., p. 249.

86. Louis S. Greenbaum, "Nurses and Doctors in Conflict: Piety and Medicine in the Paris Hôtel-Dieu on the Eve of the French Revolution," *Clio Medica,* 1978, *13,* 247–67 [248].

87. Ibid., p. 254.

88. Ibid., p. 259.

89. Dora B. Weiner, "The Brothers of Charity and the Mentally Ill in Pre-Revolutionary France," *Soc. Hist. of Med.,* 1989, *2,* 321–37 [324–25].

90. Ibid., p. 327–28.

91. Jan Goldstein, *Console and Classify: The French Psychiatric Profession in the Nineteenth Century* (Cambridge: Cambridge University Press, 1987), pp. 197–98.

92. P. J. G. Cabanis, *Sketch of the Revolutions of Medical Science, and Views Relating to Its Reform,* trans. and ed. A. Henderson (London: Johnson, Murray and Constable, 1806), p. 385.

93. Ibid., pp. 384–85.

94. Philippe Pinel, "Reflections médicales sur l'état monastique," *Journal Gratuit,* 9th Class: Health (1790): 81–93. Translated and quoted by Goldstein (n. 91), *Console and Classify,* p. 212.

95. Philippe Pinel, *The Clinical Training of Doctors: An Essay of 1793,* ed. and trans. Dora B. Weiner (Baltimore, Md.: Johns Hopkins University Press, 1980), p. 48.

96. Philippe Pinel, "Recherches et observations sur le traitement moral des aliénés," in Philippe Pinel, *Mémoire, recherches, observations, résultats* (Nendeln, Liechtenstein: Kraus Reprint, 1978), pp. 1–42 (Reprinted from *Mém. Soc. Méd. d'Emulation,* Year VII (1798–1799), 2, 215–55). p. 1.

97. Ibid., pp. 5, 10, 12, 14.

98. Ibid., pp. 8, 14, 33, 36, 37.

99. Ibid., p. 33. Jean-Baptiste Pussin, "superintendent" of the insane at Bicêtre, worked closely with Pinel from the time of the latter's appointment there in 1793. Pinel deeply respected Pussin's capabilities in his work with insane patients and learned much from him.

100. Philippe Pinel, *A Treatise on Insanity . . . ,* trans. D. D. Davis (Sheffield: Cadell and Davies, 1806), p. 100.

101. Ibid., p. 102.

102. Goldstein (n. 91), *Console and Classify.* The members of the nursing orders were primarily concerned with the patient's soul rather than with the body. They manifested this concern through a variety of religious exercises, and through comforting and consoling the person. Still, though, they attended to the patient's physical well-being with

a profound dedication that stemmed from being enjoined to see Christ in every sick person and from carrying out their duties with a view to ultimate spiritual rewards for their efforts.

103. Ibid., p. 5.

104. Ibid., p. 202. Here Goldstein drew on the contributions in seven installments of Paul Sérieux. "Le traitement des maladies mentales dans les maisons d'aliénés du XVIIIe siècle," *Archives internationales de neurologie*, 1924–25, *17th ser.*, 2 and *18th ser.*, 1; and on Hélène Bonnafous-Sérieux, *La Charité de Senlis . . .* (Paris: Presses Universitaires de France, 1936).

105. Goldstein (n. 91), *Console and Classify*, pp. 200–210.

106. Ibid., p. 113.

107. Ibid., pp. 204–5.

108. Ibid., pp. 206–7. Here Goldstein drew on Tissot, *Mémoire en faveur des aliénés* (Lyon: Pelagaud, Lesne et Crozet, 1837). Eccentric and colorful, Tissot named himself Frère Hilarion, apparently after St. Hilarion (ca. 291–371).

109. Scipion Pinel, *Traité complet du régime sanitaire des aliénés, ou manuel des établissemens qui leur sont consacrés* (Paris: Mauprivez, 1836), p. v.

110. Goldstein (n. 91), *Console and Classify*, p. 216.

111. Nancy Tomes, *A Generous Confidence: Thomas Story Kirkbride and the Art of Asylum-Keeping, 1840–1883* (Cambridge: Cambridge University Press, 1984).

112. Ibid., pp. 213–34.

113. Jules Claretie, "Charcot le consolateur," *Les Annales Politiques et Littéraires*, vol. 41, no. 1056 (Sept. 20, 1903), pp. 179–80.

114. See Chapter 3

115. See Worthington Hooker's *Physician and Patient* for a discussion of the sustaining and comforting functions often associated with the physician's role. *Physician and Patient; or, a Practical View of the Mutual Duties, Relations and Interests of the Medical Profession and the Community* (New York: Baker and Scribner, 1849), esp. chaps. 16 and 18.

116. James (n. 2), p. 73.

117. Walter Bromberg, *Man Above Humanity: A History of Psychotherapy* (Philadelphia: Lippincott, 1954), p. 273.

118. Jaekle and Clebsch (n. 34), *Pastoral Care*, pp. 8–9.

119. Howard J. Clinebell, Jr., *Basic Types of Pastoral Counseling* (Nashville, Tenn.: Abingdon Press, 1966).

120. See Chapter 3 and Francis W. Peabody, *Doctor and Patient* (New York: Macmillan, 1930); Oglesby Paul, *The Caring Physician: The Life of Dr. Francis W. Peabody* (Boston: Francis A. Countway Library of Medicine and Harvard Medical Alumni Association, 1991).

121. Maurice Levine, *Psychotherapy in Medical Practice* (New York: Macmillan, 1947), pp. 40–42.

122. Lewis R. Wolberg, *The Technique of Psychotherapy*, 2nd ed., 2 vols. (New York: Grune & Stratton, 1967), 1: 80.

123. Ibid., 2: 800.

124. Paul C. Horton, *Solace: The Missing Dimension in Psychiatry* (Chicago: University of Chicago Press, 1981).

125. Erich Lindemann, "Symptomatology and Management of Acute Grief," *Am. J. Psychiat.,* 1944, *101,* 141–48.

126. Colin Murray Parkes, *Bereavement: Studies of Grief in Adult Life* (New York: International Universities Press, 1972); Beverley Raphael, *The Anatomy of Bereavement* (New York: Basic Books, 1983).

127. Raphael (n. 126), *Anatomy of Bereavement,* pp. 356–61.

128. This phrase and its variations have a long history in Christian writings, with the implication that God had withdrawn or departed from the deserted soul, which was then left alone, sorrowing, and desolate.

129. Dating back to at least the fifteenth century, this adage is inscribed on Gutzon Borghum's statue of Edward Livingston Trudeau, M.D. (1849–1915) at Saranac Lake, New York.

Chapter 9: The Use of the Passions

1. Robert Burton, *The Anatomy of Melancholy,* ed. Floyd Dell and Paul Jordan-Smith (New York: Tudor, 1948), p. 467.

2. Ibid., p. 477.

3. L. J. Rather, *Mind and Body in Eighteenth Century Medicine: A Study Based on Jerome Gaub's De regimine mentis* (Berkeley: University of California Press, 1965), p. 236. Rather was here making use of an enlarged and revised edition of a work originally published in 1601. Thomas Wright, *The Passions of the Minde in Generall, in Sixe Bookes, corrected, enlarged, and with sundry new discourses augmented* (London: Anne Helme, 1621).

4. Hippocrates, *Works of Hippocrates,* trans. and ed. W. H. S. Jones and E. T. Withington, 4 vols. (Cambridge: Harvard University Press, 1923–1931), 1: xlvii.

5. Hippocrates, *Hippocratic Writings,* trans. J. Chadwick and W. N. Mann, I. M. Lonie, E. T. Withington, ed. and intro. G. E. R. Lloyd (London: Penguin, 1978), p. 33.

6. Ibid., p. 266.

7. Mary Smith, "The Nervous Temperament," *Brit. J. Med. Psychol.,* 1930, *10,* 99–174 [105–6]; Galen, *De temperamentis,* in Claudii Galeni, *Opera omnia,* 20 vols. in 22, ed. Carolus Gottlob Kühn (Leipzig: Cnobloch, 1821–1833), 1: 509–694.

8. Galen, *On the Natural Faculties,* trans. and ed. A. J. Brock (Cambridge: Harvard University Press, 1963), p. 199.

9. Galen, *Method of Physick,* trans. P. English (Edinburgh: George Suintoun & James Glen, 1656), pp. 49–51, 226–28.

10. Soranus, *Soranus' Gynecology,* trans. and intro. Owsei Temkin (Baltimore, Md.: Johns Hopkins University Press, 1956), p. xxxii; Caelius Aurelianus, *On Acute Diseases* and *On Chronic Diseases,* ed. and trans. I. E. Drabkin (Chicago: University of Chicago Press, 1950), p. xvii.

11. Ibid., pp. 547–49.

12. H. M. Gardiner, Ruth Clark Metcalf, and John G. Beebe-Center, *Feelings and Emotion: A History of Theories* (New York: American Book Company, 1937), pp. 10–25.

13. Ibid., pp. 26–57.

14. Ibid., pp. 64–68.

15. Ibid., p. 75.

16. L. J. Rather, "The 'Six Things Non-Natural': A Note on the Origins and Fate of a Doctrine and a Phrase," *Clio Medica,* 1968, *3,* 337–47 [337].

17. Ibid., p. 341.

18. Jerome J. Bylebyl, "Galen on the Non-Natural Causes of Variation in the Pulse," *Bull. Hist. Med.,* 1971, *45,* 482–85.

19. Peter H. Niebyl, "The Non-Naturals," *Bull. Hist. Med.,* 1971, *45,* 486–92.

20. Aristotle, *The Complete Works of Aristotle,* ed. Jonathan Barnes, 2 vols. (Princeton, N.J.: Princeton University Press, 1984), 2: 1378a20–1388b30.

21. Soranus (n. 10), *Acute Diseases and Chronic Diseases,* pp. 547–49.

22. Galen, *On the Passions and Errors of the Soul,* trans. Paul W. Harkins, intro. Walther Riese (Columbus: Ohio State University Press, 1963), p. 46.

23. Ibid., p. 125.

24. John T. McNeill, "Medicine for Sin as Prescribed in the Penitentials," *Church Hist.,* 1932, *l,* 14–26; John T. McNeill and Helena M. Gamer, *Medieval Handbooks of Penance: A Translation of the Principal "Libri poenitentiales" and Selections from Related Documents* (New York: Columbia University Press, 1938).

25. Ibid., pp. 92–93.

26. John Cassian, *The Conferences,* trans. and ed. Edgar C. S. Gibson, in Philip Schaff and Henry Wace (eds.), *A Select Library of the Nicene and Post-Nicene Fathers of the Christian Church,* 2nd ser., 14 vols. (Grand Rapids, Mich.: Eerdmans, 1955), 11: 495.

27. McNeill (n. 24), "Medicine for Sin," p. 17.

28. John T. McNeill, *A History of the Cure of Souls* (New York: Harper & Row, 1951), p. 114.

29. Haly filius Abbas, *Liber totius medicine . . . ,* trans. Stephen the Philosopher, ed. Michael de Capella (Lyons: 1523), book 5, chap. 38, p. 69.

30. J. Ch. Bürgel, "Psychosomatic Methods of Cures in the Islamic Middle Ages," *Humaniora Islamica,* 1973, *l,* 157–72.

31. Nancy G. Siraisi, *Taddeo Alderotti and His Pupils: Two Generations of Italian Medical Learning* (Princeton, N.J.: Princeton University Press, 1981), p. 226. Here Siraisi drew on Turisanus, *Turisani monaci plusquam commentum in Microtegni Galieni* (Venice, 1552).

32. Ibid., p. 229.

33. Henry Cornelius Agrippa, *Three Books of Occult Philosophy,* trans. J. F. (London: Gregory Moule, 1651), p. 145.

34. T. Bright, *A Treatise of Melancholie* (London: Thomas Vautrollier, 1586), pp. 255–56.

35. Felix Plater, Abdiah Cole, Nich. Culpeper, *A Golden Practice of Physick . . .* (London: Peter Cole, 1662), pp. 36–37.

36. Thomas Wright, *The Passions of the Minde in Generalle,* reprint based on 1604 ed., intro. Thomas O. Sloan (Urbana: University of Illinois Press, 1971), p. 94.

37. Ibid., p. 84.

38. Burton (n. 1), *Anatomy of Melancholy,* pp. 217–82.

39. Ibid., pp. 467–87.

40. Edward Reynolds, *A Treatise of the Passions and Faculties of the Soule of Man . . .* (London: Robert Bostock, 1640), pp. 52–54.

41. Thomas Willis, *Two Discourses Concerning the Soul of Brutes Which Is that of the Vital and Sensitive of Man,* trans. [from the Latin] S. Pordage (London: Thomas Dring, Ch. Harper, and John Leigh, 1683), pp. 193–94.

42. Gerard van Swieten, *The Commentaries upon the Aphorisms of Dr. Herman Boer-haave,* 11 vols. (London: John and Paul Knapton, 1754–1759), 1: 277–78.

43. Ibid., 1: 279–80.

44. Ibid., 11: 118.

45. Ibid., 11: 120–21.

46. An interesting contemporary expression of this theme employed a metaphor that nicely reflected the mechanical orientation which characterized the era's medicine and for which Boerhaave was a leading exponent. "They are by Nature ballanced against each other, like the *Antagonist Muscles* of the Body; either of which separately would have occasioned *Distortion* and irregular *Motion,* yet jointly they form a Machine, most accurately subservient to the *Necessities, Convenience, and Happiness* of a *rational System.*" [Francis Hutcheson], *An Essay on the Nature and Conduct of the Passions and Affections . . .* (London: John Smith and William Bruce, 1728), p. 181.

47. Robert James, *A Medicinal Dictionary . . . ,* 3 vols. (London: Osborne, 1743–1745), vol. 2: *Mania.*

48. William Battie, *A Treatise on Madness* (London: Whiston and White, 1758), pp. 84–85.

49. Rather (n. 3), *Mind and Body.* In this work, Rather included his translations of Gaub's *De regimine mentis,* editions of 1747 and 1763.

50. Ibid., pp. 14–15.

51. Francis de Valangin, *Treatise on Diet, or the Management of Human Life; By Physicians called the Six Non-Naturals . . .* (London: the Author, 1768), p. 320.

52. Ibid., p. 325.

53. Ibid., p. 336.

54. William Falconer, *A Dissertation on the Influence of the Passions upon Disorders of the Body,* 2nd ed. (London: Dilly, 1791).

55. C. J. Tissot, *De l'influence des passions de l'âme dans les maladies, et des moyens d'en corriger les mauvais effets* (Paris: Amand-Koenig, 1798).

56. For example, Joseph Parrish, *An Inaugural Dissertation on the Influence of the Passions upon the Body, in the Production and Cure of Diseases* (Philadelphia: for the author, 1805); E. Esquirol, *Des passions, considérées comme causes, symptômes et moyens curatifs de l'aliénation mentale* (Paris: Didot Jeune, 1805); Peter S. Townsend, *A Dissertation on the Influence of the Passions in the Production and Modification of Disease* (New York: for the author, 1816).

57. Lewis White Beck, *Early German Philosophy: Kant and His Predecessors* (Cambridge: Belknap Press of Harvard University Press, 1969), pp. 287–88, 328–29, 415–18.

58. Ibid., pp. 497–98.

59. Ibid.; Ernest R. Hilgard, "The Trilogy of Mind: Cognition, Affection, Conation," *J. Hist. Behav. Sci.,* 1980, *16,* 107–17.

60. This point is brought out nicely by G. E. Berrios in "The Psychopathology of Affectivity: Conceptual and Historical Aspects," *Psychol. Med.*, 1985, *15*, 745–58. With regard to melancholia and depression, this has been traced in Stanley W. Jackson, *Melancholia and Depression: From Hippocratic Times to Modern Times* (New Haven, Conn.: Yale University Press, 1986), chap. 8.

61. Philippe Pinel, *A Treatise on Insanity . . .*, trans. D. D. Davis (Sheffield, England: Todd, 1806), p. 19.

62. Ibid., p. 135.

63. Ibid., p. 150. It should be noted that I have here changed Davis's translation, by substituting "the affective faculties" for his "the active faculties." The phrase in the original French (1801) was "les facultés affectives."

64. Ibid., pp. 228–34 [228].

65. Esquirol (n. 56), *Des passions*.

66. E. Esquirol, *Mental Maladies: A Treatise on Insanity,* trans., with additions, E. K. Hunt (Philadelphia: Lea and Blanchard, 1845), pp. 228–29.

67. Eric T. Carlson and Norman Dain have taken note of this developmental trend in "The Psychotherapy that was Moral Treatment," *Am. J. Psychiat.*, 1960, *117*, 519–24. It has also been recognized by Jan Goldstein in *Console and Clarify: The French Psychiatric Profession in the Nineteenth Century* (New York: Cambridge University Press, 1987), pp. 87–88, 97–99. In addition, she has identified the influence of Rousseau in Pinel's endeavors, and, by implication, accorded him an influence in the changing status of emotion and in the nineteenth-century recognition of the possibility of primary affective disorders.

68. Johann Christian Heinroth, *Textbook of Disturbances of Mental Life: Or Disturbances of the Soul and Their Treatment,* 2 vols., trans. J. Schmorak, intro. George Mora (Baltimore, Md.: Johns Hopkins University Press, 1975), pp. 190–91.

69. Ibid., p. 250.

70. J.-B.-F. Descuret, *La médecine des passions, ou les passions considérées dans leur rapports avec les maladies, les lois et la religion,* 4th ed. (Liège: Lardinois, 1844), pp. 106, 138–45.

71. Ernst von Feuchtersleben, *The Principles of Medical Psychology . . .*, trans. H. Evans Lloyd, rev. and ed. B. G. Babington (London: Sydenham Society, 1847), p. 328.

72. Ibid., p. 332.

73. W. C. Dendy, "Psychotherapeia, or the Remedial Influence of Mind," *J. Psychol. Med. and Ment. Pathology,* 1853, *6*, 268–74 [270].

74. John Charles Bucknill and Daniel H. Tuke, *A Manual of Psychological Medicine* (Philadelphia: Blanchard and Lea, 1858), p. 488.

75. Daniel Hack Tuke, *Illustrations of the Influence of the Mind upon the Body in Health and Disease, Designed to Elucidate the Action of the Imagination,* 2nd ed. (Philadelphia: Henry C. Lea's Son, 1884), pp. 141–350.

76. Ibid., pp. 384–418.

77. Ibid., pp. 419–54.

78. Charles Baudouin, *Suggestion and Autosuggestion . . .*, trans. Eden and Cedar Paul (London: George Allen & Unwin, 1920), chaps. 4, 5.

79. Josef Breuer and Sigmund Freud, *Studies on Hysteria* (1895), in *The Standard*

Edition of the Complete Psychological Works of Sigmund Freud, trans. and ed. James Strachey, Anna Freud, et al., 24 vols. (London: Hogarth Press, 1953–1974), vol. 2 chap. 4.

80. Freud, "Freud's Psycho-Analytic Procedure" (1904), in *Standard Edition* (n. 79), 7: 249–54.

81. Jerome D. Frank, *Persuasion and Healing: A Comparative Study of Psychotherapy,* rev. ed. (Baltimore, Md.: Johns Hopkins University Press, 1973), pp. 249–53, 257–60.

82. Toksoz B. Karasu, "The Specificity Versus Nonspecificity Dilemma: Toward Identifying Therapeutic Change Agents," *Am. J. Psychiat.,* 1986, *143,* 687–95.

83. Donald J. Carek, "Affect in Psychodynamic Psychotherapy," *Am. J. Psychother.,* 1990, *44,* 274–82 [276, 278].

Chapter 10: The Use of the Imagination

1. Jeanne Achterberg, *Imagery in Healing* (Boston: New Science Library, 1985), chap. 1.

2. Anees A. Sheikh, Robert G. Kunzendorf, and Katharina S. Sheikh, "Healing Images: From Ancient Wisdom to Modern Science," in Anees A. Sheikh and Katharina S. Sheikh (eds.), *Eastern and Western Approaches to Healing: Ancient Wisdom and Modern Knowledge* (New York: John Wiley & Sons, 1989), pp. 475–82.

3. Andreas Laurentius, *A Discourse of the Preservation of Sight: of Melancholike Diseases; of Rheumes, and of Old Age,* trans. Richard Surphlet (London: Ralph Iacson, 1599), p. 73.

4. Aristotle had a crucial role in the emergence of this theory of psychic functions or faculties. Aristotle, "On the Soul" and "On Memory," in *The Complete Works of Aristotle,* 2 vols., rev. Oxford trans., ed. Jonathan Barnes (Princeton, N.J.: Princeton University Press, 1984), 1: 402a–435b, 449b4–453b11.

5. Joseph B. Juhasz, "Greek Theories of Imagination," *J. Hist. Behav. Sci.,* 1971, *7,* 39–58; Harry Austryn Wolfson, "The Internal Senses in Latin, Arabic, and Hebrew Philosophical Texts," *Harvard Theol. Rev.,* 1935, *28,* 69–133; Murray Wright Bundy, *The Theory of Imagination in Classical and Mediaeval Thought* (Urbana: University of Illinois Press, 1927); E. Ruth Harvey, *The Inward Wits: Psychological Theory in the Middle Ages and the Renaissance* (London: Warburg Institute, University of London, 1975). It should be noted that, in these contexts, the *common sense* was the faculty that combined the various sensations from the external senses to form integrated wholes which then became images attended to by the imagination.

6. Walter Pagel, "Medieval and Renaissance Contributions to Knowledge of the Brain and Its Functions," in *The History and Philosophy of Knowledge of the Brain and Its Functions,* ed. F. N. L. Poynter (Oxford: Blackwell, 1958), pp. 95–114; Edwin Clarke and C. D. O'Malley, *The Human Brain and Spinal Cord: A Historical Study Illustrated by Writings from Antiquity to the Twentieth Century* (Berkeley: University of California Press, 1968), pp. 461–69; Edwin Clarke and Kenneth Dewhurst, *An Illustrated History of Brain Function* (Oxford: Sandford, 1972), pp. 10–48.

7. In a topic somewhat apart from the theme of this study, many concerned themselves with the alleged power of the imagination to mark a fetus with birth defects that were said to be reflections of the mother's fantasies, yearnings, or even briefly held images.

8. Robert Burton, *The Anatomy of Melancholy,* ed. Floyd Dell and Paul Jordan-Smith (New York: Tudor, 1948), p. 224.

9. L. J. Rather, "Thomas Fienus' (1567–1631) Dialectical Investigation of the Imagination as Cause and Cure of Bodily Disease," *Bull. Hist. Med.,* 1967, *41,* 349–67 [356].

10. Ibid., p. 358.

11. Ibid., p. 362.

12. Ibid., pp. 363–67.

13. Stanley W. Jackson, "Robert Burton and Psychological Healing," *J. Hist. Med. & All. Sci.,* 1989, *44,* 160–78.

14. Burton (n. 8). *Anatomy of Melancholy,* pp. 467–72.

15. Ibid., p. 470.

16. Ibid., p. 473.

17. Ibid., pp. 477–78. These "artificial inventions," and Burton's discussion thereof, are dealt with in detail in Chapter 13.

18. [William Vaughan], *Directions for Health, Naturall and Artificiall: Derived from the best Physicians, as well Moderne as Antient,* 7th ed. (London: Thomas Harper, 1633), p. 130 (1st ed. 1600).

19. [Pierre] Charron, *Of Wisdom. Three Books,* trans. George Stanhope, 2 vols. (London: Gillyflower, 1697), 1: 158–60. The original, *De la Sagesse,* was published in 1601.

20. Burton (n. 6), *Anatomy of Melancholy,* p. 220.

21. Keith Thomas, *Religion and the Decline of Magic: Studies in Popular Beliefs in Sixteenth and Seventeenth Century England* (London: Weidenfeld and Nicolson, 1971), chap. 7.

22. C. E. McMahon, "The Role of Imagination in the Disease Process: Pre-Cartesian History" *Psychol. Med.,* 1976, *6,* 179–84.

23. Ibid., pp. 183–84.

24. Theodore M. Brown, "Descartes, Dualism, and Psychosomatic Medicine," in *The Anatomy of Madness: Essays in the History of Psychiatry,* 2 vols., ed. W. F. Bynum, Roy Porter, and Michael Shepherd (London and New York: Tavistock, 1985), 1: 40–62.

25. Ibid., p. 41.

26. George Baglivi, *The Practice of Physick* . . . (London: Andr. Bell, 1704), pp. 177–80, 183.

27. Brown (n. 24), p. 44. Brown cites several relevant passages from Friedrich Hoffman, *Fundamenta medicinae,* intro. and trans. Lester S. King (London: MacDonald, 1971), pp. 47, 55, 108.

28. See Gaub's *De regimine mentis* of 1763, trans., ed., and annot. Leland Rather, *Mind and Body in Eighteenth Century Medicine: A Study Based on Jerome Gaub's De regimine mentis* (Berkeley and Los Angeles: University of California Press, 1965), pp. 115–204, 218–42.

29. Ibid., p. 10.

30. Ibid., p. 17.

31. Peter Shaw, *The Reflector: Representing Human Affairs, as They Are; and May Be Improved* (London: Longmans, 1750), pp. 227–30.

32. William Battie, *A Treatise on Madness* (London: Whiston and White, 1758), pp. 5–6.

33. [James Boswell], *Boswell's Life of Johnson* . . . , ed. George Birkbeck Hill, 6 vols. (Oxford: Clarendon Press, 1887), 4: 208.

34. Michael V. DePorte, *Nightmares and Hobbyhorses: Swift, Sterne, and Augustan Ideas of Madness* (San Marino: Huntington Library, 1974), chap. 1.

35. Mesmer's work will be dealt with in greater detail in Chapter 11.

36. Alfred Binet and Charles Féré. *Animal Magnetism* (New York: Appleton, 1888), pp. 1–26; Henri F. Ellenberger, *The Discovery of the Unconscious: The History and Evolution of Dynamic Psychiatry* (New York: Basic Books, 1970), pp. 57–69. For Mesmer's own accounts of his work, see F. A. Mesmer, *Mesmerism: A Translation of the Original Scientific and Medical Writings of F. A. Mesmer,* trans. and ed. George Bloch, intro. E. R. Hilgard (Los Altos, Calif.: William Kaufmann, 1980).

37. *Rapport des commissaires, chargés par le roi, de l'examen du magnétisme animal* (Paris: Moutard, 1784), p. 53.

38. Ibid., p. 62.

39. Ibid., p. 74.

40. John Haygarth, *Of the Imagination, as a Cause and as a Cure of Disorders of the Body* . . . (Bath: Cruttwell, 1801), p. 15.

41. Ibid., p. 4.

42. Ibid., p. 28. Dr. Falconer, also of Bath, had written a prize-winning essay in the 1780s, in response to the following question proposed by the Medical Society of London: "What diseases may be mitigated or cured, by exciting particular affections or passions of the mind?" William Falconer, *A Dissertation on the Influence of the Passions upon Disorders of the Body,* 2nd ed. (London: Dilly, 1791). Further, Haygarth had discussed his investigative plan with Falconer; Falconer participated in the therapeutic trials; and Haygarth dedicated the resulting volume to Falconer. Falconer's dissertation, the question put to him by the Medical Society, and Haygarth's work reflected convictions and practices of the day to the effect that the mind had a significant influence on the body, and that the imagination and the passions could influence bodily conditions for good or for ill.

43. Haygarth (n. 40), *Imagination,* p. 32.

44. *Rapport . . . magnétisme animal* (n. 37), p. 74.

45. Jan Goldstein, *Console and Classify: The French Psychiatric Profession in the Nineteenth Century* (Cambridge: Cambridge University Press, 1987), pp. 52–54.

46. Ibid., pp. 78–79.

47. Robley Dunglison, *General Therapeutics, or, Principles of Medical Practice* . . . (Philadelphia: Carey, Lea and Blanchard, 1836), pp. 51–59.

48. Jonathan Pereira, *The Elements of Materia Medica and Therapeutics,* 3rd Am. ed., ed. Joseph Carson (Philadelphia: Blanchard and Lea, 1852), pp. 65–70.

49. Daniel Hack Tuke, *Illustrations of the Influence of the Mind upon the Body in Health and Disease, Designed to Elucidate the Action of the Imagination,* 2nd ed. (Philadelphia: Henry C. Lea's Son, 1884), pp. 1–28.

50. Binet and Féré (n. 36), *Animal Magnetism,* pp. 352–55.

51. Charles Féré, *La médecine d'imagination* (Paris: Progrès Medical, 1886).

52. Alfred T. Schofield, *The Unconscious Mind* (New York: Funk and Wagnalls, 1901), pp. 371–72.

53. C. G. Jung, *Memories, Dreams, Reflections,* ed. Aniela Jaffé, trans. Richard and Clara Winston (New York: Pantheon, 1961), pp. 170–99.

54. Ibid., p. 177.

55. C. G. Jung, *The Collected Works of C. G. Jung,* 20 vols. in 21, eds. Gerhard Adler, Michael Fordham, Herbert Read, and William McGuire, trans. R. F. C. Hull (Princeton, N.J.: Princeton University Press, 1953–1979), 8: 317.

56. Ibid., 9(1): 190.

57. Edward S. Casey, *Imagining: A Phenomenological Study* (Bloomington: Indiana University Press, 1976), p. 213.

58. Ibid., p. 214.

59. Mardi Jon Horowitz, *Image Formation and Cognition* (New York: Appleton-Century-Crofts, 1970), p. 289.

60. For greater detail on these matters, the following authorities are suggested, authorities to whom this account is indebted and among whom several have been themselves significant contributors to more recent developments in the field. Horowitz (n. 59), *Image Formation;* Jerome L. Singer, *Imagery and Daydream Methods in Psychotherapy and Behavior Modification* (New York: Academic Press, 1974); Jerome L. Singer and Kenneth S. Pope (eds.), *The Power of Human Imagination: New Methods in Psychotherapy* (New York: Plenum, 1978); A. A. Sheikh (ed.), *Imagery: Current Theory, Research, and Application* (New York: Wiley, 1983); Anees A. Sheikh (ed.), *Imagination and Healing* (Farmingdale, N.Y.: Baywood, 1984); Casey (n. 57), *Imagining.*

61. Sheikh (n. 60), *Imagination and Healing,* p. 6.

62. Singer and Pope (n. 60), *Human Imagination.*

Chapter 11: *Animal Magnetism, Mesmerism, and Hypnosis*

1. Franz Anton Mesmer, "Dissertation on the Discovery of Animal Magnetism," in *Mesmerism: A Translation of the Original Scientific and Medical Writings of F.A. Mesmer,* intro. E. R. Hilgard, trans. and ed. George Bloch (Los Altos, Calif.: William Kaufmann, 1980), p. 48).

2. Ibid., pp. 48–49.

3. Ibid., p. 46.

4. Ibid., p. 51.

5. Ibid., p. 56.

6. Ibid., p. 57.

7. Henri F. Ellenberger, *The Discovery of the Unconscious: The History and Evolution of Dynamic Psychiatry* (New York: Basic Books, 1970), pp. 62–64. In addition to Ellenberger's valuable account of the emergence and development of mesmerism and animal magnetism, I am indebted to two excellent, more recent studies: Alan Gauld, *A History of Hypnotism* (Cambridge: Cambridge University Press, 1992) and Adam Crabtree, *From Mesmer to Freud: Magnetic Sleep and the Roots of Psychological Healing* (New Haven, Conn.: Yale University Press, 1993).

8. Ellenberger (n. 7), *Discovery of the Unconscious,* pp. 91–103.

9. For the more significant of these reports, from the Academy of Sciences, see

Rapport des commissaires, chargés par le roi, de l'examen du magnétisme animal (Paris: Moutard, 1784). Regarding the role of the imagination, see Chapter 10.

10. Maxime de Puységur, *Rapport des cures opérées à Bayonne par le magnétisme animal* . . . (Bayonne: Prault, 1784); M. de Puységur, *Report of Cures by Animal Magnetism Occurring at Bayonne with Verifications,* trans. J. J. Slay, in Maurice M. Tinterow, *Foundations of Hypnosis: From Mesmer to Freud* (Springfield, Ill.: Charles C Thomas, 1970).

11. Ibid., p. 64.

12. Ibid., p. 65.

13. Armand Marie Jacques Chastenet de Puységur, *Mémoires pour servir à l'histoire et à l'établissement du magnétisme animal* (Paris: Dentu, 1784); Ellenberger (n. 7), *Discovery of the Unconscious,* pp. 70–72; Gauld (n. 7), *History of Hypnotism,* pp. 41–42; Crabtree (n. 7) *From Mesmer to Freud,* pp. 38–43.

14. Armand Marie Jacques Chastenet de Puységur, *Suite des mémoires pour servir à l'histoire et à l'établissement du magnétisme animal* (Paris: n.p, 1785).

15. Armand Marie Jacques Chastenet de Puységur, *Du magnétisme animal, considéré dans ses rapports avec diverses branches de la physique générale* (Paris: Desenne, 1807); Ellenberger (n. 7), *Discovery of the Unconscious,* p. 72; Gauld (n. 7), *History of Hypnotism,* p. 47.

16. Puységur (n. 15), *Du magnétisme animal;* Puységur, *Recherches, expériences et observations physiologiques* . . . (Paris: Dentu, 1811); Puységur, *Les fous, les insensés, les maniaques et les frénétiques* . . . (Paris: Dentu, 1812); and later editions of Puységur (n. 13), *Mémoires.*

17. J.-P.-F. Deleuze, *Histoire critique du magnétisme animal,* 2 vols. (Paris: Mame, 1813).

18. J.-P.-F. Deleuze, *Instruction pratique sur le magnétisme animal* (Paris: Dentu, 1825).

19. Deleuze noted that he was using the word *pass,* "which is common to all magnetizers," to signify "all the movements made by the hand in *passing* over the body, whether by slightly touching, or at a distance." J.-P.-F. Deleuze, *Practical Instruction in Animal Magnetism,* 2nd ed., trans. Thomas C. Hartshorn (Providence, R.I.: Cranston, 1837), p. 21.

20. Ibid., chaps. 2, 3.

21. Abbé de Faria, *De la cause du sommeil lucide, ou Etude de la nature de l'homme* (Paris: Mme. Horiac, 1819); Ellenberger (n. 7), *Discovery of the Unconscious,* p. 75; Gauld (n. 7) *History of Hypnotism,* p. 274; Crabtree (n. 7) *From Mesmer to Freud,* p. 123.

22. Pierre Janet, *Psychological Healing: A Historical and Clinical Study,* 2 vols., trans. Eden and Cedar Paul (New York: Macmillan, 1925), 1: 154–60; George W. Jacoby, *Suggestion and Psychotherapy* (New York: Charles Scribner's Sons, 1912), pp. 197–200; Ellenberger (n. 7), *Discovery of the Unconscious,* pp. 75–76.

23. John Elliotson, *Numerous Cases of Surgical Operations Without Pain in the Mesmeric State:* . . . (London: Baillière, 1843); *The Zoist,* 1843–1856, vols. 1–13; John Elliotson, *The Harveian Oration,* . . . *Royal College of Physicians, London, June 27th, 1846* (London: Baillière, 1846).

24. James Esdaile, *Mesmerism in India, and Its Practical Application in Surgery and Medicine* (Hartford, Conn.: Silas Andrus and Son, 1847).

25. James Braid, *Satanic Agency and Mesmerism Reviewed*, . . . (Manchester, England: Sims and Dinham, and Galt and Anderson, 1842); Tinterow (n. 10), *Foundations of Hypnosis*, pp. 320–23.

26. Ibid., p. 326–28.

27. James Braid, *Neurypnology: or, the Rationale of Nervous Sleep, Considered in Relation with Animal Magnetism* (London: John Churchill, Adam & Charles Black, 1843), pp. 12–13.

28. Ibid., pp. 4–6, 21, 24, 26–30, 19.

29. James Braid, *Braid on Hypnotism: Neurypnology* . . . , ed. Arthur Edward Waite (London: George Redway, 1899), pp. 26, 333.

30. Ibid., pp. 65–66. For a more detailed account of Braid and suggestion, see Chapter 12.

31. Ellenberger (n. 7), *Discovery of the Unconscious*, p. 85.

32. Ambroise Auguste Liébeault, *Du sommeil et des états analogues considérés surtout au point de vue de l'action du moral sur le physique* (Paris and Nancy: Victor Masson et fils and Nicolas Grosjean, 1866).

33. J. Milne Bramwell, *Hypnosis: Its History, Practice and Theory* (Philadelphia: Lippincott, 1903), pp. 30–33, 41–42; Ellenberger (n. 7), *Discovery of the Unconscious*, pp. 85–86; Gauld (n. 7), *History of Hypnotism*, pp. 319–24; Crabtree (n. 7), *From Mesmer to Freud*, pp. 163–64.

34. Hippolyte Bernheim, *De la suggestion dans l'état hypnotique* . . . (Paris: Octave Doin, 1884); Bernheim, *De la suggestion et de ses applications à la thérapeutique* (Paris: Octave Doin, 1886); Bernheim, *Suggestive Therapeutics: A Treatise on the Nature and Uses of Hypnotism*, trans. Christian A. Herter (New York: London Book Co., 1947).

35. Bernheim, *Suggestive Therapeutics*, pp. 15–16, 1–4, 210, 404–7.

36. Ibid., part 2, chap. 1.

37. Janet (n. 22), *Psychological Healing*, 1: 165–71; Georges Guillain, *J.-M. Charcot, 1825–1893: His Life — His Work*, ed. and trans. Pearce Bailey (New York: Paul B. Hoeber, 1959), chap. 15; Ellenberger (n. 7), *Discovery of the Unconscious*, pp. 89–101.

38. Jean-Martin Charcot, "Sur les divers états nerveux déterminés par l'hypnotisation chez les hystériques," *Comptes-rendus hebdomadaires des séances de l'Académie des Sciences*, 1882, *94*, 403–5.

39. J.-M. Charcot, *Clinical Lectures on Diseases of the Nervous System delivered at the Infirmary of la Salpêtrière*, 3 vols., trans. George Sigerson (vols. 1 and 2) and Thomas Savill (vol. 3) (London: New Sydenham Society, 1877–89), 3: 252–316.

40. Robert G. Hillman, "A Scientific Study of Mystery: The Role of the Medical and Popular Press in the Nancy-Salpêtrière Controversy on Hypnotism," *Bull. Hist. Med.*, 1965, *39*, 163–82.

41. Gauld (n. 7), *History of Hypnotism*, pp. 327–42; Crabtree (n. 7), *From Mesmer to Freud*, pp. 164–68.

42. Max Dessoir, *Bibliographie des modernen Hypnotismus* (Berlin: Carl Düncker, 1888); Dessoir, *Erster Nachtrag zur Bibliographie des modernen Hypnotismus* (Berlin: Carl Düncker, 1890).

43. Janet (n. 22), *Psychological Healing,* 1: 194–98; Ellenberger (n. 7), *Discovery of the Unconscious,* pp. 87–89; Gauld (n. 7), *History of Hypnotism,* pp. 336–42.

44. August Forel, *Der Hypnotismus* (Stuttgart: Ferdinand Enke, 1889); Forel, *Hypnotism, or, Suggestion and Psychotherapy: A Study of the Psychological, Psycho-Physiological and Therapeutic Aspects of Hypnotism,* trans. H. W. Armit (New York: Rebman, 1907); Janet (n. 22), *Psychological Healing,* 1: 195; Ellenberger (n. 7), *Discovery of the Unconscious,* pp. 88, 285; Gauld (n. 7), *History of Hypnotism,* pp. 341–42.

45. Albert Moll, *Der Hypnotismus* (Berlin: Kornfeld, 1889); Moll, *Hypnotism,* 2nd ed. (London: Walter Scott, 1891); Janet (n. 22), *Psychological Healing,* 1: 195; Gauld (n. 7), *History of Hypnotism,* pp. 341–42.

46. C. Lloyd Tuckey, *Psycho-Therapeutics: or, Treatment by Hypnotism and Suggestion,* 3rd ed. (London: Baillière, Tindall and Cox, 1891).

47. Bramwell (n. 33), *Hypnosis.*

48. J. Milne Bramwell, *Hypnotism and Treatment by Suggestion* (London: Cassell, 1909), p. 164.

49. Janet (n. 22), *Psychological Healing,* 1: 197.

50. Ibid., 1: 198.

51. Pierre Janet, *L'automatisme psychologique: Essai de psychologie expérimentale sur les formes inférieures de l'activité humaine,* 6th ed. (Paris: Félix Alcan, 1910).

52. Throughout this section on Janet, the author is indebted to Henri Ellenberger's detailed account of Janet's life and work (n. 7), *Discovery of the Unconscious,* chap. 6.

53. Ibid., p. 374.

54. Ibid., p. 386.

55. Janet (n. 22), *Psychological Healing,* 1: chaps. 9–11.

56. Ibid., 1: 197–203.

57. Ibid., 1: 207.

58. Erna Lesky, *The Vienna Medical School of the 19th Century,* trans. L. Williams and I. S. Levij (Baltimore, Md.: Johns Hopkins University Press, 1976), p. 352; Albrecht Hirschmüller, *The Life and Work of Josef Breuer: Physiology and Psychoanalysis* (New York: New York University Press, 1989), p. 93.

59. See acccounts in Chapters 5 and 6.

60. Sigmund Freud, "Report on My Studies in Paris and Berlin," in *Standard Edition of the Complete Psychological Works of Sigmund Freud,* trans. and ed. James Strachey, Anna Freud, et al., 24 vols. (London: Hogarth Press, 1953–74), 1: 4 (editor's note).

61. Breuer and Freud *Standard Edition* (n. 60), 2: xi.

62. Freud, "Extracts from Freud's Footnotes to His Translation of Charcot's *Tuesday Lectures*" *Standard Edition* (n. 60), 1: 141.

63. Hirschmüller (n. 58), *Josef Breuer,* p. 142.

64. Freud, "Review of August Forel's *Hypnotism*" *Standard Edition* (n. 60), 1: 101.

65. Freud, "Hypnosis" *Standard Edition* (n. 60), 1: 105–14, quotation on p. 111.

66. Freud *Standard Edition* (n. 60), 1: 66 (editor's introduction).

67. Breuer and Freud *Studies on Hysteria* in *Standard Edition* (n. 60), 2: 255.

68. Freud, "On Psychotherapy" *Standard Edition* (n. 60), 7: 261.

69. Freud, "Five Lectures on Psychoanalysis" *Standard Edition* (n. 60), 11: 22.

70. Freud, "An Autobiographical Study" *Standard Edition* (n. 60), 20: 27.

71. Léon Chertok and Raymond de Saussure, *The Therapeutic Revolution: From Mesmer to Freud,* trans. R. H. Ahrenfeldt (New York: Brunner/Mazel, 1979), pp. 124–26. See also, Léon Chertok, "The Discovery of the Transference: Towards an Epistemological Interpretation," *Int. J. Psycho-Anal.,* 1968, 49, 560–77.

72. Bernheim (n. 34). *Suggestive Therapeutics,* p. x.

73. Janet (n. 22), *Psychological Healing,* 1: 203.

74. Paul Dubois, *The Psychic Treatment of Nervous Disorders: The Psychoneuroses and Their Moral Treatment,* trans. and ed. Smith Ely Jelliffe and William A. White (New York: Funk & Wagnalls, 1907), p. 108. This work is considered in detail in Chapter 13.

75. William Brown, "The Revival of Emotional Memories and Its Therapeutic Value," *Brit. J. Psychol., Medical Section,* 1920, 1, 16–19; Brown, *Psychology and Psycho-Therapy* (London: Edward Arnold, 1922); Brown, *Suggestion and Mental Analysis: An Outline of the Theory and Practice of Mind Cure,* 2nd ed. (London: University of London Press, 1922).

76. J. A. Hadfield, "Hypnotism," in H. Crichton-Miller (ed.), *Functional Nerve Disease: An Epitome of War Experience for the Practitioner* (London: Oxford University Press, 1920); Hadfield, "Treatment by Suggestion and Hypno-Analysis," in Emanuel Miller (ed.), *The Neuroses in War* (New York: Macmillan, 1940).

77. Ernst Simmel, *Kriegsneurosen und psychische Trauma* (Munich: Nemnich, 1918); Simmel, "War Neuroses," in Sandor Lorand (ed.), *Psychoanalysis Today* (New York: International Universities Press, 1944), pp. 227–48. See Chapter 6 for a more detailed context for these references to catharsis.

78. Lewis R. Wolberg, *Medical Hypnosis,* 2 vols. (New York: Grune & Stratton, 1948), 1: 13.

79. H. E. Wingfield, *An Introduction to the Study of Hypnotism: Experimental and Therapeutic,* 2nd ed. (London: Baillière, Tindall and Cox, 1920).

80. Henry Yellowlees, *A Manual of Psychotherapy for Practitioners and Students* (London: Black, 1923), pp. 80, 98–99.

81. William McDougall, *Outline of Abnormal Psychology* (New York: Charles Scribner's Sons, 1926), pp. 464–66, 472.

82. Paul Schilder and Otto Kanders, *Hypnosis,* trans. Simon Rothenberg (New York: Nervous and Mental Disease Publishing, 1927), pp. 95–102.

83. Wolberg (n. 78), *Medical Hypnosis,* 1: 13.

84. E.g., Charles Fisher, "Hypnosis in Treatment of Neuroses Due to War and to Other Causes," *War Medicine,* 1943, 4, 565–76; John G. Watkins, *Hypnotherapy of War Neuroses: A Clinical Psychologist's Casebook* (New York: Ronald Press, 1949); Jacob H. Conn, "Hypnosynthesis: III. Hypnotherapy of Chronic War Neuroses with a Discussion of the Value of Abreaction, Regression, and Revivication," *J. Clin. & Experimental Hypnosis,* 1953, 1, 29–43.

85. Margaret Brenman and Merton M. Gill, *Hypnotherapy* (New York: Josiah Macy, Jr., Foundation, 1944); Brenman and Gill, *Hypnotherapy: A Survey of the Literature* (New York: International Universities Press, 1947). See also their later work, Merton M. Gill and Margaret Brenman, *Hypnosis and Related States: Psychoanalytic Studies in Regression* (New York: International Universities Press, 1959).

86. Lewis R. Wolberg, *Hypnoanalysis* (New York: Grune & Stratton, 1945); Wolberg

(n. 78), *Medical Hypnosis;* Jerome M. Schneck (ed.), *Hypnosis in Modern Medicine* (Springfield, Ill.: Charles C Thomas, 1953); Jay Haley (ed.), *Advanced Techniques of Hypnosis and Therapy: The Selected Papers of Milton H. Erickson, M.D.* (New York: Grune & Stratton, 1967); Milton H. Erikson, *The Collected Papers of Milton H. Erickson on Hypnosis,* 4 vols., ed. E. L. Rossi (New York: Irvington, 1980).

87. Lewis R. Wolberg, *The Technique of Psychotherapy,* 2 vols., 2nd ed. (New York: Grune & Stratton, 1972), 2: 889–901; David Spiegel and Herbert Spiegel, "Hypnosis," in Harold K. Kaplan and Benjamin J. Sadock, eds., *Comprehensive Textbook of Psychiatry,* 2 vols, 4th ed. (Baltimore, Md.: Williams & Wilkins, 1985), 2: 1389–1403.

88. Ibid., 2: 1389.

89. Ibid.

90. Ibid.

Chapter 12: Suggestion

1. James A. H. Murray et al. (eds.), *A New English Dictionary . . .* , 13 vols. (Oxford: Clarendon Press, 1888–1933), 9, pt. 2: 119.

2. Leland E. Hinsie and Robert J. Campbell, *Psychiatric Dictionary,* 3rd ed. (New York: Oxford University Press, 1960), p. 702.

3. Horace B. English and Ava Champney English, *A Comprehensive Dictionary of Psychological and Psychoanalytical Terms* (New York: Longmans, Green, 1958), p. 535.

4. Murray (n. 1), *OED,* 9. pt. 2: 119.

5. Mary Hamilton, *Incubation, or the Cure of Diseases in Pagan Temples and Christian Churches* (St. Andrews, Scotland/London: W. C. Henderson & Son and Simpkin, Marshall, Hamilton, Kent & Co., 1906); Emma J. Edelstein and Ludwig Edelstein, *Asclepius: A Collection and Interpretation of the Testimonies,* 2 vols. (Baltimore, Md.: Johns Hopkins Press, 1945).

6. E. A. Wallis Budge, *Amulets and Talismans,* (New Hyde Park, N.Y.: University Books, 1961); George Barton Cutten, *Three Thousand Years of Mental Healing* (New York: Charles Scribner's Sons, 1911); C. J. S. Thompson, *Magic and Healing* (London: Rider, 1946); James J. Walsh, *Psychotherapy* (New York: Appleton, 1912), chap. 8.

7. Thompson (n. 6), *Magic and Healing;* Cutten (n. 6), *Three Thousand Years of Mental Healing;* Keith Thomas, *Religion and the Decline of Magic* (London: Weidenfeld and Nicolson, 1971), chap. 7; Marc Bloch, *The Royal Touch: Sacred Monarchy and Scrofula in England and France* (London/Montreal: Routledge & Kegan Paul and McGill-Queens University Press, 1973).

8. Cutten (n. 6), *Three Thousand Years of Mental Healing;* Louis Rose, *Faith Healing,* ed. Bryan Morgan (Harmondsworth, England: Penguin Books, 1971); Thomas (n. 7), *Religion and the Decline of Magic.*

9. Leslie D. Weatherhead, *Psychology, Religion and Healing,* rev. ed. (London: Hodder and Stoughton, 1952), pp. 51–60.

10. Murray (n. 1), *OED,* 4: 31.

11. Anne H. Soukhanov et al. (eds.), *The American Heritage Dictionary of the English Language,* 3rd ed. (Boston: Houghton Mifflin, 1992), p. 656.

12. Weatherhead (n. 9), *Psychology, Religion and Healing,* p. 432.

13. Elwood Worcester, "Suggestion," in Elwood Worcester, Samuel McComb, and Isador H. Coriat, *Religion and Medicine: The Moral Control of Nervous Disorders* (New York: Moffat, Yard & Company, 1908), pp. 43–92 [44].

14. Samuel McComb, "Faith and Its Therapeutic Power," in Worcester, McComb, and Coriat (n. 13), *Religion and Medicine,* p. 293.

15. W. H. R. Rivers, "Psycho-Therapeutics," in James Hastings et al. (eds.), *Encyclopaedia of Religion and Ethics,* 13 vols. (New York: Charles Scribner's Sons, 1909–1927), 10: 433–40 [434].

16. Ibid., pp. 436–37.

17. Rose (n. 8), *Faith Healing,* p. 127.

18. William Osler, "Medicine in the Nineteenth Century," in *Aequanimitas: With Other Addresses, to Medical Students, Nurses, and Practitioners of Medicine,* 3rd ed. (Philadelphia: Blakiston, 1945), pp. 219–62 [258–59]. Paper originally presented at Johns Hopkins Historical Club, January 1901 and first published in the *Sun,* New York, January 27, 1901.

19. John Cotta, *A Short Discoverie of the Unobserved Dangers of Severall Sorts of Ignorant and Unconsiderate Practisers of Physicke in England*(London: William Jones and Richard Boyle, 1612), pp. 51–52.

20. Ibid., p. 54.

21. Robert Burton, *The Anatomy of Melancholy,* eds. Floyd Dell and Paul Jordan-Smith (New York: Tudor Publishing Co., 1948), pp. 221–23 (part 1, sec. 2, mem. 3, subs. 2).

22. Michael MacDonald, *Mystical Bedlam: Madness, Anxiety, and Healing in Seventeenth-Century England* (Cambridge: Cambridge University Press, 1981), p. 182.

23. See Chapter 10 for a detailed account of these and the following observations on the imagination as cause and cure of illnesses.

24. L. J. Rather, "Thomas Fienus' (1567–1631) Dialectical Investigation of the Imagination as Cause and Cure of Bodily Disease," *Bull. Hist. Med.,* 1967, *41,* 349–67; Burton (n. 21), *Anatomy of Melancholy,* pp. 220–24 (part 1, sec. 2, memb. 3, subs. 2).

25. Thomas (n. 7), *Religion and the Decline of Magic,* chap. 7.

26. See Chapter 11 for a detailed account of the matters dealt with here and for the emergence of suggestion as the successor to imagination in explanations.

27. James Braid, *Braid on Hypnotism: The Beginnings of Modern Hypnosis,* rev. ed., ed. Arthur Edward Waite, foreword J. H. Conn (New York: Julian Press, 1960), pp. 337–39.

28. Ibid., pp. 26, 333–37.

29. James Braid, *Hypnotic Therapeutics, Illustrated by Cases* . . . ([London]: n.p., 1853), p. 8 (reprinted from *Monthly Journal of Medical Science,* 1853, *17,* 14–47).

30. Braid (n. 27), *Braid on Hypnotism,* pp. 65–66.

31. Daniel Hack Tuke, *Illustrations of the Influence of the Mind upon the Body in Health and Disease: Designed to Elucidate the Action of the Imagination,* 2nd ed. (Philadelphia: Henry C. Lea's Sons & Co., 1884), p. 382.

32. Ibid., p. 419.

33. Alfred Binet and Charles Féré, *Animal Magnetism* (New York: Appleton, 1888), pp. 352–55.

34. Charles Féré. *La médicine d'imagination* (Paris: Progrès Medical, 1886).

35. For a more detailed account of the contributions of Liébeault and Bernheim to the development of hypnotism, see Chapter 11.

36. Hippolyte Bernheim, *De la suggestion dans l'état hypnotique et dans l'état de veille* (Paris: Octave Doin, 1884); Bernheim, *De la suggestion et de ses applications à la thérapeutique* (Paris: Octave Doin, 1886); Bernheim, *Suggestive Therapeutics: A Treatise on the Nature and Uses of Hypnotism,* trans. from 2nd and rev. French ed. Christian A. Herter (New York: London Book, 1947).

37. Bernheim, *Suggestive Therapeutics,* p. 15.

38. Ibid., pp. 1–4.

39. Ibid., part 2, chap. 1.

40. Hippolyte Bernheim, *Hypnotisme, suggestion, psychothérapie: Etudes nouvelles* (Paris: Octave Doin, 1891).

41. Hippolyte Bernheim, *Bernheim's New Studies in Hypnotism,* trans. and intro. Richard S. Sandor (New York: International Universities Press, 1980), pp. xv–xvi.

42. Ibid., pp. 1–7.

43. Ibid., p. 69. And Bernheim defined *suggestion* as "the act by which an idea is introduced into the brain and accepted by it." He thought, in rather mechanistic terms, of a reflex arc: "Every idea comes to the brain through the senses"; in the centripetal phase, the impression becomes an idea and is accepted by the brain; in the centrifugal phase, the suggested idea becomes an action. He referred to this scheme as a "fundamental law . . . the *law of ideodynamism.*" In referring to this theory, others came to use terms such as *ideomotor force* and *ideomotor theory* (ibid., pp. 18–32).

44. The following is a representative sample of this literature: C. Lloyd Tuckey, *Psycho-Therapeutics: or, Treatment by Hypnotism and Suggestion,* 3rd ed. (London: Baillière, Tindall and Cox, 1891); Wilhelm M. Wundt, *Hypnotismus und Suggestion* (Leipzig: Wilhelm Engelmann, 1892); Alexandre Cullere, *La thérapeutique suggestive . . .* (Paris: Librairie J.-B. Baillière et Fils, 1893); E. Virgil Neal and Charles S. Clark (eds.), *Hypnotism and Hypnotic Suggestion,* 5th ed. (Rochester, N.Y.: State Publishing, 1900); Joseph Grasset, *L'hypnotisme et la suggestion* (Paris: Octave Doin, 1903); J. Milne Bramwell, *Hypnotism and Treatment by Suggestion* (London: Cassell, 1909); Charles F. Winbigler, *Suggestion: Its Law and Application, or The Principle and Practice of Psycho-Therapeutics* (Washington/London: Spencer A. Lewis/Fowler, 1909); George W. Jacoby, *Suggestion and Psychotherapy* (New York: Charles Scribner's Sons, 1912); Emile Coué, *De la suggestion et de ses applications . . .* (Chaumont: Andriot Moissonnier, 1912).

45. Francis X. Dercum, *Rest, Mental Therapeutics, Suggestion* (Philadelphia: Blakiston's Sons, 1911), pp. 249–318; Walsh (n. 6), *Psychotherapy,* chaps. 3, 7.

46. Hugo Münsterberg, *Psychotherapy* (New York: Moffat, Yard, 1909).

47. See Chapter 13 for a more detailed account of persuasion therapy in this era.

48. Emile Coué, *Self Mastery Through Conscious Autosuggestion* (New York: American Library Service, 1922); Coué, *How to Practice Suggestion and Autosuggestion,* preface Charles Baudouin (New York: American Library Service, 1923); Charles Baudouin, *Suggestion and Autosuggestion,* trans. Eden and Cedar Paul (London: George Allen & Unwin, 1920).

49. William Brown, *Psychology and Psychotherapy* (London: Edward Arnold, 1921), p. 133.

50. Ibid.

51. Ibid., chaps. 6, 8, 9.

52. Ibid., p. 151.

53. Ibid., pp. 102–4, 151–52.

54. Ibid., pp. 108–11.

55. Ibid., p. 100.

56. William Brown, *Suggestion and Mental Analysis,* 2nd ed. (London: University of London Press, 1922), p. 7.

57. Ibid., pp. 17–18.

58. William Brown, *Psychological Methods of Healing: An Introduction to Psycho-therapy* (London: University of London Press, 1938), pp. 114–22; Edmund Jacobson, *Progressive Relaxation* (Chicago: University of Chicago Press, 1929).

59. Brown (n. 58), *Psychological Methods of Healing,* p. 207.

60. Henry Yellowlees, *A Manual of Psychotherapy for Practitioners and Students* (London: Black, 1923), p. 65.

61. Ibid., pp. 65–70.

62. Ibid., p. 72.

63. Ibid., pp. 106–7. These views are akin to those held by William Brown, and they appear to be derived from Ernest Jones, "The Action of Suggestion in Psychotherapy," in Ernest Jones, *Papers on Psycho-Analysis,* 2nd ed. (London: Baillière, Tindall and Cox, 1920), pp. 318–59; this paper was originally published in *J. Abnorm. Psychol.,* 1910–11, 5, 217–54.

64. Yellowlees (n. 60), *Manual of Psychotherapy,* p. 111.

65. Although the terms *direct suggestion* and *indirect suggestion* date back to the work of Boris Sidis (1867–1923), *The Psychology of Suggestion* (New York: Appleton, 1899), it is only since World War II that they have acquired the meanings assumed here. A direct suggestion involves a direct statement of the desired response, whether to a patient under hypnosis or in the waking state. In the case of an indirect suggestion, the desired response is only implied, whether wittingly or unwittingly, through subtle implication, placebo, faradization, etc.

66. Maurice Levine, *Psychotherapy in Medical Practice* (New York: Macmillan, 1947), chaps. 2, 3.

67. Ibid., pp. 61–62.

68. Ibid., pp. 62–63.

69. Emanuel Miller (ed.), *The Neuroses in War* (New York: Macmillan, 1940), p. vii.

70. J. A. Hadfield, "Treatment by Suggestion and Hypno-Analysis," in Miller (n. 69), *Neuroses in War,* pp. 128–49.

71. See Chapter 6.

72. Roy R. Grinker and John P. Spiegel, *War Neuroses* (Philadelphia: Blakiston, 1945), pp. 77–86—this work had been published originally in 1943 as *War Neuroses in North Africa,* but with a very restricted circulation; Grinker and Spiegel, *Men Under Stress* (Philadelphia: Blakiston, 1945), chaps. 7, 16, 17.

73. John G. Watkins, *Hypnotherapy of War Neuroses* (New York: Ronald Press, 1949), pp. 77–79.

74. Sigmund Freud, *The Origins of Psycho-Analysis: Letters to Wilhelm Fliess, Drafts,*

and Notes: 1887–1902, ed. Marie Bonaparte, Anna Freud, Ernst Kris, trans. Eric Mosbacher and James Strachey, intro. Ernst Kris (New York: Basic Books, 1954), p. 53.

75. Sigmund Freud, "Preface to the Translation of Bernheim's *Suggestion,*" in *The Standard Edition of the Complete Psychological Works of Sigmund Freud,* 24 vols., trans. and ed., James Strachey, Anna Freud, et al. (London: Hogarth Press, 1955–1974), 1: 75–85. Charcot had argued that the hypnotic state was *not* the result of suggestion. For more detail on Charcot's views, see Chapter 11.

76. Ibid., p. 83. The term *autosuggestion* and this manner of using it were not new, having been employed by both Charcot and Bernheim. J. M. Charcot, *Clinical Lectures on Diseases of the Nervous System,* vol. 3, trans. Thomas Savill (London: New Sydenham Society, 1889), pp. 345, 384; Bernheim (n. 36), *Suggestive Therapeutics,* pp. 102, 214.

77. Breuer and Freud, *Studies on Hysteria,* in *Standard Edition* (n. 75) 2: 270–72.

78. Freud, "Freud's Psycho-Analytic Procedure" and "On Psychotherapy," in *Standard Edition* (n. 75), vol. 7.

79. Jones (n. 63), *Papers on Psycho-Analysis,* p. 346.

80. Freud, "Lines of Advance in Psycho-Analytic Therapy" in *Standard Edition* (n. 75), 17: 168.

81. Freud, *Introductory Lectures on Psycho-Analysis* in *Standard Edition* (n. 75), 16: 451.

82. Freud, *The Question of Lay Analysis* in *Standard Edition* (n. 75), 20: 190, 225.

83. Freud, "Two Encyclopaedia Articles," in *Standard Edition* (n. 75), 18: 250–51.

84. Sandor Ferenczi, "Introjection and Transference," in Sandor Ferenczi, *Sex in Psychoanalysis,* trans. Ernest Jones, intro. Clara Thompson (New York: Basic Books, 1950), pp. 35–93 [67].

85. Jones (n. 63), *Papers on Psycho-Analysis,* pp. 324, 358–59.

86. Freud, *Introductory Lectures,* in *Standard Edition* (n. 75), 16: 446.

87. Freud, *An Autobiographical Study,* in *Standard Edition,* (n. 75), 20: 42.

88. Freud, "Psycho-Analysis," in *Standard Edition* (n. 75), 20: 268.

89. Freud, *Introductory Lectures,* in *Standard Edition* (n. 75), 16: 453.

90. Arthur K. Shapiro, "Placebo Effects in Medicine, Psychotherapy, and Psychoanalysis," in Allen E. Bergin and Sol L. Garfield (eds.), *Handbook of Psychotherapy and Behavior Change: An Empirical Analysis* (New York: John Wiley & Sons, 1971), p. 440.

91. Arthur K. Shapiro, "A Historic and Heuristic Definition of the Placebo," *Psychiatry,* 1964, *27,* 52–58 [52–53].

92. Ibid.

93. Hinsie and Campbell (n. 2), *Psychiatric Dictionary,* p. 563.

94. Arthur K. Shapiro, "The Placebo Effect in the History of Medical Treatment (Implications for Psychiatry), *Am. J. Psychiat.,* 1953, *116,* 298–304 [303].

95. Hippocrates, *Hippocratic Writings,* vol. 7, ed. and trans., Wesley D. Smith (Cambridge: Harvard University Press, 1994), p. 257 [*Epidemics* 6.5.8.].

96. Seneca, "On Mercy," in *Moral Essays,* 3 vols., trans. John W. Basore (Cambridge: Harvard University Press, 1965–1975), 1: 407 [bk. I: xvii].

97. Judith Wilcox and John M. Riddle, "Qusṭā ibn Lūqā's *Physical Ligatures* and the Recognition of the Placebo Effect," *Medieval Encounters,* 1994, *1,* 1–48, 2, 15, 18.

98. Kenneth M. Calestro, "Psychotherapy, Faith Healing, and Suggestion," *Int. J. Psychiat.*, 1972, *10*, 83–113 [105–6].

99. T. X. Barber, "Medicine, Suggestive Therapy, and Healing," in R. J. Kastenbaum, T. X. Barber, S. C. Wilson, B. L. Ryder, and L. B. Hathaway (eds.), *Old, Sick, and Helpless: When Therapy Begins* (Cambridge, Mass.: Ballinger, 1981), pp. 7–56; Mark Lipkin, "Suggestion and Healing," *Perspectives in Biology and Medicine*, 1984, *28*, 121–26.

100. Shapiro (n. 90), p. 444.

101. Arthur K. Shapiro, "A Contribution to a History of the Placebo Effect," *Behav. Sci.*, 1960, *5*, 109–35 [126–29].

102. Shapiro (n. 90), pp. 447, 450–52.

103. Edward Bibring, "Psychoanalysis and the Dynamic Psychotherapies," *J. Am. Psychoanal. Assoc.*, 1954, *2*, 745–70, pp. 745–46.

104. Ibid., p. 747.

105. E.g., Calestro (n. 98); Barber (n. 99); Lipkin (n. 99).

106. Ari Kiev, "The Study of Folk Psychiatry," in Ari Kiev (ed.), *Magic, Faith, and Healing: Studies in Primitive Psychiatry Today* (New York: Free Press, 1964), pp. 3–35; Raymond Prince, "Indigenous Yoruba Psychiatry," in Ari Kiev (ed.), *Magic, Faith, and Healing: Studies in Primitive Psychiatry Today* (New York: Free Press, 1964), pp. 84–120; Calestro (n. 98).

107. Prince (n. 106), p. 110.

108. Calestro (n. 98), pp. 101–2, 107.

109. Lewis R. Wolberg, *The Technique of Psychotherapy*, 2nd ed., 2 vols. (New York: Grune & Stratton, 1967), p. 30.

110. Milton R. Erickson, *Advanced Techiques of Hypnosis and Therapy: The Selected Papers of Milton R. Erickson, M.D.*, ed. Jay Haley (New York: Grune & Stratton, 1967); *American Journal of Clinical Hypnosis.*

111. Wolberg (n. 109), *Technique of Psychotherapy*, 1: 30, 80–83. The term *prestige suggestion* appears to have been introduced by William McDougall before World War I to refer to instances where the knowledge, experience, status, manner, or otherwise impressive nature of the source of the suggestion plays a significant role in its being influential; William McDougall, *An Introduction to Social Psychology* (Boston: John W. Luce, 1909), pp. 98–99.

112. D. H. Malan, *A Study of Brief Psychotherapy* (London: Tavistock Publications, 1963); Leopold Bellak and Leonard Small, *Emergency Psychotherapy and Brief Psychotherapy* (New York: Grune & Stratton, 1965); Lewis R. Wolberg (ed.), *Short-Term Psychotherapy* (New York: Grune & Stratton, 1965); Peter E. Sifneos, *Short-Term Psychotherapy and Emotional Crisis* (Cambridge: Harvard University Press, 1972); James Mann, *Time-Limited Psychotherapy* (Cambridge: Harvard University Press, 1973).

113. Paul A. Dewald, *Psychotherapy: A Dynamic Approach*, 2nd ed. (New York: Basic Books, 1969), pp. 190–93; David S. Werman, *The Practice of Supportive Psychotherapy* (New York: Brunner/Mazel, 1984).

114. In the late eighteenth and early nineteenth centuries, in the work of some of the Scottish philosophers of the mind, the term *suggestion* was used in quite a different way from that which became common in the late nineteenth century. Thomas Reid (1710–

1796) used *suggestion* rather than *association* in discussing the nature of the connections between mental elements in sequences of such elements in a person's mind (*An Inquiry into the Human Mind . . .* , 2nd ed. [Edinburgh: Millar and Kincaid and Bell, 1765], pp. 49–50). Thomas Brown (1778–1820) argued at some length for the use of *suggestion* rather than *association*. Rather than being connected by associational linkages as the associationists would have it, mental elements, in Brown's view, arise in the human mind as the result of the suggestive influence of preceding elements; and "association of ideas" was too limited a notion, as much more than ideas was involved in any sequence of mental elements (*Lectures on the Philosophy of the Human Mind,* 4 vols. [Edinburgh: Tait, 1820], 2: lectures 33–40).

Chapter 13: Persuasion

1. James A. H. Murray et al. (eds.), *A New English Dictionary . . .* , 13 vols. (Oxford: Clarendon Press, 1888–1933), 7: 733.

2. Horace B. English and Ava Champney English, *A Comprehensive Dictionary of Psychological and Psychoanalytical Terms* (New York: Longmans, Green, 1958), p. 385.

3. Leland E. Hinsie and Robert Jean Campbell, *Psychiatric Dictionary,* 3rd ed. (New York: Oxford University Press, 1960), p. 548.

4. Erling Eng, "Modern Psychotherapy and Ancient Rhetoric," *Psychother. Psychosom.,* 1974, 24, 493–96.

5. Ibid., p. 495.

6. Pedro Laín Entralgo, *The Therapy of the Word in Classical Antiquity,* ed. and trans. L. J. Rather and John M. Sharp (New Haven, Conn.: Yale University Press, 1970), pp. 23, 25, 64, 66, 29–30, 67–68, 91, 93, 97, 104.

7. Bernard Weinberg, "Rhetoric After Plato," in Philip P. Wiener (ed.), *Dictionary of the History of Ideas: Studies of Selected Pivotal Ideas,* 5 vols. (New York: Charles Scribner's Sons, 1968–1974), 4: 167–73 [167].

8. Aristotle, "Rhetoric," in *The Complete Works of Aristotle,* 2 vols., ed. Jonathan Barnes (Princeton, N.J.: Princeton University Press, 1984), 2: 1355b27–28.

9. Ibid., 2: 1355a4–5.

10. Ibid., 2: 1356a3–14, 1377b 15–1378a20.

11. Ibid., 2: 1356a3–4, 23–25, 1378a21–1388b31.

12. Ibid., 2: 1356a19–21.

13. Ibid., 2: 1356a22–24.

14. Weinberg (n. 7), p. 172.

15. Andrea A. Lunsford and Lisa S. Ede, "On Distinctions Between Classical and Modern Rhetoric," in Robert J. Connors, Lisa S. Ede, and Andrea A. Lunsford (eds.), *Essays on Classical Rhetoric and Modern Discourse* (Carbondale: Southern Illinois University Press, 1984), pp. 37–49.

16. Brian Vickers, "On the Practicalities of Renaissance Rhetoric," in Brian Vickers (ed.), *Rhetoric Revalued: Papers from the International Society for the History of Rhetoric* (Binghamton, N.Y.: Center for Medieval & Early Renaissance Studies, 1982), pp. 133–41 [136].

17. Brian Vickers, "Introduction," in Vickers, *Rhetoric Revalued* (n. 16), p. 25.

18. See Chapters 9 and 10.

19. Vickers (n. 16), p. 21.

20. Ibid., p. 19.

21. Francis Bacon. *The Works of Francis Bacon,* 7 vols., eds. James Spedding, Robert Leslie Ellis, and Douglas Denon Heath (New York: Garrett Press, 1968), 4: 455. This edition was reprinted from the Longmans edition, London, 1857–1874.

22. Ibid., 4: 456.

23. Ibid., 3: 383.

24. Ibid., 4: 456–57.

25. Robert Burton, *The Anatomy of Melancholy,* eds. Floyd Dell and Paul Jordan-Smith (New York: Tudor, 1948), pp. 473, 475–76.

26. Ibid., pp. 477–78. These matters are dealt with in some detail later in this chapter.

27. Ibid., pp. 491–557. See Chapter 8 for Burton's work on consolation.

28. See Chapters 9 and 10.

29. Samuel Johnson, *A Dictionary of the English Language . . . ,* 2 vols. (London: Knapton, 1755), vol. 2.

30. Stanley W. Jackson, "Introduction," in William Pargeter, *Observations on Maniacal Disorders* (1792), ed. and intro. Stanley W. Jackson (London: Routledge, 1988) pp. ix–xl.

31. Eric T. Carlson and Meribeth M. Simpson, "Moral Persuasion as Therapy," in J. H. Masserman (ed.), *Current Psychiatric Therapies,* vol. 4 (New York: Grune & Stratton, 1964), pp. 13–24.

32. Ibid., p. 13.

33. Ibid., pp. 15–18. Benjamin Rush outlined these stages in *Medical Inquiries and Observations, upon the Diseases of the Mind* (Philadelphia: Kimber & Richardson, 1812), pp. 208–9.

34. A detailed account of the history of the latter two is included in Chapter 9.

35. Carlson and Simpson (n. 31), pp. 21–23.

36. This is quoted from George Campbell, *The Philosophy of Rhetoric* (London: Strahan, 1776), by James Engell, "The New Rhetoricians: Psychology, Semiotics, and Critical Theory," in Christopher Fox (ed.), *Psychology and Literature in the Eighteenth Century* (New York: AMS Press, 1987), pp. 277–302 [p. 284].

37. Philippe Pinel, *A Treatise on Insanity . . . ,* trans. D. D. Davis (Sheffield: Cadell and Davies, 1806), pp. 100, 228–34.

38. Kathleen M. Grange, "Pinel and Eighteenth-Century Psychiatry," *Bull. Hist. Med.,* 1961, *35,* 442–53.

39. Pinel (n. 37) *Treatise on Insanity,* pp. 61–63, 224–28.

40. Ibid., pp. 68, 95–98. We seem to have here the first two of Rush's three stages, perhaps even the source from which he developed his own scheme.

41. Celsus, *De medicina,* 3 vols., trans. W. G. Spencer (Cambridge: Harvard University Press, 1953–1961), 1: 295 (bk. III.18).

42. A. J. Brock, *Greek Medicine: Being Extracts Illustrative of Medical Writers from Hippocrates to Galen* (London: Dent & Sons, 1929), p. 214.

43. Alexander of Tralles, *Oeuvres médicales d'Alexandre de Tralles,* 4 vols., ed. F. Brunet (Paris: Geuthner, 1933–1937), 2: 231–32.

44. Andreas Laurentius, *A Discourse of the Preservation of the Sight: of Melancholike Diseases; of Rheumes, and of Old Age,* trans. Richard Surphlet (London: Richard Iacson, 1599), pp. 101–3.

45. Robert Burton, *The Anatomy of Melancholy,* eds. Floyd Dell and Paul Jordan-Smith (New York: Tudor, 1948), pp. 477–78 (part 2, sect. 2, memb. 6, subs. 2).

46. J. Ch. Bürgel, "Psychosomatic Methods of Cures in the Islamic Middle Ages," *Humaniora Islamica,* 1973, *1,* 157–72; Bürgel, "Secular and Religious Features of Medieval Arabic Medicine," in Charles Leslie (ed.), *Asian Medical Systems: A Comparative Study* (Berkeley: University of California Press, 1976), p. 52.

47. [Michael Ettmüller] *Etmullerus Abridg'd: Or, A Compleat System of the Theory and Practice of Physic* . . . (London: Harris, Hubbard, and Bell, 1699), p. 546.

48. Denis Diderot and Jean le Rond d'Alembert, eds. *Encyclopédie* . . . , 3rd ed., 36 vols. (Geneva/Neufchatel: Jean-Léonard Pellet/Société Typographique, 1778–1779), 21: 433–37.

49. Ibid., pp. 435–36.

50. Murray (n. 1), *OED* 4: 516.

51. Joseph Addison, Richard Steele, et al., *The Spectator,* new edition, with the *Lives of the Authors* by Robert Bisset, 8 vols. (London: Jordan, 1794), 6: 183.

52. Voltaire, *Philosophical Dictionary,* trans. and intro. Peter Gay (New York: Basic Books, 1962), 1: 279–83. Though missing from a number of other translations, the subtitle is present in various editions from the 1760s: "S'il faut user de fraudes pieuses avec le peuple?"

53. Ibid., pp. 279–81.

54. Eric T. Carlson and Norman Dain, "The Psychotherapy that Was Moral Treatment," *Am. J. Psychiatry,* 1960, *117,* 519–24 [522].

55. John Haslam, *Observations on Madness and Melancholy* . . . , 2nd ed. (London: Callow, 1809), pp. 304–5.

56. Pinel (n. 37), *Treatise on Insanity,* pp. 224–28.

57. Ibid., p. 98. See, Philippe Pinel, *Traité médico-philosophique sur l'aliénation mentale, ou la manie* (Paris: Richard, Caille et Ravier, 1801), p. 95.

58. John Ferriar, *Medical Histories and Reflections,* 3 vols. (Warrington: Cadell, 1792–1798), 2: 109.

59. Benjamin Rush, *Medical Inquiries and Observations, upon the Diseases of the Mind* (Philadelphia: Kimber and Richardson, 1812), pp. 108–11.

60. John Charles Bucknill and Daniel H. Tuke, *A Manual of Psychological Medicine* . . . (Philadelphia: Blanchard and Lea, 1858), pp. 496–97.

61. Paul Dubois, *The Psychic Treatment of Nervous Disorders (The Psychoneuroses and Their Moral Treatment),* trans. and ed. Smith Ely Jelliffe and William A. White (New York: Funk & Wagnalls, 1907), p. 108.

62. Ibid., p. 216.

63. Ibid., pp. 106–19.

64. Ibid., p. 35.

65. J. Déjerine and E. Gauckler, *The Psychoneuroses and Their Treatment by Psychotherapy,* trans. Smith Ely Jelliffe, 2nd ed. (Philadelphia: Lippincott, 1915), p. 283.

66. Ibid., pp. vii–viii.

67. Ibid., p. 284.

68. Dubois (n. 61), *Psychic Treatment,* p. 35.

69. Ernst von Feuchtersleben. *The Principles of Medical Psychology,* trans. H. Evans Lloyd, rev. and ed. B. G. Babington (London: Sydenham Society, 1847), pp. 319–68.

70. Pierre Janet, *Psychological Healing: A Historical and Clinical Study,* 2 vols., trans. Eden and Cedar Paul (New York: Macmillan, 1925), 2: 710–87.

71. Morton Prince, *The Unconscious: The Fundamentals of Human Personality Normal and Abnormal* (New York: Macmillan, 1914), pp. 288–89.

72. Morton Prince, "The Educational Treatment of Neurasthenia and Certain Hysterical States," in Morton Prince, *Psychotherapy and Multiple Personality: Selected Essays,* ed. and intro. Nathan G. Hale, Jr. (Cambridge: Harvard University Press, 1975), p. 100. Originally published in *Boston Med. Surg. J.,* 1898, *139,* 332–37.

73. Ibid, p. 104.

74. Henry Yellowlees, *A Manual of Psychotherapy for Practitioners and Students* (London: Black, 1923), pp. 72–73.

75. Maurice Levine, *Psychotherapy in Medical Practice* (New York: Macmillan, 1942) pp. 125–33.

76. Lewis R. Wolberg, *The Technique of Psychotherapy* (New York: Grune & Stratton, 1954), p. 24. So-called supportive psychotherapy crucially involves contributions from the bedrock of psychological healing: the healer-sufferer relationship, listening, and talking. In addition, there tends to be varying admixtures of persuasion, suggestion, and conditioning; and any of our other basic elements may occasionally be a factor.

77. Ibid., pp. 24–25.

78. Ibid., p. 27.

79. Ibid.

80. Ibid., p. 534.

81. Lewis R. Wolberg, *The Technique of Psychotherapy,* 2 vols., 2nd ed. (New York: Grune & Stratton, 1972), 1: 103–72.

82. Patrick J. Mahony, "Freud in the Light of Classical Rhetoric," *J. Hist. Behav. Sci.,* 1974, *10,* 413–25 [413].

83. Ibid., p. 416.

84. Ibid., pp. 424–25.

85. Ibid., p. 413.

86. Gene M. Abroms "Persuasion in Psychotherapy," *Am. J. Psychiat.,* 1968, *124,* 1212–19 [1213]. See Jerome D. Frank, *Persuasion and Healing: A Comparative Study of Psychotherapy,* rev. ed. (Baltimore, Md.: Johns Hopkins University Press, 1973); Jay Haley, *Strategies of Psychotherapy* (New York: Grune & Stratton, 1963).

87. Abroms (n. 86), pp. 1212–13.

88. Ibid., p. 1212.

89. Susan R. Glaser, "Rhetoric and Psychotherapy," in Michael J. Mahoney (ed.), *Psychotherapy Process: Current Issues and Future Directions* (New York: Plenum Press, 1980), pp. 313–33.

90. Robert Spillane, "Rhetoric as Remedy: Some Philosophical Antecedents of Psychotherapeutic Ethics," *Brit. J. Med. Psychol.,* 1987, *60,* 217–24.

91. Jerome D. Frank, "Psychotherapy, Rhetoric, and Hermeneutics: Implications for

Practice and Research," *Psychotherapy,* 1987, 24, 293–302; Jerome D. Frank and Julia B. Frank, *Persuasion and Healing: A Comparative Study of Psychotherapy,* 3rd ed. (Baltimore, Md.: Johns Hopkins University Press, 1991), pp. 65–70.

Chapter 14: Conditioning and Reward or Punishment

1. Ernest R. Hilgard, *Theories of Learning,* 2nd ed. (New York: Appleton-Century-Crofts, 1956), p. 3.

2. Gregory A. Kimble, *Hilgard and Marquis' Conditioning and Learning,* 2nd ed. (New York: Appleton-Century-Crofts, 1961); Hilgard (n. 1), *Theories of Learning.*

3. Sue Walrond-Skinner, *Dictionary of Psychotherapy* (London: Routledge & Kegan Paul, 1986), p. 69.

4. R. W. Burchfield (ed.), *A Supplement to the Oxford English Dictionary,* 4 vols. (Oxford: Clarendon Press, 1972–1986), 1: 606.

5. James Mark Baldwin (ed.), *Dictionary of Philosophy and Psychology,* 3 vols. (1901), new edition with corrections (Gloucester, Mass. Peter Smith, 1960), 1: 435–36.

6. Leo Postman, "Rewards and Punishments in Human Learning," in Leo Postman (ed.), *Psychology in the Making: Histories of Selected Research Problems* (New York: Knopf, 1964), p. 331.

7. Philippe Ariès, *Centuries of Childhood: A Social History of Family Life,* trans. Robert Baldick (New York: Knopf, 1962); David Hunt, *Parents and Children in History: The Psychology of Family Life in Early Modern France* (New York: Basic Books, 1970); Lloyd deMause, "The Evolution of Childhood," in Lloyd deMause (ed.), *The History of Childhood* (New York: The Psychohistory Press, 1974).

8. Alan E. Kazdin and Joan L. Pulaski, "Joseph Lancaster and Behavior Modification in Education," *J. Hist. Behav. Sci.,* 1977, 13, 261–66. See Joseph Lancaster, *Improvements in Education, as It Respects the Industrious Classes of the Community* (London: Darton and Harvey, 1805).

9. Kazdin and Pulaski (n. 8), p. 261.

10. Paul T. Mountjoy, James H. Bos, Michael O. Duncan, and Robert B. Verplank, "Falconry: Neglected Aspect of the History of Psychology," *J. Hist. Behav. Sci.,* 1969, 5, 59–67 [59].

11. Solomon Diamond (ed.), *The Roots of Psychology: A Sourcebook in the History of Ideas* (New York: Basic Books, 1974), pp. 302, 309–11.

12. Kenelme Digby, *Two Treatises. In the One of Which, the Nature of Bodies; in the Other, the Nature of Mans Soule; Is looked into: in Way of Discovery, of the Immortality of Reasonable Soules* (Paris: Gilles Blaizot, 1644), p. 334.

13. Robert Burton, *The Anatomy of Melancholy,* ed. Floyd Dell and Paul Jordan-Smith (New York: Tudor Publishing, 1948) p. 474.

14. Mark A. Stewart, "Psychotherapy by Reciprocal Inhibition," *Am. J. Psychiat.,* 1961, 118, 175–77. The treatment discussed here was carried out at the Bicêtre in 1843 and reported in a paper read at the Académie royale de Médicine in 1845, which was then published in 1846: F. Leuret, *Des indications à suivre dans le traitement moral de la folie* (Paris: Librairie V le Normant, 1846), pp. 61–76 [reprinted, Nendeln, Liechtenstein, KTO Press, 1978]. Wolpe's work is discussed later in this chapter.

15. Eric T. Carlson and Norman Dain, "The Psychotherapy that Was Moral Treat-

ment," *Am. J. Psychiat.*, 1960, *117*, 519–24; Anne Digby, *Madness, Morality, and Medicine: A Study of the York Retreat, 1796–1914* (Cambridge: Cambridge University Press, 1985).

16. Horace B. English and Ava Champney English, *A Comprehensive Dictionary of Psychological and Psychoanalytical Terms* (New York: Longmans, Green, 1958), p. 107.

17. Ivan P. Pavlov, *Conditioned Reflexes: An Investigation of the Physiological Activity of the Cerebral Cortex,* trans. and ed. G. V. Anrep (Oxford: Oxford University Press, 1927); Pavlov, *Lectures on Conditioned Reflexes,* trans. W. Horsley Gantt (New York: International Publishers, 1928).

18. W. Horsley Gantt, "Conditional or Conditioned, Reflex or Response?" *Conditional Reflex,* 1966, *1,* 69–73; Cyril M. Franks, "Behavior Therapy and Its Pavlovian Origins: Review and Perspectives," in Cyril M. Franks (ed.), *Behavior Therapy: Appraisal and Status* (New York: McGraw-Hill, 1969), pp. 7–8.

19. Kimble (n. 2), *Hilgard and Marquis' Conditioning and Learning,* pp. 21–22. See V. M. Bekhterev, *General Principles of Human Reflexology: An Introduction to the Objective Study of Personality,* trans. E. Murphy and W. Murphy (London: Jarrolds, 1933).

20. Richard J. Herrnstein and Edwin G. Boring (eds.), *A Source Book in the History of Psychology* (Cambridge: Harvard University Press, 1965), p. 534.

21. Robert I. Watson, *The Great Psychologists: Aristotle to Freud* (Philadelphia: Lippincott, 1963), chap. 18; Raymond E. Fancher, *Pioneers of Psychology* (New York: Norton, 1979), pp. 314–38.

22. J. B. Watson, "Psychology as the Behaviorist Views It," *Psychol. Rev.,* 1913, *20,* 158–77.

23. John B. Watson, *Behavior: An Introduction to Comparative Psychology* (New York: Holt, 1914); Watson, *Psychology from the Standpoint of a Behaviorist* (Philadelphia: Lippincott, 1919) — the work was revised in 1924 and again in 1929.

24. English and English (n. 16), *Dictionary of Psychological and Psychoanalytical Terms,* p. 107.

25. B. F. Skinner, *The Behavior of Organisms: An Experimental Analysis* (New York: Appleton-Century-Crofts, 1938).

26. Alan E. Kazdin, *History of Behavior Modification: Experimental Foundations of Contemporary Research* (Baltimore, Md.: University Park Press, 1978), pp. 92–93.

27. Ibid., pp. 97–101.

28. See, e.g., Duane P. Schultz, *A History of Modern Psychology* (New York: Academic Press, 1969), chap. 11.

29. Carol R. Glass and Diane B. Arnkoff, "Behavior Therapy," in Donald K. Freedheim et al. (eds.), *History of Psychotherapy: A Century of Change* (Washington: American Psychological Association, 1992), p. 587.

30. Joseph Wolpe, "Conditioning Is the Basis of All Psychotherapeutic Change," in Arthur Burton (ed.), *What Makes Behavior Change Possible?* (New York: Brunner/Mazel, 1976), p. 58. See also Joseph Wolpe, *Psychotherapy by Reciprocal Inhibition* (Stanford, Calif.: Stanford University Press, 1958); Joseph Wolpe, Andrew Salter, and L. J. Reyna (eds.), *The Conditioning Therapies: The Challenge in Psychotherapy* (New York: Holt, Rinehart and Winston, 1964); Joseph Wolpe, *The Practice of Behavior Therapy* (New York: Pergamon, 1969).

31. Daniel B. Fishman and Cyril M. Franks, "Evolution and Differentiation Within

Behavior Therapy: A Theoretical and Epistemological Review," in Freedheim (n. 29), *History of Psychotherapy*, p. 172.

32. Cyril M. Franks (ed.), *Conditioning Techniques in Clinical Practice and Research* (New York: Springer, 1964), p. 12.

33. Joseph Wolpe, "Psychotherapy: The Nonscientific Heritage and the New Science," *Behav. Res. Ther.*, 1963, *1*, 23–28 [23].

34. Ibid.

35. Although they are usually ignored in accounts of the history of conditioning therapies or behavior therapy, a good argument has been made for the relevance of several clinical endeavors based on Pavlovian conditioning that were undertaken during the first two decades of the twentieth century — see E. J. Freedberg, "Behaviour Therapy: A Comparison Between Early (1890–1920) and Contemporary Techniques," *Canadian Psychologist*, 1973, *14*, 225–40.

36. John B. Watson and Rosalie Rayner, "Conditioned Emotional Reactions," *J. Experimental Psychol.*, 1920, *3*, 1–14.

37. Mary Cover Jones, "The Elimination of Children's Fears," *J. Experimental Psychol.*, 1924, *7*, 383–90; Jones, "A Laboratory Study of Fear: The Case of Peter," *Pedagogical Seminary*, 1924, *31*, 308–15.

38. Clark L. Hull, *Principles of Behavior* (New York: Appleton-Century-Crofts, 1943).

39. Skinner (n. 25), *Behavior of Organisms*.

40. O. H. Mowrer and W. M. Mowrer, "Enuresis: A Method for Its Study and Treatment," *Am. J. Orthopsychiat.*, 1938, *8*, 436–59.

41. Kazdin (n. 26), *History of Behavior Modification*, pp. 152–59.

42. Ogden R. Lindsley and B. F. Skinner, "A Method for the Experimental Analysis of Behavior of Psychotic Patients," *Am. Psychol.*, 1954, *9*, 419–20.

43. Charles B. Ferster and Marian K. DeMyer, "The Development of Performances in Autistic Children in an Automatically Controlled Environment," *J. Chronic Dis.*, 1961, *13*, 312–45.

44. Andrew Salter, *Conditioned Reflex Therapy: The Direct Approach to the Reconstruction of Personality* (New York: Creative Age Press, 1949).

45. Kazdin (n. 26), *History of Behavior Modification*, pp. 246–73.

46. T. Ayllon and N. H. Azrin, *The Token Economy: A Motivational System for Therapy and Rehabilitation* (New York: Appleton-Century-Crofts, 1968); Robert P. Liberman, "Behavioral Modification of Schizophrenia: A Review," *Schizophrenia Bulletin*, issue 6, Fall 1972, pp. 37–48; Alan E. Kazdin, *The Token Economy: A Review and Evaluation* (New York/London: Plenum Press, 1977).

47. Jules M. Masserman, *Behavior and Neurosis: An Experimental Psycho-Analytic Approach to Psychobiologic Principles* (Chicago: University of Chicago Press, 1943).

48. Kazdin (n. 26), *History of Behavior Modification*, pp. 152–59.

49. Arnold A. Lazarus, "New Methods in Psychotherapy: A Case Study," *South African Med. J.*, 1958, *32*, 660–64.

50. Wolpe (n. 30), *Psychotherapy by Reciprocal Inhibition*.

51. Wolpe (n. 30), *The Practice of Behavior Therapy*, pp. 91–168.

52. H. J. Eysenck, *Behaviour Therapy and the Neuroses* (Oxford: Pergamon, 1960);

Eysenck (ed.), *Experiments in Behaviour Therapy: Readings in Modern Methods of Treatment of Mental Disorders Derived from Learning Theory* (New York: Macmillan, 1964).

53. H. J. Eysenck, "Learning Theory and Behaviour Therapy," *J. Ment. Sci.,* 1959, *105,* 61–75 [66].

54. Ibid., pp. 64–66.

55. Hilgard (n. 1), *Theories of Learning,* p. 8.

56. To some degree, though not necessarily in terms designed to suit the cognitive learning theorist, these matters are dealt with in Chapters 15 and 16.

57. Edward J. Kempf, "A Study of the Anaesthesia, Convulsions, Vomiting, Visual Constriction, Erythema and Itching of Mrs. V. G.," *J. Abnorm. Psychol.,* 1917, *12,* 3–26. This example and others are to be found in Edward J. Kempf, *Selected Papers,* ed. Dorothy Clarke Kempf and John C. Burnham (Bloomington: Indiana University Press, 1974).

58. Franz Alexander, "The Dynamics of Psychotherapy in the Light of Learning Theory," *Am. J. Psychiat.,* 1963, *120,* 441–48 [446–47].

59. Judd Marmor, "Psychoanalytic Therapy as an Educational Process," in Jules Masserman (ed.), *Science and Psychoanalysis,* vol. 5 (New York: Grune & Stratton, 1962).

60. Judd Marmor, "Psychoanalytic Therapy and Theories of Learning," in *Psychiatry in Transition: Selected Papers of Judd Marmor, M.D.* (New York: Brunner/Mazel, 1974). Originally published in Jules Masserman (ed.), *Science and Psychoanalysis,* vol. 7 (New York: Grune & Stratton, 1964),.

61. Ibid., pp. 216–17.

62. Ibid., p. 223.

63. Judd Marmor, "The Nature of the Psychotherapeutic Process Revisited," *Can. Psychiat. Assoc. J.,* 1975, *20,* 557–65 [560].

64. Saul Rosenzweig, "Some Implicit Common Factors in Diverse Methods of Psychotherapy," *Am. J. Orthopsychiat.,* 1936, *6,* 412–15.

65. Allen E. Bergin and Hans S. Strupp, "Some Empirical and Conceptual Bases for Coordinated Research in Psychotherapy: A Critical Review of Issues, Trends, and Evidence," *Int. J. Psychiat.,* 1969, *7,* 18–90 — see p. 24.

Chapter 15: Explanation and Interpretation

1. Aristotle. *Metaphysics,* in *The Complete Works of Aristotle,* 2 vols., rev. Oxford trans., ed. Jonathan Barnes (Princeton, N.J.: Princeton University Press, 1984), 2: 980a22.

2. Jonathan Lear, *Aristotle: The Desire to Understand* (Cambridge: Cambridge University Press, 1988), pp. 3, 6, 117.

3. H. Tristram Engelhardt, Jr., "The Concepts of Health and Disease," in H. Tristram Engelhardt, Jr., and Stuart F. Spicker (eds.), *Evaluation and Explanation in the Biomedical Sciences* (Dordrecht: Reidel, 1975), p. 136.

4. Henry E. Sigerist, *A History of Medicine,* vol. 1 (New York: Oxford University Press, 1951), p. 180.

5. James A. H. Murray et al. (eds.), *A New English Dictionary . . . ,* 13 vols. (Oxford: Clarendon Press, 1888–1933), 5: 415–16.

6. Rudolf Ekstein, "Thoughts Concerning the Nature of the Interpretive Process," in Morton Levitt (ed.), *Readings in Psychoanalytic Psychology* (New York: Appleton-Century-Crofts, 1959), p. 223.

7. James Dimon, "Interpretation: Review of the Literature," *Psychoanalytic Inquiry,* 1992, *12,* 182–95 [182–83].

8. Sigmund Freud, *The Interpretation of Dreams* (1900), vols. 4 and 5 in *The Standard Edition of the Complete Psychological Works of Sigmund Freud,* 24 vols., trans. and ed. James Strachey, Anna Freud, et al. (London: Hogarth Press, 1955–1974), 4: 11.

9. Ibid., 4: 96.

10. Ibid., 4: 10.

11. Freud, "Freud's Psycho-Analytic Procedure" (1904), in *Standard Edition* (n. 8), 7: 252.

12. Freud, "On Beginning the Treatment (Further Recommendations on the Technique of Psycho-Analysis I)" (1913), in *Standard Edition* (n. 8) 12: 139–44.

13. J. Laplanche and J.-B. Pontalis, *The Language of Psycho-Analysis,* trans. Donald Nicholson-Smith (New York: Norton, 1973), p. 228.

14. James Strachey, "The Nature of the Therapeutic Action of Psycho-Analysis," *Int. J. Psycho-Anal.,* 1934, *15,* 127–59.

15. Rudolph M. Loewenstein, "The Problem of Interpretation," *Psychoanal. Quart.,* 1951, *20,* 1–14 [4].

16. Ibid., pp. 1–3.

17. Ralph R. Greenson, *The Technique and Practice of Psychoanalysis,* vol. 1 (New York: International Universities Press, 1967), pp. 37–42.

18. Ibid., pp. 97–98.

19. Harold P. Blum, "The Position and Value of Extratransference Interpretation," *J. Am. Psychoanal. Assoc.,* 1983, *31,* 587–617 [588, 592, 589, 614–15].

20. Karl A. Menninger and Philip S. Holzman, *Theory of Psychoanalytic Technique,* 2nd ed. (New York: Basic Books, 1973), p. 138.

21. Franz Alexander and Thomas Morton French, *Psychoanalytic Therapy: Principles and Application* (New York: Ronald Press, 1946).

22. Edward Bibring, "Psychoanalysis and the Dynamic Psychotherapies," *J. Am. Psychoanal. Assoc.,* 1954, *2,* 745–70 [752, 763].

23. Hans W. Loewald, "On the Therapeutic Action of Psycho-Analysis," *Int. J. Psycho-Anal.,* 1960, *41,* 16–33.

24. Steven T. Levy and Lawrence B. Inderbitzin, "Interpretation," in Alan Sugarman, Robert A. Nemiroff, and Daniel P. Greenson (eds.), *The Technique and Practice of Psychoanalysis, Volume II: A Memorial Volume to Ralph R. Greenson* (Madison, Conn.: International Universities Press, 1992), p. 101.

25. Laplanche and Pontalis (n. 13), *Language of Psycho-Analysis,* p. 227.

26. Greenson (n. 17), *Technique and Practice of Psychoanalysis,* p. 39.

27. Ekstein (n. 6), p. 232.

28. Stephen A. Appelbaum, "The Idealization of Insight," *Int. J. Psychoanal. Psychother.,* 1975, *4,* 272–302.

29. Steven T. Levy, *Principles of Interpretation* (Northvale, N.J.: Jason Aronson, 1990), p. 185.

30. Carl R. Rogers, *Counseling and Psychotherapy: Newer Concepts in Practice* (Boston: Houghton Mifflin, 1942), p. 40.

31. Ibid., pp. 174–75, 177, 194–96.

32. Ibid., pp. 195–96.

33. Carl R. Rogers, *Client-Centered Therapy: Its Current Practice, Implications, and Theory* (Boston: Houghton Mifflin, 1951), p. 289.

34. Carl R. Rogers, "The Necessary and Sufficient Conditions of Therapeutic Personality Change," *J. Consult. Psychol.,* 1957, *21,* 95–103.

35. E.g., Edward J. Kempf, "A Study of the Anaesthesia, Convulsions, Vomiting, Visual Constriction, Erythema, and Itching of Mrs. V. G.," *J. Abnorm. Psychol.,* 1917. *12,* 3–26; Franz Alexander, "The Dynamics of Psychotherapy in the Light of Learning Theory," *Am. J. Psychiat.,* 1963, *120,* 440–48; Judd Marmor, "Psychoanalytic Therapy and Theories of Learning," in Jules Masserman (ed.), *Science and Psychoanalysis,* vol. 7 (New York: Grune & Stratton, 1964); Marmor, "Dynamic Psychotherapy and Behavior Therapy," *Arch. Gen. Psychiat.,* 1971, *24,* 22–28; Paul L. Wachtel, *Psychoanalysis and Behavior Therapy: Toward an Integration* (New York: Basic Books, 1977). See Chapter 14 for an extended discussion of these matters.

36. Judd Marmor, "The Nature of the Psychotherapeutic Process Revisited," *Can. Psychiat. Assoc. J.,* 1975, *20,* 557–65 [562].

37. Jerry A. Greenwald, "The Ground Rules in Gestalt Therapy," in Chris Hatcher and Philip Himelstein (eds.), *The Handbook of Gestalt Therapy* (New York: Jason Aronson, 1976), p. 275.

38. Frederick S. Perls, "Four Lectures," in Joen Fagan and Irma Lee Shepherd (eds.), *Gestalt Therapy Now: Theory, Techniques, Applications* (New York: Harper Colophon Books, 1971), p. 27.

39. Claudio Naranjo, "Present-Centeredness: Technique, Prescription, and Ideal," in Fagan and Shepherd (n. 38), *Gestalt Therapy Now,* p. 57.

40. Stephen A. Appelbaum, *Out in Inner Space: A Psychoanalyst Explores the New Therapies* (New York: Anchor Press/Doubleday, 1979), pp. 433, 476–77.

41. Ibid., pp. 476–77.

42. Saul Rosenzweig, "Some Implicit Common Factors in Diverse Methods of Psychotherapy," *Am. J. Orthopsychiat.,* 1936, *6,* 412–15.

43. Allen E. Bergin and Hans S. Strupp, "Some Empirical and Conceptual Bases for Coordinated Research in Psychotherapy: A Critical Review of Issues, Trends, and Evidence," *Int. J. Psychiat.,* 1969, *7,* 18–90 [24].

44. Marmor (n. 36), pp. 560, 562.

45. Robert L. Woolfolk, Louis A. Sass, Stanley B. Messer, "Introduction to Hermeneutics," in Stanley B. Messer, Louis A. Sass, and Robert L. Woolfolk (eds.), *Hermeneutics and Psychological Theory: Interpretive Perspectives on Personality, Psychotherapy, and Psychopathology* (New Brunswick, N.J.: Rutgers University Press, 1988), p. 2.

46. W. Dilthey, *Selected Writings,* ed., trans., and intro. H. P. Rickman (Cambridge: Cambridge University Press, 1976), pp. 226–31, 247–63; H. P. Rickman, "Wilhelm Dilthey," in Paul Edwards (ed.), *The Encyclopedia of Philosophy,* 8 vols. (New York: Macmillan and Free Press, 1967), 2: 403–6. See also H. A. Hodges, *The Philosophy of Wilhelm Dilthey* (Westport, Conn.: Greenwood Press, [1952] 1974).

47. Richard D. Chessick, *What Constitutes the Patient in Psychotherapy: Alternative Approaches to Understanding Humans* (Northvale, N.J.: Jason Aronson, 1992), pp. xix, 39–57.

48. Ibid., pp. 42, 45. Here Chessick draws on Hans-Georg Gadamer, *Truth and Method*, 2nd rev. ed., ed. Joel Weinsheimer and Donald G. Marshall (New York: Crossroad, 1991).

49. Chessick (n. 47), *What Constitutes the Patient in Psychotherapy*, p. 50. Here Chessick draws on Hans-Georg Gadamer, *Philosophical Hermeneutics*, trans. D. Linge (Berkeley: University of California Press, 1977).

50. Richard J. Bernstein, "Interpretation and Its Discontents: The Choreography of Critique," in Messer, Sass, and Woolfolk (n. 52), *Hermeneutics and Psychological Theory*, p. 88.

Chapter 16: Self-Understanding and Insight

1. James A. H. Murray et al. (eds.), *A New English Dictionary . . .* , 13 vols. (Oxford: Clarendon Press, 1888–1933), 5: 337.

2. Joseph M. Patwell et al. (eds.), *The American Heritage Dictionary of the English Language,* 3rd ed. (Boston: Houghton Mifflin, 1992), p. 934.

3. Horace B. English and Ava Champney English, *A Comprehensive Dictionary of Psychological and Psychoanalytical Terms* (New York: Longmans, Green, 1958), p. 264.

4. N. G. L. Hammond and H. H. Scullard (eds.), *The Oxford Classical Dictionary,* 2nd ed. (Oxford: Clarendon Press, 1970), pp. 322–23.

5. Ibid., pp. 81–82.

6. Ibid., pp. 129–30.

7. Helen North, *Sophrosyne: Self-Knowledge and Self-Restraint in Greek Literature* (Ithaca, N.Y.: Cornell University Press, 1966), p. 380.

8. Plato, *The Republic,* in *The Dialogues of Plato,* 2 vols., trans. B. Jowett (New York: Random House, 1937), 1: 591–879 [682–710] [*Republic,* bk. IV].

9. Plato, *Charmides* in *Works* (n. 8), 1: 14 [*Charmides,* 164–65].

10. Plato, *Phaedrus,* in *Works* (n. 8), 1: 235 [*Phaedrus,* 229–30].

11. Plato, *Alcibiades I,* in *Works* (n. 8), 2: 757, 763–64, 768–69 [*Alcibiades I,* 124, 129, 132–33]. Whether or not this dialogue was written by Plato, it would appear to be relevant here.

12. Cicero, *De inventione,* trans. H. M. Hubbell, in *Works,* 28 vols. (Cambridge/London: Harvard University Press/William Heinemann, 1914–1949), 2: II. 54. 164; Cicero, *De officiis,* trans. Walter Miller, in *Works,* 21: I. 27. 93.

13. Cicero, *Tusculan Disputations,* trans. J. E. King, 2nd ed. (Cambridge/London: Harvard University Press/William Heinemann, 1966), V. 24–25. 68–70.

14. Ibid., I. 22. 52.

15. Cicero, *De legibus,* trans. Clinton Walker Keyes, in (n. 12) *Works,* 16: 289–519, I. 22. 58–59.

16. Cicero (n. 13), *Tusculan Disputations,* bk. III.

17. North (n. 7), *Sophrosyne,* pp. 312–79.

18. Clement of Alexandria, *Christ the Educator* [*Paedagogus*], trans. Simon P. Wood (New York: Fathers of the Church, Inc., 1954), p. 199 [bk. III, chap. 1].

19. North (n. 7), *Sophrosyne*, p. 332. See Plato, *Theaetetus,* in (n. 8) *The Dialogues of Plato,* 2: 178 [*Theaetetus,* 176]; Plato, *Laws,* in (n. 8) *The Dialogues of Plato,* 2: 488 [*Laws,* bk. IV, 716].

20. North (n. 7), *Sophrosyne,* pp. 237–39.

21. Plotinus, *The Enneads,* trans. Stephen MacKenna (Burdett, N.Y.: Larson Publications, 1992), pp. 439–50 [V. 3. 10]; Philip Merlan, "Plotinus," in *The Encyclopedia of Philosophy,* ed. Paul Edwards, 8 vols. (New York: Macmillan and Free Press, 1967), 6: 351–59.

22. Augustine, *The Soliloquies* [*Soliloquia*], in *Augustine: Earlier Writings,* trans. and intro. John H. S. Burleigh (Philadelphia: Westminster Press, 1953), p. 41 [*Soliloquia,* II, 1,1].

23. Augustine, *Confessions,* trans., intro., and annot. Henry Chadwick (Oxford: Oxford University Press, 1991); Augustine, *The Trinity* [*De Trinitate*], in *Augustine: Later Works,* trans. and intro. John Burnaby (Philadelphia: Westminster Press, 1955), bks. IX–X.

24. R. A. Markus, "Augustine: Reason and Illumination," in *The Cambridge History of Later Greek and Early Medieval Philosophy,* ed. A. H. Armstrong (Cambridge: Cambridge University Press, 1967), p. 373.

25. Augustine (n. 23), *The Trinity,* p. 60 [bk. IX, 4, iv].

26. Ibid., pp. 77–80 [bk. X, 5, iii–6, iv].

27. Ibid., p. 80 [bk. X, 7, v].

28. Boethius, *The Consolation of Philosophy,* intro. Irwin Edman (New York: Modern Library, 1943), p. 9.

29. Ibid., pp. 18–19.

30. Eliza Gregory Wilkins, *The Delphic Maxims in Literature* (Chicago: University of Chicago Press, 1929), pp. 74–75.

31. Ibid., pp. 76–78.

32. Ibid., p. 78.

33. Ibid., p. 85.

34. Ibid., pp. 85–115; Richard Baxter, *The Mischiefs of Self-Ignorance and the Benefits of Self-Acquaintance* (London: Tyton, 1662).

35. Wilkins (n. 30), *Delphic Maxims,* p. 100.

36. Ibid., p. 113.

37. Ibid., pp. 116–33.

38. Ibid., p. 133.

39. Ibid., chaps. 8–10.

40. Samuel Taylor Coleridge, *Biographia Literaria,* or *Biographical Sketches of My Literary Life and Opinions,* ed. James Engell and W. Jackson Bate (Princeton, N.J.: Princeton University Press, 1983), 1: 252.

41. William A. Knight, *Varia, Studies on Problems of Philosophy and Ethics* (London: John Murray, 1901), p. 165.

42. Bennett Simon, *Mind and Madness in Ancient Greece: The Classical Roots of Modern Psychiatry* (Ithaca, N.Y.: Cornell University Press, 1978), p. 273.

43. Ibid., p. 186.

44. Josef Breuer and Sigmund Freud, *Studies on Hysteria,* in *The Standard Edition of the Complete Psychological Works of Sigmund Freud,* 24 vols., trans. and ed. James Strachey, Anna Freud, et al. (London: Hogarth Press, 1955–1974), 2: 6.

45. The word *insight* is not indexed anywhere in the *Standard Edition* of Freud's works. Nevertheless, it is used with some frequency in the text — usually to mean "understanding," and only occasionally to mean "self-understanding." The same is true for the equivalent German word *Einsicht* in Freud's *Gesammelte Werke.* In the latter, *Krankheitseinsicht* is indexed, but it tends to have the meaning "awareness of illness" — that is, "insight" in the sense in which it was used in twentieth-century general psychiatry. See later in this chapter for an account of this usage.

46. Freud *Standard Edition* (n. 44), 2: chap. 4.

47. Sigmund Freud, "On Beginning the Treatment (Further Recommendations on the Technique of Psycho-Analysis I)" in *Standard Edition* (n. 44), 12: 141–42.

48. Samuel Slipp (ed.), *Curative Factors in Dynamic Psychotherapy* (New York: McGraw-Hill, 1982), pp. 2–3.

49. Harold P. Blum, "The Curative and Creative Aspects of Insight," *J. Am. Psychoanal. Assoc.,* 1979, 27 (Suppl.), 41–69 [41].

50. Ibid., p. 47.

51. Lloyd H. Silverman, "The Unconscious Fantasy as Therapeutic Agent in Psychoanalytic Treatment," in Slipp (n. 48), *Curative Factors,* p. 199.

52. Gregory Zilboorg, "The Emotional Problem and the Therapeutic Role of Insight," *Psychoanal. Quart.,* 1952, 21, 1–24.

53. E.g., Robert L. Hatcher, "Insight and Self-Observation," in Slipp (n. 48), *Curative Factors,* pp. 72–74.

54. James Strachey, "The Nature of the Therapeutic Action of Psycho-Analysis," *Int. J. Psycho-Anal.,* 1934, 15, 127–59 [141–50].

55. Jerome Richfield, "An Analysis of the Concept of Insight," *Psychoanal. Quart.,* 1954, 23, 390–408 [404–5].

56. Ibid., p. 400.

57. John R. Reid and Jacob E. Finesinger, "The Role of Insight in Psychotherapy," *Am. J. Psychiat.,* 1951–1952, 108, 726–34.

58. Hans. W. Loewald, "On the Therapeutic Action of Psychoanalysis," *Int. J. Psycho-Anal.,* 1960, 41, 16–33 [24].

59. Hans. W. Loewald, "Psychoanalysis as an Art and the Fantasy Character of the Psychoanalytic Situation," *J. Am. Psychoanal. Assoc.,* 1975, 23, 277–99 [287].

60. Franz Alexander and Thomas Morton French, *Psychoanalytic Therapy: Principles and Application* (New York: Ronald Press, 1946). For an elaborated presentation of this notion, in tandem with vigorous attention to the arguments of his critics, see Franz Alexander, *Psychoanalysis and Psychotherapy: Developments in Theory, Technique and Training* (New York: Norton, 1956). For more on Alexander's views regarding insight, see next section of this chapter.

61. Heinz Kohut, *How Does Analysis Cure?* ed. Arnold Goldberg and Paul E. Stepansky (Chicago: University of Chicago Press, 1984), p. 56.

62. Robert S. Wallerstein, "How Does Self Psychology Differ in Practice?" *Int. J. Psycho-Anal.,* 1985, 66, 391–404 [397].

63. Ibid., p. 402.

64. Kohut (n. 61), *How Does Analysis Cure?* p. 66.

65. Ibid., p. 77.

66. Allen Wheelis, "Will and Psychoanalysis," *Am. J. Psychoanal.,* 1956, 4, 285–303.

67. Allen Wheelis, "The Place of Action in Personality Change," *Psychiatry,* 1950, *13,* 135–48.

68. Allen Wheelis, *How People Change* (New York: Harper & Row, 1973), pp. 17, 101–2. Emphasis added.

69. Arthur F. Valenstein, "The Psycho-Analytic Situation: Affects, Emotional Reliving, and Insight in the Psycho-Analytic Process," *Int. J. Psycho-Anal.,* 1962, 43, 315–24 [323].

70. Arthur F. Valenstein, "Working Through and Resistance to Change: Insight and the Action System," *J. Am. Psychoanal. Assoc.,* 1983, *31,* 353–73, quotation on p. 362.

71. Edward Bibring, "Psychoanalysis and the Dynamic Psychotherapies," *J. Am. Psychoanal. Assoc.,* 1954, 2, 745–70.

72. Judd Marmor, "Psychoanalytic Therapy as an Educational Process," in *Psychiatry in Transition: Selected Papers of Judd Marmor, M.D.* (New York: Brunner/Mazel, 1974); Marmor, "Psychoanalytic Therapy and Theories of Learning," in *Psychiatry in Transition.* Further, for all the differences in the manifest content of their formulations, practitioners of these various approaches tend to employ notions that reflect "a central core of common reality." Ibid., p. 214.

73. Alexander and French (n. 60), *Psychoanalytic Therapy,* p. 102.

74. Ibid., pp. 126–27.

75. Ibid., p. 128.

76. Ibid., p. 130.

77. Franz Alexander, "The Dynamics of Psychotherapy in the Light of Learning Theory," *Am. J. Psychiat.,* 1963, *120,* 440–48 [447].

78. Bibring (n. 71), p. 768.

79. William Brown, *Psychology and Psychotherapy* (London: Edward Arnold, 1921), pp. 102, 103.

80. W. H. R. Rivers, "Psycho-Therapeutics," in James Hastings et al. (eds.), *Encyclopaedia of Religion and Ethics,* 13 vols. (New York: Charles Scribner's Sons, 1908–1927), vol. 10, p. 437.

81. Carl R. Rogers, *Counseling and Psychotherapy: Newer Concepts in Practice* (Boston: Houghton Mifflin, 1942), p. 40.

82. Ibid., pp. 174–75.

83. See discussion of Rogers' views on interpretation in Chapter 15.

84. Rogers (n. 82), *Counseling and Psychotherapy,* p. 196.

85. Ibid., pp. 206–7.

86. Ibid., p. 255.

87. Leland E. Hinsie and Jacob Shatzky, *Psychiatric Dictionary* (London: Oxford University Press, 1940), p. 296. This definition continued to appear in later editions of this dictionary.

88. Zilboorg (n. 52), p. 2.

89. Emil Kraepelin, *Psychiatrie: Ein Lehrbuch für Studierende und Ärzte,* 5th ed. (Leipzig: Johann Ambrosius Barth, 1896) pp. 214–15.

90. Emil Kraepelin, *Psychiatrie: Ein Lehrbuch für Studierende und Ärzte,* 2 vols., 6th ed. (Leipzig: Johann Ambrosius Barth, 1899); Kraepelin, *Psychiatrie . . . ,* 2 vols., 7th ed. (Leipzig: Johann Ambrosius Barth, 1903–1904); Kraepelin, *Psychiatrie . . . ,* 4 vols., 8th ed. (Leipzig: Johann Ambrosius Barth, 1909–1915).

91. E.g., C. G. Jung, "On Manic Mood Disorder" (1903), in *The Collected Works of C. G. Jung,* 20 vols. in 21, trans. R. F. C. Hull, ed. Herbert Read, Michael Fordham, et al. (Princeton, N.J.: Princeton University Press, 1957–1979), vol. 1, pp. 118–26; Jung, "The Content of the Psychoses" (1908), in *Works,* 3: 166.

92. Adolf Meyer, "Notes of Clinics in Psychopathology," in *The Collected Papers of Adolf Meyer,* 4 vols., ed. Eunice E. Winters (Baltimore, Md.: Johns Hopkins University Press, 1950–1952), 3: 142.

93. D. K. Henderson and R. D. Gillespie, *A Text-Book of Psychiatry for Students and Practitioners* (London: Oxford University Press, 1927), p. 80.

94. Ibid., p. 89.

95. Karl Jaspers, *General Psychopathology,* trans. J. Hoenig and Marian W. Hamilton (Chicago: University of Chicago Press, 1963), pp. 414–19.

96. Ibid., pp. 419–22.

97. Ibid., pp. 422–24.

98. E.g., see Karl Jaspers, *Allgemeine Psychopathologie: Für Studierende, Ärzte und Psychologen,* 3rd ed. (Berlin: Julius Springer, 1923), pp. 261–65.

Chapter 17: Self-Observation and Introspection

1. See Chapter 16.

2. Robert I. Watson, *The Great Psychologists: Aristotle to Freud* (Philadelphia: Lippincott, 1963), p. 19. The intimate connection between self-examination and the acquisition of self-understanding has been pointed out by Bennett Simon and Herbert Weiner, "Models of Mind and Mental Illness in Ancient Greece: I. The Homeric Model of Mind," *J. Hist. Behav. Sci.,* 1966, 2, 303–14 [308]. See also the attention to this connection evident in Georg Misch, *A History of Autobiography in Antiquity,* 2 vols. (Westport, Conn.: Greenwood Press, 1973).

3. Watson (n. 2), *The Great Psychologists,* pp. 85–88.

4. Augustine, *Confessions,* trans., introd., and annot. Henry Chadwick (Oxford: Oxford University Press, 1991), p. 180.

5. Ibid., pp. xxi, xxv.

6. Ibid., p. 123.

7. Ibid., p. 120.

8. Ibid., pp. 179–220 [bk. X].

9. Augustine, *The Trinity* [*De Trinitate*], in *Augustine: Later Works,* trans. and intro. John Burnaby (Philadelphia: Westminster Press, 1955), p. 72 [bk. X].

10. Ibid., p. 80 [bk. X, 7, v].

11. See Chapter 16.

12. Paul Oskar Kristeller, *Renaissance Thought II: Papers on Humanism and the Arts* (New York: Harper Torchbooks, 1965), pp. 65–67.

13. Petrarch [Francesco Petrarca], *Petrarch's Secret, or the Soul's Conflict with Passion,*

trans. William H. Draper (London: Chatto and Windus, 1911); Davy A. Carozza and H. James Shey, *Petrarch's* Secretum *with Introduction, Notes, and Critical Anthology* (New York: Peter Lang, 1989); Petrarch, *Letters from Petrarch,* trans. Morris Bishop (Bloomington: Indiana University Press, 1966).

14. Carozza and Shey (n. 13), *Petrarch's* Secretum, p. 5.

15. Morris Bishop, foreword to Petrarch (n. 13), *Letters from Petrarch,* p. v.

16. P. Mansell Jones, *French Introspectives: From Montaigne to André Gide* (Port Washington, N.Y.: Kennikat Press, 1970), pp. 37–38. And John E. Gedo and Ernest S. Wolf have discoursed at some length on Montaigne as an "introspective psychologist": see "From the History of Introspective Psychology: The Humanist Strain," in John E. Gedo and George H. Pollock (eds.), *Freud: The Fusion of Science and Humanism* (New York: International Universities Press, 1976) [*Psychological Issues,* Monograph 34/35].

17. Michel de Montaigne, *The Essays of Michel de Montaigne,* trans. and ed. M. A. Screech (London: Penguin Press, 1991), p. 424 [II, 6].

18. Ibid., p. 1217 [III, 13].

19. Robert Boyle, *The Christian Virtuoso: The Second Part,* in *The Works of the Honourable Robert Boyle,* 5 vols., ed. Thomas Birch (London: Millar, 1744), 5: 708 [sect. 2, aphorisms to subsec. 2].

20. John Locke, *An Essay Concerning Human Understanding,* 2 vols., ed. Alexander Campbell Fraser (New York: Dover, 1959), 1: 122–24 [bk. II, chap. 1, 2–4].

21. Matthew Hale, *The Primitive Origination of Mankind, Considered and Examined According to the Light of Nature* (London: William Shrowsbery, 1677), pp. 21–22.

22. Ibid, p. 55.

23. Samuel Johnson, *A Dictionary of the English Language: . . . ,* 2 vols. (London: Knapton, 1755), vol. 1.

24. G. S. Brett, *Brett's History of Psychology,* ed. R. S. Peters, rev. and abridged (London: George Allen & Unwin, 1962), pp. 417–78; Edwin G. Boring, *A History of Experimental Psychology,* 2nd ed. (New York: Appleton-Century-Crofts, 1957), chaps. 10–12.

25. Thomas Reid, *An Inquiry into the Human Mind, on the Principles of Common Sense* (Edinburgh: Millar, Kincaid and Bell, 1764), pp. ix, 5–6, 11.

26. *Lamentations* 3:40.

27. *II Corinthians* 13:5.

28. *I Corinthians* 11:28.

29. William A. Clebsch and Charles R. Jaekle, *Pastoral Care in Historical Perspective* (New York: Jason Aronson, 1975), pp. 296–97, 306; John T. McNeill, *A History of the Cure of Souls* (New York: Harper & Row, 1951), pp. 287–89. Clebsch and Jaekle drew particularly from a translation of *Le manuel des confesseurs* (1837) by Abbé Jean Joseph Gaume (1802–1879). Gaume, in turn, had drawn from the works of the great Roman Catholic masters of spiritual direction; and his book went through many editions in the nineteenth century. As Gaume's work illustrates, self-examination was considered an integral element in the preparation for and in the process of confession. Edward Bouverie Pusey, a leading figure in the Oxford Movement, translated Gaume's book in 1877, and it became influential for the Church of England. *Advice for Those Who Exercise the Ministry of Reconciliation Through Confession and Absolution . . . ,* abridged, condensed, and

adapted to the use of the English Church, trans. Rev. E. B. Pusey (London: Innes, 1893). While abridging, Dr. Pusey added 174 pages of preface that included comments on the importance of self-examination and self-knowledge.

30. *The Canons and Dogmatic Decrees of the Council of Trent,* A.D. 1563, trans. J. Waterworth, in Philip Schaff, *The Creeds of Christendom, with a History and Critical Notes,* 3 vols. (Grand Rapids, Mich.: Baker Book House 1969), 2: 77–206, pp. 147–48.

31. Henry Charles Lea, *A History of Auricular Confession and Indulgences in the Latin Church,* 3 vols. (New York: Greenwood Press, 1968), 2: 413 and n.

32. John T. McNeill, "Medicine for Sin as Prescribed in the Penitentials," *Church History,* 1932, *1,* 14–26; John T. McNeill and Helena M. Gamer, *Medieval Handbooks of Penance: A Translation of the Principle* libri poenitentiales *from Related Documents* (New York: Octagon Books, [1938] 1979).

33. McNeill (n. 29), *History of the Cure of Souls.*

34. Ibid., p. 220.

35. McNeill (n. 29), *History of the Cure of Souls;* E. Brooks Holifield, *A History of Pastoral Care in America: From Salvation to Self-Realization* (Nashville: Abingdon Press, 1983), pp. 25–29.

36. Jonathan Edwards, *Christian Cautions: or, the Necessity of Self-Examination,* in *The Works of Jonathan Edwards, A.M.,* ed. Edward Hicknan, 2 vols., 10th ed. (London: Henry G. Bohn, 1865), 2: 173–85.

37. James A. H. Murray et al. (eds.), *A New English Dictionary . . . ,* 13 vols. (Oxford: Clarendon Press, 1888–1933), 5: 441.

38. Watson (n. 2), *The Great Psychologists,* pp. 241–54. For more detail on the history of introspection in experimental psychology, see Edwin G. Boring, "A History of Introspection," in Edwin G. Boring, *Psychologist at Large: An Autobiography and Selected Essays* (New York: Basic Books, 1961); Kurt Danziger, "The History of Introspection Reconsidered," *J. Hist. Behav. Sci.,* 1980, *16,* 241–62. Danziger extends the discussion and modifies Boring's views somewhat, especially regarding Wundt. Danziger points out that Wundt carefully differentiated self-observation (*Selbstbeobachtung*) from inner perception (*innere Wahrnehmung*) and concentrated his investigative efforts on a quite narrowed version of inner perception; but some have blurred this distinction by using the English term *introspection* for both Wundt's German terms.

39. William James, *The Principles of Psychology,* 2 vols. (New York: Henry Holt, 1890), 1: 185.

40. Watson (n. 2), *The Great Psychologists,* pp. 358–69.

41. Wilhelm Wundt, *Principles of Physiological Psychology,* vol. 1, trans. Edward Bradford Titchener, from 5th German ed. (London/New York: Swan Sonnenschein/Macmillan, 1904); Wundt, *Outlines of Psychology,* 3rd English ed., trans. Charles Hubbard Judd, from 7th German ed. (London/New York: Williams & Norgate/G. E. Stechert, 1907); Edward Bradford Titchener, *A Text-Book of Psychology,* 2 vols. (New York: Macmillan, 1909–1910).

42. Titchener (n. 41), *A Text-Book of Psychology,* 1: 30.

43. Horace B. English and Ava Champney English, *A Comprehensive Dictionary of Psychological and Psychoanalytical Terms* (New York: Longmans, Green, 1958), p. 276.

44. Boring (n. 38), *Psychologist at Large,* p. 219.

45. Danziger (n. 38), pp. 255–58.

46. John B. Watson, "Psychology as the Behaviorist Views It," *Psychol. Rev.,* 1913, 20, 158–77 [158].

47. Edwin G. Boring, "Introspection," in *Encyclopaedia Britannica,* 24 vols. (Chicago: William Benton, 1956), 12: 542.

48. Peter McKellar, "The Method of Introspection," in Jordan M. Scher (ed.), *Theories of the Mind* (New York: Free Press of Glencoe, 1962), pp. 619–44 [621].

49. Ibid., pp. 622–25.

50. Ibid., p. 626.

51. Ibid., pp. 628–34.

52. Ibid., p. 627.

53. Sigmund Freud, *The Interpretation of Dreams,* in *The Standard Edition of the Complete Psychological Works of Sigmund Freud,* 24 vols., ed. and trans. James Strachey et al. (London: Hogarth Press, 1955–1974), vols. 4&5, 4: 101–2.

54. Sigmund Freud, "On Beginning the Treatment (Further Recommendations on the Technique of Psycho-Analysis)," in *Standard Edition* (n. 53), 12: 134.

55. Sigmund Freud, *Introductory Lectures on Psycho-Analysis,* in *Standard Edition* (n. 53), 16: 287.

56. E.g., Hans W. Loewald, "Psychoanalytic Theory and the Psychoanalytic Process," in Hans W. Loewald, *Papers on Psychoanalysis* (New Haven, Conn.: Yale University Press, 1980), pp. 285–86.

57. Robert L. Hatcher, "Insight and Self-Observation," *J. Am. Psychoanal. Assoc.,* 1973, 21, 377–98 [387].

58. Freud, *Interpretation of Dreams,* in *Standard Edition* (n. 53), 4: 101–2.

59. Hatcher (n. 58), pp. 389–94.

60. Heinz Kohut, "Introspection, Empathy, and Psychoanalysis," *J. Am. Psychoanal. Assoc.,* 1959, 7, 459–83 [459–60].

61. Ibid., p. 464.

62. Anna Robeson Burr, *Religious Confessions and Confessants: With a Chapter on the History of Introspection* (Boston: Houghton Mifflin, 1914), p. 87.

63. Holifield (n. 35) *History of Pastoral Care in America,* p. 29.

Chapter 18: Overview and Afterthoughts

1. I borrow this term from Paul R. Fleischman, *The Healing Zone: Religious Issues in Psychotherapy* (New York: Paragon House, 1989).

2. Franz Alexander, "Psychological Aspects of Medicine," *Psychosomatic Medicine,* 1939, 1, 7–18 [7].

3. Judd Marmor, "The Nature of the Psychotherapeutic Process Revisited," *Can. Psychiat. Assoc. J.,* 1975, 20, 557–65.

4. See Chapter 15.

5. See Chapter 13, n. 84.

References

Abroms, Gene M. "Persuasion in Psychotherapy." *Am. J. Psychiat.*, 1968, *124,* 1212–19.

Achtenberg, Jeanne. *Imagery in Healing* (Boston: New Science Library, 1985).

Addison, Joseph, Richard Steele, et al. *The Spectator,* new edition, with the *Lives of the Authors,* by Robert Bisset, 8 vols. (London: Jordan, 1794).

Aeschylus. *Prometheus Bound,* trans. David Grene. In *The Complete Greek Tragedies,* 4 vols., ed. David Grene and Richmond Lattimore (Chicago: University of Chicago Press, 1959), vol. 1

Agrippa, Henry Cornelius. *Three Books of Occult Philosophy,* trans. J. F. (London: Gregory Moule, 1651).

Alexander of Tralles. *Oeuvres médicales d'Alexandre de Tralles,* 4 vols., ed. F. Brunet (Paris: Geuthner, 1933–1937).

Alexander, Franz. "Psychological Aspects of Medicine." *Psychosomatic Medicine,* 1939, *1,* 7–18.

Alexander, Franz. *Psychoanalysis and Psychotherapy: Developments in Theory, Technique and Training* (New York: Norton, 1956).

Alexander, Franz. "The Problem of Psychoanalytic Technique." In Franz Alexander, *The Scope of Psychoanalysis, 1921–1961: Selected Papers of Franz Alexander* (New York: Basic Books, 1961).

Alexander, Franz. "The Dynamics of Psychotherapy in the Light of Learning Theory." *Am. J. Psychiat.,* 1963, *120,* 441–48.

Alexander, Franz, and Thomas Morton French. *Psychoanalytic Therapy: Principles and Application* (New York: Ronald Press, 1946).

Amundsen, Darrel W., "The Medieval Catholic Tradition." In Ronald L. Numbers and Darrel W. Amundsen (eds.), *Caring and Curing: Health and Medicine in the Western Religious Traditions* (New York: Macmillan, 1986).

Amundsen, Darrel W., and Gary B. Ferngren. "Philanthropy in Medicine: Some Historical Perspectives." In Earl E. Shelp (ed.), *Beneficence and Health Care* (Dordrecht: Reidel, 1982).

Amundsen, Darrel W., and Gary B. Ferngren. "Evolution of the Patient-Physician Relationship: Antiquity Through the Renaissance." In Earl E. Shelp (ed.), *The Clinical Encounter: The Moral Fabric of the Patient-Physician Relationship* (Dordrecht: Reidel, 1983).

Appelbaum, Stephen A. "The Idealization of Insight." *Int. J. Pschoanal. Psychother.,* 1975, 4, 272–302.

Appelbaum, Stephen A. *Out in Inner Space: A Psychoanalyst Explores the New Therapies* (New York: Doubleday, 1979).

Ariès, Philippe. *Centuries of Childhood: A Social History of Family Life,* trans. Robert Baldick (New York: Knopf, 1962).

Aristotle. *On the Soul.* In *The Complete Works of Aristotle,* 2 vols., rev. Oxford trans., ed. Jonathan Barnes (Princeton, N.J.: Princeton University Press, 1984), vol. 1.

Aristotle. *Sense and Sensibilia.* In *Works,* vol. 1.

Aristotle. *On Memory.* In *Works,* vol. 1.

Aristotle. *Metaphysics.* In *Works,* vol. 2.

Aristotle. *Politics.* In *Works,* vol. 2.

Aristotle. *Rhetoric.* In *Works,* vol. 2.

Aristotle. *Poetics.* In *Works,* vol. 2.

Arnould, E. J. *Le manuel des péchés: Etude de littérature religieuse anglo-normande (XIIIe siècle)* (Paris: Librairie Droz, 1940a).

Arnould, E. J. (ed.). *Le Livre de Seyntz Medicines, The Unpublished Devotional Treatise of Henry of Lancaster* (Oxford: Blackwell, 1940b).

Augustine. *The Soliloquies [Soliloquia].* In *Augustine: Earlier Writings,* trans. and intro. John H. S. Burleigh (Philadelphia: Westminster Press, 1953).

Augustine. *The Trinity [De trinitate].* In *Augustine: Later Works,* trans. and intro. John Burnaby (Philadelphia: Westminster Press, 1955).

Augustine. *Concerning the City of God Against the Pagans,* ed. and intro. David Knowles, trans. Henry Bettenson (Harmondsworth: Pelican Classics, 1972).

Augustine. *Confessions,* trans., intro., and annot. Henry Chadwick (Oxford: Oxford University Press, 1991).

Ayllon, T., and N. H. Azrin. *The Token Economy: A Motivational System for Therapy and Rehabilitation* (New York: Appleton-Century-Crofts, 1968).

Bacon, Francis. *The Essayes: Or Counsels Civill and Morall of Francis Bacon* (New York: Heritage Press, 1944).

Bacon, Francis. *The Works of Francis Bacon,* 7 vols., eds. James Spedding, Robert Leslie Ellis, and Douglas Denon Heath (New York: Garrett Press, 1968).

Baglivi, George. *The Practice of Physick . . .* (London: Andr. Bell, 1704).

Baldwin, James Mark (ed.). *Dictionary of Philosophy and Psychology,* 2 vols. (New York: Macmillan, 1901).

Balint, Michael. *The Doctor, His Patient and the Illness,* 2nd ed. (London: Pitman Medical, 1968).

Ballester, Luis García. "Diseases of the Soul (Nosemata tes Psyches) in Galen: The Impossibility of Galenic Psychotherapy." *Clio Medica,* 1974, 9, 35–43.

Barber, T. X. "Medicine, Suggestive Therapy, and Healing." In R. J. Kastenbaum, T. X. Barber, S. C. Wilson, B. L. Ryder, and L. B. Hathaway (eds.), *Old, Sick, and Helpless: When Therapy Begins* (Cambridge, Mass.: Ballinger, 1981).

Barclay, James R. *Foundations of Counseling Strategies* (New York: John Wiley & Sons, 1971).

Baron, Richard J. "Bridging Clinical Distance: An Empathic Rediscovery of the Known." *J. Med. & Philosophy,* 1981, 6, 5–23.

Basch, Michael Franz. "Empathic Understanding: A Review of the Concept and Some Theoretical Considerations." *J. Am. Psychoanal. Assoc.,* 1983, 31, 101–26.

Bate, Walter Jackson. "The Sympathetic Imagination in Eighteenth-Century English Criticism." *English Literary History,* 1945, 12, 144–66.

Battie, William. *A Treatise on Madness* (London: Whiston and White, 1758).

Baudouin, Charles. *Suggestion and Autosuggestion . . . ,* trans. Eden and Cedar Paul (London: George Allen & Unwin, 1920).

Baxter, Richard. *The Mischiefs of Self-Ignorance and the Benefits of Self-Acquaintance* (London: Tyton, 1662).

Baxter, Richard. *Gildas Salvianus: The Reformed Pastor,* ed. and intro. John T. Wilkinson (London: Epworth Press, 1939).

Beall, Thomas J. "The Physician's Calling." M.D. thesis, University of Pennsylvania, 1858.

Beattie, James. *Essays on Poetry and Music, as They Affect the Mind . . . ,* 3rd ed. (London: Dilly and Creech, 1779).

Beck, Lewis White. *Early German Philosophy: Kant and His Predecessors* (Cambridge: Belknap Press of Harvard University Press, 1969).

Behr, C. A. *Aelius Aristides and the Sacred Tales* (Amsterdam: Adolf M. Hakkert, 1968).

Bekhterev, V. M. *General Principles of Human Reflexology: An Introduction to the Objective Study of Personality,* trans. E. Murphy and W. Murphy (London: Jarrolds, 1933).

Bellak, Leopold, and Leonard Small. *Emergency Psychotherapy and Brief Psychotherapy* (New York: Grune & Stratton, 1965).

Bergin, Allen E., and Hans S. Strupp. "Some Empirical and Conceptual Bases for Coordinated Research in Psychotherapy: A Critical Review of Issues, Trends, and Evidence." *Int. J. Psychiat.,* 1969, 7, 18–90.

Berkowitz, Leonard. "The Case for Bottling Up Rage." *Psychology Today,* 1973, 7, 24–31.

Bernays, Jakob. *Grundzüge der verlorenen Abhandlung des Aristoteles über Wirkung der Tragödie* (Breslau: Eduard Trewendt, 1857).

Bernays, Jakob. *Zwei Abhandlungen über die Aristotelische Theorie des Dramas* (Berlin: Wilhelm Hertz, 1880).

Bernheim, Hippolyte. *De la suggestion dans l'état hypnotique et dans l'état de veille* (Paris: Octave Doin, 1884).

Bernheim, Hippolyte. *De la suggestion et de ses applications à la thérapeutique* (Paris: Octave Doin, 1886).

Bernheim, Hippolyte. *Hypnotisme, suggestion, psychothérapie: Etudes nouvelles* (Paris: Octave Doin, 1891).

Bernheim, Hippolyte. *Suggestive Therapeutics: A Treatise on the Nature and Uses of Hypnotism,* trans. Christian A. Herter (New York: London Book, 1947).

Bernheim, Hippolyte. *Bernheim's New Studies in Hypnotism,* trans. Richard S. Sandor (New York: International Universities Press, 1980).

Bernstein, Richard J. "Interpretation and Its Discontents: The Choreography of Critique." In Stanley B. Messer, Louis A. Sass, and Robert L. Woolfolk (eds.), *Hermeneutics and Psychological Theory: Interpretive Perspectives on Personality, Psychotherapy, and Psychopathology* (New Brunswick, N.J.: Rutgers University Press, 1988).

Berrios, G. E. "The Psychopathology of Affectivity: Conceptual and Historical Aspects." *Psychol. Med.,* 1985, *15,* 745–58.

Beyenka, Sister Mary Melchior. *Consolation in Saint Augustine* (Washington, D.C.: Catholic University of America Press, 1950).

Bibring, Edward. "Psychoanalysis and the Dynamic Psychotherapies." *J. Am. Psychoanal. Assoc.,* 1954, 2, 745–70.

Binet, Alfred. *Les altérations de la personnalité* (Paris: Germer Baillière, 1892).

Binet, Alfred, and Charles Féré. *Animal Magnetism* (New York: Appleton, 1888).

Binstock, William A. "Purgation Through Pity and Terror." *Int. J. Psycho-Anal.,* 1973, *54,* 499–504.

Bird, Brian. *Talking with Patients,* 2nd ed. (Philadelphia: Lippincott, 1973).

Bloch, Marc. *The Royal Touch: Sacred Monarchy and Scrofula in England and France* (London/Montreal: Routledge & Kegan Paul and McGill-Queens University Press, 1973).

Blum, Harold P. "The Curative and Creative Aspects of Insight." *J. Am. Psychoanal. Assoc..* 1979, 27 (suppl.), 41–69.

Blum, Harold P. "The Position and Value of Extratransference Interpretation." *J. Am. Psychoanal. Assoc.,* 1983, *31,* 587–617.

Boethius. *The Consolation of Philosophy,* intro. Irwin Edman (New York: Modern Library, 1943).

Boethius. *The Consolation of Philosophy,* trans., ed., and intro. Richard Green (Indianapolis, Ind.: Bobbs-Merrill, 1962).

Boethius, Anicius Manlius Severinus. *The Consolation of Philosophy,* trans. I. T., ed. and intro. William Anderson (Carbondale: Southern Illinois University Press, 1963).

Bonhoeffer, Dietrich. *Life Together,* trans. and intro. John W. Doberstein (New York: Harper & Row, 1954).

Boring, Edwin G. "Introspection." In *Encyclopaedia Britannica,* 24 vols. (Chicago: William Benton, 1956), 12: 542.

Boring, Edwin G. *A History of Experimental Psychology,* 2nd ed. (New York: Appleton-Century-Crofts, 1957).

Boring, Edwin G. "A History of Introspection." In Edwin G. Boring, *Psychologist at Large: An Autobiography and Selected Essays* (New York: Basic Books, 1961).

Boswell, James. *Boswell's Life of Johnson* . . . , ed. George Birkbeck Hill, 6 vols. (Oxford: Clarendon Press, 1887).

Bourru, H., and P. Burot, "Un cas de neurasthénie hystérique avec double personnalité." *First International Congress of Experimental and Therapeutic Hypnotism* (Paris: Doin, 1889).

Boyle, Robert. *The Christian Virtuoso: The Second Part.* In *The Works of the Honourable Robert Boyle,* 5 vols., ed. Thomas Birch (London: Millar, 1744), vol. 5.

Braid, James. *Neurypnology: or, the Rationale of Nervous Sleep, Considered in Relation with Animal Magnetism* (London: John Churchill, Adam & Charles Black, 1843).

Braid, James. *Hypnotic Therapeutics, Illustrated by Cases.* . . . (London: n.p., 1853). Reprinted from *Monthly Journal of Medical Science,* 1853, *17,* 14–47.

Braid, James. *Braid on Hypnotism: Neurypnology* . . . , ed. Arthur Edward Waite (London: George Redway, 1899).

Braid, James. *Satanic Agency and Mesmerism Reviewed,* . . . . In Maurice M. Tinterow (ed.), *Foundations of Hypnosis: From Mesmer to Freud* (Springfield, Ill.: Charles C Thomas, 1970).

Bramwell, J. Milne. *Hypnosis: Its History, Practice and Theory* (Philadelphia: Lippincott, 1903).

Bramwell, J. Milne. *Hypnotism and Treatment by Suggestion* (London: Caswell, 1909).

Brenman, Margaret, and Merton M. Gill. *Hypnotherapy* (New York: Josiah Macy, Jr., Foundation, 1944).

Brenman, Margaret, and Merton M. Gill. *Hypnotherapy: A Survey of the Literature* (New York: International Universities Press, 1947).

Breuer, Josef, and Sigmund Freud. *Studies on Hysteria (1895).* In *The Standard Edition of the Complete Psychological Works of Sigmund Freud,* 24 vols., trans. and ed. James Strachey, Anna Freud, et al. (London: Hogarth Press, 1955–1974), vol. 2.

Bright, T. *A Treatise of Melancholie* (London: Thomas Vautrollier, 1586).

Brock, Arthur J. *Greek Medicine: Being Extracts Illustrative of Medical Writers from Hippocrates to Galen* (London: Dent & Sons, 1929).

Bromberg, Walter. *Man Above Humanity: A History of Psychotherapy* (Philadelphia: Lippincott, 1954).

Brown, Theodore M. "Descartes, Dualism, and Psychosomatic Medicine." In *The Anatomy of Madness: Essays in the History of Psychiatry.* 2 vols., ed. W. F. Bynum, Roy Porter, and Michael Shepherd (London: Tavistock Publications, 1985) 1: 40–62.

Brown, Thomas. *Lectures on the Philosophy of the Human Mind,* 4 vols. (Edinburgh: Tait, 1820).

Brown, William. "The Revival of Emotional Memories and Its Therapeutic Value (I)." *Brit. J. Psychol., Medical Section,* 1920, *1,* 16–19.

Brown, William. *Psychology and Psycho-Therapy* (London: Edward Arnold, 1922a).

Brown, William. *Suggestion and Mental Analysis: An Outline of the Theory and Practice of Mind Cure,* 2nd ed. (London: University of London Press, 1922b).

Brown, William. *Psychological Methods of Healing: An Introduction to Psychotherapy* (London: University of London Press, 1938).

Browne, W. A. F. *What Asylums Were, Are, and Ought to Be* (Edinburgh: Adam and Charles Black, 1837).

Brunius, Teddy. *Inspiration and Katharsis: The Interpretation of Aristotle's The Poetics VI, 1449 b 26* (Uppsala, Sweden: 1966).

Brunius, Teddy. "Catharsis." In Philip P. Wiener (ed.), *Dictionary of the History of Ideas,* 4 vols. (New York: Charles Scribner's Sons, 1968–1973), 1: 264–70.

Brunner, José. "Psychiatry, Psychoanalysis, and Politics During the First World War." *J. Hist. Behav. Sci.,* 1991, *27,* 352–65.

Bucknill, John Charles, and Daniel H. Tuke. *A Manual of Psychological Medicine* (Philadelphia: Blanchard and Lea, 1858).

Budge, E. A. Wallis. *Amulets and Talismans* (New Hyde Park, N.Y.: University Books, 1961).

Bundy, Murray Wright. *The Theory of Imagination in Classical and Mediaeval Thought* (Urbana: University of Illinois Press, 1927).

Burchfield, R. W. (ed.), *A Supplement to the Oxford English Dictionary,* 4 vols. (Oxford: Clarendon Press, 1972–1986).

Bürgel, J. Ch., "Psychosomatic Methods of Cures in the Islamic Middle Ages." *Humaniora Islamica,* 1973, *1,* 157–72.

Bürgel, J. Ch. "Secular and Religious Features of Medieval Arabic Medicine." In Charles Leslie (ed.), *Asian Medical Systems: A Comparative Study* (Berkeley: University of California Press, 1976).

Burr, Anna Robeson. *Religious Confession and Confessants: With a Chapter on the History of Introspection* (Boston: Houghton Mifflin, 1914).

Burton, Robert. *The Anatomy of Melancholy,* eds. Floyd Dell and Paul Jordan-Smith (New York: Tudor, 1948).

Bylebyl, Jerome J. "Galen on the Non-Natural Causes of Variation in the Pulse." *Bull. Hist. Med.,* 1971, *45,* 482–85.

Cabanis, Pierre-Jean-Georges. *Coup d'oeil sur les révolutions et sur la réforme de la médicine* (Paris: Crapart, Caille et Ravier, 1804).

Cabanis, Pierre-Jean-Georges. *Sketch of the Revolutions of Medical Science, and Views Relating to its Reform,* ed. and trans. A. Henderson (London: Johnson, Murray, and Constable, 1806).

Cabanis, Pierre-Jean-Georges. *On the Relations Between the Physical and Moral Aspects of Man,* 2 vols., trans. Margaret Duggan Saidi, ed. George Mora, intros. Sergio Moravia and George Mora (Baltimore, Md.: Johns Hopkins University Press, 1981).

Caelius Aurelianus. *On Acute and on Chronic Diseases,* ed. and trans. I. E. Drabkin (Chicago: University of Chicago Press, 1950).

Calestro, Kenneth M. "Psychotherapy, Faith Healing, and Suggestion," *Int. J. Psychiat.,* 1972, *10,* 83–113.

Campbell, George. *The Philosophy of Rhetoric* (London: Strahan, 1776).

The Canons and Dogmatic Decrees of the Council of Trent. A.D. 1563, trans. J. Waterworth. In Philip Schaff, *The Creeds of Christendom, with a History and Critical Notes,* 3 vols. (Grand Rapids, Mich.: Baker Book House, 1969), 2: 77–206.

Carek, Donald J. "Affect in Psychodynamic Psychotherapy." *Am. J. Psychother.,* 1990, *44,* 274–82.

Carlson, Eric T., and Norman Dain. "The Psychotherapy that Was Moral Treatment." *Am. J. Psychiat.,* 1960, *117,* 519–24.

Carlson, Eric T., and Meribeth M. Simpson. "Moral Persuasion as Therapy." In Jules H. Masserman (ed.), *Current Psychiatric Therapies,* vol. 4 (New York: Grune & Stratton, 1964).

Carozza, Davy A., and H. James Shey. *Petrarch's* Secretum *with Introduction, Notes, and Critical Anthology* (New York: Peter Lang, 1989).

Casey, Edward S. *Imagining: A Phenomenological Study* (Bloomington: Indiana University Press, 1976).

Cassian, John. *The Conferences,* ed. and trans. Edgar C. S. Gibson. In Philip Schaff and Henry Wace (eds.), *A Select Library of the Nicene and Post-Nicene Fathers of the Christian Church,* 2nd ser., 14 vols. (Grand Rapids, Mich.: Eerdmans, 1955), vol. 11.

Cassiodorus Senator. *An Introduction to Divine and Human Readings,* trans. and annot. Leslie Webber Jones (from *Institutiones Divinarum et Saecularium Litterarum,* ed. R. A. B. Mynors) (New York: Columbia University Press, 1946).

Celsus. *De medicina,* 3 vols., trans. W. G. Spencer (Cambridge: Harvard University Press, 1935–1938).

Charcot, Jean-Martin. *Clinical Lectures on Diseases of the Nervous System Delivered at the Infirmary of La Salpêtrière,* 3 vols., trans. George Sigerson (vols. 1 and 2), Thomas Savill (vol. 3) (London: New Sydenham Society, 1877–1889).

Charcot, Jean-Martin. "Sur les divers états nerveux déterminés par l'hypnotisation chez les hystériques." *Comptes-rendus hebdomadaires des séances de l'Académie des Sciences,* 1882, 94, 403–5.

Charron, [Pierre]. *Of Wisdom: Three Books,* trans. George Stanhope, 2 vols. (London: Gillyflower, 1697).

Chertok, L. "On the Discovery of the Cathartic Method." *Int. J. Psycho-Anal.,* 1961, 42, 284–87.

Chertok, Léon, and Raymond de Saussure. *The Therapeutic Revolution: From Mesmer to Freud,* trans. R. H. Ahrenfeldt (New York: Brunner/Mazel, 1979).

Chessick, Richard D. *The Technique and Practice of Intensive Psychotherapy* (New York: Jason Aronson, 1974).

Chessick, Richard D. *Great Ideas in Psychotherapy* (New York: Jason Aronson, 1977).

Chessick, Richard D. "Socrates: First Psychotherapist." *Am. J. Psychoanal.,* 1982, 42, 71–83.

Chessick, Richard D. *The Technique and Practice of Listening in Intensive Psychotherapy* (Northvale, N.J.: Jason Aronson, 1989).

Chisholm, Hugh, et al. (eds.). *The Encyclopaedia Britannica . . . ,* 11th ed., 29 vols. (New York: Encyclopaedia Britannica, 1910–1911).

Chrysostom, John. "The Homilies on the Statues," trans. W. R. W. Stephens. In *Nicene and Post-Nicene Fathers,* 14 vols., ed. Philip Schaff (New York: Christian Literature, 1886–1889), First Series, 9:315–489.

Chrysostom, John. "Letter to a Young Widow." In *Nicene and Post-Nicene Fathers,* 14 vols., ed. Philip Schaff (New York: Christian Literature, 1886–1889), First Series, 9:121–28.

Cicero. *Tusculan Disputations,* trans. J. E. King (Cambridge: Harvard University Press, 1966).

Cicero. *De inventione,* trans. H. M. Hubbell. In *Works,* 28 vols. (Cambridge/London: Harvard University Press/William Heinemann, 1914–1949), vol. 2.

Cicero, *De legibus,* trans. Clinton Walter Keyes. In *Works,* 28 vols. (Cambridge/London: Harvard University Press/William Heinemann, 1914–1949), vol. 16.

Cicero, *De officiis,* trans. Walter Miller. In *Works,* 28 vols. (Cambridge/London: Harvard University Press/William Heinemann, 1914–1949), vol. 21.

Claretie, Jules. "Charcot le consolateur." *Les annales politiques et littéraires,* Sept. 20, 1903, pp. 179–80.

Clark, Donald Lemen. *Rhetoric in Greco-Roman Education* (New York: Columbia University Press, 1957).

Clarke, Edwin, and Kenneth Dewhurst. *An Illustrated History of Brain Function* (Oxford: Sandford, 1972).

Clarke, Edwin, and C. D. O'Malley. *The Human Brain and Spinal Cord: A Historical Study Illustrated by Writings from Antiquity to the Twentieth Century* (Berkeley: University of California Press, 1968).

Clebsch, William A., and Charles R. Jaekle. *Pastoral Care in Historical Perspective* (New York: Jason Aronson, 1975).

Clement of Alexandria. *Christ the Educator [Paedagogus],* trans. Simon P. Wood (New York: Fathers of the Church, 1954).

Clements, Forest E. "Primitive Concepts of Disease." *University of California Publications in American Archeology and Ethnology,* 1932, 32 (2), 185–252.

Clifford, Samuel. *The Signs and Causes of Melancholy . . . Collected out of the Works of Mr. Richard Baxter . . .* (London: Cruttenden and Cox, 1716).

Clinebell, Howard J., Jr. *Basic Types of Pastoral Counseling* (Nashville, Tenn.: Abingdon Press, 1966).

Cobbe, Frances Power. "Faith Healing and Fear Killing," *Contemporary Review,* 1887, 51, 794–813.

Coleridge, Samuel T. *Table Talk of Samuel Taylor Coleridge . . . ,* intro. Henry Morley (London: George Routledge and Sons, 1884).

Coleridge, Samuel Taylor. *Biographia Literaria, or Biographical Sketches of My Literary Life and Opinions,* 2 vols. in 1, eds. James Engell and W. Jackson Bate (Princeton, N.J.: Princeton University Press, 1983).

Coltrera, Joseph T., and Nathaniel Ross. "Freud's Psychoanalytic Technique — From the Beginnings to 1923." In Benjamin B. Wolman (ed.), *Psychoanalytic Techniques: A Handbook for the Practicing Psychoanalyst* (New York: Basic Books, 1967).

Conn, Jacob H. "Hypnosynthesis: III. Hypnotherapy of Chronic War Neuroses with a Discussion of the Value of Abreaction, Regression, and Revivification," *J. Clin. & Experimental Hypnosis,* 1953, *1,* 29–43.

Cooley, Charles Horton. *Sociological Theory and Social Research,* intro. and annot. Robert Cooley Angell (New York: Henry Holt, 1930).

Copleston, Frederick. *A History of Philosophy,* 8 vols. (Westminster, Md.: Newman Press, 1946–1966).

Cotta, John. *A Short Discoverie of the Unobserved Dangers of Severall Sorts of Ignorant and Unconsiderate Practisers of Physicke in England . . .* (London: William Jones and Richard Boyle, 1612).

Coué, Emile. *De la suggestion et de ses applications* . . . (Chaumont: Andriot Moissonier, 1912).

Coué, Emile. *Self Mastery Through Conscious Autosuggestion* (New York: American Library Service, 1922).

Coué, Emile. *How to Practice Suggestion and Autosuggestion,* preface Charles Baudouin (New York: American Library Service, 1923).

Crabtree, Adam. *Animal Magnetism, Early Hypnotism, and Psychical Research, 1766–1925: An Annotated Bibliography* (White Plains, N.Y.: Kraus International Publications, 1988).

Crabtree, Adam. *From Mesmer to Freud: Magnetic Sleep and the Roots of Psychological Healing* (New Haven, Conn.: Yale University Press, 1993).

Cross, F. L., and E. A. Livingstone (eds.). *The Oxford Dictionary of the Christian Church,* 2nd ed. (Oxford: Oxford University Press, 1974).

Cullere, Alexandre. *La thérapeutique suggestive* . . . (Paris: Baillière et Fils, 1893).

Cutten, George Barton. *Three Thousand Years of Mental Healing* (New York: Charles Scribner's Sons, 1911).

Danziger, Kurt. "The History of Introspection Reconsidered." *J. Hist. Behav. Sci.,* 1980, *16,* 241–62.

Darlington, H. S. "The Confession of Sins." *Psychoanal. Rev.,* 1937, 24, 150–64.

Déjerine, J., and E. Gauckler. *The Psychoneuroses and Their Treatment by Psychotherapy,* 2nd ed., trans. Smith Ely Jelliffe (Philadelphia: Lippincott, 1915).

Delatte, Paul. *The Rule of St. Benedict: A Commentary,* trans. Justin McCann (London: Burns Oates & Washbourne, 1921).

Delboeuf, J. R. L. *Le magnétisme animal* (Paris: Germer Baillière, 1889).

Deleuze, J.-P.-F. *Histoire critique du magnétisme animal,* 2 vols. (Paris: Mame, 1813).

Deleuze, J.-P.-F. *Instruction pratique sur le magnétisme animal* (Paris: Dentu, 1825).

Deleuze, J.-P.-F. *Practical Instruction in Animal Magnetism,* 2nd ed., trans. Thomas C. Hartshorn (Providence, R.I.: Cranston, 1837).

DeMause, Lloyd (ed.). *The History of Childhood* (New York: Psychohistory Press, 1974).

Dendy, W. C. "Psychotherapeia, or the Remedial Influence of Mind." *J. Psychol. Med. & Ment. Pathology,* 1853, 6, 268–74.

DePorte, Michael V. *Nightmares and Hobbyhorses: Swift, Sterne, and Augustan Ideas of Madness* (San Marino, Calif.: Huntington Library, 1974).

Dercum, Francis X. *Rest, Mental Therapeutics, Suggestion* (Philadelphia: Blakiston's Sons, 1911).

Descuret, J.-B.-F. *La médecine des passions, ou les passions considérées dans leur rapports avec les maladies, les lois et la religion,* 4th ed. (Liège: Lardinois, 1844).

Dessoir, Max. *Bibliographie des modernen Hypnotismus* (Berlin: Carl Düncker, 1888).

Dessoir, Max. *Erster Nachtrag zur Bibliographie des modernen Hypnotismus* (Berlin: Carl Düncker, 1890).

Deutsch, Helene. "Occult Processes Occurring During Psychoanalysis." In George Devereux (ed.), *Psychoanalysis and the Occult* (New York: International Universities Press, 1953).

Dewald, Paul A. *Psychotherapy: A Dynamic Approach,* 2nd ed. (New York: Basic Books, 1969).

Dewald, Paul A. *The Psychoanalytic Process: A Case Illustration* (New York: Basic Books, 1972).

Diamond, Solomon (ed.). *The Roots of Psychology: A Sourcebook in the History of Ideas* (New York: Basic Books, 1974).

Diderot, Denis, and Jean le Rond d'Alembert (eds.). *Encyclopédie . . . ,* 3rd ed., 36 vols. (Geneva/Neufchatel: Jean-Léonard Pellet/Société Typographique, 1778–1779).

Digby, Anne. *Madness, Morality, and Medicine: A Study of the York Retreat, 1796–1914* (Cambridge: Cambridge University Press, 1985).

Digby, Kenelme. *Two Treatises. In the One of Which, the Nature of Bodies; in the Other, the Nature of Mans Soule; Is looked into: in Way of Discovery, of the Immortality of Reasonable Soules* (Paris: Gilles Blaizot, 1644).

Dilthey, W. *Selected Writings,* ed., trans., and intro. H. P. Rickman (Cambridge: Cambridge University Press, 1976).

Dimon, James. "Interpretation: Review of the literature." *Psychoanalytic Inquiry,* 1992, 12, 182–95.

D'Irsay, Stephen. "Patristic Medicine." *Ann. Med. Hist.,* 1927, 9, 364–78.

Dodds, E. R. *The Greeks and the Irrational* (Boston: Beacon Press, 1957).

Dodds, E. R. *Pagan and Christian in an Age of Anxiety* (Cambridge: Cambridge University Press, 1965).

Donoghue, Quentin, and Linda Shapiro. *Bless Me, Father, For I Have Sinned: Catholics Speak Out About Confession* (New York: Donald I. Fine, 1984).

Dube, K. C. "Nosology and Therapy of Mental Illness in *Ayurveda.*" *Comparative Medicine East and West,* 1978, 6, 209–28.

Dubois, Paul. *The Psychic Treatment of Nervous Disorders: The Psychoneuroses and Their Moral Treatment,* trans. and ed. Smith Ely Jelliffe and William A. White (New York: Funk & Wagnalls, 1907).

Dunglison, Robley. *General Therapeutics, or, Principles of Medical Practice . . .* (Philadelphia: Carey, Lea and Blanchard, 1836).

Edelstein, Emma J., and Ludwig Edelstein. *Asclepius: A Collection and Interpretation of the Testimonies,* 2 vols. (Baltimore, Md.: Johns Hopkins Press, 1945).

Edelstein, Ludwig. "The Professional Ethics of the Greek Physician." In *Ancient Medicine: Selected Papers of Ludwig Edelstein,* ed. Owsei Temkin and C. Lilian Temkin, trans. C. Lilian Temkin (Baltimore, Md.: Johns Hopkins Press, 1967).

Edwards, Jonathan. *Christian Cautions: or, the Necessity of Self-Examination.* In *The Works of Jonathan Edwards, A.M.,* ed. Edward Hicknan, 2 vols., 10th ed. (London: Henry G. Bohn, 1865), 2: 173–85.

Ehrenwald, Jan (ed.). *The History of Psychotherapy: From Healing Magic to Encounter* (New York: Jason Aronson, 1976).

Ekstein, Rudolf. "Thoughts Concerning the Nature of the Interpretive Process." In Morton Levitt (ed.), *Readings in Psychoanalytic Psychology* (New York: Appleton-Century-Crofts, 1959).

Ell, Stephen R. "Concepts of Disease and the Physician in the Early Middle Ages." *Janus,* 1978, 65, 153–65.

Ellenberger, Henri F. "The Pathogenic Secret and Its Therapeutics." *J. Hist. Behav. Sci.,* 1966, 2, 29–42.

Ellenberger, Henri F. *The Discovery of the Unconscious: The History and Evolution of Dynamic Psychiatry* (New York: Basic Books, 1970).

Ellenberger, Henri F. "The Story of 'Anna O.': A Critical Review with New Data." *J. Hist. Behav. Sci.*, 1972, 8, 267–79.

Elliotson, John. *Numerous Cases of Surgical Operations Without Pain in the Mesmeric State: . . .* (London: Baillière, 1843).

Elliotson, John. *The Harveian Oration, . . . Royal College of Physicians, London, June 27th, 1846* (London: Baillière, 1846).

Encyclopaedia Britannica, 11th ed., 29 vols. (New York: Encyclopaedia Britannica, 1910–1911).

Encyclopaedia Britannica, 14th ed., 24 vols. (Chicago: William Benton, 1956).

Eng, Erling. "Modern Psychotherapy and Ancient Rhetoric." *Psychother. Psychosom.*, 1974, 24, 493–96.

Engelhardt, H. Tristram, Jr. "The Concepts of Health and Disease." In H. Tristram Engelhardt, Jr. and Stuart F. Spicker (eds.), *Evaluation and Explanation in the Biomedical Sciences* (Dordrecht: Reidel, 1975).

Engell, James. "The New Rhetoricians: Psychology, Semiotics, and Critical Theory." In Christopher Fox (ed.), *Psychology and Literature in the Eighteenth Century* (New York: AMS Press, 1987).

English, Horace B., and Ava Champney English. *A Comprehensive Dictionary of Psychological and Psychoanalytical Terms* (New York: Longmans, Green, 1958).

Entralgo, Pedro Laín. *Doctor and Patient*, trans. Frances Partridge (London: World University Library/Weidenfeld and Nicolson, 1968).

Entralgo, Pedro Laín. *The Therapy of the Word in Classical Antiquity*, trans. L. J. Rather and John M. Sharp (New Haven, Conn.: Yale University Press, 1970).

Erickson, Milton H. *The Collected Papers of Milton H. Erickson on Hypnosis*, 4 vols., ed. E. L. Rossi (New York: Irvington, 1980).

Esdaile, James. *Mesmerism in India, and Its Practical Application in Surgery and Medicine* (Hartford, Conn.: Silas Andrus and Son, 1847).

Esquirol, E. *Des passions, considérées comme causes, symptômes et moyens curatifs de l'aliénation mentale* (Paris: Didot Jeune, 1805).

Esquirol, E. *Mental Maladies: A Treatise on Insanity*, trans. E. K. Hunt (Philadelphia: Lea and Blanchard, 1845).

[Ettmüller, Michael]. *Etmullerus Abridg'd: Or, A Compleat System of the Theory and Practice of Physic . . .* (London: Harris, Hubbard, and Bell, 1699).

Eysenck, H. J. "Learning Theory and Behaviour Therapy." *J. Ment. Sci.*, 1959, 105, 61–75.

Eysenck, H. J. *Behaviour Therapy and the Neuroses* (Oxford: Pergamon, 1960).

Eysenck, H. J. (ed.). *Experiments in Behaviour Therapy: Readings in Modern Methods of Treatment of Mental Disorders Derived from Learning Theory* (New York: Macmillan, 1964).

Fagan, Joen, and Irma Lee Shepherd (eds.). *Gestalt Therapy Now: Theory, Techniques, Applications* (New York: Harper Colophon, 1971).

Falconer, William. *A Dissertation on the Influence of the Passions upon Disorders of the Body*, 2nd ed. (London: Dilly, 1791).

Fancher, Raymond E. *Pioneers of Psychology* (New York: Norton, 1979).

Faria, José Custodio de. *De la cause du sommeil lucide, ou étude de la nature de l'homme,* intro. D. G. Dalgado (Paris: Henri Jouve, 1906). Originally published in Paris in 1819.

Féré, Charles. *La médecine d'imagination* (Paris: Progrès Medical, 1886).

Ferenczi, Sandor. "Introjection and Transference." In Sandor Ferenczi, *Sex in Psycho-analysis,* trans. Ernest Jones, intro. Clara Thompson (New York: Basic Books, 1950).

Ferenczi, Sandor. "The Elasticity of Psycho-Analytic Technique." In Sandor Ferenczi, *Final Contributions to the Problems and Methods of Psycho-Analysis,* ed. Michael Balint, trans. Eric Mosbacher et al., intro. Clara Thompson (New York: Basic Books, 1955a).

Ferenczi, Sandor. "The Principle of Relaxation and Neo-Catharsis." In Sandor Ferenczi, *Final Contributions to the Problems and Methods of Psycho-Analysis,* ed. Michael Balint, trans. Eric Mosbacher et al., intro. Clara Thompson (New York: Basic Books, 1955b).

Ferrara, Kathleen Warden. *Therapeutic Ways with Words* (New York: Oxford University Press, 1994).

Ferriar, John. *Medical Histories and Reflections,* 3 vols. (Warrington: Cadell, 1792–1798).

Ferster, Charles B., and Marian K. DeMyer. "The Development of Performances in Autistic Children in an Automatically Controlled Environment." *J. Chronic Dis.,* 1961, *13,* 312–45.

Feuchtersleben, Ernst von. *The Principles of Medical Psychology* . . . , trans. H. Evans Lloyd, rev. and ed. B. G. Babington (London: Sydenham Society, 1847).

Fiering, Norman S. "Irresistible Compassion: An Aspect of Eighteenth-Century Sympathy and Humanitarianism," *J. Hist. Ideas,* 1976, *37,* 195–218.

Fine, Reuben. *A History of Psychoanalysis* (New York: Columbia University Press, 1979).

Fisher, Charles. "Hypnosis in Treatment of Neuroses Due to War and to Other Causes." *War Medicine,* 1943, *4,* 565–76.

Fishman, Daniel B., and Cyril M. Franks. "Evolution and Differentiation Within Behavior Therapy: A Theoretical and Epistemological Review." In Donald K. Freedheim et al. (eds.), *History of Psychotherapy: A Century of Change* (Washington, D.C.: American Psychological Association, 1992).

Fleischman, Paul R. *The Healing Zone: Religious Issues in Psychotherapy* (New York: Paragon House, 1989).

Fliess, Robert. "Metapsychology of the Analyst." *Psychoanal. Quart.,* 1942, *11,* 211–27.

Fliess, Robert. "Countertransference and Counteridentification." *J. Am. Psychoanal. Assoc.,* 1953, *1,* 268–84.

Forel, August. *Der Hypnotismus* . . . (Stuttgart: Enke, 1889).

Forel, August. *Hypnotism, or, Suggestion and Psychotherapy: A Study of the Psychological, Psycho-Physiological and Therapeutic Aspects of Hypnotism,* trans. H. W. Armit (New York: Rebman, 1907).

Foucault, Michel. *The Birth of the Clinic: An Archaeology of Medical Perception,* trans. A. M. Sheridan Smith (New York: Pantheon Books, 1973).

Frank, Jerome D. "The Dynamics of the Psychotherapeutic Relationship: Determinants and Effects of the Therapist's Influence." *Psychiatry,* 1959, 22, 17–39.

Frank, Jerome D. "The Role of Hope in Psychotherapy." *Int. J. Psychiat.,* 1968, 5, 383–95.

Frank, Jerome D. *Persuasion & Healing: A Comparative Study of Psychotherapy,* rev. ed. (Baltimore, Md.: Johns Hopkins University Press, 1973).

Frank, Jerome D. "Psychotherapy: The Restoration of Morale." *Am. J. Psychiat.,* 1974, 131, 271–74.

Frank, Jerome D. "Therapeutic Components of Psychotherapy." *J. Nerv. Ment. Dis.,* 1974, 159, 325–42.

Frank, Jerome D. "Psychotherapy, Rhetoric, and Hermeneutics: Implications for Practice and Research." *Psychotherapy,* 1987, 24, 293–302.

Frank, Jerome D., and Julia B. Frank. *Persuasion and Healing: A Comparative Study of Psychotherapy,* 3rd ed. (Baltimore, Md.: Johns Hopkins University Press, 1991).

Frank, Jerome D., Lester H. Gliedman, Stanley D. Imber, Anthony R. Stone, and Earl H. Nash. "Patients' Expectancies and Relearning as Factors Determining Improvement in Psychotherapy." *Am. J. Psychiat.,* 1959, 115, 961–68.

Franks, Cyril M. *Conditioning Techniques in Clinical Practice and Research* (New York: Springer, 1964).

Franks, Cyril M. "Behavior Therapy and Its Pavlovian Origins: Review and Perspectives." In Cyril M. Franks (ed.), *Behavior Therapy: Appraisal and Status* (New York: McGraw-Hill, 1969).

Freedberg, E. J. "Behavior Therapy: A Comparison Between Early (1890–1920) and Contemporary Techniques." *Canadian Psychologist,* 1973, 14, 225–40.

Freedheim, Donald K. (ed.). *History of Psychotherapy: A Century of Change* (Washington, D.C.: American Psychological Association, 1992).

French, Thomas M. *The Integration of Behavior,* 3 vols. (Chicago: University of Chicago Press, 1952–1958).

Freud, Sigmund. *The Origins of Psycho-Analysis: Letters to Wilhelm Fliess, Drafts and Notes: 1887–1902,* ed. Marie Bonaparte, Anna Freud, Ernst Kris, trans. Eric Mosbacher and James Strachey, intro. Ernst Kris (New York: Basic Books, 1954).

Freud, Sigmund. "Papers on Hypnotism and Suggestion" (1888–1892). In *The Standard Edition of the Complete Psychological Works of Sigmund Freud,* 24 vols., trans. and ed. James Strachey, Anna Freud, et al. (London: Hogarth Press, 1955–1974), vol. 1.

Freud, Sigmund. "Psychical (or Mental) Treatment" (1890). in *Standard Edition,* vol. 7.

Freud, Sigmund. "The Neuro-Psychoses of Defence" (1894). In *Standard Edition,* vol. 3.

Freud, Sigmund. "Sexuality in the Aetiology of the Neuroses" (1898). In *Standard Edition,* vol. 3.

Freud, Sigmund. *Interpretation of Dreams* (1900). In *Standard Edition,* vols. 4–5.

Freud, Sigmund. "Freud's Psycho-Analytic Procedure" (1904). In *Standard Edition,* vol. 7.

Freud, Sigmund. "Fragment of an Analysis of a Case of Hysteria" (1905a). In *Standard Edition,* vol. 7.

Freud, Sigmund. *Jokes and Their Relation to the Unconscious* (1905b). In *Standard Edition,* vol. 8.

Freud, Sigmund. "On Psychotherapy" (1905c). In *Standard Edition*, vol. 7.

Freud, Sigmund. *Three Essays on the Theory of Sexuality* (1905d). In *Standard Edition*, vol. 7.

Freud, Sigmund. *Delusions and Dreams in Jensen's* Gradiva (1907). In *Standard Edition*, vol. 9.

Freud, Sigmund. "Five Lectures on Psycho-Analysis" (1910a). In *Standard Edition*, vol. 11.

Freud, Sigmund. "The Future Prospects of Psycho-Analytic Therapy" (1910b). In *Standard Edition*, vol. 11.

Freud, Sigmund. "The Dynamics of Transference" (1912a). In *Standard Edition*, vol. 12.

Freud, Sigmund. "Recommendations to Physicians Practising Psycho-Analysis" (1912b). In *Standard Edition*, vol. 12.

Freud, Sigmund. "On Beginning the Treatment (Further Recommendations on the Technique of Psycho-Analysis I")" (1913). In *Standard Edition*, vol. 12.

Freud, Sigmund. "Observations on Transference-Love: Further Recommendations on the Technique of Psycho-Analysis III" (1915). In *Standard Edition*, vol. 12.

Freud, Sigmund. *Introductory Lectures on Psycho-Analysis* (1916–1917). In *Standard Edition*, vols. 15–16.

Freud, Sigmund. "Lines of Advance in Psycho-Analytic Therapy" (1919). In *Standard Edition*, vol. 17.

Freud, Sigmund. *Group Psychology and the Analysis of the Ego* (1921). In *Standard Edition*, vol. 18.

Freud, Sigmund. "Two Encyclopaedia Articles" (1923). In *Standard Edition*, vol. 18.

Freud, Sigmund. "A Short Account of Psycho-Analysis" (1924). In *Standard Edition*, vol. 19.

Freud, Sigmund. *An Autobiographical Study* (1925). In *Standard Edition*, vol. 20.

Freud, Sigmund. "Psycho-Analysis" (1926a). In *Standard Edition*, vol. 20.

Freud, Sigmund. *The Question of Lay Analysis* (1926b). In *Standard Edition*, vol. 20.

Friedman, Lawrence. *The Anatomy of Psychotherapy* (Hillsdale, N.J.: Analytic Press, 1988).

Fromm-Reichmann, Frieda. *Principles of Intensive Psychotherapy* (Chicago: University of Chicago Press, 1950).

Gadamer, Hans-Georg. *Philosophical Hermeneutics,* trans. D. Linge (Berkeley: University of California Press, 1977).

Gadamer, Hans-Georg. *Truth and Method,* 2nd ed., ed. Joel Weinsheimer and Donald G. Marshall (New York: Crossroad, 1991).

Galen. *Method of Physick,* trans. P. English (Edinburgh: George Suintoun & James Glen, 1656).

Galen. "De temperamentis." In Galen, *Opera omnia,* 22 vols., ed. Carolus Gottlob Kühn (Leipzig: Cnobloch, 1821–1833), vol. 1.

Galen. "Quod optimus medicus sit quoque philosophus." In *Opera omnia,* vol. 1.

Galen. *On the Natural Faculties,* trans. and ed. A. J. Brock (Cambridge: Harvard University Press, 1963a).

Galen. *On the Passions and Errors of the Soul,* trans. Paul W. Harkins, ed. and intro. Walther Riese (Columbus: Ohio State University Press, 1963b).

Gantt, W. Horsley. "Conditional or Conditioned, Reflex or Response?" *Conditional Reflex*, 1966, *1*, 69–73.

Gardiner, H. M., Ruth Clark Metcalf, and John G. Beebe-Center. *Feeling and Emotion: A History of Theories* (New York: American Book, 1937).

Gauld, Alan. *A History of Hypnotism* (Cambridge: Cambridge University Press, 1992).

Gaume, Jean Joseph. *Advice for Those Who Exercise the Ministry of Reconciliation Through Confession and Absolution . . .*, abridged, condensed, and adapted to the use of the English Church, trans. Rev. E. B. Pusey (London: Innes, 1893).

Gauss, Charles Edward. "Empathy." In Philip P. Wiener (ed.), *Dictionary of the History of Ideas*, 5 vols. (New York: Charles Scribner's Sons, 1973–1974), vol. 2.

Gay, Peter. *Freud: A Life for our Time* (New York: Norton, 1988).

Gedo, John E., and Ernest S. Wolf. "From the History of Introspective Psychology: The Humanist Strain." In John E. Gedo and George H. Pollock (eds.), *Freud: The Fusion of Science and Humanism* (New York: International Universities Press, 1976).

Gill, Christopher. "Ancient Psychotherapy." *J. Hist. Ideas*, 1985, *46*, 307–25.

Gill, Merton M., and Margaret Brenman. *Hypnosis and Related States: Psychoanalytic Studies in Regression* (New York: International Universities Press, 1959).

Gilman, Sandor L. (ed.). *The Face of Madness: Hugh W. Diamond and the Origin of Psychiatric Photography*, intro. Eric T. Carlson (New York: Brunner/Mazel, 1976).

Gitelson, Maxwell. "The Curative Factors in Psycho-Analysis: I. The First Phase of Psycho-Analysis." *Int. J. Psycho-Anal.*, 1962, *43*, 194–205.

Glaser, Susan R. "Rhetoric and Psychotherapy." In Michael J. Mahoney (ed.), *Psychotherapy Process: Current Issues and Future Directions* (New York: Plenum Press, 1980).

Glass, Carol R., and Diane B. Arnkoff. "Behavior Therapy." In Donald K. Freedheim (ed.), *History of Psychotherapy: A Century of Change* (Washington, D.C.: American Psychological Association, 1992).

Goldstein, Jan. *Console and Classify: The French Psychiatric Profession in the Nineteenth Century* (Cambridge: Cambridge University Press, 1987).

Grange, Kathleen. "Pinel and Eighteenth-Century Psychiatry." *Bull. Hist. Med.*, 1961, *35*, 442–53.

Grasset, Joseph. *L'hypnotisme et la suggestion* (Paris: Doin, 1903).

Greenbaum, Louis S. "Nurses and Doctors in Conflict: Piety and Medicine in the Paris Hôtel-Dieu on the Eve of the French Revolution." *Clio Medica*, 1978, *13*, 247–67.

Greene, William Chase. *Moira: Fate, Good, and Evil in Greek Thought* (New York: Harper Torchbooks, 1963).

Greenson, Ralph R. "Empathy and Its Vicissitudes." *Int. J. Psycho-Anal.*, 1960, *41*, 418–24.

Greenson, Ralph R. *The Technique and Practice of Psychoanalysis* (New York: International Universities Press, 1967).

Greenson, Ralph R., and Milton Wexler. "The Non-Transference Relationship in the Psychoanalytic Situation." *Int. J. Psycho-Anal.*, 1969, *50*, 27–39.

Greenwald, Jerry A. "The Ground Rules in Gestalt Therapy." In Chris Hatcher and Philip Himelstein (eds.), *The Handbook of Gestalt Therapy* (New York: Jason Aronson, 1976).

Gregg, Robert C. *Consolation Philosophy: Greek and Christian Paideia in Basil and the Two Gregories* (Cambridge, Mass.: Philadelphia Patristic Foundation, 1975).

Gregory, John. *Lectures on the Duties and Qualifications of a Physician* (London: Strahan and Cadell, 1772).

Grinker, Roy R., and John P. Spiegel. *Men Under Stress* (Philadelphia: Blakiston, 1945a).

Grinker, Roy R., and John P. Spiegel. *War Neuroses* (Philadelphia: Blakiston, 1945b).

Grosseteste, Robert. *Templum Dei,* ed. Joseph Goering and F. A. C. Mantello (Toronto: Pontifical Institute of Mediaeval Studies, 1984).

Guillain, Georges. *J.-M. Charcot, 1825–1893: His Life — His Work,* ed. and trans. Pearce Bailey (New York: Paul Hoeber, 1959).

Hadfield, J. A. "Hypnotism." In H. Crichton-Miller (ed.), *Functional Nerve Disease: An Epitome of War Experience for the Practitioner* (London: Oxford University Press, 1920).

Hadfield, J. A. "Treatment by Suggestion and Hypno-Analysis." In Emanuel Miller (ed.). *The Neuroses in War* (New York: Macmillan, 1940).

Haldipur, C. V. "Madness in Ancient India: Concept of Insanity in *Charaka Samhita* (First century A.D.)." *Comprehensive Psychiatry,* 1984, 25, 335–44.

Hale, Matthew. *The Primitive Origination of Mankind, Considered and Examined According to the Light of Nature* (London: William Shrowsbery, 1677).

Haley, Jay. *Strategies of Psychotherapy* (New York: Grune & Stratton, 1963).

Haley, Jay (ed.). *Advanced Techniques of Hypnosis and Therapy: The Selected Papers of Milton H. Erickson, M.D.* (New York: Grune & Stratton, 1967).

Haly filius Abbas. *Liber totius medicine* . . . , trans. Stephen the Philosopher, ed. Michael de Capella (Lyons: 1523).

Hamilton, Mary. *Incubation, or the Cure of Disease in Pagan Temples and Christian Churches* (London: Henderson, 1906).

Hammond, N. G. L., and H. H. Scullard (eds.). *The Oxford Classical Dictionary,* 2nd ed. (Oxford: Clarendon Press, 1970).

Hartley, Percival Horton-Smith, and Harold Richard Aldridge. *Johannes de Mirfeld of St. Bartholomew's, Smithfield: His Life and Works* (Cambridge: Cambridge University Press, 1936).

Harvey, E. Ruth. *The Inward Wits: Psychological Theory in the Middle Ages and the Renaissance* (London: Warburg Institute, University of London, 1975).

Haslam, John. *Observations on Madness and Melancholy* . . . , 2nd ed. (London: Callow, 1809).

Hastings, James, et al. (eds.) *A Dictionary of the Bible* . . . , 5 vols. (New York: Charles Scribner's Sons, 1902–1919).

Hatcher, Chris, and Philip Himelstein (eds.). *The Handbook of Gestalt Therapy* (New York: Jason Aronson, 1976).

Hatcher, Robert L. "Insight and Self-Observation." *J. Am. Psychoanal. Assoc.,* 1973, 21, 377–98.

Haygarth, John. *Of the Imagination, as a Cause and as a Cure of Disorders of the Body* . . . (Bath: Cruttwell, 1801).

Heimann, Paula. "On Counter-Transference." *Int. J. Psycho-Anal.,* 1950, 31, 81–84.

Heinroth, Johann Christian. *Textbook of Disturbances of Mental Life: Or Disturbances of the Soul and Their Treatment,* 2 vols., trans. J. Schmorak, intro. George Mora (Baltimore, Md.: Johns Hopkins University Press, 1975).

Henderson, D. K., and R. D. Gillespie. *A Text-Book of Psychiatry for Students and Practitioners* (London: Oxford University Press, 1927).

Herbert, George. *A Priest to the Temple, or, the Country Parson.* In *The Works of George Herbert,* ed. F. E. Hutchinson (Oxford: Clarendon Press, 1970).

Herrnstein, Richard J., and Edwin G. Boring (eds.). *A Source Book in the History of Psychology* (Cambridge: Harvard University Press, 1965).

Hilgard, Ernest R. *Theories of Learning,* 2nd ed. (New York: Appleton-Century-Crofts, 1956).

Hilgard, Ernest R. "The Trilogy of Mind: Cognition, Affection, Conation." *J. Hist. Behav. Sci.,* 1980, *16,* 107–17.

Hillman, Robert G. "A Scientific Study of Mystery: The Role of the Medical and Popular Press in the Nancy-Salpêtrière Controversy on Hypnotism." *Bull. Hist. Med.,* 1965, *39,* 163–82.

Hinsie, Leland E., and Robert J. Campbell. *Psychiatric Dictionary,* 3rd ed. (New York: Oxford University Press, 1960).

Hinsie, Leland E., and Jacob Shatzky. *Psychiatric Dictionary* (London: Oxford University Press, 1940).

Hippocrates. *Hippocratic Writings,* trans. J. Chadwick and W. N. Mann, I. M. Lonie, E. T. Withington, ed. and intro. G. E. R. Lloyd (Harmondsworth: Penguin, 1978).

Hippocrates. *Works of Hippocrates,* vols.1–4, ed. and trans. W. H. S. Jones and E. T. Withington (Cambridge: Harvard University Press, 1923–1931).

Hippocrates. *Works of Hippocrates,* vols. 5–8, ed. and trans. Paul Potter and Wesley D. Smith (Cambridge: Harvard University, 1988–1995).

Hirschmüller, Albrecht. *The Life and Work of Josef Breuer: Physiology and Psychoanalysis* (New York: New York University Press, 1989).

Hodges, H. A. *The Philosophy of Wilhelm Dilthey* (London/Westport, Conn.: Routledge & Kegan Paul/Greenwood Press, 1952/1974).

Hoek, A. *Eenvoudige mededeelingen aagaande de genezing van eene krankzinnige door het levens-magnetismus* ('s Gravenhage, The Netherlands: De Gebroeders van Cleef, 1868).

Hoffman, Friedrich. *Fundamenta medicinae,* intro. and trans. Lester S. King (London: MacDonald, 1971).

Holifield, E. Brooks. *A History of Pastoral Care in America: From Salvation to Self-Realization* (Nashville, Tenn.: Abingdon Press, 1983).

Hooker, Worthington. *Physician and Patient; or, a Practical View of the Mutual Duties, Relations, and Interests of the Medical Profession and the Community* (New York: Baker and Scribner, 1849).

Hordern, Anthony. "The Response of the Neurotic Personality to Abreaction." *J. Ment. Sci.,* 1952, *98,* 630–39.

Horowitz, Mardi Jon. *Image Formation and Cognition* (New York: Appleton-Century-Crofts, 1970).

Horsley, J. S. "Narco-Analysis." *J. Ment. Sci.,* 1936, *82,* 416–22.

Horton, Paul C. *Solace: The Missing Dimension in Psychiatry* (Chicago: University of Chicago Press, 1981).

Hull, Clark L. *Principles of Behavior* (New York: Appleton-Century-Crofts, 1943).

Hume, David. *A Treatise of Human Nature,* ed. L. A. Selby-Bigge (Oxford: Clarendon Press, 1964).

Hunsdahl, Jørgen B. "Concerning Einfühlung (Empathy): A Concept Analysis of Its Origin and Early Development." *J. Hist. Behav. Sci.,* 1967, *3,* 180–91.

Hunt, David. *Parents and Children in History: The Psychology of Family Life in Early Modern France* (New York: Basic Books, 1970).

Hunter, Richard, and Ida Macalpine. *Three Hundred Years of Psychiatry, 1535–1860* (London: Oxford University Press, 1963).

Hutcheson, Francis. *An Essay on the Nature and Conduct of the Passions and Affections* . . . (London: John Smith and William Bruce, 1728).

Hutcheson, Francis. *A System of Moral Philosophy,* 2 vols. . . . [ed.] Francis Hutcheson, M.D. . . . (London: Millar and Longman, 1755).

Ihde, Don. *Listening and Voice: A Phenomenology of Sound* (Athens: Ohio State University Press, 1976).

Jackson, Stanley W. *Melancholia and Depression: From Hippocratic Times to Modern Times* (New Haven, Conn.: Yale University Press, 1986).

Jackson, Stanley W. "Introduction." In William Pargeter, *Observations on Maniacal Disorders* (1792), ed. Stanley W. Jackson (London: Routledge, 1988).

Jackson, Stanley W. "Robert Burton and Psychological Healing." *J. Hist. Med. Allied Sci.,* 1989, *44,* 160–78.

Jacobson, Edmund. *Progressive Relaxation* (Chicago: University of Chicago Press, 1929).

Jacoby, George W. *Suggestion and Psychotherapy* (New York: Charles Scribner's Sons, 1912).

James, Robert. *A Medicinal Dictionary* . . . , 3 vols. (London: Osborne, 1743–1745).

James, William. *The Principles of Psychology,* 2 vols. (New York: Henry Holt, 1890).

Janet, Pierre. "Les actes inconscients et le dédoublements de la personnalité pendant le somnambulisme provoqué." *Revue Philosophique,* 1886, *22,* 577–92.

Janet, Pierre. *L'automatisme psychologique: Essai de psychologie expérimentale* . . . (Paris: Alcan, 1889).

Janet, Pierre. *L'automatisme psychologique: Essai de psychologie expérimentale* . . . , 6th ed. (Paris: Félix Alcan, 1910).

Janet, Pierre. *Les médications psychologiques,* 2 vols. (Paris: Alcan, 1919).

Janet, Pierre. *Psychological Healing: A Historical and Clinical Study,* 2 vols., trans. Eden and Cedar Paul (New York: Macmillan, 1925).

Janet, Pierre. *Principles of Psychotherapy,* trans. H. M. and E. R. Guthrie (London: George Allen & Unwin, 1925).

Janov, Arthur. *The Primal Scream, Primal Therapy: The Cure for Neurosis* (New York: Putnam's Sons, 1970).

Jaspers, Karl. *Allgemeine Psychopathologie: Für Studierende, Ärzte und Psychologen,* 3rd ed. (Berlin: Julius Springer, 1923).

Jaspers, Karl. *General Psychopathology,* trans. J. Hoenig and Marian W. Hamilton (Chicago: University of Chicago Press, 1963).

Jewson, N. D. "The Disappearance of the Sick-Man from Medical Cosmology." *Sociology,* 1976, *10,* 225–40.

Johnson, Samuel. *A Dictionary of the English Language . . . ,* 2 vols. (London: Knapton, Longman, Hitch and Hawes; Millar, and Dodsley, 1755).

Johnson, Wendell. *Your Most Enchanted Listener.* (New York: Harper, 1956).

Jones, Ernest. "The Action of Suggestion in Psychotherapy." In Ernest Jones, *Papers on Psycho-Analysis,* 2nd ed. (London: Baillière, Tindall and Cox, 1920).

Jones, Ernest. *The Life and Work of Sigmund Freud,* 3 vols. (New York: Basic Books, 1953–1957).

Jones, Mary Cover. "The Elimination of Children's Fears." *J. Experimental Psychol.,* 1924a, 7, 383–90.

Jones, Mary Cover. "A Laboratory Study of Fear: The Case of Peter." *Pedagogical Seminary,* 1924b, *31,* 308–15.

Jones, P. Mansell. *French Introspectives: From Montaigne to André Gide* (Port Washington, N.Y.: Kennikat Press, 1970).

Juhasz, Joseph B. "Greek Theories of Imagination." *J. Hist. Behav. Sci.,* 1971, 7, 39–58.

Jung, C. G. "On Manic Mood Disorder." In Herbert Read, Michael Fordham, Gerhard Adler, and William McGuire (eds.), *The Collected Works of C. G. Jung,* 20 vols. in 21 (Princeton, N.J.: Princeton University Press, 1953–1979), 1: 109–34.

Jung, C. G. "The Content of the Psychoses." In *Works,* 3: 155–78.

Jung, C. G. "The Therapeutic Value of Abreaction." In *Works,* 16: 129–38.

Jung, C. G. "Problems of Modern Psychotherapy." In *Works,* 16: 53–75.

Jung, C. G. "Psychotherapists or the Clergy." In *Works,* 11: 327–47.

Jung, C. G. "Yoga and the West." In *Works,* 11: 529–37.

Jung, C. G. "The Psychological Foundations of Belief in Spirits." In *Works,* 8: 301–18.

Jung, C. G. "The Psychological Aspects of the Kore." In *Works,* 9(1): 182–203.

Jung, C. G. *Memories, Dreams, Reflections,* ed. Aniela Jaffé, trans. Richard and Clara Winston (New York: Pantheon, 1961).

Kazdin, Alan E. *The Token Economy: A Review and Evaluation* (New York: Plenum, 1977).

Kazdin, Alan E. *History of Behavior Modification: Experimental Foundations of Contemporary Research* (Baltimore, Md.: University Park Press, 1978).

Kazdin, Alan E., and Joan L. Pulaski. "Joseph Lancaster and Behavior Modification in Education." *J. Hist. Behav. Sci.,* 1977, *13,* 261–66.

Kelly, Gerald. *The Good Confessor* (New York: Sentinel Press, 1951).

Kemp, Charles F. *Physicians of the Soul: A History of Pastoral Counseling* (New York: Macmillan, 1947).

Kemp, Simon. *Medieval Psychology* (Westport, Conn.: Greenwood Press, 1990).

Kempf, Edward J. "A Study of the Anaesthesia, Convulsions, Vomiting, Visual Constriction, Erythema and Itching of Mrs. V. G." *J. Abnorm. Psychol.,* 1917, *12,* 3–26.

Kempf, Edward J. *Selected Papers,* ed. Dorothy Clarke Kempf and John C. Burnham (Bloomington: Indiana University Press, 1974).

Kennedy, George A. *The Art of Persuasion in Greece* (Princeton, N.J.: Princeton University Press, 1963).

Kennedy, George A. *Greek Rhetoric Under Christian Emperors* (Princeton, N.J.: Princeton University Press, 1983).

Kerferd, G. B. "Katharsis." In Paul Edwards (ed.), *The Encyclopedia of Philosophy,* 8 vols. (New York: Macmillan and Free Press, 1967), 4: 326–27.

Kiev, Ari. "The Study of Folk Psychiatry." In Ari Kiev (ed.), *Magic, Faith, and Healing: Studies in Primitive Psychiatry Today* (New York: Free Press, 1964).

Kiev, Ari (ed.). *Magic, Faith, and Healing: Studies in Primitive Psychiatry Today* (New York: Free Press, 1964).

Kimble, Gregory A. *Hilgard and Marquis's Conditioning and Learning,* 2nd ed. (New York: Appleton-Century-Crofts, 1961).

King, Lester S. *The Road to Medical Enlightenment, 1650–1695* (London/New York: Macdonald/American Elsevier, 1970).

Kleinman, Arthur. *The Illness Narratives: Suffering, Healing, and the Human Condition* (New York: Basic Books, 1988a).

Kleinman, Arthur. *Rethinking Psychiatry: From Cultural Category to Personal Experience* (New York: Free Press, 1988b).

Knight, Robert P. "Psychotherapy of an Adolescent Catatonic Schizophrenic with Mutism: A Study in Empathy and Establishing Contact." *Psychiatry,* 1946, 9, 323–39.

Knight, William A. *Varia, Studies on Problems of Philosophy and Ethics* (London: John Murray, 1901).

Kohut, Heinz. "Introspection, Empathy, and Psychoanalysis." *J. Am. Psychoanal. Assoc.,* 1959, 7, 459–83.

Kohut, Heinz. *How Does Analysis Cure?* ed. Arnold Goldberg and Paul E. Stepansky (Chicago: University of Chicago Press, 1984).

Kraepelin, Emil. *Psychiatrie: Ein Lehrbuch für Studierende und Ärzte,* 5th ed. (Leipzig: Johann Ambrosius Barth, 1896).

Kraepelin, Emil. *Psychiatrie . . . ,* 2 vols. 6th ed. (Leipzig: Johann Ambrosius Barth, 1899).

Kraepelin, Emil. *Psychiatrie . . . ,* 2 vols., 7th ed. (Leipzig: Johann Ambrosius Barth, 1903–1904).

Kraepelin, Emil. *Psychiatrie . . . ,* 4 vols., 8th ed. (Leipzig: Johann Ambrosius Barth, 1909–1915).

Kristeller, Paul Oskar. *Renaissance Thought II: Papers on Humanism and the Arts* (New York: Harper Torchbooks, 1965).

La Barre, Weston, "Confession as Cathartic Therapy in American Indian Tribes." In Ari Kiev (ed.), *Magic, Faith, and Healing: Studies in Primitive Psychiatry Today* (New York: Free Press, 1964).

Labov, William, and David Fanshel. *Therapeutic Discourse: Psychotherapy as Conversation* (New York: Academic Press, 1977).

Lancaster, Joseph. *Improvements in Education, as It Respects the Industrious Classes of the Community* (London: Darton and Harbey, 1805).

Langston, A. D. Beach. "Tudor Books of Consolation," Ph.D. dissertation, University of North Carolina, 1940.

Laplanche, J., and J.-B. Pontalis. *The Language of Psycho-Analysis,* trans. Donald Nicholson-Smith (New York: Norton, 1973).

Laurentius, Andreas. *A Discourse of the Preservation of Sight: of Melancholike Diseases; of Rheumes, and of Old Age,* trans. Richard Surphlet (London: Ralph Iacson, 1599).

Lazarus, Arnold A. "New Methods in Psychotherapy: A Case Study." *South African Med. J.,* 1958, 32, 660–64.

Lea, Henry Charles. *A History of Auricular Confession and Indulgences in the Latin Church,* 3 vols. (New York: Greenwood Press, 1968).

Lear, Jonathan. *Aristotle: The Desire to Understand* (Cambridge: Cambridge University Press, 1988).

Lear, Jonathan. *Love and Its Place in Nature: A Philosophical Interpretation of Freudian Psychoanalysis* (New York: Farrar, Strauss & Giroux, 1990).

Leigh, Denis, C. M. B. Pare, and John Marks (eds.). *A Concise Encyclopaedia of Psychiatry* (Lancaster, England: MTP Press, 1977).

Leonardo da Vinci. *Selections from the Notebooks of Leonardo da Vinci,* ed. Irma A. Richter (London: Oxford University Press, 1952).

Lesky, Erna. *The Vienna Medical School of the 19th Century,* trans. L. Williams and I. S. Levij (Baltimore, Md.: Johns Hopkins University Press, 1976).

Leuret, F. *Des indications à suivre dans le traitement moral de la folie* (Paris: Librairie 5e le Normant, 1846) [Reprinted, Nendeln, Liechtenstein: KTO Press, 1978].

Levine, Maurice. *Psychotherapy in Medical Practice* (New York: Macmillan, 1947).

Levy, Steven T. *Principles of Interpretation* (Northvale, N.J.: Jason Aronson, 1990).

Levy, Steven T., and Lawrence B. Inderbitzin. "Interpretation." In Alan Sugarman, Robert A. Nemiroff, and Daniel P. Greenson (eds.), *The Technique and Practice of Psychoanalysis, Vol. II: A Memorial Volume to Ralph R. Greenson* (Madison, Conn.: International Universities Press, 1992).

Liberman, Robert P. "Behavioral Modification of Schizophrenia: A Review." *Schizophrenia Bulletin,* issue 6, Fall 1972, pp. 37–48.

Liébeault, Ambroise Auguste. *Du sommeil et des états analogues considérés surtout au point de vue de l'action du moral sur le physique* (Paris: Victor Masson et fils and Nicolas Grosjean, 1866).

Lindemann, Erich. "Symptomatology and Management of Acute Grief." *Am. J. Psychiat.,* 1944, 101, 141–48.

Lindsley, Ogden R., and B. F. Skinner. "A Method for the Experimental Analysis of Behavior of Psychotic Patients." *Am. Psychol.,* 1954, 9, 419–20.

Lipkin, Mark. "Suggestion and Healing." *Perspectives in Biology and Medicine,* 1984, 28, 121–26.

Lipps, Theodor. "Empathy, Inner Imitation, and Sense-Feelings," trans. Max Schertel and Melvin M. Rader. In Melvin M. Rader (ed.), *A Modern Book of Esthetics: An Anthology* (New York: Henry Holt, 1935).

Locke, John. *An Essay Concerning Human Understanding,* 2 vols., ed. Alexander Campbell Fraser (New York: Dover, 1959).

Loewald, Hans W. "On the Therapeutic Action of Psychoanalysis." *Int. J. Psycho-Anal.,* 1960, 41, 16–33.

Loewald, Hans W. "Psychoanalysis as an Art and the Fantasy Character of the Psychoanalytic Situation." *J. Am. Psychoanal. Assoc.,* 1975, *23,* 277–99.

Loewald, Hans W. "Psychoanalytic Theory and the Psychoanalytic Process." In Hans W. Loewald, *Papers on Psychoanalysis* (New Haven, Conn.: Yale University Press, 1980).

Loewenstein, Rudolph M. "The Problem of Interpretation." *Psychoanal. Quart.,* 1951, *20,* 1–14.

Lowen, Alexander. *Bioenergetics* (New York: Coward, McCann & Geoghegan, 1975).

Lowy, Frederick H. "The Abuse of Abreaction: An Unhappy Legacy of Freud's Cathartic Method." *Can. Psychiat. Assoc. J.,* 1970, *15,* 557–65.

Lunsford, Andrea A., and Lisa S. Ede. "On Distinctions Between Classical and Modern Rhetoric." In Robert J. Connors, Lisa S. Ede, and Andrea A. Lunsford (eds.), *Essays on Classical Rhetoric and Modern Discourse* (Carbondale: Southern Illinois University Press, 1984).

Lynch, William F. *Images of Hope: Imagination as Healer of the Hopeless* (Baltimore: Helicon Press, 1965).

McClure, George William, Jr. "The Renaissance Vision of Solace and Tranquillity: Consolation and Therapeutic Wisdom in Italian Thought," Ph.D. dissertation, University of Michigan, 1981.

McClure, George William, Jr. *Sorrow and Consolation in Italian Humanism* (Princeton, N.J.: Princeton University Press, 1991).

McComb, Samuel. "Faith and Its Therapeutic Power." In Elwood Worcester, Samuel McComb, and Isador H. Coriat, *Religion and Medicine: The Moral Control of Nervous Disorders* (New York: Moffat, Yard, 1908).

MacDonald, Michael. *Mystical Bedlam: Madness, Anxiety, and Healing in Seventeenth-Century England* (Cambridge: Cambridge University Press, 1981).

MacDonald, Michael. "Religion, Social Change and Psychological Healing in England, 1600–1800." In W. J. Sheils (ed.), *The Church and Healing* (Oxford: Basil Blackwell, 1982).

McDougall, William. *An Introduction to Social Psychology* (Boston: John W. Luce, 1909).

McDougall, William. "The Revival of Emotional Memories and Its Therapeutic Value (III)." *Brit. J. Psychol., Medical Section,* 1920, *1,* 23–29.

McDougall, William. *Outline of Abnormal Psychology* (New York: Charles Scribner's Sons, 1926).

McGovern, John P., and Chester R. Burns. *Humanism in Medicine* (Springfield, Ill.: Charles C Thomas, 1973).

McKellar, Peter. "The Method of Introspection." In Jordan M. Scher (ed.), *Theories of the Mind* (New York: Free Press, 1962).

MacKinney, Loren C. "Medical Ethics and Etiquette in the Early Middle Ages: The Persistence of Hippocratic Ideals." *Bull. Hist. Med.,* 1952, *26,* 1–31.

McMahon, C. E. "The Role of Imagination in the Disease Process: Pre-Cartesian History." *Psychol. Med.,* 1976, *6,* 179–84.

McNeill, John T. "Medicine for Sin as Prescribed in the Penitentials." *Church History,* 1932, *1,* 14–26.

McNeill, John T. *A History of the Cure of Souls* (New York: Harper Torchbooks, 1965).

McNeill, John T., and Helena M. Gamer. *Medieval Handbooks of Penance* . . . (New York: Octagon Books, 1979).

Mahony, Patrick J. "Freud in the Light of Classical Rhetoric." *J. Hist. Behav. Sci.,* 1974, *10,* 413–25.

Mahony, Patrick. "The Boundaries of Free Association." *Psychoanalysis and Contemporary Thought,* 1979, 2, 151–98.

Malan, D. H. *A Study of Brief Psychotherapy* (London: Tavistock Publications, 1963).

Mann, Horace, et al. *First Annual Report of the Trustees of State Lunatic Hospital,* December 1833. In *Reports and Other Documents Relating to the State Lunatic Hospital at Worcester, Mass.* (Boston: Dutton and Wentworth, Printers to the State, 1837).

Mann, James. *Time-Limited Psychotherapy* (Cambridge: Harvard University Press, 1973).

Mannyng, Robert, of Brunne. *Handlyng Synne,* ed. Idelle Sullens (Binghamton, N.Y.: Medieval & Renaissance Texts & Studies, 1983).

Markus, R. A. "Augustine: Reason and Illumination." In *The Cambridge History of Later Greek & Early Medieval Philosophy,* ed. A. H. Armstrong (Cambridge: Cambridge University Press, 1967).

Marmor, Judd. "Psychoanalytic Therapy as an Educational Process." In Jules Masserman (ed.), *Science and Psychoanalysis,* vol. 5 (New York: Grune & Stratton, 1962).

Marmor, Judd. "Psychoanalytic Therapy and Theories of Learning." In Jules Masserman (ed.), *Science and Psychoanalysis,* vol. 7 (New York: Grune & Stratton, 1964).

Marmor, Judd. "Dynamic Psychotherapy and Behavior Therapy." *Arch. Gen. Psychiat.,* 1971, 24, 22–28.

Marmor, Judd. "The Nature of the Psychotherapeutic Process Revisited." *Can. Psychiat. Assoc. J.,* 1975, 20, 557–65.

Masserman, Jules M. *Behavior and Neurosis: An Experimental Psycho-Analytic Approach to Psychobiologic Principles* (Chicago: University of Chicago Press, 1943).

Matthau, Carol. *Among the Porcupines: A Memoir* (New York: Turtle Bay Books, 1992).

Mead, George H. *Mind, Self, and Society: From the Standpoint of a Social Behaviorist,* ed. and intro. Charles W. Morris (Chicago: University of Chicago Press, 1934).

Menninger, Karl. *Theory of Psychoanalytic Technique* (New York: Basic Books, 1958).

Menninger, Karl A., and Philip S. Holzman. *Theory of Psychoanalytic Technique,* 2nd ed. (New York: Basic Books, 1973).

Merlan, Philip. "Plotinus." In *The Encyclopedia of Philosophy,* ed. Paul Edwards, 8 vols. (New York: Macmillan and Free Press, 1967), 6: 351–59.

Mesmer, F. A. *Dissertation on the Discovery of Animal Magnetism.* In *Mesmerism:* . . . *Original Scientific and Medical Writings of F. A. Mesmer,* trans. and ed. George Bloch (Los Altos, Calif.: William Kaufmann, 1980a).

Mesmer, F. A. *Mesmerism: A Translation of the Original Scientific and Medical Writings of F. A. Mesmer,* intro. E. R. Hilgard, trans. and ed. George Bloch (Los Altos, Calif.: William Kaufmann, 1980b).

Meyer, Adolf. "Notes of Clinics in Psychopathology." In *The Collected Papers of Adolf Meyer,* 4 vols., ed. Eunice E. Winters (Baltimore, Md.: Johns Hopkins Press, 1950–1952), 3: 139–223.

Misch, Georg. *A History of Autobiography in Antiquity,* 2 vols. (Westport, Conn.: Greenwood Press, 1973).

Mitchell, Kenneth R., and Herbert Anderson. *All Our Losses, All Our Griefs: Resources for Pastoral Care* (Philadelphia: Westminster Press, 1983).

Moll, Albert. *Der Hypnotismus* (Berlin: Fischer, 1889).

Moll, Albert. *Hypnotism,* 2nd ed. (London: Walter Scott, 1891).

Moll, Albert. *Der Rapport in der Hypnose . . .* (Leipzig, Abel, 1892).

Montaigne, Michel de. *The Essays of Michel de Montaigne,* trans. and ed. M. A. Screech (London: Penguin, 1991).

Moody, W. A. "The Responsibility and Duty of the Physician." M.D. thesis, University of Nashville, Tenn., 1851.

Morantz-Sanchez, Regina Markell. *Sympathy and Science: Women Physicians in American Medicine* (New York: Oxford University Press, 1985).

More, Ellen Singer, and Maureen A. Milligan (eds.). *The Empathic Practitioner: Empathy, Gender and Medicine* (New Brunswick, N.J.: Rutgers University Press, 1994).

Moreno, J. L. *Psychodrama* (New York: Beacon House, 1946).

Moreno, J. L. "Psychodrama." In Silvano Arieti (ed.), *American Handbook of Psychiatry,* 3 vols. (New York: Basic Books, 1959–1966), 2: 1375–96.

Morrill, Henry Edwin. "Formation of Character." M.D. thesis, University of Pennsylvania, 1840.

Mountjoy, Paul T., James H. Bos, Michael O. Duncan, and Robert B. Verplank. "Falconry: Neglected Aspect of the History of Psychology." *J. Hist. Behav. Sci.,* 1969, *5,* 59–67.

Mowrer, O. H., and W. M. Mowrer, "Enuresis: A Method for Its Study and Treatment." *Am. J. Orthopsychiat.,* 1938, *8,* 436–59.

Münsterberg, Hugo. *Psychotherapy* (New York: Moffat, Yard, 1909).

Murray, James A. H., et al. (eds.). *A New English Dictionary . . . ,* 13 vols. (Oxford: Clarendon Press, 1888–1933).

Naranjo, Claudio. "Present-Centeredness: Technique, Prescription, and Ideal." In Joen Fagan and Irma Lee Shepherd (eds.). *Gestalt Therapy Now: Theory, Techniques, Applications* (New York: Colophon Books, 1971).

Neal, E. Virgil, and Charles S. Clark (eds.). *Hypnotism and Hypnotic Suggestion,* 5th ed. (Rochester, N.Y.: State Publishing, 1900).

Nichols, Michael P., and Melvin Zax. *Catharsis in Psychotherapy* (New York: Gardner Press, 1977).

Niebyl, Peter H. "The Non-Naturals." *Bull. Hist. Med.,* 1971, *45,* 487–92.

North, Helen. *Sophrosyne: Self-Knowledge and Self-Restraint in Greek Literature* (Ithaca, N.Y.: Cornell University Press, 1966).

Numbers, Ronald L., and Darrell W. Amundsen (eds.). *Caring and Curing: Health and Medicine in the Western Religious Traditions* (New York: Macmillan, 1986).

Nussbaum, Martha C. *The Therapy of Desire: Theory and Practice in Hellenistic Ethics* (Princeton, N.J.: Princeton University Press, 1994).

Oates, Whitney J. (ed.). *The Stoic and Epicurean Philosophers* (New York: Modern Library, 1940).

Olden, Christine. "On Adult Empathy with Children." *Psychoanalytic Study of the Child,* 1953, *8,* 11–26 (New York: International Universities Press, 1953).

Olden, Christine. "Notes on the Development of Empathy." *Psychoanalytic Study of the Child,* 1958, *13,* 505–18 (New York: International Universities Press, 1958).

Orr, Douglass. "Transference and Countertransference: A Historical Survey." *J. Am. Psychoanal. Assoc.,* 1954, 2, 621–70.

Osler, William. *Aequanimitas,* 3rd ed. (Phildelphia: Blakiston, 1945).

Osler, William. *The Collected Essays of Sir William Osler,* 3 vols., ed. intro. John P. McGovern and Charles G. Roland (Birmingham: Classics of Medicine Library, 1985).

Pagel, Walter. "Medieval and Renaissance Contributions to Knowledge of the Brain and Its Functions." In *The History and Philosophy of Knowledge of the Brain and Its Functions,* ed. F. N. L. Poynter (Oxford: Blackwell, 1958).

Paracelsus. *Selected Writings,* ed. and intro. Jolande Jacobi, trans. Norbert Guterman (New York: Pantheon Books, 1951).

Parkes, Colin Murray. *Bereavement: Studies of Grief in Adult Life* (New York: International Universities Press, 1972).

Parrish, Joseph. *An Inaugural Dissertation on the Influence of the Passions upon the Body, in the Production and Cure of Diseases* (Philadelphia: for the author, 1805).

Patch, Howard Rollin. *The Tradition of Boethius: A Study of His Importance in Medieval Culture* (New York: Oxford University Press, 1935).

Paul, Oglesby. *The Caring Physician: The Life of Dr. Francis W. Peabody* (Boston: Francis A. Countway Library of Medicine and Harvard Medical Alumni Association, 1991).

Pavlov, Ivan P. *Conditioned Reflexes: An Investigation of the Physiological Activity of the Cerebral Cortex,* trans. and ed. G. V. Anrep (Oxford: Oxford University Press, 1927).

Pavlov, Ivan P. *Lectures on Conditioned Reflexes,* trans. W. Horsley Gantt (New York: International Publishers, 1928).

Peabody, Francis Weld. "The Care of the Patient." *J. Amer. Med. Assoc.,* 1927, 88, 877–82.

Peabody, Francis Weld. *Doctor and Patient: Papers on the Relationship of the Physician to Men and Institutions* (New York: Macmillan, 1930).

Pennebaker, James W. "Confession, Inhibition, and Disease." In L. Berkowitz (ed.), *Advances in Experimental Social Psychology,* vol. 22 (New York: Academic Press, 1989).

Pereira, Jonathan. *The Elements of Materia Medica and Therapeutics,* 3rd Am. ed., ed. Joseph Carson (Philadelphia: Blanchard and Lea, 1852).

Perls, Frederick S. "Four Lectures." In Joen Fagan and Irma Lee Shepherd (eds.), *Gestalt Therapy Now: Theory, Techniques, Applications* (New York: Harper Colophon Books, 1971).

Perls, Frederick, Ralph E. Hefferline, and Paul Goodman. *Gestalt Therapy: Excitement and Growth in the Human Personality* (New York: Dell, 1951).

Pernick, Martin S. *A Calculus of Suffering: Pain, Professionalism, and Anesthesia in Nineteenth-Century America* (New York: Columbia University Press, 1985).

Peters, R. S. (ed.). *Brett's History of Psychology* (London: George Allen & Unwin, 1962).

Petrarch. *Petrarch's Secret, or the Soul's Conflict with Passion: Three Dialogues Between Himself and S. Augustine,* trans. William H. Draper (London: Chatto and Windus, 1911).

Petrarch. *Letters from Petrarch,* trans. Morris Bishop (Bloomington: Indiana University Press, 1966).

Petrarch. *Petrarch's Remedies for Fortune Fair and Foul,* trans. and commentary Conrad H. Rawski, 5 vols. (Bloomington: Indiana University Press, 1991).

Pettazzoni, Raffaele. *La confessione dei peccati,* 3 vols. (Bologna: Zanichelli, 1929–1936).

Pettazzoni, Raffaele. *La confession des péchés,* 2 vols., trans. R. Monnot (Paris: Librairie Ernest Leroux, 1931–1932).

Pettazzoni, Raffaele. "Confession of Sins and the Classics." *Harvard Theological Review,* 1937, 30, 1–14.

Pettazzoni, Raffaele. "Confession of Sins: An Attempted General Interpretation." In Raffaele Pettazzoni, *Essays on the History of Religions,* trans. H. J. Rose (Leiden: Brill, 1954).

Pinel, Philippe. "Réflexions médicales sur l'état monastique." *Journal gratuit* (1790), 81–93.

Pinel, Philippe. *Traité médico-philosophique sur l'aliénation mentale, ou la manie* (Paris: Richard, Caille et Ravier, 1801).

Pinel, Philippe *A Treatise on Insanity . . . ,* trans. D. D. Davis (Sheffield, England: Cadell and Davies, 1806).

Pinel, Philippe "Recherches et observations sur le traitement moral des aliénés." In P. Pinel, *Mémoire, recherches, observations, résultats* (Nendeln, Liechtenstein: Kraus Reprint, 1978).

Pinel, Philippe. *The Clinical Training of Doctors: An Essay of 1793,* ed., trans., and intro. Dora B. Weiner (Baltimore, Md.: Johns Hopkins University Press, 1980).

Pinel, Scipion. *Traité complet du régime sanitaire des aliénés, ou manuel des établissements qui leur sont consacrés* (Paris: Mauprivez, 1836).

Plater, Felix, Abdiah Cole, Nicholas Culpeper. *A Golden Practice of Physick . . .* (London: Peter Cole, 1662).

Plato. *Charmides.* In *The Dialogues of Plato,* 2 vols., trans. B. Jowett, intro. Raphael Demos (New York: Random House, 1937), vol. 1.

Plato. *The Dialogues of Plato,* 2 vols., trans. B. Jowett, intro. Raphael Demos (New York: Random House, 1937).

Plotinus, *The Enneads,* trans. Stephen MacKenna (Burdett, N.Y.: Larson Publications, 1992).

Plutarch. "Lives of the Ten Orators." In *Plutarch's Moralia,* 15 vols., trans. Frank Cole Babbitt et al. (Cambridge: Harvard University Press, 1949–1976), vol. 10.

Polster, Erving, and Miriam Polster. *Gestalt Therapy Integrated: Contours of Theory and Practice* (New York; Brunner/Mazel, 1973).

Porter, Roy. *Mind-Forg'd Manacles: A History of Madness in England from the Restoration to the Regency* (Cambridge: Harvard University Press, 1987).

Postman, Leo. "Rewards and Punishments in Human Learning." In Leo Postman (ed.), *Psychology in the Making; Histories of Selected Research Problems* (New York: Knopf, 1964).

Prince, Morton. *The Unconscious: The Fundamentals of Human Personality, Normal and Abnormal* (New York: Macmillan, 1914).

Prince, Morton. "The Educational Treatment of Neurasthenia and Certain Hysterical States." in Morton Prince, *Psychotherapy and Multiple Personality: Selected Essays,* ed. and intro. Nathan G. Hale, Jr. (Cambridge: Harvard University Press, 1975). Originally published in *Boston Med. Surg. J.*, 1898, *139*, 332–37.

Prince, Raymond. "Indigenous Yoruba Psychiatry." In Ari Kiev (ed.), *Magic, Faith, and Healing: Studies in Primitive Psychiatry Today* (New York: Free Press, 1964).

Puységur, Armand Marie Jacques de Chastenet, marquis de. *Mémoires pour servir à l'histoire et à l'établissement du magnétisme animal* (Londres, n. p., 1785). Originally published in Paris in 1784.

Puységur, Armand Marie Jacques de Chastenet, marquis de. *Suite des mémoires pour servir à l'histoire et à l'établissement du magnétisme animal* (Londres: n.p., 1785).

Puységur, A. M. J. de Chastenet, Marquis de. *Du magnétisme animal, considéré dans ses rapports avec diverses branches de la physique générale* (Paris: Imprimerie de Cellot, 1807).

Puységur, Armand Marie Jacques de Chastenet, marquis de. *Recherches, expériences et observations physiologiques* ... (Paris: Dentu, 1811).

Puységur, Armand Marie Jacques de Chastenet, marquis de. *Les fous, les insensés, les maniaques et les frénétiques* ... (Paris: Dentu, 1812).

Puységur, Jacques Maxime Paul de Chastenet, comte de. *Rapport des cures opérées à Bayonne par le magnétisme animal* ... (Bayonne: Prault, 1784).

Puységur, Maxime de. *Report of Cures by Animal Magnetism Occurring at Bayonne with Verifications,* trans. J. J. Slay. In Maurice M. Tinterow (ed.), *Foundations of Hypnosis: From Mesmer to Freud* (Springfield, Ill.: Charles C Thomas, 1970).

Raphael, Beverley. *The Anatomy of Bereavement* (New York: Basic Books, 1983).

Raphael, D. D. (ed.). *British Moralists, 1650–1800*, 2 vols. (Oxford: Clarendon Press, 1969).

Rapport des commissaires, chargés par le roi, de l'examen du magnétisme animal (Paris: Moutard, 1784).

Rather, L. J. *Mind and Body in Eighteenth Century Medicine: A Study Based on Jerome Gaub's* De regimine mentis (Berkeley: University of California Press, 1965).

Rather, L. J. "Thomas Fienus' (1567–1631) Dialectical Investigation of the Imagination as Cause and Cure of Bodily Disease." *Bull. Hist. Med.*, 1967, *41*, 349–67.

Rather, L. J. "The 'Six Things Non-Natural': A Note on the Origins and Fate of a Doctrine and a Phrase." *Clio Medica*, 1968, *3*, 337–47.

Ratzan, Richard M., and Gary B. Ferngren. "A Greek Progymnasma on the Physician-Poisoner." *J. Hist. Med. Allied Sci.*, 1993, *48*, 157–70.

Reich, Wilhelm. *Character-Analysis* (New York: Orgone Institute Press, 1949).

Reich, Wilhelm. *Selected Writings: An Introduction to Orgonomy* (New York: Farrar, Straus and Cudahy, 1960).

Reid, John R., and Jacob E. Finesinger. "The Role of Insight in Psychotherapy." *Am. J. Psychiat.*, 1951–1952, *108*, 726–34.

Reid, Thomas. *An Inquiry into the Human Mind, on the Principles of Common Sense* (Edinburgh: Millar, and Kincaid & Bell, 1764).

Reik, Theodor. *Listening with the Third Ear: The Inner Experience of a Psychoanalyst* (Garden City, N.Y.: Garden City Books, 1951).

Reynolds, Edward. *A Treatise of the Passions and Faculties of the Soule of Man* ... (London: Robert Bostock, 1640).

Richfield, Jerome. "An Analysis of the Concept of Insight." *Psychoanal. Quart.*, 1954, 23, 390–408.

Rickman, H. P. "Wilhelm Dilthey." In Paul Edwards (ed.), *The Encyclopedia of Philosophy*, 8 vols. (New York: Macmillan and Free Press, 1967), 2: 403–06.

Ricoeur, Paul. *Freud and Philosophy: An Essay on Interpretation*, trans. Denis Savage (New Haven, Conn.: Yale University Press, 1970).

Rivers, W. H. R. "Psycho-therapeutics." In James Hastings et al. (eds.), *Encyclopaedia of Religion and Ethics*, 13 vols. (New York: Charles Scribner's Sons, 1909–1927), 10: 433–40.

Roeggl, Aloysius. *The Confessional*, 6th ed., trans. Augustine Wirth (New York: Benziger, 1882).

Rogers, Carl R. *Counseling and Psychotherapy: Newer Concepts in Practice* (Boston: Houghton Mifflin, 1942).

Rogers, Carl R. *Client-Centered Therapy: Its Current Practice, Implications, and Theory* (Boston: Houghton Mifflin, 1951).

Rogers, Carl R. "The Necessary and Sufficient Conditions of Therapeutic Personality Change." *J. Consult. Psychol.*, 1957, 21, 95–103.

Rogers, Spencer L. "Egyptian Psychotherapy." *Ciba Symposia*, 1947, 9, 617–22.

Rogerson, C. H. "Narco-Analysis with Nitrous Oxide." *Brit. Med. J.*, 1944, 1, 811–12.

Rose, Louis. *Faith Healing*, ed. Bryan Morgan (Harmondsworth: Penguin, 1971).

Rosenzweig, Saul. "Some Implicit Common Factors in Diverse Methods of Psychotherapy." *Am. J. Orthopsychiat.*, 1936, 6, 412–15.

Rush, Benjamin. *Medical Inquiries and Observations, upon the Diseases of the Mind* (Philadelphia: Kimber & Richardson, 1812.)

Salter, Andrew. *Conditioned Reflex Therapy: The Direct Approach to the Reconstruction of Personality* (New York: Creative Age Press, 1949).

Sandler, Joseph, Christopher Dare, and Alex Holder. *The Patient and the Analyst: The Basis of the Psychoanalytic Process* (New York: International Universities Press, 1973).

Sarton, George. *Galen of Pergamon* (Lawrence: University of Kansas Press, 1954).

Schafer, Roy. "Generative Empathy in the Treatment Situation." *Psychoanal. Quart.*, 1959, 28, 342–73.

Scheff. T. J. *Catharsis in Healing, Ritual, and Drama* (Berkeley: University of California Press, 1979).

Schilder, Paul, and Otto Kanders. *Hypnosis*, trans. Simon Rothenberg (New York: Nervous and Mental Disease Publishing, 1927).

Schneck, Jerome M. (ed.). *Hypnosis in Modern Medicine* (Springfield, Ill.: Charles C Thomas, 1953).

Schofield, Alfred T. *The Unconscious Mind* (New York: Funk and Wagnalls, 1901).

Schopenhauer, Arthur. *On the Basis of Morality*, trans. E. F. J. Payne, intro. Richard Taylor (Indianapolis, Ind.: Bobbs-Merrill, 1965).

Schroeder, H. J. *Disciplinary Decrees of the General Councils: Text, Translation, and Commentary* (St. Louis: Herder, 1937).

Schroeder, Theodore. "The Psycho-Analytic Method of Observation." *Int. J. Psycho-Anal.*, 1925, 6, 155–70.

Schultz, Duane P. *A History of Modern Psychology* (New York: Academic Press, 1969).

Schwaber, Evelyne. "Narcissism, Self Psychology, and the Listening Perspective." *Annual of Psychoanalysis,* 1981, *9,* 115–32 (New York: International Universities Press, 1981a).

Schwaber, Evelyne. "Empathy: A Mode of Analytic Listening." *Psychoanal. Inquiry,* 1981b, *1,* 357–92.

Schwaber, Evelyne. "A Particular Perspective on Analytic Listening." *Psychoanalytic Study of the Child,* 1983, *38,* 519–46 (New Haven, Conn.: Yale University Press, 1983).

Seneca. *Moral Essays,* 3 vols., trans. John W. Basore (Cambridge: Harvard University Press, 1965–1975).

Seneca. *Ad Lucilium epistulae morales,* 3 vols., trans. Richard M. Gummere (Cambridge: Harvard University Press, 1967–1971).

Shapiro, Arthur K. "The Placebo Effect in the History of Medical Treatment: Implications for Psychiatry." *Am. J. Psychiat.,* 1959, *116,* 298–304.

Shapiro, Arthur K. "A Contribution to the History of the Placebo Effect." *Behav. Sci.,* 1960, *5,* 109–35.

Shapiro, Arthur K. "A Historic and Heuristic Definition of the Placebo." *Psychiatry,* 1964, *27,* 52–58.

Shapiro, Arthur K. "Placebo Effects in Medicine, Psychotherapy, and Psychoanalysis." In Allen E. Bergin and Sol L. Garfield (eds.), *Handbook of Psychotherapy and Behavior Change: An Empirical Analysis* (New York: John Wiley & Sons, 1971).

Shapiro, Arthur K., and Louis A. Morris. "The Placebo Effect in Medical and Psychological Therapies." In Sol L. Garfield and Allen E. Bergin (eds.), *Handbook of Psychotherapy and Behavior Change: An Empirical Analysis,* 2nd ed. (New York: John Wiley & Sons, 1978).

Shaw, Peter. *The Reflector: Representing Human Affairs, as They Are; and May Be Improved* (London: Longmans, 1750).

Sheikh, A. A. (ed.). *Imagery: Current Theory, Research, and Application* (New York: Wiley, 1983).

Sheikh, Anees A. (ed.). *Imagination and Healing* (Farmingdale, N.Y.: Baywood, 1984).

Sheikh, Anees A., Robert G. Kunzendorf, and Katharina S. Sheikh. "Healing Images: From Ancient Wisdom to Modern Science." In Anees A. Sheikh and Katharina S. Sheikh (eds.), *Eastern and Western Approaches to Healing: Ancient Wisdom and Modern Knowledge* (New York: John Wiley & Sons, 1989).

Sheils, W. J. (ed.). *The Church and Healing* (Oxford: Basil Blackwell, 1982).

Shorter, Edward. *Bedside Manners: The Troubled History of Doctors and Patients* (Harmondsworth, England: Viking, 1986).

Shorvon, H. J., and William Sargant. "Excitatory Abreaction: With Special Reference to Its Mechanism and the Use of Ether." *J. Ment. Sci.,* 1947, *93,* 709–32.

Sidis, Boris. *The Psychology of Suggestion* (New York: Appleton, 1899).

Siegel, Rudolph E. *Galen on Psychology, Psychopathology, and Function and Diseases of the Nervous System* (Basel: Karger, 1973).

Sifneos, Peter E. *Short-Term Psychotherapy and Emotional Crisis* (Cambridge: Harvard University Press, 1972).

Sigerist, Henry E, *A History of Medicine,* vol. 1 (New York: Oxford University Press, 1951).

Silverman, Lloyd H. "The Unconscious Fantasy as Therapeutic Agent in Psychoanalytic Treatment." In Samuel Slipp (ed.), *Curative Factors in Dynamic Psychotherapy* (New York: McGraw-Hill, 1982).

Simmel, Ernst. *Kriegsneurosen und psychische Trauma* (Munich: Nemnich, 1918).

Simmel, Ernst. "War Neuroses." In Sandor Lorand (ed.), *Psychoanalysis Today* (New York: International Universities Press, 1944).

Simon, Bennett. *Mind and Madness in Ancient Greece: The Classical Roots of Modern Psychiatry* (Ithaca, N.Y.: Cornell University Press, 1978).

Simon, Bennett, and Herbert Weiner. "Models of Mind and Mental Illness in Ancient Greece: I. The Homeric Model of Mind." *J. Hist. Behav. Sci.,* 1966, *2,* 303–14.

Singer, Jerome L. *Imagery and Daydream Methods in Psychotherapy and Behavior Modification* (New York: Academic Press, 1974).

Singer, Jerome L., and Kenneth Pope (eds.). *The Power of Human Imagination: New Methods in Psychotherapy* (New York: Plenum, 1978).

Siraisi, Nancy G. *Taddeo Alderotti and His Pupils: Two Generations of Italian Medical Learning* (Princeton, N.J.: Princeton University Press, 1981).

Skinner, B. F. *The Behavior of Organisms: An Experimental Analysis* (New York: Appleton-Century-Crofts, 1938).

Slipp, Samuel (ed.). *Curative Factors in Dynamic Psychotherapy* (New York: McGraw-Hill, 1982).

Smith, Adam. *The Theory of Moral Sentiments,* ed. D. D. Raphael and A. L. Macfie (Oxford: Clarendon Press, 1991).

Smith, Mary, "The Nervous Temperament." *Brit. J. Med. Psychol.,* 1930, *10,* 99–174.

Soranus. *Soranus' Gynecology,* trans. and intro. Owsei Temkin (Baltimore, Md.: Johns Hopkins Press, 1956).

Soukhanov, Anne H., et al. (eds.). *The American Heritage Dictionary of the English Language,* 3rd ed. (Boston: Houghton Mifflin, 1992).

Spiegel, David, and Herbert Spiegel. "Hypnosis." In Harold K. Kaplan and Benjamin J. Sadock (eds.), *Comprehensive Textbook of Psychiatry IV,* 2 vols., 4th ed. (Baltimore: Williams & Wilkins, 1985).

Spillane, Robert. "Rhetoric as Remedy: Some Philosophical Antecedents of Psychotherapeutic Ethics." *Brit. J. Med. Psychol.,* 1987, *60,* 217–24.

Spiro, Howard. *Doctors, Patients, and Placebos* (New Haven, Conn.: Yale University Press, 1986).

Spiro, Howard, et al. (eds.). *Empathy and the Practice of Medicine: Beyond Pills and the Scalpel* (New Haven, Conn.: Yale University Press, 1993).

Staum, Martin S. *Cabanis: Enlightenment and Medical Philosophy in the French Revolution* (Princeton, N.J.: Princeton University Press, 1980).

Stern, Adolph. "On the Counter-Transference in Psychoanalysis." *Psychoanal. Rev.,* 1924, *11,* 166–74.

Stewart, Mark A. "Psychotherapy by Reciprocal Inhibition." *Am. J. Psychiat.,* 1961, *118,* 175–77.

Stone, Martin. "Shellshock and the Psychologists." In W. F. Bynum, Roy Porter, and

Michael Shepherd (eds.), *The Anatomy of Madness: Essays in the History of Psychiatry,* 2 vols. (London: Tavistock Publications, 1985), 2: 242–71.

Stotland, Ezra. *The Psychology of Hope* (San Francisco: Jossey-Bass, 1969).

Strachey, James. "The Nature of the Therapeutic Action of Psycho-Analysis." *Int. J. Psycho-Anal.,* 1934, *15,* 127–59.

Strauss, Maurice B. (ed.). *Familiar Medical Quotations* (Boston: Little, Brown, 1968).

Strupp, Hans H. "Psychotherapy Research and Practice: An Overview." In Sol L. Garfield and Allen E. Bergin (eds.), *Handbook of Psychotherapy and Behavior Change: An Empirical Analysis,* 2nd ed. (New York: John Wiley & Sons, 1978).

Strupp, Hans H., and Suzanne W. Hadley. "Specific vs Non-Specific Factors in Psychotherapy: Controlled Study of Outcome." *Arch. Gen. Psychiat.,* 1979, *36,* 1125–36.

Sullivan, Lawrence E. (ed.). *Healing and Restoring: Health and Medicine in the World's Religious Traditions* (New York: Macmillan, 1989).

Sym, John. *Lifes Preservative Against Self-Killing . . .* (London: Dawlman and Fawne, 1637).

Sym, John. *Lifes Preservative Against Self-Killing . . .,* ed. and intro. Michael MacDonald (London: Routledge, 1988).

Symonds, Percival M. "A Comprehensive Theory of Psychotherapy." *Am. J. Orthopsychiat.,* 1954, *24,* 697–712.

Tannenbaum, Rebecca J. "Earnestness, Temperance, Industry: The Definition and Uses of Professional Character Among Nineteenth-Century American Physicians." *J. Hist. Med. Allied Sci.,* 1949, *49,* 251–83.

Temkin, Owsei. *Galenism: Rise and Decline of a Medical Philosophy* (Ithaca, N.Y.: Cornell University Press, 1973).

Temkin, Owsei. *Hippocrates in a World of Pagans and Christians* (Baltimore, Md.: Johns Hopkins University Press, 1991).

Tentler, Thomas N. *Sin and Confession on the Eve of the Reformation* (Princeton, N.J.: Princeton University Press, 1977).

Thomas, Keith. *Religion and the Decline of Magic: Studies in Popular Beliefs in Sixteenth and Seventeenth Century England* (London: Weidenfeld and Nicolson, 1971).

Thompson, C. J. S. *Magic and Healing* (London: Rider, 1946).

Tinterow, Maurice M. (ed.). *Foundations of Hypnosis: From Mesmer to Freud* (Springfield, Ill.: Charles C Thomas, 1970).

Tissot, C. J. *De l'influence des passions de l'âme dans les maladies, et des moyens d'en corriger les mauvais effets* (Paris: Amand-Koenig, 1798).

Titchener, Edward B. *A Text-Book of Psychology,* 2 vols. (New York: Macmillan, 1909–1910).

Titchener, Edward B. *Lectures on the Experimental Psychology of Thought-Processes* (New York: Macmillan, 1926).

Tolstoy, Leo. *War and Peace,* trans. Louise and Aylmer Maude, foreword Clifton Fadiman (New York: Simon and Schuster, 1942).

Tomes, Nancy. *A Generous Confidence: Thomas Story Kirkbride and the Art of Asylum-Keeping, 1840–1883* (Cambridge: Cambridge University Press, 1984).

Torrey, E. Fuller. *Witchdoctors and Psychiatrists: The Common Roots of Psychotherapy and Its Future* (Northvale, N.J.: Jason Aronson, 1986).

Townsend, Peter S. *A Dissertation on the Influence of the Passions in the Production and Modification of Disease* (New York: for the author, 1816).

Trinkaus, Charles. *The Poet as Philosopher: Petrarch and the Formation of Renaissance Consciousness* (New Haven, Conn.: Yale University Press, 1979).

Tuckey, C. Lloyd. *Psycho-Therapeutics; or Treatment by Sleep and Suggestion* (London: Baillière, Tindall and Cox, 1889).

Tuckey, C. Lloyd. *Psycho-Therapeutics: or, Treatment by Hypnotism and Suggestion,* 3rd ed. (London: Baillière, Tindall and Cox, 1891).

Tuke, Daniel Hack. *Illustrations of the Influence of the Mind upon the Body in Health and Disease . . .* (London: Churchill, 1872).

Tuke, Daniel Hack. *Illustrations of the Influence of the Mind upon the Body in Health and Disease . . . ,* 2nd ed. (Philadelphia: Henry C. Lea's Sons, 1884).

Tuke, D. Hack (ed.). *Dictionary of Psychological Medicine,* 2 vols. (Philadelphia: Blakiston, Son, 1892).

Twyne, Thomas. *Phisicke against Fortune . . .* Written in Latine by Frauncis Petrarch (London: Richard Watkyns, 1579).

Valangin, Francis de. *Treatise on Diet, or the Management of Human Life; By Physicians called the Six Non-Naturals . . .* (London: the Author, 1768).

Valenstein, Arthur F, "The Psycho-Analytic Situation: Affects, Emotional Reliving, and Insight in the Psycho-Analytic Process." *Int. J. Psycho-Anal.,* 1962, *43,* 315–24.

Valenstein, Arthur F, "Working Through and Resistance to Change: Insight and the Action System." *J. Am. Psychoanal. Assoc.,* 1983, *31,* 353–73.

Van der Hart, Onno, and Kees van der Velden. "The Hypnotherapy of Dr. Andries Hoek: Uncovering Hypnotherapy Before Janet, Breuer, and Freud." *Am. J. Clin. Hypn.,* 1987, *29,* 264–71,

Van Eeden, [Frederik]. "The Theory of Psycho-Therapeutics," *Medical Magazine,* 1895, *1,* 232–57.

Van Eeden, Frederik. *Happy Humanity* (Garden City, N.Y.: Doubleday, Page, 1912).

Van Eeden, Frederik, and Albert Willem van Renterghem. *Clinique de psychothérapie suggestive fondée à Amsterdam* (Brussels: Manceaux, 1889).

Van Helmont, Franciscus Mercurius. *The Spirit of Disease; or, Diseases from the Spirit: Laid open in some Observations Concerning Man, and his Diseases. Wherein is showed how much the Mind influenceth the Body in causing and curing of Diseases . . .* (London: Sarah Howkins, 1694).

Van Renterghem, Albert Willem, and Frederik van Eeden, *Psycho-thérapie: Communications statistiques, observations cliniques nouvelles. Compte rendu des résultats obtenus dans la clinique de psycho-thérapie suggestive d'Amsterdam, pendant la deuxième période* (Paris: Sociétés d'Editions Scientifiques, 1894).

Van Swieten, Gerard. *The Commentaries upon the Aphorisms of Dr. Herman Boerhaave,* 11 vols. (London: John and Paul Knapton, 1754–1759).

[Vaughan, William]. *Directions for Health, Naturall and Artificiall: Derived from the best Physicians, as well Moderne as Antient,* 7th ed. (London: Thomas Harper, 1633).

Vickers, Brian. "Introduction" and "On the Practicalities of Renaissance Rhetoric." In Brian Vickers (ed.), *Rhetoric Revalued: Papers from the International Society for the*

History of Rhetoric (Binghamton, N.Y.: Center for Medieval & Early Renaissance Studies, 1982).

Vietor, Agnes C. (ed.). *A Woman's Quest: The Life of Marie E. Zakrzewska, M.D.* (New York: Appleton, 1924).

Voltaire. *Philosophical Dictionary,* 2 vols., trans. and intro. Peter Gay (New York: Basic Books, 1962).

Von Staden, Heinrich. *Herophilus: The Art of Medicine in Early Alexandria* (Cambridge: Cambridge University Press, 1989).

Wachtel, Paul L. *Psychoanalysis and Behavior Therapy: Toward an Integration* (New York: Basic Books, 1977).

Walker, Nigel. *A Short History of Psychotherapy: Its Theory and Practice* (London: Routledge & Kegan Paul, 1957).

Wallerstein, Robert S. "How Does Self Psychology Differ in Practice?" *Int. J. Psycho-Anal.,* 1985, *66,* 391–404.

Wallerstein, Robert S. *The Talking Cures: The Psychoanalyses and the Psychotherapies* (New Haven, Conn.: Yale University Press, 1995).

Walrond-Skinner, Sue. *Dictionary of Psychotherapy.* (London: Routledge & Kegan Paul, 1986).

Walsh, James J. *Psychotherapy: Including the History of the Use of Mental Influence, Directly and Indirectly, in Healing and the Principles for the Application of Energies Derived from the Mind to the Treatment of Disease* (New York: Appleton, 1912).

Watkins, John G. *Hypnotherapy of War Neuroses: A Clinical Psychologist's Casebook* (New York: Ronald Press, 1949).

Watson, J. B. "Psychology as the Behaviorist Views It." *Psychol. Rev.,* 1913, *20,* 158–77.

Watson, John B. *Behavior: An Introduction to Comparative Psychology* (New York: Holt, 1914).

Watson, John B. *Psychology from the Standpoint of a Behaviorist* (Philadelphia: Lippincott, 1919).

Watson, John B., and Rosalie Rayner. "Conditioned Emotional Reactions." *J. Experimental Psychol.,* 1920, *3,* 1–14.

Watson, Robert I. *The Great Psychologists: Aristotle to Freud* (Philadelphia: Lippincott, 1963).

Weatherhead, Leslie D. *Psychology, Religion, and Healing* (London: Hodder and Stoughton, 1951).

Weinberg, Bernard. "Rhetoric After Plato." In Philip P. Weiner (ed.), *Dictionary of the History of Ideas: Studies of Selected Pivotal Ideas,* 5 vols. (New York: Charles Scribner's Sons, 1968–1974), 4: 167–73.

Weiner, Dora B. "The Brothers of Charity and the Mentally Ill in Pre-Revolutionary France." *Soc. Hist. of Med.,* 1989, *2,* 321–37.

Werman, David S. *The Practice of Supportive Psychotherapy* (New York: Brunner/Mazel, 1984).

Wheelis, Allen. "The Place of Action in Personality Change." *Psychiatry,* 1950, *13,* 135–48.

Wheelis, Allen. "Will and Psychoanalysis." *Am. J. Psychoanal.,* 1956, *4,* 285–303.

Wheelis, Allen. *How People Change* (New York: Harper & Row, 1973).

Wilcox, Judith, and John M. Riddle. "Qusṭā ibn Lūqā's *Physical Ligatures* and the Recognition of the Placebo Effect," *Medieval Encounters*, 1994, *1*, 1–48.

Wilkins, Eliza Gregory. *The Delphic Maxims in Literature* (Chicago: University of Chicago Press, 1929).

Willis, Thomas. *Two Discourses Concerning the Soul of Brutes Which is that of the Vital and Sensitive of Man*, trans. S. Pordage (London: Thomas Dring, Ch. Harper, and John Leigh, 1683).

Winbigler, Charles F. *Suggestion: Its Law and Application, or The Principle and Practice of Psycho-Therapeutics* (Washington/London: Spencer A. Lewis/Fowler, 1909).

Wingfield, H. E. *An Introduction to the Study of Hypnotism: Experimental and Therapeutic*, 2nd ed. (London: Baillière, Tindall and Cox, 1920).

Wispé, Lauren G. "Sympathy and Empathy." In David L. Sills (ed.), *International Encyclopedia of the Social Sciences*, 17 vols. (New York: Macmillan and Free Press, 1968), vol. 15.

Wolberg, Lewis R. *Hypnoanalysis* (New York: Grune & Stratton, 1945).

Wolberg, Lewis R. *Medical Hypnosis*, 2 vols. (New York: Grune & Stratton, 1948).

Wolberg, Lewis R. *The Technique of Psychotherapy* (New York: Grune & Stratton, 1954).

Wolberg, Lewis R. *The Technique of Psychotherapy*, 2nd ed., 2 vols. (New York: Grune & Stratton, 1972).

Wolberg, Lewis R. (ed.). *Short-Term Psychotherapy* (New York: Grune & Stratton, 1965).

Wolfson, Harry Austryn. "The Internal Senses in Latin, Arabic, and Hebrew Philosophical Texts." *Harvard Theol. Rev.*, 1935, *28*, 69–133.

Wolpe, Joseph. *Psychotherapy by Reciprocal Inhibition* (Stanford, Calif.: Stanford University Press, 1958).

Wolpe, Joseph. "Psychotherapy: The Nonscientific Heritage and the New Science." *Behav. Res. Ther.*, 1963, *1*, 23–28.

Wolpe, Joseph. *The Practice of Behavior Therapy* (New York: Pergamon, 1969).

Wolpe, Joseph. "Conditioning Is the Basis of All Psychotherapeutic Change." In Arthur Burton (ed.), *What Makes Behavior Change Possible?* (New York: Brunner/Mazel, 1976).

Wolpe, Joseph, Andrew Salter, L. J. Reyna (eds.). *The Conditioning Therapies: The Challenge in Psychotherapy* (New York: Holt, Rinehart and Winston, 1964).

Woolfolk, Robert L., Louis A. Sass, Stanley B. Messer. "Introduction to Hermeneutics." In Stanley B. Messer, Louis A. Sass, and Robert L. Woolfolk (eds.), *Hermeneutics and Psychological Theory: Interpretive Perspectives on Personality, Psychotherapy and Psychopathology* (New Brunswick, N.J.: Rutgers University Press, 1988).

Worcester, Elwood. "Suggestion." In Elwood Worcester, Samuel McComb, Isador H. Coriat, *Religion and Medicine: The Moral Control of Nervous Disorders* (New York: Moffat, Yard, 1908).

Wright, Thomas. *The Passions of the Minde in Generall*, in Six Bookes, . . . (London: Anne Helme, 1621).

Wright, Thomas. *The Passions of the Minde in Generalle,* reprint based on 1604 ed., intro. Thomas O. Sloan (Urbana: University of Illinois Press, 1971).

Wundt, Wilhelm M. *Hypnotismus und Suggestion* (Leipzig: Wilhelm Engelmann, 1892).

Wundt, Wilhelm. *Principles of Physiological Psychology,* vol. 1, trans. Edward Bradford Titchener, from 5th German ed. (London/New York: Swan Sonnenschein/Macmillan, 1904).

Wundt, Wilhelm. *Outlines of Psychology,* 3rd English ed., trans. Charles Hubbard Judd, from 7th German ed. (London/New York: Williams & Norgate/Stechert, 1907).

Wyss, Dieter. *Depth Psychology: A Critical History,* trans. Gerald Onn (New York: Norton, 1966).

Yellowlees, Henry. *A Manual of Psychotherapy for Practitioners and Students* (London: Black, 1923).

Zilboorg, Gregory. "The Emotional Problem and the Therapeutic Role of Insight." *Psychoanal. Quart.,* 1952, 21, 1–24.

Zimmerman, Leo M. "Surgery." In Allen G. Debus (ed.), *Medicine in Seventeenth Century England* (Berkeley: University of California Press, 1974).

Zysk, Kenneth G. *Religious Healing in the Veda* (Philadelphia: American Philosophical Society, 1985).

Index

Abreaction. *See* Catharsis
Abroms, Gene M., 306
Affects. *See* Passions
Alexander, Franz, 130–31, 320–32, 335, 354, 356–57, 385
Alexander of Tralles, 295–97
Alternative medicine, 391–92
Anna O., 85–86, 105–6, 256
Antiphon, 21, 100, 167, 288–89
Appelbaum, Stephen, 336, 338
Aristotle, 22, 30–31, 81, 102, 118–19, 120, 205, 207, 222, 289–90
Artificial inventions. *See* Pious frauds
Augustine, 172–73, 346–47, 366–67
Ayurvedic medicine, 33

Bacon, Francis, 155, 156, 291
Balint, Michael, 76–77
Battie, William, 213–14, 228
Baxter, Richard, 184–85, 348
Beattie, James, 51–52
Behavior therapy, 110, 315–19, 387. *See also* Conditioning

Bekhterev, Vladimir M., 313
Benedict of Nursia, 45
Benedikt, Moritz, 152, 256
Bereavement studies, 195
Bernays, Jacob, 123
Bernheim, Hippolyte, 8, 249–52, 253, 257, 258–59, 270–71, 278, 279
Bertrand, Alexandre, 245, 286
Bibring, Edward, 136, 283–84, 335, 356
Binet, Alfred, 127, 232, 270
Binstock, William A., 131, 137
Bioenergetics, and catharsis, 137–38
Bird, Brian, 112–13
Blum, Harold, 334, 352
Boerhaave, Herman, 212–13
Boethius, 173–74, 347
Bonhoeffer, Dietrich, 80
Boyle, Robert, 368
Braid, James, 246–48, 269, 286
Bramwell, J. Milne, 253
Breuer, Josef, 6, 85–86, 105–7, 123–25, 126, 127, 131–32, 157, 255–58
Bromberg, Walter, 192–93